Staged Diabetes Management

Second Edition

Staged Diabetes Management

A Systematic Approach

Second Edition

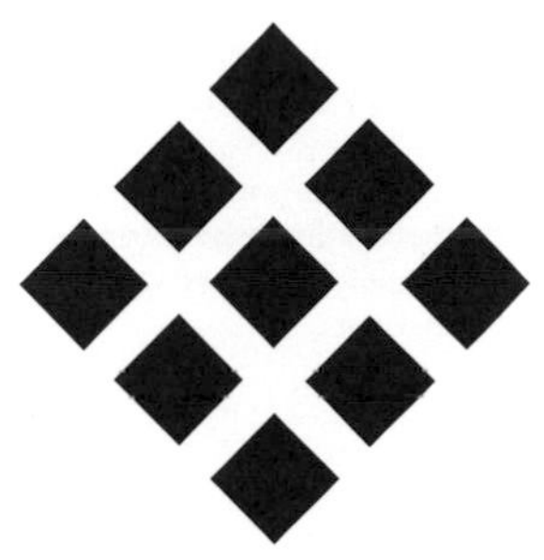

Mazze, Strock, Simonson, Bergenstal
International Diabetes Center

John Wiley & Sons, Ltd

Staged Diabetes Management™ was developed by the International Diabetes Center with the support of unrestricted educational and research grants from BD (Becton Dickinson and Company)

Matrex is a joint venture of BD and the International Diabetes Center

MATREX
PROVEN PATHWAYS FOR ENHANCED CARE
A JOINT VENTURE OF BD AND THE INTERNATIONAL DIABETES CENTER

Published 2004 John Wiley & Sons, Ltd.
The Atrium, Southern Gate, Chichester,
West Sussex PO19 8SQ, England

Telephone (+44) 1243 779777

Email (for orders and customer service enquiries): cs-books@wiley.co.uk
Visit our Home Page on www.wileyeurope.com or www.wiley.com

Other Wiley Editorial Offices

John Wiley & Sons Inc., 111 River Street, Hoboken, NJ 07030, USA

Jossey-Bass, 989 Market Street, San Francisco, CA 94103-1741, USA

Wiley-VCH Verlag GmbH, Boschstr. 12, D-69469 Weinheim, Germany

John Wiley & Sons Australia Ltd., 33 Park Road, Milton, Queensland 4064, Australia

John Wiley & Sons (Asia) Pte Ltd., 2 Clementi Loop #02-01, Jin Xing Distripark, Singapore 129809

John Wiley & Sons Canada Ltd., 22 Worcester Road, Etobicoke Rexdale, Ontario, Canada M9W 1L1

Wiley also publishes its books in a variety of electronic formats. Some content that appears in print may not be available in electronic books.

Library of Congress Cataloging-in-Publication Data

Staged diabetes management : a systematic approach / by Roger S. Mazze...
[et al.] (International Diabetes Center).
p. ; cm.
Includes bibliographical references and index.
ISBN 0-470-86576-8 (cloth : alk. paper)
1. Diabetes. 2. Medical protocols. 3. Evidence-based medicine. I. Mazze, R. S. II. International Diabetes Center.
[DNLM: 1. Diabetes Mellitus–therapy. 2. Diabetes Mellitus–diagnosis.
WK 815 S779 2004]
RC660.S67 2004
616.4′62–dc22

2004007053

British Library Cataloguing in Publication Data

A catalogue record for this book is available from the British Library

ISBN 0-470-86576-8

Typeset in 11/13.5pt Times by Keytec Typesetting Ltd, Bridport, Dorset
Printed and bound in Great Britain by Antony Rowe Ltd, Chippenham, Wilts
This book is printed on acid-free paper responsibly manufactured from sustainable forestry in which at least two trees are planted for each one used for paper production.

Dedicated to the Memory Of Dr. Donnell D. Etzwiler

Donnell Etzwiler was a man of ideas and vision. He believed that the patient was part of a team that included all healthcare professionals working in concert to provide the best care and education.

He dared to dream that others would share his vision. For 30 years he was President of the International Diabetes Center; always challenging those he worked with to do their best. He tirelessly shared his ideas and vision with thousands of health professionals from around the world.

More than once, Donnell Etzwiler was willing to subject each of his ideas to the rigors of scientific inquiry and criticism. He accepted the notion that as scientists we are fallible, that we learn from each discovery, and that indeed we may be mistaken.

Donnell Etzwiler filled every moment with the joys of discovery, with commitment to his skills as a physician, with teaching his colleagues, with caring for all of us, and most important with devotion to family.

We owe it as friends and colleagues, as witnesses to his generosity of spirit, to dedicate this book to his memory.

Roger S. Mazze, Ellie Strock, Gregg Simonson and Richard Bergenstal

Contents

About the Authors

Roger S. Mazze, PhD, Chief Academic Officer, International Diabetes Center, Vice President, Park Nicollet Institute. Director, World Health Organization Collaborating Center at International Diabetes Center and Clinical Professor of Family Practice and Community Health, University of Minnesota Medical School. Formerly, Professor of Biostatistics, Epidemiology and Community Health, and Executive Director and Co-Principal Investigator of the Diabetes Research and Training Center, Albert Einstein College of Medicine and Distinguished Visiting Scientist to the United States Centers for Disease Control. Past Co-Chairperson, American Diabetes Association Council on Health Care Delivery.

Ellie S. Strock, RN, BC, ANP, CDE, Chief of Professional Services, International Diabetes Center, Vice President, Park Nicollet Institute. Chief Education Director, World Health Organization Collaborating Center at International Diabetes Center. Board Certified Adult Nurse Practitioner, Department of Endocrinology, Park Nicollet Health Services.

Gregg D. Simonson, PhD, Director, Program Research and Implementation and Chief Research Officer, World Health Organization Collaborating Center at International Diabetes Center. Adjunct Assistant Professor, Department of Family Practice and Community Health, University of Minnesota Medical School. Formerly, Post-Doctoral Fellow, Juvenile Diabetes Foundation, Department of Pediatrics, University of Wisconsin.

Richard M. Bergenstal, MD, Executive Director, International Diabetes Center and Clinical Professor of Medicine in Endocrinology, University of Minnesota Medical School. Consultant, Department of Endocrinology, Park Nicollet Health Services. Formerly, Assistant Professor of Medicine, University of Chicago. Past Member, National Board of Directors, American Diabetes Association.

Staged Diabetes Management: A Systematic Approach (2nd Edition) R. S. Mazze, E. S. Strock, G. D. Simonson and R. M. Bergenstal
 ISBN: 0 470 86576 8

Acknowledgments

The authors would like to recognize the expert review and contributions to specific chapters provided by the following individuals:

Chapter 2: The Implementation of Staged Diabetes Management

Renea Bradley, MSN, ARNP, CDE, International Diabetes Center

Rachel Robinson, PHN, CDE, MPH, International Diabetes Center

Chapter 3: Therapeutic Principles for the Treatment of Diabetes

David Kendall, MD, International Diabetes Center

Chapter 4: Type 2 Diabetes

Nancy Cooper, RD, LD, CDE, International Diabetes Center

Marion Franz, MS, RD, LD, CDE

Manuel Idrogo, MD, University of Minnesota

Chapter 5: Type 2 Diabetes and Insulin Resistance Syndrome in Children and Adolescents

Rachel Robinson, PHN, CDE, MPH, International Diabetes Center

Stephanie Gerken, RD, CDE, International Diabetes Center

Martha Spencer, MD, International Diabetes Center

Stephen Ponder, MD, Driscoll Childrens Hospital

Manuel Idrogo, MD, University of Minnesota

Chapter 6: Type 1 Diabetes

Martha Spencer, MD, International Diabetes Center

Chapter 7: Pregestational and Gestational Diabetes

Janet Davidson, BSN, RN, CDE, International Diabetes Center

Diane Reader, RD, LD, CDE, International Diabetes Center

Chapter 8: Macrovascular Complications

William Keane, MD, Hennepin County Medical Center

David Kendall, MD, International Diabetes Center

Chapter 9: Microvascular Complications

Ronald Klein, MD, MPH, University of Wisconsin Medical School

Marvin Levin, MD, Washington School of Medicine

Michael Pfeifer, MD, East Carolina University School of Medicine

Steven Rith-Najarian, MD, MPH, Indian Health Service

Chapter 10: Hospitalization

Irl Hirsch, MD, University of Washington

The authors would like to acknowledge the following individuals:

Kelly Acton, MD
Sandie Anderson, RN, CDE
Barbara Barry, MS, RD, CDE
Renea Bradley, MSN, ARNP, CDE
Rahim Bassiri, MD
Evan Benjamin, MD
Brenda Broussard, MPH, MBA, RD
Tish Callahan, BS, RN, CDE
Gay Castle, RD, LD, CDE
Nancy Cooper, RD, LD, CDE
Andrew Crighton, MD
Norma Curtis, RN
Larry Deeb, MD
Marcie Draheim, RN, CDE
Lisa Fish, MD
Stephanie Gerken, RD, CDE
Joseph Giangola, MD
Barry Ginsberg, MD, PhD
Dorothy Gohdes, MD
Mary Greeley, MS, RD, CDE
Broatch Haig, RD, CDE
Ronald Harris, MD
Bruce Henson, MD
Priscilla Hollander, MD, PhD
Joe Humphry, MD
Manuel Idrogo, MD
Ronald Iverson, MD
Joel Jahraus, MD
Mary Johnson, RN, CDE
David Kendall, MD
Elizabeth Kern, MD
Annie Kontos, DO
Oded Langer, MD
Deborah Lippert, BSN, RN, CDE
Michele Malone, BSN, RN
Kempei Matsuoka, MD
Michael Miller, MD
Arlene Monk, RD, LD, CDE
Karen Moulton, CFNP, MHS, CDE
Kathryn Mulcahy, MSN, RN, CDE
Joseph Nelson, MA, LP
Jan Pearson, BAN, RN, CDE
Alan Peiris, MD, PhD
Jan Perloff, MD
Stephan Ponder, MD, FAAP, CDE
Kate Raines, MSN, RN, CDE
Terry Raymer, MD, CDE
Patti Rickheim, MS, RN, CDE
Steve Rith-Najarian, MD
Rachel Robinson, PHN, MPH, CDE
Suzanne Rogacz, MD
Muriel Sorbel, MA, RN, CDE
Helen Stover, RN, CDE
Ken Strauss, MD
Stuart Sundem, MPH
Meng Tan, MD
Sandra Thurm, BSN, RN, CDE
Timothy Wahl, MD

PART ONE

STAGED DIABETES MANAGEMENT IN PRACTICE

1 Introduction to Staged Diabetes Management

The underlying principle in managing diabetes has undergone several important changes over the last two decades. Diabetes was once believed to be a disease with inevitable microvascular and macrovascular complications. Current approaches to management, however, recognize the benefit of maintaining tight glycemic control and addressing associated metabolic disorders. The focus in diabetes management has shifted to include the importance of achieving blood pressure and lipid targets along with conventional blood glucose control. In fact, any improvement in these physiologic markers is seen as a means to prevent or slow the progression of microvascular and macrovascular complications.[1–4] Most individuals with diabetes and its associated disorders require a variety of therapies to treat, delay, or prevent complications. High-quality care is dependent on understanding which therapies are appropriate and when to use them.

The majority of individuals with diabetes have their first contact with a primary care provider (family practitioner, pediatrician, internist, nurse practitioner, physician assistant, or obstetrician). Only a small proportion (estimated, overall, at less than 10 per cent of all people with diabetes) are initially seen and regularly followed by a specialist (either an endocrinologist in the United States or a diabetologist or endocrinologist in other countries). Primary care providers have expressed the desire for guidelines to ensure that they are conforming to current good practices. Typically, primary care providers have had an inconsistent approach to diabetes screening, diagnosis, treatment, and management of complications. This inconsistency may be traced to the lack of ample, persuasive scientific evidence available in the primary care setting showing that improved diabetes management through metabolic control and intensive therapies are necessary to prevent the short and long term complications of diabetes. With the expansion of diabetes to encompass attention to related metabolic disorders, including metabolic syndrome, the inconsistency in treatment approaches has become more problematic. In short, primary care providers need a carefully developed set of clinical guidelines and algorithms that can be realistically implemented, tested, and shown to be efficacious and cost effective.[5]

> Primary care is that care provided by physicians specifically trained for and skilled in comprehensive first contact and continuing care for persons with any undiagnosed sign, symptom, or health concern not limited by problem origin, organ system, gender, or diagnosis. Primary care includes health promotion, disease prevention, health maintenance, counseling, patient education, diagnosis and treatment of acute and chronic illness in a variety of health care settings. Primary care is performed and managed by a personal physician, utilizing other health professionals,

Staged Diabetes Management: A Systematic Approach (2nd Edition) R. S. Mazze, E. S. Strock, G. D. Simonson and R. M. Bergenstal
© 2004 Matrex ISBN: 0 470 86576 8

> consultation and/or referral as appropriate. Primary care provides patient advocacy in the health care system to accomplish cost-effective care by coordination of health care services.
>
> —The American Academy of Family Physicians

Staged Diabetes Management (SDM) is a systematic approach to preventing, detecting, and treating diabetes, metabolic syndrome, and associated disorders using practice guidelines and clinical pathways (algorithms) that reflect the changing responsibilities of the primary care provider and the primary care team.

The purpose of SDM is to:

- provide a systematic, data-based approach for clinical decision making
- provide a consistent set of scientifically based practice guidelines that can be adapted by a community according to its resources
- identify appropriate criteria for initiating and altering therapies during three treatment phases: Start, Adjust, and Maintain
- provide a common customized Master DecisionPath for each type of diabetes and metabolic syndrome that both patients and providers can use to understand treatment options, to enhance communication, and to optimize therapies
- facilitate the detection and treatment of diabetes, insulin resistance, and their complications by primary care providers, in consultation with specialists.
- foster a patient centered team approach to the management of diabetes and associated complications

The development of Staged Diabetes Management

The idea for SDM stems from the need to provide a systematic approach to disease prevention, detection, and treatment using methodologies that are easily applicable to the primary care setting. To accomplish this, a team of endocrinologists, family physicians, clinical nurse specialists, dietitians, and community health specialists joined together in 1988 to identify the therapeutic principles that lie at the core of diabetes management. Specialists joined the team as needed, including perinatologists, epidemiologists, and psychologists, among others. The team investigated approaches to the treatment of type 1 diabetes, type 2 diabetes, and diabetes in pregnancy as well as their associated complications and co-morbidities. At biweekly conferences over a period of 5 months, each step in diagnosing and treating each type of diabetes was carefully delineated.

Key decision points were placed on algorithms termed "DecisionPaths." These DecisionPaths contained the following:

- treatment modalities
- criteria for initiating treatment
- criteria for changing treatment
- key clinical decision points
- metabolic targets, including reasonable timelines to achieve target
- recommended follow-up

Since its initiation in 1988, SDM has undergone clinical trials and implementation studies in more than 800 sites worldwide. The results have led to changes in the original design of SDM and are reflected in this text. Nevertheless, the basic principles upon which SDM is founded remain intact.

To continue to refine this systematic approach to clinical decision-making, the records of randomly selected patients with diabetes or at risk for developing diabetes are periodically evaluated. These are supplemented by research data from SDM sites as well as a comprehensive review of relevant literature.

In type 1 diabetes, this review and update process focuses on:

- criteria for selecting an appropriate insulin regimen
- criteria for prescribing insulin analogues
- criteria for administering insulin pump therapy
- medical nutrition therapy (meal planning and exercise)
- patient education
- assessment of inhaled insulin and other newer therapies

For each of these subjects, where possible, metabolic markers such as sequential glycosylated hemoglobin (HbA_{1c}) and verified self-monitored blood glucose data are obtained. Short- and long-term outcomes, such as metabolic control, complications surveillance, and microvascular and macrovascular complications, are tracked. Recently, cost and patient satisfaction factors have been added to the analysis.

For type 2 diabetes, the focus has changed from concentration on criteria for initiation of medical nutrition therapy, oral agent, combination, and insulin therapies to prevention, screening, early detection, and intensive multi-dimensional therapies. Treatment components such as patient education, nutritional interventions, and psychosocial counseling are also examined. Diabetes is examined as part of the metabolic syndrome, with attention to obesity, hypertension, dyslipidemia, and renal disease.

In type 2 diabetes, data are organized to address the following.

- Treatment modalities: medical nutrition therapy, oral agent monotherapies (alpha-glucosidase inhibitors, biguanides, meglitinides, sulfonylureas, nateglinides, and thiazolidinediones), oral agent combination therapies, insulin and oral agent combination therapies, insulin, and insulin analogues
- Criteria for initiating treatment: factors to consider in selecting the first treatment modality
- Criteria for changing treatment: factors to consider for selecting subsequent treatment modalities
- Information about establishing, monitoring, and evaluating therapies: details related to any of the decisions, treatments, or actions. (This includes information to be collected by either the patient or the physician to evaluate how effective the treatment is in meeting therapeutic goals. It also encompasses monitoring associated with the schedule of provider and patient data collection, including the timing of laboratory tests and the frequency of self-monitoring of blood glucose.)

For gestational diabetes (GDM), the focus now includes an examination of the association between GDM, insulin resistance, and type 2 diabetes. Criteria for initiation of medical nutrition, glyburide, and insulin therapies are carefully evaluated against the short- and long-term outcomes of pregnancy (including neonatal size, childhood and adult obesity for the offspring, maternal metabolic complications, and the development of type 2 diabetes, hypertension, and dyslipidemia).

Complications have been divided into those associated with the metabolic syndrome (obesity, hypertension, and dyslipidemia) and those more closely associated with microvascular disease (renal, retinal, and neurological disorders). For each complication general practice guidelines, stipulating screening and diagnostic criteria, treatment options, targets, monitoring, and follow-up, have been developed. Additionally, hospitalization for acute metabolic complications of diabetes and management of diabetes during surgery and other inter-current events are addressed.

Developed for the primary care setting, the material on complications serves as a basis for clinical decision-making. As with all of SDM, referral to a specialist is advised whenever the complexities of the disease exceed the resources available in the primary care setting. Each complication practice guideline is followed by DecisionPaths, which outline screening, diagnosis, therapy selection, and follow-up procedures. Most sections also include a table that addresses the changes in treatment for diabetes in the presence of the complication.

The structure of Staged Diabetes Management

Staged Diabetes Management is a systematic approach to the prevention, detection, and treatment of diabetes and metabolic syndrome and their complications that organizes care in terms of stages and phases.[6] Stages refer to type of treatment, with the underlying concept that there should be a consistency in the use of treatment modalities: for example, the notion that medical nutrition therapy is a critical element in the goal of managing blood glucose and blood pressure. Thinking in terms of stages also helps to understand the universal role, independent of type of diabetes, that insulin plays in establishing and maintaining glycemic control. Most important, however, is the concept that stages are dynamic, subject to initiation, adjustment, maintenance, and abandonment. Care of a chronic illness such as diabetes or hypertension is, after all, a continuum. It begins with diagnosis and/or initiation of a therapy (starting phase), and then moves to the adjusting phase until the targets are reached, at which point the current therapy is maintained. Therefore, we have chosen to conceptualize care by way of the concepts of stage, delineating therapy, and phase, delineating progress.

Stages of therapy for diabetes

Diabetes care is undergoing a revolution in terms of available therapies. During the past decade more than seven new classifications of medications (both oral agents and insulin) have been introduced. We chose to call each therapy a stage to enable us to demonstrate how they have an impact on diabetes management. The medical nutrition and activity therapy stage, formerly known simply as diet and exercise, constitutes within SDM the use of a food and activity plan to help patients achieve their metabolic targets. Oral agents, both nonhypoglycemic and hypoglycemic, constitute the oral agent stage. Finally, insulin (rapid, short, intermediate, and long acting) constitutes our insulin stages 1 through 4 plus pump therapy. Within insulin therapies, stage numbers refer to the number of insulin injections administered per day. All insulin therapy is also considered from the perspective of providing basal (or background) and bolus (or pre-meal) requirements.

Phases of therapy

Approaching the treatment of any disease without a structure in mind is akin to driving with a final destination in mind, but without a map to follow. To make certain that we have a map and that we know where we are on the map, we divided care into three phases: start phase, adjust phase, and maintain phase. This approach suggests that treatment is dynamic. It reflects actual practice. At any point in treatment the individual is in one of these three phases. Knowing the phase is analogous to knowing one's place on the map. It is possible to see instantaneously both where one has been and where one is headed.

Start phase

The start treatment phase refers to the collection of data upon which to base diagnosis and initiate treatment. Ideally, diabetes care and management of complications begin with baseline data from which the practitioner can assess a patient's clinical status. Each type of diabetes, associated complication, or co-morbidity requires different data for diagnosis and clinical decision-making. In type 1 diabetes, for example, clinical symptoms, blood glucose values, urine ketones, serum pH, age, and body weight serve as critical starting points. In type 2 diabetes, blood glucose values, HbA_{1c}, body mass index, markers of insulin resistance, and co-morbidities are critical elements in understanding the nature of this disease.

Adjust phase

During the adjust treatment phase, changes in therapy—whether in insulin dose or regimen, food plan, exercise/activity, or oral agent—are made to optimize metabolic control. Lasting anywhere from days to months, this phase is marked by substantial patient involvement in collecting data upon which to decide on medication changes and to judge the effects of the alterations in therapy. The principles by which major alterations in food plan, exercise/activity, oral agent, or insulin dose, mapped out in the Master DecisionPaths, are provided in greater detail in the Start and Adjust DecisionPaths for each stage (therapy) of diabetes management. For the purpose of routine diabetes management, a single standard or guideline for glucose control is highly desirable. The results of the Diabetes Control and Complications Trial[1] in type 1 diabetes and the United Kingdom Diabetes Prospective Study[7] in type 2 diabetes have demonstrated the desirability of one standard of glucose control. It should be understood that the glycemic goals for type 2 diabetes uncomplicated by pregnancy are the same as those for type 1 diabetes, specifically between 70 and 140 mg/dL (3.9 and 7.8 mmol/L), pre-meal. However, target blood glucose ranges should then be determined individually. For diabetes complicated by pregnancy, blood glucose levels ranging from 60 to 120 mg/dL (3.3 to 6.7 mmol/L) should serve as a guide. Glycosylated hemoglobin A_{1G} (HbA_{1c}) should be used to verify overall blood glucose control. Therefore, as a general guide, HbA_{1c} levels within one percentage point of the upper limit of normal should be the goal in type 1 and type 2 diabetes. For diabetes in pregnancy, HbA_{1c} values should be within normal range. If this goal is not met within a specified period of time, the therapy should be adjusted or changed. It is this last point that underlines the need for thinking about diabetes in terms of phases. The goal should be to move the patient from adjust to maintain as quickly and as safely as is reasonable. Patients in the adjust phase are at higher risk for complications. It is not until they reach the maintain phase that the risk of complications is substantially lowered.

Maintain phase

This phase begins when the patient has reached and is involved in maintaining the target blood glucose goals associated with the long-term prevention of complications. Patients are expected to move in and out of this phase independent of the type of treatment, based on such factors as changes in lifestyle, compliance with regimen, psychological and social adjustment to diabetes, willingness to achieve tighter control, and natural progression of diabetes. Thus, some changes in therapy are expected in this phase, but they are related more to fine-tuning than to major alterations in dose of medication.

Phases in the treatment of insulin resistance and complications

As with the treatment of diabetes, management of insulin resistance related disorders such as hypertension can be seen as divided into start, adjust, and maintain therapy. Naturally, for each disorder the object is to restore normal or near-normal status, when possible. In many cases, due to preexisting co-morbidities, the objective is to prevent further progression of the complication.

Practice guidelines

Staged Diabetes Management relies on practice guidelines to lay the foundation for treatment and on DecisionPaths to provide the means. Thus, SDM consists of a set of practice guidelines for the three types of diabetes, for metabolic syndrome, and for other complications. Practice guidelines are structured to address prevention, screening and diagnosis, treatment options, metabolic targets, monitoring, and follow-up. Figure 1.1 shows the Type 2 Diabetes Practice Guidelines.

For over a decade the Institute of Medicine (IOM) has been evaluating the characteristics of practice guidelines that contribute to successful implementation. Defined by the IOM, practice guidelines are "systematically developed statements to assist practitioner and patient in decisions about appropriate health care for specific clinical circumstances."[8] Incorporating science and clinical judgment, practice guidelines are meant to improve the quality of care by ensuring consistency in the delivery of health care services. Quality of care has been directly associated with reduced variation in medical practice. A common practice guideline accepted by all health care providers removes inconsistencies in the diagnosis and treatment of medical conditions and results in more effective use of health care resources, improved outcomes, cost savings, and reduced risk of legal liability for negligent care.

> Scientific evidence and clinical judgment can be systematically combined to produce clinically valid, operational recommendations for appropriate care that can and will be used to persuade clinicians, patients and others to change their practices in ways that lead to better health outcomes and lower health care costs.
>
> —Guidelines for Clinical Practice, The Institute of Medicine[8]

Valid practice guidelines facilitate consistent, effective, and efficient medical care and ultimately lead to improved outcomes for patients. To accomplish this, guidelines must contain sufficient detail to have measurable clinical outcomes. For best results, practice guidelines should be specific, comprehensive, and accepted by the community of physicians and all other medical team members. Guidelines need to be flexible enough for everyday use in clinical practice and must reflect the available community resources.

The first principle of practice guidelines is that they are based on sound scientific findings. Staged Diabetes Management Practice Guidelines are based on the recommendations of the American Diabetes Association (ADA), the National Diabetes Data Group, the International Diabetes Federation (IDF), the World Health Organization (WHO), American Association of Diabetes Educators (AADE), and other diabetes organizations representing several countries outside of the United States. These organizations have reviewed the current scientific data and many have reached consensus on major elements of diabetes care:

- diagnostic criteria and classification
- treatment options
- therapeutic targets for blood glucose, HbA_{1c}, blood pressure, and lipids
- frequency of blood glucose, urine ketones, and HbA_{1c} monitoring
- complication surveillance (eye and foot exams, screening for microalbuminuria)
- medical follow-up recommendations
- need to identify and treat complications of diabetes as early as possible

These organizations have also addressed insulin

Screening

Screen all patients every 3 years starting at age 45; if risk factors present, start earlier and screen annually

Risk Factors

- BMI > 25 kg/m^2 (especially waist-to-hip ratio > 1)
- Family history of type 2 diabetes (especially first-degree relatives)
- Age (risk increases with age)
- Hypertension (≥140/90 mm Hg)
- Dyslipidemia (HDL ≤ 35 mg/dL [0.90 mmol/L] and/or triglyceride ≥ 250 mg/dL [2.8 mmol/L])
- Previous impaired fasting glucose (IFG) with fasting plasma glucose 100–125 mg/dL (5.6–6.9 mmol/L)
- Previous impaired glucose tolerance (IGT) with oral glucose tolerance test (OGTT) 2 hour glucose value 140–199 mg/dL (7.8–11 mmol/L)
- Previous gestational diabetes: macrosomic or large-for-gestational age infant
- Polycystic ovary syndrome
- Acanthosis Nigricans
- American Indian or Alaska Native; African-American; Asian; Native Hawaiian or Other Pacific Islander; Hispanic

Diagnosis

Plasma Glucose Casual ≥ 200 mg/dL (11.1 mmol/L) plus symptoms, fasting ≥ 126 mg/dL (7.0 mmol/L), or 75 gram oral glucose tolerance test (OGTT) 2 hour glucose value ≥ 200 mg/dL (11.1 mmol/L); if positive, confirm diagnosis within 7 days unless evidence of metabolic decompensation

Symptoms Often none

Common: blurred vision; urinary tract infection; yeast infection; dry, itchy skin; numbness or tingling in extremities; fatigue

Occasional: increased urination, thirst, and appetite; nocturia; weight loss

Urine Ketones Usually negative

Treatment Options

Medical nutrition therapy; oral agent (α-glucosidase inhibitor, metformin, repaglinide, nateglinide, sulfonylurea, thiazolidinedione); combination therapy (oral agents, oral agent–insulin); Insulin: Stages 2, 3, 4

Targets

Self-Monitored Blood Glucose (SMBG)

- More than 50% of SMBG values within target range
- Pre-meal; 70–140 mg/dL (3.9–7.8 mmol/L)
- Post-meal (2 hours after start of meal): < 160 mg/dL (8.9 mmol/L)
- Bedtime: 100–160 mg/dL (5.6–8.9 mmol/L)
- No severe (assisted) or nocturnal hypoglycemia

  Adjust pre-meal target upwards if decreased life expectancy; frail elderly; cognitive disorders; or other medical concerns (cardiac disease, stroke, hypoglycemia unawareness, end-stage renal disease)

Hemoglobin HbA_{1c}

- Within 1.0 percentage point of upper limit of normal (e.g., normal 6.0%; target < 7.0%)
- Frequency: 3–4 times per year
- Use HbA_{1c} to verify SMBG data

Monitoring

SMBG 2 4 times per day (e.g., before meals, 2 hours after start of meal, bedtime); may be modified due to cost, technical ability, availability of meters; if on insulin, check 3 AM SMBG as needed

Method Meter with memory and log book

Follow-up

Monthly Office visit during adjust phase (weekly phone contact may be necessary)

Every 3 Months Hypoglycemia; medications; weight or BMI; medical nutrition therapy; BP; SMBG data (download meter); HbA_{1c}; eye screen; foot screen; diabetes/nutrition continuing education; smoking cessation counseling, aspirin therapy

Yearly In addition to the 3 month follow-up, complete the following: history and physical; fasting lipid profile; albuminuria screen; dilated eye examination; dental examination; neurologic assessment; complete foot examination (pulses, nerves, ankle-branchial index and inspection); immunizations

Complications Surveillance

Cardiovascular, renal, retinal, neurological, foot, oral, and dermatological

See *Chronic Complications MasterDecisionPath*

Figure 1.1 Type 2 Diabetes Practice Guidelines

resistance and many have reached a working consensus that:

- relates insulin resistance to hyperglycemia, hypertension, dyslipidemia, central obesity and renal disease
- recognizes the need to intensively treat each condition
- recognizes the increased risk of developing one condition when another exists
- sets general targets

The second principle of practice guidelines is that they contain sufficient specificity to allow for their implementation. The SDM Master and Specific DecisionPaths aid in implementing the practice guidelines.

The third principle of practice guidelines is that they are adapted to the community, adopted by the health care providers, and reflect the specific resources of the community. The key components of this process include:

- community needs assessment
- orientation to SDM
- adaptation and adoption of practice guidelines by health care professionals
- implementation plan for SDM
- plan for short-term and long-term outcome assessment:

Master DecisionPaths

The SDM Master DecisionPaths outline the therapeutic stages for each type of diabetes and show the most effective route for attaining metabolic control. Each stage represents a therapeutic regimen. Stages include medical nutrition and activity therapy, oral agent, combination therapy, and insulin.

The Master DecisionPaths guide the selection of an initial treatment for diabetes based on the current plasma glucose and/or HbA_{1c} at diagnosis. They also help in setting the level of blood glucose control and HbA_{1c} targets with their patients. If a therapy fails, the Master DecisionPaths guide the progression to other stages of therapy. The Type 2 Diabetes Master DecisionPath is shown in Figure 1.2 as an example.

Access to the Master DecisionPath takes place through the rounded rectangular shapes, which contain the entry criteria. Each rectangular shape defines a particular therapeutic stage, the timeline within which to reach target, and guidelines for moving to another stage of therapy if targets are not met. All Master DecisionPaths follow the same format.

The "shorthand" notations within the rectangles represent the therapy and depict the four times for administering a pharmacologic agent: AM (fasting), Midday (before the Midday meal), PM (before the evening meal), and BT (bedtime, or at least 2 to 3 hours after the evening meal). Letters are written for each time period to indicate which medication is administered, or a "0" (zero) is written to indicate when no medication is given at that time. Thus, Insulin Stage 2 is written as "R/N–0–R/N–0," referring to the short-acting regular insulin (R) mixed with N insulin injected before breakfast and again before the evening meal. No medication is taken at midday or at bedtime. Note that rapid-acting (RA) Lispro or Aspart insulin can be substituted for regular insulin in most insulin regimens. For Insulin Stage 2, the resulting shorthand is "RA/N–0–RA/N–0."

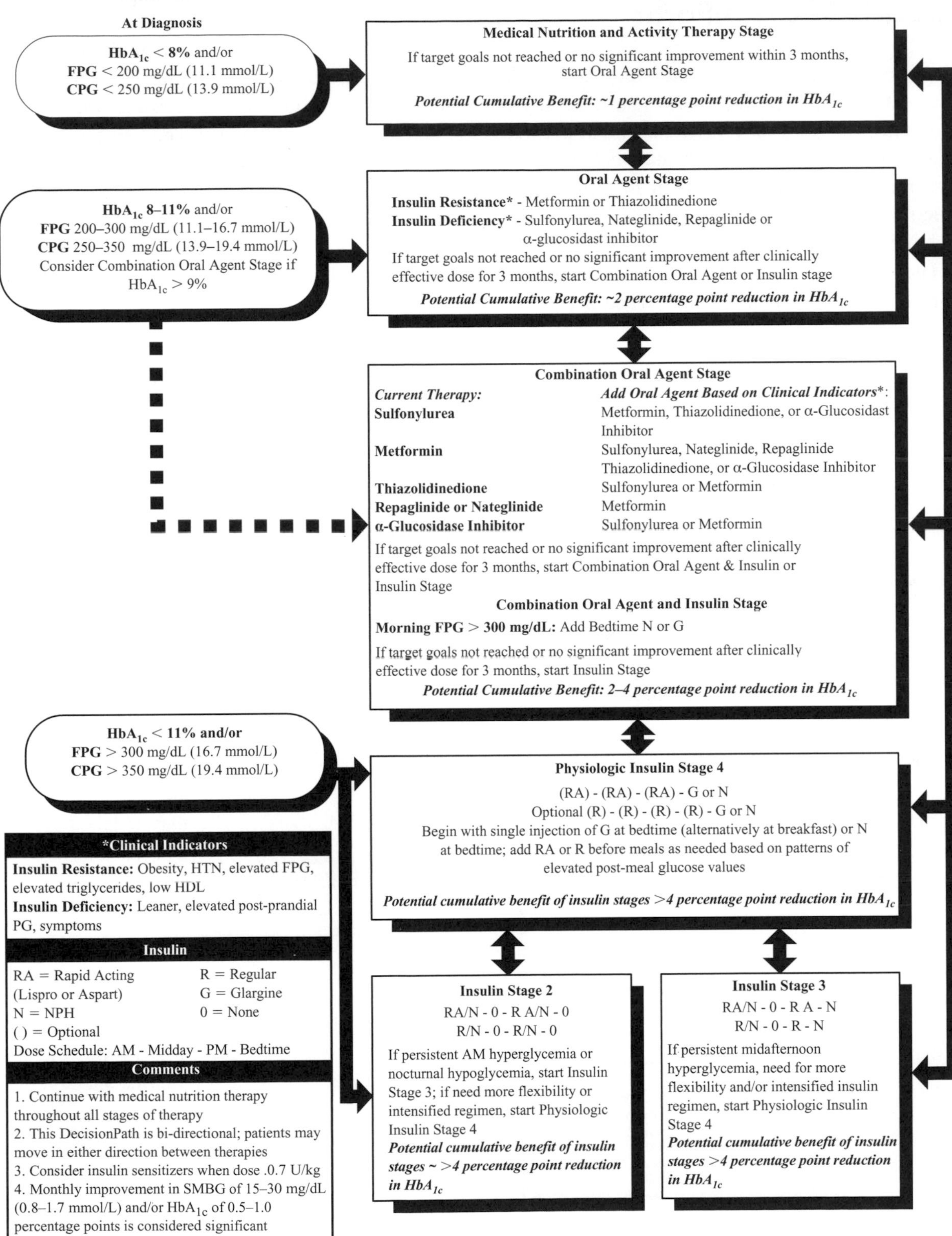

Figure 1.2 Type-2 Diabetes Master DecisionPath

Specific DecisionPaths

The heart of the DecisionPath approach is the intersection of stage and phase (start, adjust, or maintain). Staged Diabetes Management provides a DecisionPath for each such intersection, which describes the action to be taken in terms of the specific therapy and also indicates the general path being followed and the progress being made.

There are two types of Specific DecisionPath: start and adjust/maintain. Using Type 2 Diabetes Insulin Stage 2 as an example (see Figure 1.3), note that the structure of the Start DecisionPath begins with the entry criteria (blood glucose at diagnosis or failure of a previous therapy). It then moves to the medical visit and the blood glucose targets and is followed by notes related to starting the treatment. After the "how to start" comes the follow-up information. The same structure is used for all Start DecisionPaths.

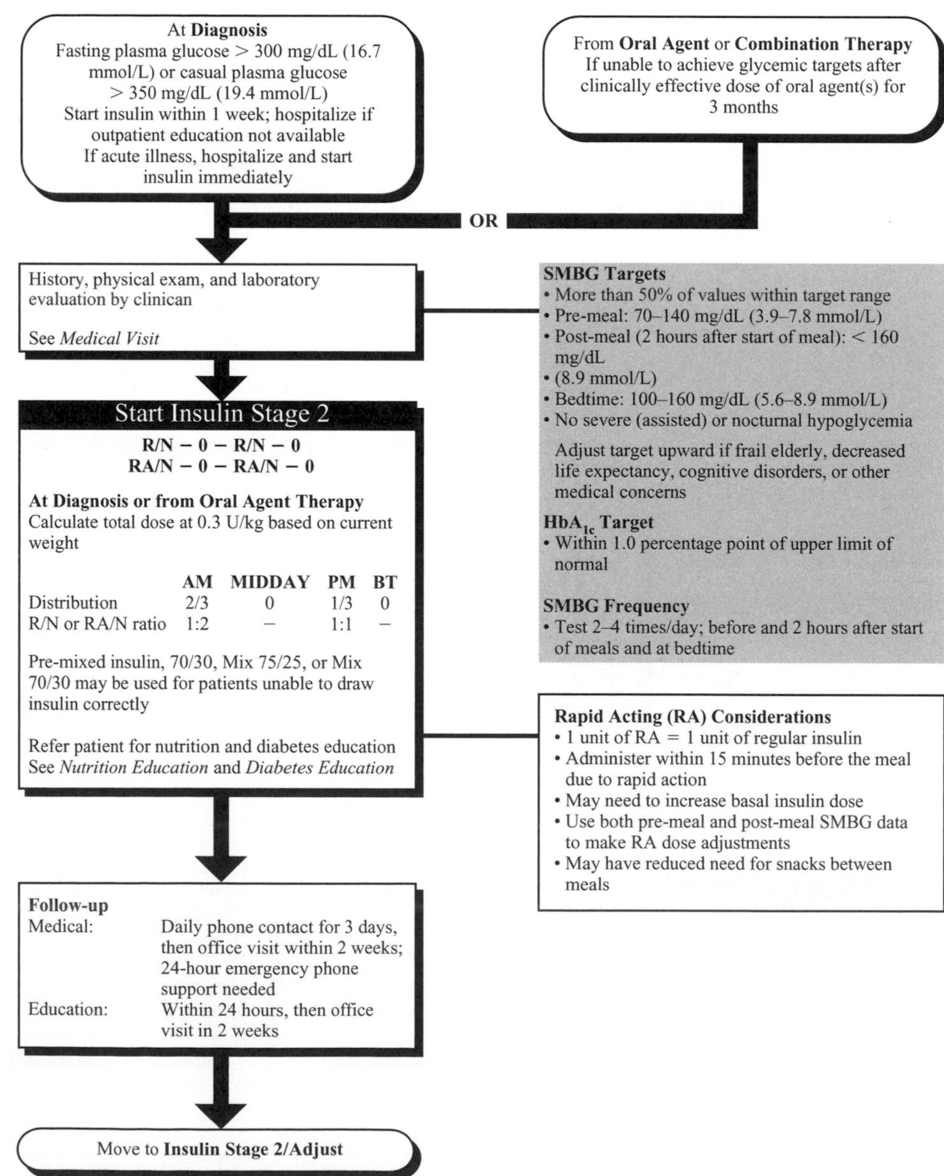

Figure 1.3 Type 2 Diabetes Insulin Stage 2/Start DecisionPath

A second type of Specific DecisionPath relates to adjusting and maintaining the current therapy. As shown in the Metformin/Adjust DecisionPath (Figure 1.4), the DecisionPath begins with a brief review of key data and a reminder of the target levels. These data (current medications, diabetes control, adherence, weight change, and hypo/hyperglycemic events) are common for all forms of diabetes. This is followed by a closer evaluation of current glycemic control.

When glycemic target levels are reached, the patient enters the maintain phase. The DecisionPaths for adjusting therapy (i.e., Figure 1.4 Metformin/Adjust) contain guidelines for routine follow-up, which are consistent with the standards of practice recommended by national diabetes organizations. These include the frequency of visits and the period of time between visits. If the target blood glucose level has not been reached, the next step is to determine why. Many

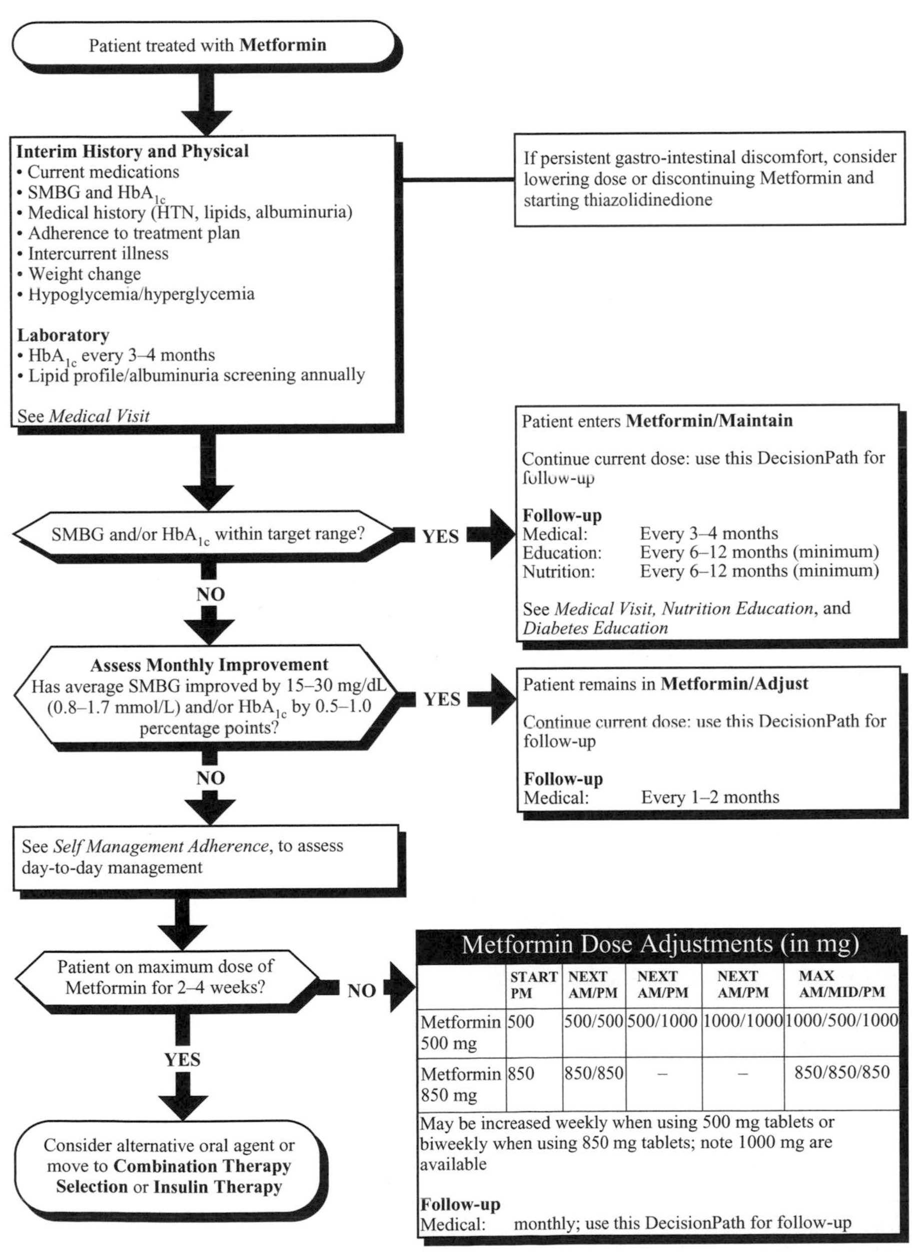

	START PM	NEXT AM/PM	NEXT AM/PM	NEXT AM/PM	MAX AM/MID/PM
Metformin 500 mg	500	500/500	500/1000	1000/1000	1000/500/1000
Metformin 850 mg	850	850/850	–	–	850/850/850
May be increased weekly when using 500 mg tablets or biweekly when using 850 mg tablets; note 1000 mg are available					
Follow-up Medical: monthly; use this DecisionPath for follow-up					

Figure 1.4 Metformin/Adjust DecisionPath

practitioners blame a lack of patient adherence. When this is the case, the Ancillary DecisionPaths entitled "Psychological and Social Assessment" and "Diabetes Management Adherence Assessment" are used to address issues related to adherence. However, *an underlying principle of SDM is that therapies, not patients, fail.* Thus, if adherence is not the problem, the next step is to assess whether any improvement has occurred. Over the period of 1 month the average self-monitored blood glucose (SMBG) should drop by 15–30 mg/dL (0.8–1.7 mmol/L), which corresponds to a drop in the HbA_{1c} of 0.5–1 percentage point. If this is occurring, the current treatment is continued without any adjustment. If these criteria are not met, further adjustment is necessary.

Each pharmacological agent has a maximum safe and effective dose. For oral agents, SDM utilizes maximum dose criteria provided in the package insert, but also reports the clinically effective dose, which sometimes is well below the maximum recommended dose. For example, the clinically effective dose of sulfonylureas is approximately two-thirds the maximum dose. For insulin, in general, between 1 and 1.5 U/kg (depending on the type of diabetes and the age of the patient) is considered the maximum safe dose. Exceeding this range requires a re-evaluation of the therapy. Staged Diabetes Management provides similar criteria for each adjust phase, and also provides reasons for moving from one stage to the next. For example, the choice of combination or insulin therapy is based on whether the lack of improvement is due primarily to fasting hyperglycemia or postprandial hyperglycemia. For insulin Stage 2, the criteria for moving to Insulin Stage 3 are persistent fasting hyperglycemia, nocturnal hypoglycemia, or insufficient improvement in HbA_{1c}.

Criteria for adjusting and changing therapy

The underlying principle in SDM is that there is a rational and consistent set of criteria that can be applied when considering moving a patient from one therapy (stage) to another. Part of the principle is that the decision be founded on (but not limited to) verified SMBG data and HbA_{1c} values. The therapeutic goal is to achieve a change of 0.5 to 1.0 percentage point in HbA_{1c} each month with a parallel improvement in average blood glucose as measured by reduction in SMBG of 15–30 mg/dL (0.8–1.7 mmol/L). To achieve this therapeutic goal, current therapy must be reconsidered frequently. Assessing the patient's adherence to the treatment plan includes reviewing blood glucose monitoring technique and records, food plan and activity record keeping, and consistency in following the pharmacologic regimen.

The first step to assess the current therapy is to ensure that a sufficient number of SMBG tests are performed. Generally, this requires a minimum of four tests each day at specified times, such as: before meals, 2 hours post-meal, bedtime, and 3 AM as required. If patterns of SMBG data confirm blood glucose levels consistently greater than target, consider *adjusting* the therapy. If no improvement is noted, consider *changing* to an alternative therapy. The change to more complex therapies permits greater flexibility in reaching a particular blood glucose target.

Diabetes Management Assessment DecisionPaths

Diabetes Management Assessment DecisionPaths provide specific information for initial and follow-up medical visits, psychological and social evaluation, treatment and prevention of hypoglycemia, illness assessment and management, diabetes and nutrition education, exercise, and adherence assessment. For example, the Diabetes Education DecisionPath shown in Figure 1.5 lists the data the educator needs prior to seeing the patient as well as the length of time each visit requires and the topics to be covered. Nutrition and exercise DecisionPaths follow the same format. Adherence assessment covers both metabolic parameters and behavioral cues that may explain poor adherence. The therapeutic DecisionPaths refer as needed to the Diabetes Management Assessment DecisionPaths.

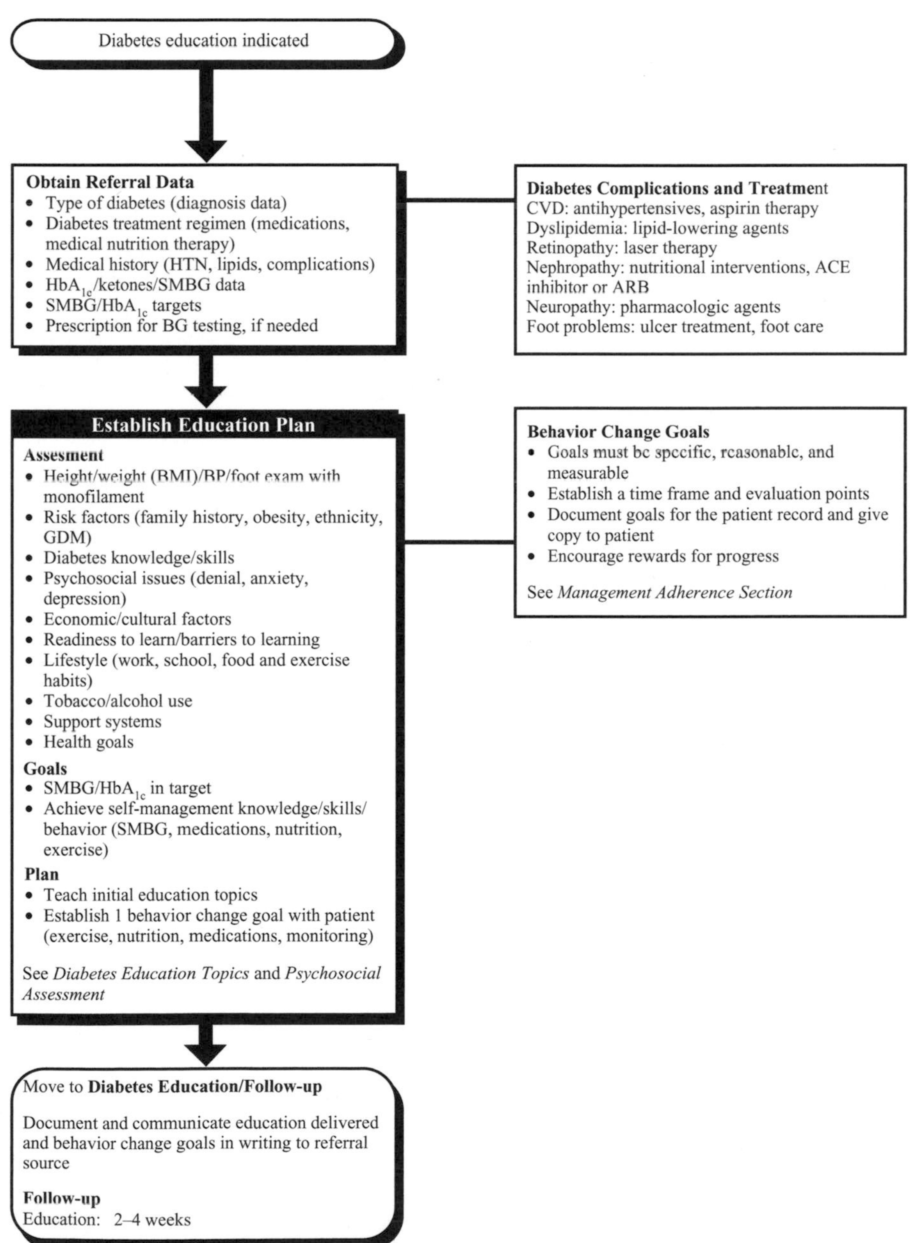

Figure 1.5 Diabetes Education/Initial DecisionPath

Metabolic syndrome, complications, and hospitalization DecisionPaths

The DecisionPaths for vascular complications, nephropathy, retinopathy, neuropathy, and foot disease generally follow the same format as those for treatment of diabetes. They differ in terms of

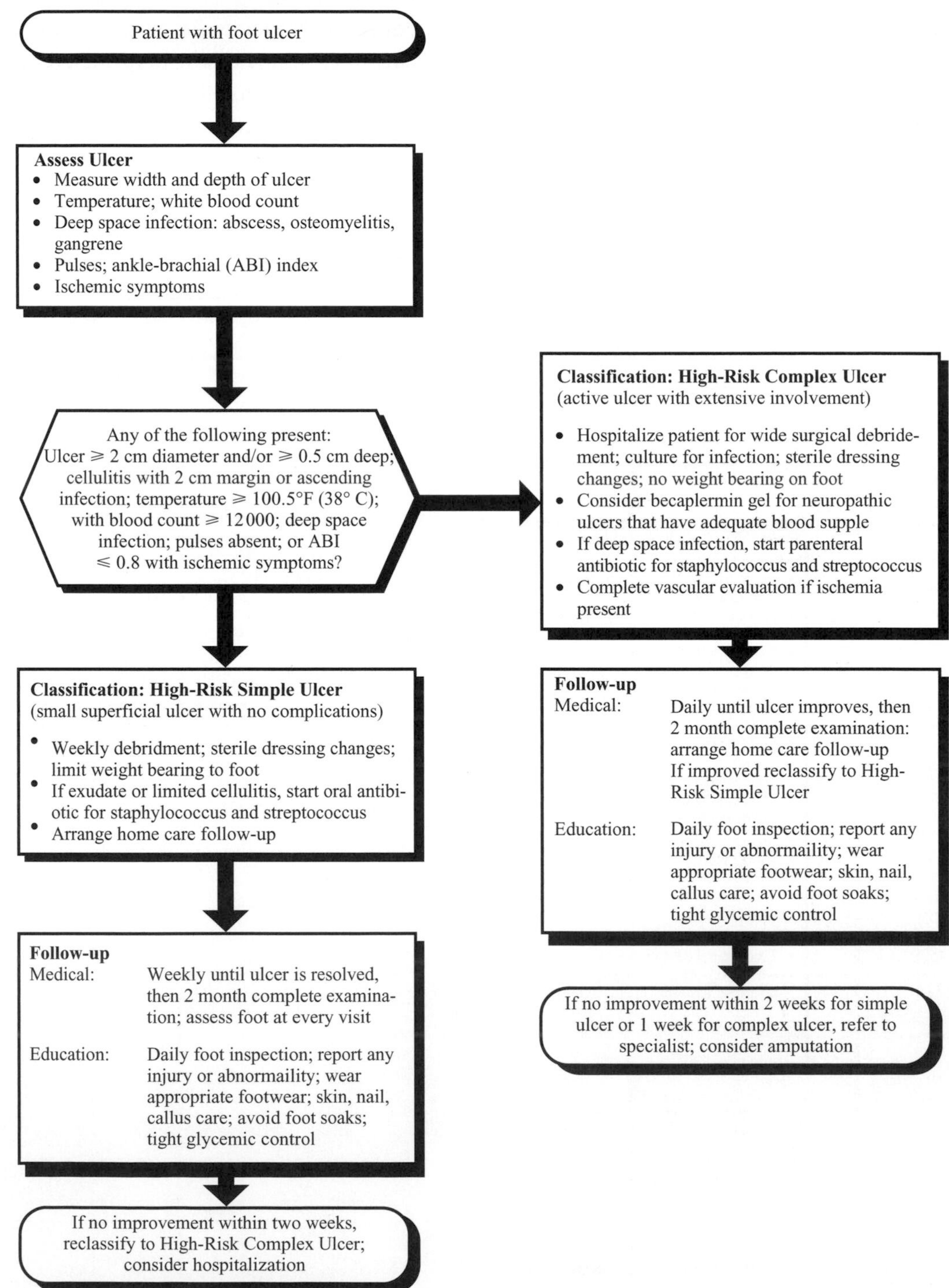

Figure 1.6 Foot Ulcer Treatment DecisionPath

their subject matter. They address prevention, screening, and diagnosis as well as starting and adjusting therapy (see Figure 1.6).

The patient and Staged Diabetes Management

Because patient participation is an integral part of SDM, they should be provided with a brief version of the Master DecisionPath to familiarize them with available therapeutic options. Along with the Master DecisionPath, the patient should be aware of the tests that are generally performed (such as HbA_{1c}). One approach is to provide patients with booklets that provide places to record blood glucose and HbA_{1c} targets along with actual values.

Additionally, SDM encourages the use of a progress record, which is a tool that allows patients and providers to track the course of treatment over time. The progress record provides the history of care at a glance, allowing both patient and provider to see where they have been and where they are going. This is a valuable aid in teaching and in maintaining adherence to complex therapies. The patient is kept informed and involved at every step. Figure 1.7 shows an example of a progress record for type 2 diabetes and illustrates how it is used.

Progress Record

							✔ Your Phase of Treatment		
Date	**Your Blood Glucose Range** (mg/dL)	**Pre-Meal Blood Glucose Target** (mg/dL)	**Your HbA_{1c}**	**HbA_{1c} Target**	**Stage of Treatment**	**Medication Dose**	**Start**	**Adjust**	**Maintain**
6/1 (office)	233	70–140	9.5	less than 7.0	Glipizide	5 mg AM	✔		
6/7 (phone)	225	70–140			Glipizide	10 mg AM		✔	
6/21 (office)	205	70–140			Glipizide	10 mg AM		✔	
7/5 (phone)	210	70–140			Glipizide	15 mg AM		✔	
7/19 (office)	207	70–140			Glipizide	10 mg AM/PM		✔	
8/2 (phone)	200	70–140			Glipizide	15 mg AM/PM		✔	
8/16 (office)	180	70–140			Glipizide	20 mg AM/PM		✔	
9/7 (phone)	188	70–140			Insulin Stage 2	5/0-0-4/4-0	✔		
9/21 (office)	100-160	70–140	8.5	less than 7.0	Insulin Stage 2	7/9-0-4/4-0			✔
10/3 (phone)	90-155	70–140			Insulin Stage 2	7/9-0-5/4-0		✔	
12/2 (office)	70-140	70–140	6.9	less than 7.0	Insulin Stage 2	7/9-0-5/4-0			✔

Figure 1.7 Patient Progress Record

The diabetes care team

The concept of a diabetes care team is not new. However, the role of the patient as a member of the team is new. Because of the reliance on patient collected data combined with the need for the patient to cooperate, understand the therapies and follow complex regimens, the patient must be considered at the center of the care team. In primary care management, the team may include the physician, nurse educator, nurse practitioner, physician's assistant, pharmacist, and dietitian with the psychologist/social worker or exercise physiologist included where available. This team approach is especially needed in the absence of a diabetes specialist. If a specialist is available, the team might include both the primary care physician and a diabetes specialist. Under such circumstances the DecisionPath to be followed would include the conditions for referral and would be shared by all involved in diabetes care. DecisionPaths specify the role of each professional. The nurse and dietitian have especially unique roles to play, roles that in many instances the physician cannot assume without additional training and time. The DecisionPaths and the narratives include specific information about nutritional interventions and education. The primary care provider is specifically trained for, and skilled in, comprehensive first contact and continuing care for persons with diabetes. Responsibilities include health promotion, disease prevention, health maintenance, counseling, patient education, diagnosis, and treatment. The primary care provider coordinates the care of the individual with diabetes using other health professionals, consultation, and/or referrals as appropriate. The primary care provider serves as "patient advocate in the health care system to accomplish cost-effective care by coordination of health care services." Is the primary care physician to be considered the "diabetologist?"

"Diabetologist" is a term that is often misunderstood. In the United States, there is no such degree or board examination. A diabetologist is often considered any health professional with expertise in diabetes. However, for both legal and ethical considerations, the physician specialist in diabetes is generally referred to as a board-certified endocrinologist. This is different from those physicians whose practice concentrates on diabetes. Currently, the National Committee for Quality Assurance (NCQA) recognizes individual providers or groups of providers as a "Recognized Physician," indicating that the physician (or group of physicians) has undergone a careful evaluation of clinical practice and met specific criteria for the treatment of diabetes. This focus on assessing expertise by clinical outcomes in place of formal education is in part recognition that extensive clinical experience with beneficial outcomes is an important factor in measuring clinical ability.

The team member known as the "diabetes educator" provides initial and ongoing education related to self-management, survival skills, prevention and detection of complications, as well as diabetes skills training. Generally nurses and dietitians (recently physicians and pharmacists have taken on this role), educators have extensive knowledge of diabetes medical management and ample experience in self-management education. Like the NCQA Physician Recognition program, national organizations certify the expertise of the educator by making certain that they have provided at least 1000 hours of diabetes patient education and passed a national examination. Upon completion the health care professional is awarded certification as a Certified Diabetes Educator (CDE).

The registered dietitian is responsible for assessing the dietary needs of the individual and helping develop a food plan consistent with the nutrient requirements for growth and development in children and sustained good health in adults. Often a CDE as well, the dietitian addresses eating habits, suggests changes in behavior, and designs a course of action to optimize the nutritional component of diabetes care. Dietitians will also work with patients to establish an activity and/or exercise plan.

The psychologist/social worker assesses the

individual's initial and ongoing emotional adjustment to diabetes as well as the family's adjustment. Recently, as patients are more involved in clinical decisions and day-to-day therapy adjustments, the psychologist's role as a force for empowering patients to participate in their own care has received renewed emphasis.

Other team members include the pharmacist, podiatrist, exercise physiologist, and such specialists as cardiologists, neurologists, and nephrologists. The underlying concept of team care is that all health care providers and the patient agree in advance as to the course of treatment. This avoids both misunderstandings and counterproductive treatment. More important, it significantly reduces error.

The changing perspective of diabetes care: DCCT and UKPDS

Two long-term clinical trials between 1977 and 1998 were designed to determine whether glycemic control was associated with the onset and progression of complications of diabetes. The Diabetes Control and Complications Trial (DCCT), conducted in the United States and Canada, and the United Kingdom Prospective Diabetes Study (UKPDS), conducted in centers through the United Kingdom concluded that glycemic control was a critical factor in the development and progression of microvascular complications and that treatment should be targeted to explicit metabolic markers such as blood glucose and blood pressure.[1,7]

The DCCT began in 1983 with a fundamental question: does improvement in glycemic control prevent the onset of and/or slow the progression of microvascular complications in the individual with newly detected type 1 diabetes? While the primary focus of the study was on retinal and renal complications, the research question expanded to include other microvascular complications (neuropathies) as well as macrovascular complications (hypertension and cardiovascular disease) and psychosocial disorders. The DCCT was completed in June 1993. Over the period of the study, 1441 patients entered the study, and less than 1 per cent dropped out. Twenty-seven clinical centers and two satellites in the United States and Canada participated. Patients were randomly assigned to conventional treatment, usually two injections of mixed (intermediate- and short-acting) insulin per day with the expectation of an $HbA_{1c} > 8.5$ per cent or to intensive treatment, usually three or more injections per day with the goal of $HbA_{1c} < 7$ per cent. Patients in the intensively treated group were followed monthly, whereas those in the conventional group were seen at three-month intervals. Eye examinations, renal function assessment, neurological evaluation, blood pressure measurement, and neurobehavioral assessment along with metabolic measurements were completed on 95 per cent of the patients throughout the study period. The results are summarized in Table 1.1.

Table 1.1 DCCT study results: complications risk reduction for intensively treated group

Condition	% Risk Reduction
Retinopathy	76
Neuropathy	60
Nephropathy (macroalbuminuria)	54

Following completion of the DCCT several centers agreed to follow the participants from both the conventional and intensive control groups to determine the long-term risk of developing complications as part of the Epidemiology of Diabetes Interventions and Complications (EDIC) study.[10] The patients in the DCCT conventional therapy group were offered intensive therapy and all patients (including the intensive therapy group) were placed under the care of their physician and diabetes team. The study is still ongoing; however, interim outcomes show that there continues to be a close association between the development and progression of complications and level of glycemic control throughout the DCCT study period. Patients from the intensive therapy group continue to have significantly reduced risk of retinopathy and nephropathy compared to patients from the conventional therapy group several years after the termination of the DCCT.[11]

The results of both the DCCT and EDIC require a thoughtful process of integration into current practice in terms of the treatment of type 1 diabetes. The intensively treated group did not suffer adversely (except for a threefold risk of hypoglycemia principally at the beginning of the study and marginal weight gain) when glycemic control was tightened. At the onset of the study, the average HbA_{1c} was approximately 9 per cent. More than 700 patients' glycemic control had to be rapidly reduced to an HbA_{1c} of 7 per cent or less for the duration of the study. While hypoglycemia increased, once glycemic control was stabilized, these reactions were reduced in most patients. Weighing the risk of hypoglycemia against the benefit of improvement in control, study investigators concluded that, with appropriate caution taken, all but a small minority of type 1 patients would benefit from improved control. It was further noted that any improvement in glycemic control would reduce the risk of microvascular disease. An interesting finding in the intensified group was that the emphasis on more complex treatments and maintaining goals toward euglycemia did not adversely affect the patients' psychosocial well-being. This was an important finding, since many have cited the possible negative impact of intensified therapies on quality of life and psychosocial well-being.

Not all patients in the experimental group achieved tight control, and at least 20 per cent of those in the conventionally treated group had significantly improved HbA_{1c} during the study. The two questions that remain are whether the study results can be duplicated under non-study conditions and to what degree the findings remain consistent over time. Since the end of the study both questions have been addressed.

Can the intensive treatment found in the DCCT be duplicated in primary care practice? In 1993 the International Diabetes Center published its algorithms that resulted in maintaining near-normal glycemia in its cohort of DCCT patients. It showed that a systematic approach based on specific glycemic criteria for alteration of therapy significantly lowered and sustained blood glucose to levels that matched the DCCT experimental group. These protocols were used in numerous sites between 1993 and 2002 within primary care practices within the United States, Japan, Poland, Mexico, Brazil, and France. In September 2000, health professionals from around the world responsible for implementing SDM met to share implementation strategies and outcomes at an International Congress held in Puebla, Mexico.[12] The findings are summarized in Table 1.2.

Can the tight glycemic control achieved in the DCCT be sustained? Follow-up of DCCT patients for 9 years confirmed that patients who are intensively treated and maintain near-normal glycemia reduce their risk of complications. Called EDIC, the study showed that if patients are not treated intensively, even those originally in the experimental group will have deterioration in HbA_{1c}. In fact, over time, the significant difference that existed at the end of the study in HbA_{1c} levels all but disappears if patients are not treated to specific metabolic targets.

At the completion of the DCCT, and until the publication of the results of the UKPDS, the findings for type 1 diabetes served as the basis for arguments supporting the need for intensified treatment of type 2 diabetes. Ten times more prevalent than type 1 diabetes, type 2 diabetes is also associated with micro- and macrovascular complications. Within a short time after the results of the DCCT were announced, many scientists and clinicians, as well as such national organizations as the ADA, concluded that improved glycemic control in type 2 diabetes was as beneficial as in type 1 diabetes.[9] More recently this has been supported by several studies that have been conducted in Denmark, Japan, and the United Kingdom involving individuals with type 2 diabetes. The UKPDS is the largest study yet to be conducted in individuals with type 2 diabetes. It was a prospective randomized controlled trial,

Table 1.2 International SDM outcomes

Country	Outcome
France	Improved metabolic and process outcomes versus control group. SDM Group ($n = 30$) versus Standard Care ($n = 36$) • Mean decrease in HbA_{1c} of 0.8 percentage points in SDM Group versus mean increase of 0.45 percentage points in Standard Care Group, $p = 0.001$ • Microalbuminuria screening 77% in SDM Group versus 38% in Standard Care Group, $p = 0.01$ • 5.07 monofilament exam 80% in SDM Group versus 25% in Standard Care Group, $p = 0.01$ • HDL determination 53% in SDM Group versus 30% in Standard Care Group, $p = 0.01$
Germany	Patients with diabetes ($n = 196$) receiving care by physicians following SDM had significantly increased ($p < 0.001$) patient satisfaction and quality of life compared to patients receiving standard care ($n = 174$).
Japan	Patients with diabetes ($n = 76$) treated by internists following SDM showed a 1.5 percentage point reduction in HbA_{1c} from baseline while patients treated by usual care showed a 0.5 percentage point increase in HbA_{1c}.
Poland	Women with gestational diabetes mellitus (GDM) managed by physicians following SDM ($n = 205$) had significantly improved outcomes shown by reduced rates of macrosomia and fetal hypoglycemia compared with women with GDM receiving standard care ($n = 67$).

which enrolled more than 5000 individuals with newly diagnosed type 2 diabetes in 23 centers throughout the United Kingdom between 1977 and 1991.[7,13] After a 3 month diet and exercise run-in period, patients were randomized to receive either "conventional" or "intensive" treatment using sulfonylurea (chlorpropamide, glibenclamide, or glipizide), metformin, or insulin. The goal of conventional treatment was to maintain fasting plasma glucose levels < 270 mg/dL (15.0 mmol/L), while the goal of intensive treatment was to maintain fasting plasma glucose levels < 108 mg/dL (6.0 mmol/L). By the completion of the trial the intensive therapy group and conventional therapy group had a difference in mean HbA_{1c} of 0.9 per cent (7.0 versus 7.9 per cent). This difference in glycemic control was accomplished in part due to the willingness to move from monotherapies to combination therapies and the widespread introduction of insulin therapies when oral agents failed to maintain near-normal glycemia. The study resulted in a 25 per cent reduction in risk for microvascular complications ($p < 0.01$) and a 16 per cent reduction in risk for myocardial infarction ($p = 0.052$) when the intensively treated group was compared with controls. Moreover, the UKPDS provided no evidence for an increase in cardiovascular risk with either sulfonylurea or insulin therapy.

Additional UKPDS findings:

- the incidence of hypoglycemia in intensive therapies is minimal
- weight gain is not significant as patients move to insulin therapies
- overall improvement in glycemic control requires attention to the natural history of the disease
- improvement in indirect measures of macrovascular disease (hypertension and dyslipidemia) occurs with improved glycemic control, independent of the particular pharmacological agent used
- control of blood pressure is a major contributor to reduction in risk of cardiovascular and microvascular disease

Since the publication of the UKPDS numerous studies have supported the long-term benefits and risk reduction associated with improved blood glucose and blood pressure control. The current consensus is to treat the person with type 2 diabetes with the same intensity and toward the same metabolic goals as the person with type 1 diabetes.

While no such large-scale studies of diabetes in pregnancy exist, nevertheless these same principles remain intact for gestational and pregestational diabetes. Achievement of near-normal blood glucose continues to afford the best protection from both adverse maternal and perinatal morbidity and mortality. Increasingly, as the number of women with gestational diabetes and pregestational diabetes is becoming higher, the importance of detecting and vigorously treating hyperglycemia in pregnancy is becoming greater. Ample scientific evidence exists that untreated hyperglycemia in pregnancy will not only have short-term consequences for the mother and neonate, but can have long-term consequences for the newborn as well.

Metabolic syndrome (insulin resistance syndrome)

In the early 1970s a constellation of common disorders were recognized as occurring "coincidental" to type 2 diabetes. It was reported that 80 per cent of those with type 2 diabetes were overweight or obese at diagnosis; additionally, hypertension seemed present in most patients along with dyslipidemia. Many investigators found that these individuals also had hyperinsulinemia. These findings were initially presented by Gerald Reaven and associates, becoming known as Reaven's syndrome. Later it was called syndrome X, the deadly quartet, metabolic syndrome, dysmetabolic syndrome, and insulin resistance syndrome. *For purposes of clarity, SDM uses the term metabolic syndrome*. Sometime during the evolution of this syndrome, investigators found underlying renal disease to be common as well in these patients. Currently its components are believed to be related to both cellular and vascular insulin resistance. While the actual number is not certain, it has been estimated that 50 million adults in the United States have metabolic syndrome.[14]

Several organizations have created criteria for the clinical identification of metabolic syndrome. Useful criteria have been developed as part of the National Cholesterol Education Program Adult Treatment Panel III (NCEP-ATP III) guidelines.[15] Current criteria from the NCEP-ATP III guidelines *require any three* of the following risk factors to make the diagnosis of metabolic syndrome (insulin resistance syndrome):

Risk Factor	**Defining Level**
Abdominal obesity	Waist circumference > 40 in. (102 cm) men > 35 in. (88 cm) women
Fasting glucose	⩾ 110 mg/dL (6.1 mmol/L)
Blood pressure	⩾ 130/⩾85 mmHg
Triglycerides	⩾ 150 mg/dL (1.7 mmol/L)
High density lipoprotein (HDL)	< 40 mg/dL men (1.0 mmol/L) < 50 mg/dL women (1.3 mmol/L)

Children and adolescents with type 2 diabetes and/or metabolic syndrome

The traditional view is that while type 1 diabetes is a disease of childhood and adolescents, type 2 diabetes and concomitant metabolic syndrome are diseases of adults. This view is corroborated by data that show the incidence of type 1 diabetes reaches its peak during adolescence and the number of new cases of type 2 diabetes rises with age. Additionally, more than 20 per cent of those aged 65 years or older have type 2 diabetes.[16] It is only recently that type 2 diabetes and metabolic syndrome are being diagnosed in children and adolescents. This is most probably due to recognition of the strong genetic component in the etiology of diabetes. The identification of type 2 diabetes in children clusters in Hispanic, African-American, Native American, and Pacific Island peoples. Among the Pima Indians children as young as four years old have been diagnosed with type 2 diabetes. Hispanic children living near the Mexican border and in San Antonio, Texas, have been found to have a high incidence of both insulin resistance and type 2 diabetes. Along with a genetic predisposition, obesity in children and adolescents is associated with the development of type 2 diabetes at a very young age. High caloric intake from diets comprised principally of fats and carbohydrate combined with reduced activity result in an imbalance between energy intake and energy output. This results in increased obesity, further exacerbating insulin resistance. Because the identification and treatment of these children require modification from the approach to adults, a separate section is included in the text.

Common diagnostic criteria

In 1997 the American Diabetic Association (ADA) announced new fasting plasma glucose criteria for the diagnosis of diabetes to assure greater uniformity throughout the United States.[17] The new criteria were developed in response to growing evidence that the complications of diabetes begin to emerge at much lower fasting plasma glucose levels than previously thought. Thus, the fasting plasma glucose level required for diagnosis was lowered from 140 mg/dL (7.8 mmol/L) to 126 mg/dL (7.0 mmol/L). In addition, the lower fasting plasma glucose diagnostic criteria was more aligned with the criteria for casual plasma glucose – 200 mg/dL (11.1 mmol/L). Based on these criteria, the Centers for Disease Control and Prevention (CDCP) made new estimates of the incidence and prevalence of diabetes and impaired glucose homeostasis (pre-diabetes) in the United States.[16]

- The prevalence of diabetes is 17 million (11.1 million diagnosed and 5.9 million undiagnosed), representing approximately 6.2 per cent of the population.

- The prevalence of diabetes in people 65 years or older is 7.0 million (20.1 per cent of the population).

- The incidence of diabetes is 1.0 million new cases diagnosed in person aged 20 years or older.

- 16 million adults 40–74 years of age have impaired glucose tolerance (2 hour oral glucose tolerance test values of 140–199 mg/dL [7.8–11 mmol/L]) and 10 million have impaired fasting glucose (plasma glucose of 100–125 mg/dL [5.6–6.9 mmol/L].

- The incidence of gestational diabetes mellitus (GDM) is 150 000 cases/year.

- Projections to the year 2010 estimate as many as 25 million individuals in the United States will have diabetes.

The CDCP concluded that, based on these estimates, more than 450 000 people die each year with diabetes as a primary or contributing factor.

These figures highlight the significance of SDM for primary care and for those who feel that access to quality diabetes care should not be limited to those whose geographical location or economic situation allows treatment at an expert diabetes center.

Diabetes management improvement initiatives

While many organizations have developed national recommendations related to the diagnosis and treatment of diabetes and associated diseases, the American Diabetes Association is unique in having initiated a program to identify those physicians who consistently meet national standards. Currently administered by the National Committee for Quality Assurance (NCQA), the program is called the Diabetes Physician Recognition Program (DPRP). DPRP establishes clinical processes and outcomes as "benchmarks" that constitute quality care.[18] Individual physicians or groups of physicians may apply for recognition by demonstrating that they have initiated a systemic quality improvement program. DPRP is determined by chart review through a formal application process. The number of charts reviewed is based on the number of physicians in the practice (see Table 1.3). A fee is charged for the application. The NCQA argues that its recognition provides the following benefits:

- establishment of a baseline of current diabetes care allowing comparison to benchmark data
- public recognition as a quality program
- differentiation of the practice from others in the community
- designation by the NCQA as a referral site for diabetes care
- improved position for third-party reimbursement.

Table 1.3 Diabetes Physician Recognition Program benchmarks of quality diabetes care

Required Measures	Adult Benchmarks
HbA_{1c} testing*	$\geqslant$ 100%
$HbA_{1c} < 7\%$	$\geqslant$ 40%
$HbA_{1c} > 9\%$	$\leqslant$ 20%
Eye examination*	$\geqslant$ 60%
Foot examination*	$\geqslant$ 80%
Blood pressure measure*	$\geqslant$ 100%
< 140/90 mmHg	$\geqslant$ 65%
< 130/80 mmHg	$\geqslant$ 35%
Nephropathy assessment*	$\geqslant$ 80%
Lipid profile*	$\geqslant$ 85%
LDL < 130 mg/dL (3.4 mmol/L)	$\geqslant$ 63%
LDL < 100 mg/dL (2.6 mmol/L)	$\geqslant$ 36%
Optional Patient Survey	
Tobacco status and counseling	$\geqslant$ 80%
Self-management education	$\geqslant$ 90%
Medical nutrition therapy	$\geqslant$ 90%
Self-monitoring of blood glucose	
Non-insulin-treated	$\geqslant$ 50%
Insulin treated	$\geqslant$ 97%
Patient satisfaction**	
Diabetes care overall	$\geqslant$ 58%
Diabetes questions answered	$\geqslant$ 56%
Access during emergencies	$\geqslant$ 46%
Explanation of lab results	$\geqslant$ 50%
Personal manner of physician	$\geqslant$ 77%

* At least once per year.
** Rated as excellent, very good or good on a scale of excellent to poor.

References

1. Diabetes Control and Complications Trial Research Group. The effect of intensive treatment of diabetes on the development and progression of long-term complications in insulin-dependent diabetes mellitus. *N Engl J Med* 1993; **329**: 977–986.
2. Ohkubo Y, Kishikawa H and Araki E. Intensive insulin therapy prevents the progression of diabetic microvascular complications in Japanese patients with non-insulin-dependent diabetes mellitus: a randomized prospective 6-year study. *Diabetes Res Clin Pract* 1995; **28**: 103–117.
3. Meigs JB, Singer DE, Sullivan LM, *et al.* Metabolic control and prevalent cardiovascular disease in non-insulin-dependent diabetes mellitus (NIDDM): the NIDDM patient outcomes research team. *Am J Med* 1997; **102**: 38–47.
4. Turner RC, Millns H, Neil HA, *et al.* Risk factors for coronary artery disease in non-insulin dependent diabetes mellitus: United Kingdom Prospective Diabetes Study (UKPDS:23). *Br Med J* 1998; **316**: 823–828.
5. Rith-Najarian S, Branchaud C, Beaulieu O, Gohdes D, Simonson G and Mazze R. Reducing lower extremity amputation due to diabetes: application of the Staged Diabetes Management approach in a primary care setting. *J Fam Pract* 1998; **47**: 127–132.
6. Mazze RS, Etzwiler DD, Strock ES, *et al.* Staged Diabetes Management: toward an integrated model of diabetes care. *Diabetes Care* 1994; **17**: 56–66.
7. United Kingdom Prospective Diabetes Study Group. Intensive blood-glucose control with sulfonylureas or insulin compared with conventional treatment and risk of complications in patients with type 2 diabetes (UKPDS 33). *Lancet* 1998; **352**: 837–853.
8. Institute of Medicine. *Clinical Practice Guidelines.* Field MJ and Lohr KN, eds. Washington, DC: National Academy Press, 1990.
9. Nathan DM. Inferences and implications: do results from the Diabetes Control and Complications Trial apply in NIDDM? *Diabetes Care* 1995; **18**(2): 251–257.
10. Epidemiology of Diabetes Interventions and Complications (EDIC) Research Group. Epidemiology of Diabetes Interventions and Complications (EDIC): design and implementation of a long-term follow-up of the Diabetes Control and Complications Trial cohort. *Diabetes Care* 1999; **22**: 99–111.
11. Epidemiology of Diabetes Interventions and Complications (EDIC) Research Group. Retinopathy and nephropathy in patients with type 1 diabetes four years after a trial of intensive therapy. The Diabetes Control and Complications Trial/Epidemiology of Diabetes Interventions and Complications Research Group. *N Engl J Med* 2000; **342**: 381–389.
12. Mazze RS and Simonson GS. Staged Diabetes Management: a systematic evidence-based approach to the prevention and treatment of diabetes and its comorbidities. Proceedings of Staged Diabetes Management: Worldwide Outcomes 2000. *Pract Diabetes Int Suppl* 2001; **7**: S1–S16.
13. United Kingdom Prospective Diabetes Study Group. Effect of intensive blood-glucose control with metformin on complications in overweight patients with type 2 diabetes (UKPDS 34). *Lancet* 1998; **352**: 854–865.
14. Ford ES, Giles WH and Dietz WH. Prevalence of the metabolic syndrome among US adults: findings from the third National Health and Nutrition Examination Survey. *JAMA* 2002; **287**: 356–359.
15. National Cholesterol Education Adult Treatment Panel III, NIH Publication Number 01-3305, 2001.
16. Centers for Disease Control and Prevention. National diabetes fact sheet: general information and national estimates on diabetes in the United States, 2000. Atlanta, GA: US Departments of Health and Human Services, Centers for Disease Control and Prevention, 2002.
17. The Expert Committee on the Diagnosis and Classification of Diabetes Mellitus. Report of the Expert Committee on the Diagnosis and Classification of Diabetes Mellitus. *Diabetes Care* 1997; **20**: 1183–1197.
18. National Committee for Quality Assurance (NCQA) Diabetes Physician Recognition Program. 2004, www.ncqa.org/dprp.

2 The Implementation of Staged Diabetes Management

Although the key elements of the Staged Diabetes Management (SDM) program are contained in Chapters 3 through 10, to fully implement SDM requires participation in the SDM process. This entails an orientation to SDM principles as well as assessing current practices, customizing elements of SDM for the community, identifying possible obstacles to implementation, follow-up, and outcome assessment. This section describes this process in detail. For readers who are currently participating in the process, consider this text as part of the complete set of SDM materials, which also include the Quick Guides, and eSDM (electronic media). For those who are not currently participating in the SDM process, the material in this section provides a summary of all the program elements. Complete DecisionPaths are available in the Quick Guides and through eSDM. The Master DecisionPaths and Practice Guidelines will be the subject of building a consensus and through that process will be modified to reflect the unique resources of each community. Note that the examples provided in this chapter use data collected by healthcare organizations in the United States and around the world.

Commitment to improving diabetes care is crucial to the success of SDM in any community or organization, and the key is building consensus. The goal of SDM is to ensure consistent, evidence-based prevention, detection, and treatment protocols for all types of diabetes and associated complications and syndromes. To do this, all providers and diabetes team members in the community need to become acquainted with and follow the same guidelines. A process based on consensus building is used in order to optimize the adoption of SDM.

Starting and maintaining a successful SDM program requires five steps:

- community diabetes care needs assessment
- group formation
- orientation to SDM
- customization and implementation of SDM
- evaluation of SDM

Staged Diabetes Management: A Systematic Approach (2nd Edition) R. S. Mazze, E. S. Strock, G. D. Simonson and R. M. Bergenstal
 ISBN: 0 470 86576 8

Community diabetes care needs assessment

Staged Diabetes Management begins when a community understands that it needs to change the manner in which individuals with diabetes and associated diseases are being cared for and educated. Recognizing this may come as a result of a formal assessment of care and education practices, epidemiological data, or individual experience. SDM promotes a community-wide assessment of the current state of diabetes care (and may be expanded to include metabolic syndrome). This assessment provides the foundation for understanding the needs and demands of a community and its resources, and how these contribute to medical outcomes. The process also serves as the baseline against which changes in outcomes are measured.

Measurements of epidemiological data, personnel, facilities, current level of metabolic control, and complications surveillance need to be obtained to complete an analysis of care processes in any community. Estimates of these factors often are not possible. The detailed Diabetes (and Metabolic Syndrome) Needs Assessment Survey (found in the Appendix, Figure A.1) can help in the evaluation of current care, demographics, and utilization problems.

Diabetes Needs Assessment of current health care system

The areas to assess include the following:

- *Organizational information*. Name of organization, contact person, address, title, type of system (e.g., managed care organization), number and type of sites, number and type of health care providers, and chronic disease programs. This information is often already completed for in-house and public reporting. Check with the public information person at the facility (if such an individual exists).

- *Demographics.* Age, gender, reimbursement mix (Medicare, managed care organization, fee for service, out-of-pocket), ethnicity, type of diabetes, and socioeconomic background. Community-wide demographics can be obtained from many sources including state departments of health, ministries of health, and government agencies. Hospitals and clinics have periodic utilization review reports that contain this information.

- *Utilization data.* Hospitalizations, average length of stay, referrals, inpatient services, and outpatient services. Hospital utilization review records are available to the public. Use these data to complete this section. Clinic data may be available by diagnosis for billing purposes.

- *Diabetes (and related) care services.* Inpatient and outpatient care, education, number of full-time equivalents, resources (special facilities such as learning laboratories and nutrition centers), diabetes supplies, and support groups. This information is generally available from nurse educators, dietitians, and others who see large numbers of individuals with diabetes. If this is a recognized diabetes program, the annual report contains this information. *Note: as metabolic syndrome may include diabetes, it is unlikely that there are special services beyond a lipid, hypertension and/or obesity clinic. Be sure to include these elements in the assessment.*

- *Diabetes management.* Current diagnostic criteria, standard measure of patient glucose control, complications surveillance, routine screening, and referral to specialists. It may be difficult to obtain this information in a local community and often multiple sources are required to obtain the information. Once it has been obtained, it can be used for an annual comparison to evaluate the diabetes management system. *Note: the separate identification of Metabolic Syndrome as a disease is currently highly under review. If the diagnosis does exist, note the components and how care is coordinated.*

- As information is collected, also ask the following questions about the diabetes care in the community:

  1. Where is the diagnosis of diabetes made? In the physician's office? In the hospital? In a screening clinic? In another facility? Is metabolic syndrome evaluated at the same time?

  2. Who determines the initial therapy? Primary care physician? Specialist? Interdisciplinary team? Diabetes center?

  3. Who educates the patient and family? Primary care physician? Nurse educator? Dietitian? Diabetes specialist? Interdisciplinary team? Public health nurse? Certified Diabetes Educator? Other?

  4. Who is responsible for day-to-day management? Primary care physician? Nurse educator? Diabetes specialist? Interdisciplinary team? Public health nurse? Other?

  5. Who manages complications? Primary care physician? Nurse educator? Diabetes specialist? Interdisciplinary team? Public health nurse? Other?

  6. Who is responsible for nutritional assessment and follow-up? Dietitian? Primary care physician? Nurse educator? Diabetes specialist? Interdisciplinary team? Public health nurse? Other?

  7. Who is responsible for scheduling annual complication surveillance examinations? Primary care physician? Nurse educator? Diabetes specialist? Interdisciplinary team? Public health nurse? Other?

Chart audit

The chart audit has become the most common means of assessing care. Its goal is to improve the quality of disease management; and its objective is to measure quality by comparing collected data with an accepted standard. Staged Diabetes Management uses the Practice Guidelines found in this text as the standard for the chart audit in order to assess the current level of diabetes care. The SDM Practice Guidelines, which are described in detail in each of the management chapters, consist of diagnostic criteria, treatment options, targets, monitoring, and medical follow-up timelines that are consistent with benchmarks established by such national and international organizations as the American Diabetes Association, the European Association for the Study of Diabetes, and the International Diabetes Federation. A chart audit offers the following benefits:

- insight into current management of diabetes and associated disorders in terms of identifying key factors that contribute to successful treatment outcomes
- provide a real-world perspective
- identify variations in practice
- serve as a baseline measure
- comparison to accepted benchmarks
- quantify current outcomes
- document use of existing guidelines

Obtain permission

It is best to obtain a signed authorization to review charts. The person who authorizes the process may be a physician or director of medical records. The authorization should include the following information: the person(s) doing the review, the person(s) requesting the review, the purpose of the review, and how the data will be used. Be sure to state that the information will not be patient or physician specific (see sample form in Figure 2.1). Some institutions require the patient to provide informed consent if the data that are being collected will be used in future publications or public presentations.

The use of the chart audit is not internationally accepted. Many clinicians prefer that their

CONFIDENTIALITY STATEMENT
Staged Diabetes Management
Clinic Medical Record Audit

The (name of organization, group, clinic, etc.) has been requested by the physicians of the (name of facility) to provide a confidential chart audit. The purpose of this review is to understand the current quality of diabetes care and provide educational information on diabetes management to the health care providers. The chart review is an integral element of Staged Diabetes Management, which is being implemented upon the request of the physicians of the (name of facility). Staged Diabetes Management is a scientifically based model for diabetes care, which includes the implementation of practice guidelines for the improvement of standards of care in the community.

The information obtained from the audit will be summarized in a written report to the physicians of the (name of facility). The report will characterize the current basis of diabetes care provided by the physicians and the data used as a baseline of diabetes management of patients who have type 1, type 2, and gestational diabetes. All information obtained is confidential. The information summarized will not be patient- or physician-specific.

Copies of the chart audit forms are attached.
Proposed date of chart audit: ______________________
Health care organization: ______________________
Name of person providing authorization: ______________________
Signature of person providing authorization: ______________________
Name of reviewer: ______________________
Signature of reviewer: ______________________

Figure 2.1 Sample Confidentiality Statement

patient's records remain confidential. Under such circumstances how can the current practice be assessed? Regional and national epidemiological data can be helpful. Small published studies and interviews with providers are also a means of assessing current care. The underlying purpose for this step in data collection is to provide a baseline from which changes can be measured. Many providers assume that changes will take place and therefore do not feel there is a need for baseline data.

Select charts

If possible, use medical records and quality improvement departments to randomly select the charts for review. At least 35 charts of patients with diabetes for each provider should be reviewed to meet NCQA Physician Recognition criteria. If more than six providers are working in the same facility, then 210 randomly selected charts meet the criteria for NCQA Physician Recognition (see Chapter 1 for details). This provides a large enough sample from which to measure change in diabetes outcomes at a later date. If this is not the purpose, then the number of charts to be evaluated will vary depending on what kinds of change are being measured.

In large managed care organizations or clinics, chart audits for diabetes may have been completed already as part of quality improvement or certification; use these data if available. The underlying purpose is to demonstrate need and to provide a baseline against which changes may be measured (if that is necessary). It takes approximately 10–12 hours for a reviewer to audit 35 charts and another 2–4 hours to compile and summarize them. Whatever the method selected, make certain that it will meet the objective. Be careful to select charts in a random manner, such as every fourth or eighth chart for each provider. Be sure that these are active patients. Some common errors are to select the charts of deceased or inactive patients. To avoid these errors, randomly select only those patients seen at any time during the last year. Since these charts will be recalled after SDM is implemented, make certain that they are likely to remain in the community and to be seen over the next 6–12 months. Include patients in long-term care facilities or other institutional facilities.

The charts may be identified by the International Classification of Diseases, 9th edition (ICD9-CM) diagnosis codes. Some of the ICD9-CM diagnosis codes for diabetes include

250.00 Type 2 diabetes without complications

250.01 Type 1 diabetes without complications

250.02 Type 2 diabetes, uncontrolled

250.03 Type 1 diabetes, uncontrolled

250.11 Type 1 diabetes, with ketoacidosis

250.40 Type 2 diabetes with renal manifestations

250.41 Type 1 diabetes with renal manifestations

250.50 Type 2 diabetes with ophthalmic manifestations

250.51 Type 1 diabetes with ophthalmic manifestations

250.60 Type 2 diabetes with neurological manifestations

250.61 Type 1 diabetes with neurological manifestations

250.70 Type 2 diabetes with peripheral vascular disease

250.71 Type 1 diabetes with peripheral vascular disease

250.80 Type 2 diabetes with other manifestations

250.81 Type 1 diabetes with other manifestations

648.83 Gestational diabetes

277.7 Metabolic syndrome—(dysmetabolic syndrome X)

Review charts

Use the Patient Chart Audit Form (see the Appendix, Figure A.2) or other national organization's audit form for the specific type of diabetes and fill out the information requested. Sometimes it is helpful to add additional notes in the margins of particular items to be remembered. Use the progress notes, laboratory data, additional correspondence, and any other flow sheet to collect the data. Review the written progress notes of the diagnosis of diabetes and then review the last 12 months of office visits, laboratory data, and additional health care services. In the following discussion, the SDM audit form is used.

Demographic data to be collected. Review the last 12 months of the clinic chart and note the visit date, chart number (no names), date of birth, gender, race/ethnicity, year of diabetes diagnosis, and weight. Sometimes it is difficult to find year of diagnosis information, so if the chart has either a diagnosis or a medication summary in the front of the chart, use the dates there to find the date and confirm by looking at the clinic notes for the particular date. If a diagnosis or medication summary is not available, look in the laboratory section to find the first date of laboratory fasting blood glucose results $\geqslant$ 126 mg/dL (7.0 mmol/L) or casual blood glucose $\geqslant$ 200 mg/dL (11.1 mmol/L)—the diagnostic criteria for diabetes. If that cannot be found, read through the chart.

Diabetes outcome and process variable list. Review the last 12 months of the clinic chart. This section records HbA_{1c} data, annual eye and foot examinations, blood pressure, annual urine microalbuminuria screens, lipid profile, diabetes and nutrition education, whether or not the patient is self-monitoring blood glucose, SMBG target range, and whether or not the patient smokes.

Many communities document target values via a letter to the patient when reporting the HbA_{1c} results. Note whether the last HbA_{1c} and average SMBG readings are within the targeted range. If a target range has not been identified and documented, the "no" box would be checked. List date and actual value of the last HbA_{1c} and plasma glucose determinations as well as the frequency of HbA_{1c} and laboratory plasma glucose obtained in the past year. Be sure to note the laboratory normal range for HbA_{1c} and plasma glucose (due to differences in methodology, make certain to note whether plasma or whole blood analysis is used).

Check the specific complications or symptoms that have been documented by a health care provider. Note when laboratory values (such as lipids or presence of urine protein) or the physical examination findings (blood pressure) show the existence of complications but are not documented by the health care provider. Also review hospital record correspondence for the documentation of emergency room visits and hospitalizations for diabetic ketoacidosis, hyperglycomic syndrome (HHS) hyperosmolar, or hypoglycemia. Has an eye examination (with dilation) been performed within the past 12 months? This may be done by an ophthalmologist, optometrist, or primary care practitioner. Be sure to review both the progress notes and the correspondence section of the chart. Has a microalbuminuria screen been completed in the last 12 months?

Review all the laboratory data. There may also be a laboratory data flow sheet documenting dates and results. Also note how the chart documents SMBG. Is the SMBG data downloaded from a meter to a computer and the report placed in the chart? Is a copy of the patient's record book included in the chart? Is there other documentation of the SMBG values in the chart? Include documentation of diabetes and nutrition topics covered by a nurse, dietitian, or physician. Note the amount of time the patient spends in any type of education related to diabetes. Many times the actual education may be listed on a flow sheet within the chart or else in a separate chart, outside the clinic. Include the date of the last diabetes education. Be alert for patients who receive diabetes education upon diagnosis of diabetes or the initiation of a medication but receive no additional follow-up.

Diabetes therapy. This covers the last 12 months of the clinic chart. Document the patient's current therapy, whether it is medical nutrition therapy alone or in conjunction with oral agents and/or insulin. Check the type of oral medication or insulin the patient is on and record the current regimen based on the SDM model of AM–midday–PM–bedtime. If the patient has been on a particular therapy for a long period of time and has not reached the target goals, it is sometimes helpful to note the last date of the change in therapy.

Metabolic syndrome therapy. Note whether insulin resistance or related co-morbidities (hypertension, dyslipidemia, renal disease, obesity, polycystic ovary syndrome (PCOS), or Acanthosis Nigricans are recorded. Determine whether the patient is in treatment for hypertension, dyslipidemia, or any of the insulin resistance related disorders. If the patient is on a special diet for obesity or renal disease note this as well.

Summarize results

Compile the data from multiple charts into a one-page tabulated summary. This will assist in reporting to the community the current management practices.

Interview

Sometimes a chart audit misses critical points in treatment because they are not documented. It is important to determine to what extent the chart reflects actual care processes. Interview as many providers as possible to verify the chart audit findings (e.g., nurse, dietitian, physician). These findings should be included in the written report. The fact that they were uncovered only after interviews will already suggest the need for better documentation.

Write report

With the SDM Patient Chart Audit Forms completed, most communities will want a written report of the chart audit. Use the completed forms along with additional information attained by the assessment in part one to write a report for the community.

Group formation

Forming a group is a very important step in initiating SDM. The focus is to identify health professionals, institutions, and organizations with a genuine interest in using community customized Practice Guidelines to improve care and education processes. Community refers to individuals with a common interest in developing, implementing, and monitoring Practice Guidelines for diabetes and associated disorders. The community can be a managed care organization, a group practice, a primary care clinic, a medical center, a department within a medical school, or an entire region of networked physicians and other care providers. Communities can also include national organizations such as diabetes societies. The concept is the reaching of a consensus by all interested parties to assure the application of evidence based practices.

To move SDM from being just a good idea to a working system in a community, resources must be committed to adopting a new and standardized method of care. These resources can be divided into four general components: personnel, equipment and supplies, physical facilities, and finances. These are generally known as "throughputs." They serve to convert demands and needs as expressed by the people in the community into improved outcomes by providing services to people at risk for and with a disease. Central to organizing these throughputs is the "champion": an individual or individuals who support change in their community and are willing to lead this effort. This champion will need co-leaders or coordinators to help in contacting, educating, and supporting other community health care providers. Coordinators are motivated, willing to fully participate in a process that will take time and energy. Coordinators often are members of existing diabetes care and education teams and have a stake in seeing diabetes care improved in the community. Team members can include primary care physicians, diabetes nurse educators, registered dietitians, psychologists or social workers, and diabetes specialists. Although all of these types of professional may not be available in the community, the areas of education, nutrition, and psychology are important aspects of care and should be addressed, if not represented.

Once the community has been defined and the team is identified, construct the working group. This working group is comprised of the care team plus other physicians (family practitioners, pediatricians, obstetricians, and endocrinologists), health professionals (nurses, dietitians, podiatrists, pharmacists, and psychologists), as well as representatives of the administration, third-party payers, and patient groups interested and influential in the care and education of people with diabetes or associated diseases in the community. Be sure to include lay members of the local diabetes associations. These individuals and the organizations they represent can be very effective allies if, based on the group meeting, additional resources are needed to implement SDM.

The purpose of the working group is to develop an action plan that familiarizes practitioners with SDM, sets into motion modification and adoption of Practice Guidelines, and promotes constant re-evaluation of care. Take time to identify the long-term goal of SDM; this goal will affect the composition of and resources needed by the working group. It has been shown that without a vision and a plan, much of the care is merely "passing the time," failing to achieve its ultimate purpose of improving the life of the individual with diabetes. With leadership, members of the working group will reach consensus on Practice Guidelines for the care of each type of diabetes and, ultimately, will put SDM into practice and monitor its progress.

Orientation to Staged Diabetes Management

With assessment data, begin the orientation process. Start with the core care team. The presentations to the team should:

- define Staged Diabetes Management
- assess diabetes knowledge
- assess diabetes care
- establish goals

1. *What is SDM?* SDM is a process to ensure the adoption of consistent guidelines that will improve overall care.

2. *How is diabetes currently managed in the community?* On the basis of the chart audit, interview, and other data, the quality of diabetes care can be characterized as excellent, average, or poor.

3. *How will diabetes care change with SDM?* Diagnosis, classification, treatment options, and outcomes will be defined, consistently applied, and monitored.

4. *How is metabolic syndrome integrated with the traditional approach to diabetes care and education?* Because most care teams and patient education programs focus on diabetes, it will be necessary to begin the process of incorporating hypertension, dyslipidemia, renal disease, and obesity in the "routine" care and education of people with diabetes. This will necessitate a re-evaluation of current practices.

Encourage rethinking about diabetes care, and focus on broad community issues: improved care, lower costs, efficiencies of scale, organized systems, and meeting national standards. Also, review the data from the system's analysis regarding the scope and depth of diabetes in the community.

In the United States, diabetes costs over $130 billion per year, primarily due to the treatment of complications. The worldwide figures are unknown, but more than likely are 10–20 times greater. While many of the microvascular and macrovascular complications are preventable with improved control of blood glucose and blood pressure, the current situation suggests that the majority of individuals with diabetes are undertreated. Persons with type 2 diabetes, for example, have up to five times the risk of cardiovascular disease as people of the same age without diabetes. This is reflected in a five to ten times greater cost for the patient with diabetes when compared to an age and gender matched patient without diabetes. Ultimately, these costs are borne by all of society and are reflected in poor quality of life and premature death for many individuals with diabetes. It is important that the group understand the potential benefits that can be realized with the implementation of a systematic approach to early detection, intensive treatment, and close surveillance.

A key point in the presentation about SDM is that it relies on consensus. The working group must agree on the need for change, the value of a systematic approach, the need for evidence-based medicine, the desirability for approaches that treat to targets, and the need for community-wide Practice Guidelines. Consensus should be the result of full participation of all health professionals who are influential in the care and education of people with diabetes and associated disorders. The discussion should be unimpeded. Controversial issues related to roles and responsibilities, treatment options, and resource allocations should be discussed. Consensus should come by carefully evaluating data from scientific findings, national standards, and local practices. In the end, the group's efforts should produce a system that ensures a systematic approach that is not only evidence-based, but dynamic enough to undergo periodic re-evaluation and modification.

Assess diabetes knowledge

The role of the champion in developing a consensus is pivotal. It begins with an assessment of the familiarity of the working group with diabetes and insulin resistance. Since these are adult learners, testing is not advisable. The best way to assess understanding is to review their current practice and then determine how well the group understands such critical elements as diagnostic criteria, classification, treatment options, treat to target, monitoring, and surveillance for complications. National standards of classification and diagnosis of diabetes and hypertension should be reviewed. Assessment and review are important to building SDM's framework. They set the tone for using scientific information, supported by research findings and data, to establish a systematic means of treating disease. While individual clinical experience is important, SDM relies on scientific evidence to establish the common clinical pathways that guide diagnosis and treatment.

Establish goals

Once the care team and the working group are comfortable with the concept of SDM and want to implement a program tailored to their community, the next step is to set both long- and short-term goals. This gives participants a vision for the future and helps to keep the work effort on track. It is advisable to detail what will be accomplished in the next month, 6 months, 1 year, and 5 years. The long-term plan will set the stage for putting the appropriate systems in place for measuring outcomes as the team starts implementing SDM. Some typical community goals are the following.

1. Achieve consensus on screening and diagnosis of type 1, type 2, and gestational diabetes.
2. Ensure the incorporation of insulin resistance related disorders.
3. Establish common therapeutic goals and referral points in the DecisionPaths for each type of diabetes.
4. Share the customized DecisionPaths with all providers and patients.
5. Ensure that every patient's progress is documented.
6. Adopt an ongoing method for assessing outcomes.

Consensus on goals is crucial, leading to a sense of ownership and responsibility for the program. It has proven to be the critical step toward successful implementation. When the orientation is complete, the next step is to organize a working group who will participate in the review and customization of the Practice Guidelines and Master DecisionPaths.

Customization of Staged Diabetes Management

> 'Practice Guidelines must use unambiguous language, define terms precisely, and use logical and easy-to-follow modes of presentation.'
>
> —Institute of Medicine[1]

By fully participating in the customization of Practice Guidelines for the community, the participant feels some ownership of SDM. In general, the starting point is to use the national standards of practice, if they exist. Under such circumstances there are elements that cannot be customized to the community—such as the diagnostic criteria or classification system. However, there are whole sections, such as treatment options and methods of monitoring metabolic control that can be modified based on resources and local practices. There are eight steps that are designed to assist the group in adapting SDM Practice Guidelines and Master DecisionPaths to the community. In general, 4–6 hours of meeting time are required to complete the customization process. All participants should have copies of this textbook plus a set of Quick Guides.

The customization of SDM is meant to be by and for health professionals. Selection of the participants in this process requires consideration of several factors.

1. *Who are the care providers?* In general, the providers are defined as those who are responsible for all aspects of disease management, including selecting the appropriate therapy, adjusting pharmacologic agents, making a referral for diabetes and nutrition education, and managing co-morbidities. The diabetes care and education team is the starting point. There may, however, be others who play an important role, such as a pharmacist or visiting nurse.

2. *Do they operate as part of a team or as individuals?* Most groups operate as a loose confederation of individuals. This often causes confusion in medicine. A single nurse may work with five to ten physicians and receive conflicting orders. Agreement that a team approach will be used with consistency should be a goal.

3. *Can one participant represent a larger group?* In multi-site managed care organizations, a person from each site might be a member of the working group. That person would represent the site and be responsible for orienting the site after consensus is reached.

4. *Are there individuals who "must" participate to ensure acceptance of the SDM approach?* Medical directors, nursing directors, and others in administrative roles may be in critical positions to foster acceptance of SDM. Their inclusion is often necessary to ensure adequate resource allocation.

Step 1: A call to action

The first step is to review the purpose of SDM, the customization process, and the long-term goals (developed during the orientation meeting). SDM is meant to bring an evidence-based approach to disease management. Staged Diabetes Management uses DecisionPaths to guide clinical decision-making. Customizing SDM to the community allows each professional to participate in decisions on treatment. The goal is to share the same long-term vision for care in the community and the means by which the vision will be put into action. This should include such specific goals as consistent criteria for diagnosis and classification, improvement in glycemic control, and reduction in the rate of complications.

Step 2: Provide information about diabetes and insulin resistance

Staged Diabetes Management is meant for the primary care physician and team, and yet it relies on the full participation of specialists. Therefore, it is important that the individuals with expertise on diabetes, hypertension, renal disease, obesity, and other related disorders are at the meeting to provide in-depth information. Bringing specialists into the process from the onset helps in reaching a multidisciplinary consensus and ensures a consistency in approach between primary care providers and specialists. In the absence of specialists, rely on reference materials to support the need for consistency, tight metabolic control, and a multidisciplinary approach.

To assure that the scientific foundation of SDM is established SDM provides electronic media (eSDM) which includes a slide presentation produced by Flash® technology. The presentation is in modular form, covering the classification, diagnosis, pathophysiology, and natural history of each type of diabetes as well as associated disorders and complications. The presentation is periodically updated and provides a ready means for laying the scientific foundation of SDM. It is recommended that the participants in the customization process have a scientific foundation for SDM. The slide presentation assures that each participant has the opportunity to learn about the key principles of insulin resistance and insulin deficiency, treatment modalities, surveillance for complications, and other factors critical to understanding the disease process. The slides may be presented to the whole team or as self-learning modules. The presentations can be completed in 2–4 hours and should precede customization.

Step 3: Build consensus

The process of adapting Practice Guidelines and Master DecisionPaths is best accomplished through consensus building. All participants should have a chance to comment on each issue. After the discussion ends a group consensus should be possible. In the event that the group cannot decide, turn to the scientific evidence to determine whether it is a matter of insufficient data or a lack of agreement in the scientific community. Voting on an issue should be used as a last resort as it tends to leave those in the minority dissatisfied. Use the expert to try to persuade the minority to change opinions.

Step 4: Customize the Practice Guidelines

SDM is designed so that the Practice Guidelines for each type of diabetes and related disorders are structured in a similar manner. The Practice Guidelines have seven components: risk factors and screening, diagnosis, treatment options, treatment targets, monitoring, follow-up, and surveillance. In many cases certain elements of the practice guideline cannot be customized as a national or regional consensus already exists. Some examples are risk factors and diagnostic criteria.

Begin the process by selecting one practice guideline. Type 2 diabetes is often selected because of its prevalence and complexity. Start with the screening section. Many organizations have options on who to screen and how often. In the United States, individuals at high risk such as members of minority groups, people with prediabetes, and individuals with insulin resistance are generally screened independent of age. All others are generally screened after the age of 45. This may change as more epidemiological data are gathered. Each community is different based on its ethnic, racial, and age distribution. Local data on the incidence of type 2 diabetes should act as the ultimate guide. This is also a good opportunity to define the target population and high-risk groups particular to the community. The Practice Guidelines should have clinical applicability and reflect the variety of ages, ethnic, or racial groups found in the practices of clinicians in the group. Each participant should be given the opportunity to contribute to the discussion. This is the time to identify "outliers" and to make sure their concerns are factored into the customization process.

> "Clinical Applicability. Guidelines should be as inclusive as evidence and expert judgment permit, and they should explicitly state the populations to which statements apply."
>
> —Institute of Medicine[1]

A key factor to consider in customizing the Practice Guidelines is to establish a common system for classification of type 1, type 2, and gestational diabetes, especially for future coding and monitoring purposes. Too often type 2 patients are misclassified because insulin is required to achieve glycemic targets. Misclassification probably will not occur if the underlying pathophysiology of these diseases is kept in mind. Type 1 is an autoimmune disorder, type 2 results from insulin resistance coupled with relative insulin deficiency, and gestational diabetes occurs because of insulin resistance first discovered during pregnancy. The risk factors and screening criteria should take these dimensions into account.

Obesity, previous impaired glucose intolerance, family history, common insulin resistance conditions (polycystic ovary syndrome and Acanthosis Nigricans), and lack of ketones (moderate to high) are generally signs of type 2 diabetes.

Diagnosis

Inconsistencies in diagnostic criteria and inadequate documentation are among the most common problems SDM has uncovered. Therefore, the current diagnostic criteria for each type of diabetes should be reviewed. While the criteria should not be modified as they are internationally accepted, they can be clarified so as to set stricter standards. Since both fasting and casual blood glucose levels are accepted, with the latter requiring "symptoms," clarifying the symptoms and how they are to be corroborated is necessary. Stating them explicitly in the Practice Guidelines and following the Diagnosis DecisionPath assures consistency. The current standards for type 1 and type 2 diabetes are the same: fasting plasma glucose $\geqslant$ 126 mg/dL (7.0 mmol/L) or casual plasma glucose $\geqslant$ 200 mg/dL (11.1 mmol/L) with symptoms (e.g. polyuria, polydypsia, and polyphagia) both repeated on a second occasion to confirm the diagnosis. Only age and symptoms at entry may differ significantly. Alternative means (e.g. oral glucose tolerance test or, in extreme situations, C-peptide) are called for only if the group has difficulty making the diagnosis of diabetes or classifying a patient. For gestational diabetes, only the 3 hour, 100 g oral glucose tolerance test is used in the United States for diagnosis.

Note: Where controversy may exist is with hypertension and obesity. The criterion for hypertension for individuals with diabetes is a mean of two values on different occasions of $\geqslant$130/80 mmHg. This, however, has been interpreted many ways: must both the systolic and diastolic meet the conditions or either the systolic or diastolic must meet the condition? Obesity has been defined as a BMI of $\geqslant$ 30 kg/m^2. Because these differences exist, full discussion and reaching a consensus become very important.

Treatment

The group may disagree on particular approaches to disease management, but consensus on all of the therapeutic options to be offered to the patient is requisite to developing Practice Guidelines. This avoids "shopping around" by patients. Many individuals with type 2 diabetes are looking for the health care professional who will not recommend insulin. Partly based on a fear of injections and partly on the misinformation that diabetes is only serious when insulin is used, these patients often seek out health care providers who do not offer insulin treatment. A second reason for listing all available therapies is the opportunity to inventory current practice by determining the therapeutic options currently offered to patients. Finally, it presents an occasion to reinforce the scientific basis of diabetes management. By discussing the merits of each therapy and the criteria by which they are generally used in current practice, the opportunity arises to once again review the action of the various pharmacological agents. This is also an opportunity to introduce the similarities among the different types of diabetes in terms of treatments. For all forms of diabetes, medical nutrition therapy is an important part of treatment. For both type 2 diabetes and gestational diabetes, medical nutrition therapy may be the stand-alone therapy. When insulin (type 1, type 2, and gestational diabetes) or oral agents (type 2 diabetes and gestational diabetes) are selected, medical nutrition therapy is synchronized to their pharmacokinetics. Each community has its own approach to insulin therapies and its own biases on selection of oral agent administration. Nevertheless, it should be possible to agree on all of the therapeutic options or stages. Staged Diabetes Management Practice Guidelines present the most popular stages for each type of diabetes. The group may modify them. Specific DecisionPaths have been developed for all current therapies.

Treat to target

Although treatment goals currently vary among communities, there is increasing evidence of the need for near-normal control of blood glucose levels. The evidence favoring tight control in type 1, type 2, and gestational diabetes is overwhelming. Based on this evidence, many diabetes associations throughout the world have proposed blood glucose levels that are within one percentage point HbA_{1c} above normal. These are reflected in the suggested Practice Guidelines in the SDM program. Acceptance of values at or near the SDM targets is encouraged. These may be seen as long-term goals, with intermediate targets for each patient. Additionally, SDM recognizes that very young and elderly patients as well as those without economic means and those with impaired cognitive ability may require more individualized and less stringent targets.

Staged Diabetes Management uses both HbA_{1c} and SMBG to measure the level of glycemic control. Since laboratories use different assays for HbA_{1c}, SDM uses the local laboratories' normal range as the criteria for control. Setting HbA_{1c} targets helps address the need to achieve control and the probability of reaching this goal. Ranges for SMBG must be set separately from HbA_{1c} since they do not always correlate directly with HbA_{1c} (due in part to different testing patterns). The targets suggested in the SDM materials are shown in Table 2.1. The relationship between HbA_{1c} and SMBG is based on clinical studies for each type of diabetes in which patients tested at least four times per day for a period of 3 months. Use this as a general guide.

Setting goals for special circumstances is also important at this juncture. For example, HbA_{1c} should not be used in gestational diabetes since the blood glucose targets are within the normal HbA_{1c} range. Children under six years old and individuals over age 65 require slightly higher metabolic goals because of the dangers of hypoglycemia. However, for the vast majority of non-pregnant patients, targets near or within the normal ranges are appropriate.

Monitoring

Next, address a system of monitoring blood glucose. HbA_{1c} and SMBG levels provide the basis for determining whether patients have reached their target. Therefore, use these tests to develop a pattern for monitoring. Individual differences between patients may require modifications, although it is still beneficial to develop an overall rule (perhaps a minimum). As the group establishes guidelines for blood glucose monitoring and frequency of HbA_{1c} testing, keep in mind that number of tests required relates to how the data are used for decision making and monitoring.

Staged Diabetes Management uses SMBG data for two purposes: clinical decision-making and overall assessment of the therapeutic intervention. For clinical decision-making, SDM relies heavily on SMBG to detect glucose patterns in order to determine the most appropriate modifications in food plan, pharmacologic agents, and exercise/activity. The number of tests required varies throughout adjust and maintain phases. In general, four tests per day are the minimum when clinical decisions are being made (two to four tests for type 2 diabetes on medical nutrition therapy). This may be increased during the adjust phase when treatment is being changed frequently. In the maintain phase the patient has reached the glucose target and needs monitoring for confirmation and for detecting the need for further fine adjustments. It may be possible to reduce the number of tests during this phase if the SMBG data are corroborated by HbA_{1c} values. In all cases SMBG must

Table 2.1 Glycemic targets for each type of diabetes

Classification	SMBG Blood Glucose Target	HbA_{1c} Target
Type 1 diabetes	70–140 mg/dL (3.9–7.8 mmol/L) pre-meal (50%)	$< 7.0\%$
Type 2 diabetes	70–140 mg/dL (3.9–7.8 mmol/L) pre-meal (50%)	$< 7.0\%$
Gestational diabetes	60–120 mg/dL (3.3–6.7 mmol/L) (100%)	NA

have a defined purpose and the data must be acted upon. Patients will soon abandon SMBG if their health care professional ignores the results.

A general rule with SMBG is that the data should be obtained from a memory based reflectance meter. Such a meter has an onboard memory that records the blood glucose value with the corresponding time and date. The patient or health care professional can scroll through the values to determine the past several weeks' pattern. Most meters have the ability to be connected to a computer and the glucose data reported in graphic formats (which can be inserted in the chart). This reduces the likelihood of error in reporting the test results. Self-monitored blood glucose should occur at the decision-making points in the day, generally before each meal and near bedtime (3–4 hours after the end of dinner). For special circumstances, such as overnight hypoglycemia, mid-afternoon hypoglycemia, and postprandial hyperglycemia, SMBG tests can be added at the appropriate times.

HbA_{1c} is used in clinical decision-making to corroborate the metabolic control reflected in SMBG values. HbA_{1c} is a relative measure that reflects average blood glucose level for the previous 10–12 weeks. As SMBG values improve, HbA_{1c} levels will decrease. The second purpose of HbA_{1c} and SMBG is to assess whether a therapy is achieving its goal. Too often patients are maintained on unproductive therapies. The community needs criteria that any member of the health care team (or the payers) can easily use to assess progress. HbA_{1c} is an excellent measure of the overall efficacy of a therapy. If HbA_{1c} rises, therapy is not working and modification or change is necessary. Similarly, if SMBG values remain high, the current therapy is failing.

In forming the Practice Guidelines, address these five questions related to monitoring.

1. *How often should SMBG be used?* In the initial selection of treatment and in the adjust phase, at least four SMBG tests per day are needed to evaluate therapy. If therapy is failing, do more testing until the underlying problem is discovered. Then select a new therapy. In stable periods, the optimum is still four times per day, especially for those patients using insulin. Table 2.2 summarizes the testing frequency for each type of diabetes. Use this as an overall guide for all team members and patients as well. If the circumstances permit reducing SMBG, one of these alternative patterns will probably provide sufficient data:

   - 3–4/day, 2–3 days per week
   - 1–2/day, varying time of day
   - 4/day, 1 weekday, 1 weekend day

   There are many other options, but keep in mind the data must allow accurate assessment of overall glycemic control and maybe used to guide the selection of alternative therapies.

Table 2.2 Recommended SMBG testing frequency/day

	Adjust Phase			Maintain Phase		
Stage	**Type 1**	**Type 2**	**GDM**	**Type 1**	**Type 2**	**GDM**
MNT	na	2–4+	6–7	na	1–2	6-7
Oral agent	na	2–4+	na	na	1–2	na
Combination	na	2–4+	na	na	1–2	na
Insulin Stage 2	4+	4+	6–7	2–4	2–4	6–7
Insulin Stage 3	4+	4+	6–7	3–4	2–4	6–7
Physiologic Insulin Stage 4	4+	4+	6–7	4	2–4	6–7
Pump	4+	4+	6–7	4	2–4	6–7

2. *How frequently should HbA_{1c} be determined?* HbA_{1c} reflects overall control in the 10–12 weeks before the test. Optimally, HbA_{1c} values should be determined quarterly and before the patient is seen. Too often the SMBG data (especially if they are erratic) do not provide sufficient information to confirm how well the current therapy is working overall. If the HbA_{1c} is obtained before the patient is seen, these data can be compared and a more accurate assessment of control can be made. If this is not possible and there is a discrepancy between HbA_{1c} and SMBG, immediately contact the patient if change in therapy is required. If HbA_{1c} is not available, obtain a fasting plasma glucose level, which provides the best alternative overall assessment (in office) of glycemic control. Make sure to compare this test with the SMBG results, as would be done with the HbA_{1c}. An alternative test, fructosamine, which provides previous 2–3 weeks overall glycemic control, may be used in place of HbA_{1c}. However, the fructosamine comparability to HbA_{1c} has not been studied extensively.

3. *When should both HbA_{1c} and SMBG be used?* Use both when undertaking intensive therapies and when SMBG cannot be verified. Since SDM relies on sound SMBG data, confirm the SMBG values with a periodic HbA_{1c}.

4. *Who should not get an HbA_{1c}?* Since HbA_{1c} is a retrospective measure covering an extended period of time, it is generally not used in gestational diabetes except at diagnosis to determine the extent of pre-existing hyperglycemia or if there is concern that the patient has underlying type 1 or type 2 diabetes. Under such circumstances, a baseline HbA_{1c} is advisable. The range of blood glucose in pregnancy is generally 20 per cent lower than in the non-pregnant state. Even with poor management of gestational diabetes, blood glucose generally does not rise to levels that would be reflected in a significantly elevated HbA_{1c}.

5. *When and for whom should ketones be monitored?* All patients with type 1 diabetes should monitor their ketones when any two consecutive unexplained SMBG values > 240 mg/dL (13.3 mmol/L) are discovered or any illness or infection is present. For pregnant women with gestational or type 2 diabetes, monitoring ketones ensures that there is no starvation occurring. Frequency depends on the patient. In general, once per day in pregnancy is a good rule to follow.

Follow-up and surveillance

The frequency of follow-up visits is somewhat individualized. In the adjust phase, follow-up frequency will be high with weekly telephone contact and monthly office visits. In the maintain phase, frequency of visits should be routine, reflecting community practices. Three to four times a year is customary. Staged Diabetes Management provides the list of tests and procedures that generally are recommended or required (by national standards) for diabetes and co-morbidity management as well as complication surveillance. (See under each type of diabetes and the complications section.) Based on the population in any community and their particular risks, the data collected may need to be modified at each visit.

Step 5: Customize the Master DecisionPaths

After completion of the Practice Guidelines, the group should consider customization of the corresponding Master DecisionPath. It is very important to give the group the opportunity to evaluate the sequence of therapies and the criteria by which each therapy is selected. Although SDM contains the Master DecisionPaths for each type of diabetes, they are designed to be customized to represent the consensus of local practitioners. The fundamental approach throughout the customization should be to assure scientific credibility. Although SDM materials reflect the most common and current practices that have been shown to be clinically effective, limited resources may require that they be modified.

During the customization process the community should consider changing:

1. the list of treatment options
2. the order of treatment options
3. the criteria for initiating treatment
4. the criteria for moving from one therapy to the next

Note: Although in general, throughout the natural history of type 2 diabetes, patients require more complex therapies, SDM is not unidirectional. There are times when reversing the course of treatment, replacing an oral agent with medical nutrition alone, may be appropriate. This decision should be based on SMBG data confirmed by HbA_{1c}.

Before beginning customization, the group should be familiarized with the layout of the Master DecisionPath. Stages are listed along the right-hand side in rectangular shapes. Included along with the names are the conditions for moving from one stage to the next. For combination and insulin stages, the timing of the oral agent and insulin doses is also provided. For both administration of pharmacologic agents and SMBG, Staged Diabetes Management uses a premeal four-point scale: AM—fasting; Midday—approximately 4 hours after breakfast; PM—before the evening meal; and BT—3–4 hours after the evening meal or bedtime. Thus, for type 2 diabetes, OA–0–0–N indicates oral agent in the morning (AM) and NPH insulin before bedtime (BT) along with an evening snack. Physiologic Insulin Stage 4 closely mimics normal insulin secretion (hence the designation physiologic). It has several versions using a four injection regimen: R–R–R–N denotes regular insulin before each meal and NPH insulin 3 hours after the evening meal; alternatively, RA–RA–RA–G indicates the use of a rapid-action insulin analog before each meal plus a long-acting analog (glargine) at bedtime.

Therapy choices

First, look at the Master DecisionPaths provided by SDM and note the progression of therapies. Modifications in therapeutic choices or progression may be necessary based on the availability of resources or other factors. If this is so, make the changes. However, note that an expert panel reviewed the recommended therapies. They represent the simplest and most effective routes to intensive glucose control and therefore should be carefully considered by the group.

Criteria for changing therapy

Effective management requires a goal and an allowable time to meet that goal. Unfortunately, however, extended time in the adjust phase that does not lead to improvement in glycemic control is common in diabetes care. Estimates indicate that 80 per cent of all patients with diabetes stay in a therapy even when glycemic targets are not achieved. Staged Diabetes Management provides guidelines for deciding when a therapy has reached its maximum effectiveness and, therefore, should be changed. Table 2.3 summarizes these guidelines. It is strongly recommended that the community follow them in the Master DecisionPaths.

Table 2.3 Suggested timelines to reach glycemic targets

Stage	Time
Medical nutrition therapy	2–3 months
Oral agent	3 months
Insulin	6–12 months

Co-management

Staged Diabetes Management is meant to optimize primary care services without sacrificing quality. Therefore, each Master DecisionPath offers opportunities to consider expert advice. Perhaps the community does not have the resources to provide all treatment options. For example, many primary care physicians are not trained to initiate insulin pump therapy. Review the Master DecisionPaths and determine with the group which therapies should be co-managed with a specialist. In any co-management situation, the primary care provider continues as the coordinator of care. This is an opportunity to make certain that the specialist also follows the community Master DecisionPath to ensure that all team members can continue delivering consistent, quality care.

Selecting initial therapies

Staged Diabetes Management covers the therapies for a newly detected patient and the continuation of treatment for previously diagnosed cases that are to be followed according to the SDM protocols. For recently diagnosed cases the time necessary to make or confirm a diagnosis and to determine the initial treatment or stage is variable. In general, confirmation should occur within a few days. For the majority of patients no treatment need be initiated until the diagnosis is confirmed, thus the waiting period does not present a medical problem. However, for patients whose fasting or casual blood glucose at diagnosis exceeds 300 mg/dL or 16.6 mmol/L, with or without positive ketones, there is a need for immediate insulin therapy. This is especially important for individuals below the age of 30 years. The differential diagnosis between type 1 and type 2 diabetes may require extensive laboratory tests that take several days to complete. During this time the individual may develop acidosis. This could lead to diabetic ketoacidosis (DKA). To avoid this it is recommended that insulin therapy be initiated until blood glucose levels can be restored (< 200 mg/dL or 11.1 mmol/L).

For those already in treatment, the transition to SDM start phase represents the point at which a new treatment is being selected. The use of the SMBG data, laboratory plasma blood glucose, and HbA_{1c} is recommended to ensure improvement in glycemic control in as rapid and efficacious a manner as possible. For patients already self-monitoring and for whom serial HbA_{1c} values are available, the addition of a laboratory fasting plasma glucose would be helpful. These data will help differentiate between those individuals with primarily insulin deficiency and those with insulin resistance. (The natural history of type 2 diabetes suggests that relative insulin deficiency occurs 7–10 years after the onset of disease and is often accompanied by deterioration in casual plasma glucose.) Some community physicians may be reluctant to select the more complicated regimens because they believe that patients are less likely to be compliant and because they themselves may be unfamiliar with how to start, adjust, and maintain these therapies. Staged Diabetes Management provides Specific DecisionPaths for each treatment stage, which have been tested in numerous sites and reviewed by expert panels. The overwhelming evidence supports their use by primary care teams.[2]

Note: The entry plasma glucose and HbA_{1c} levels depicted on the Master DecisionPath are suggested. The group may choose to modify them. The result, however, should be one consistent set of criteria for determining which therapy is selected. This avoids confusion when several members of the health care team see the patient.

Step 6: Share Customized Practice Guidelines and Master DecisionPaths

If different members of the larger group helped modify the SDM program, determine the extent of the whole group's acceptance of the practice guideline and the Master DecisionPath for each type of diabetes. Refer to the diabetes expert if the results of any of the smaller groups' customizations seem inconsistent with the ADA or other national or international expert organizations' standards of practice. The group should adopt guidelines that are both realistic and usable. Occasionally, guidelines are too strict or too liberal. Hear all viewpoints at this juncture, be patient, and leave ample time for discussion.

Once consensus has been reached on the Practice Guidelines and Master DecisionPath, review selected Specific DecisionPaths to familiarize the group with the SDM approach. To do this, if the groups were divided according to type of diabetes, now is the time to reconvene them.

Step 7: Review Specific DecisionPaths

All treatment DecisionPaths are organized according to stage. They are self-contained with start followed by adjust/maintain. They are meant to clarify the implementation of a treatment protocol and are not meant to be modified. They follow the Food and Drug Administration guidelines and contain any contraindications or precautions.

If the Quick Guides are being used, they are color coded for each type of diabetes. Using type 2 diabetes as an example (Medical Nutrition Therapy/Start), note that the structure of the DecisionPath begins with the entry criterion (blood glucose at diagnosis). It then moves to the medical visit and the blood glucose targets. This is always followed by "how to start" the therapy along with notes related to starting the treatment. After "how to start" comes the follow-up information. This is the same structure for all start phases.

Adjust treatment

Next is the adjust/maintain phase of the DecisionPath. Once again the structure follows a set pattern. The DecisionPath begins with a brief review of key data. This is followed by an evaluation of current glycemic control. If the patient has reached the targets, they enter the maintain phase. Follow-up guidelines are detailed in the box to the right. If the patient has not reached the targets, the reason must be determined. The underlying reason is often adherence. Staged Diabetes Management provides a Specific DecisionPath to evaluate patient adherence and to identify behaviors typical of psychological or social reactions to diabetes (see the Appendix, Figures A.19 and A.24). If adherence is not the problem, the next question is whether any improvement has occurred. To determine this, a simple algorithm has been devised. If at the previous visit the SMBG or HbA_{1c} was less than twice the target, then over the period of 1 month the average SMBG should have dropped by 15 mg/dL (0.8 mmol/L) and the HbA_{1c} by 0.5 percentage points. If the SMBG and/or HbA_{1c} was greater than twice the target, the drop should have been 30 mg/dL (1.7 mmol/L) or 1.0 percentage point HbA_{1c}. If this is occurring, the current treatment is continued without any adjustment. If, however, the treatment does not meet these criteria, further adjustment is necessary. Each pharmacologic agent has a maximum safe and efficacious dose. For oral agents it is straightforward. For insulin, in general, > 1 U/kg (> 1.5 U/kg in adolescents) is considered over-insulinization and calls for a re-evaluation of the therapy. Staged Diabetes Management provides these criteria for each adjust phase, and also provides the reasons for moving from one therapy to the next. For oral agents, the choice of combination or insulin therapy is based on whether the lack of improvement is due primarily to fasting hyperglycemia or overall hyperglycemia. For Insulin Stage 2, the criteria for moving to stage 3 are persistent fasting hyperglycemia, nocturnal hypoglycemia, or insufficient improvement over the past 12 months.

Insulin adjustment guidelines

Staged Diabetes Management provides insulin adjustment guidelines according to each stage of therapy. These guidelines are meant to provide general rules for adjusting the insulin dose up or down based on the standard insulin action curves. It is highly recommended that SMBG values be the basis for the decision as to which insulin to adjust and by how much. The guideline is based on patterns of blood glucose. Make certain that a pattern is detected before beginning to make changes in the insulin dose.

Ancillary DecisionPaths

This section includes the common DecisionPaths for medical visits, hypoglycemia, illness assessment, education, nutrition, exercise, and adherence assessment. The group should review selected paths to familiarize the participants with the roles and responsibilities of team members. Begin with diabetes education. Note that the DecisionPaths list the data that the educator needs prior to seeing the patient as well as the length of time each visit requires. Nutrition and exercise follow the same format. Adherence assessment covers both the metabolic parameters and on the back side some of the behavioral cues that may explain poor adherence.

With the Specific DecisionPaths reviewed, it is time to apply these paths to actual case studies. Three or four model cases taken from the records of patients treated at the site should be summarized and used as the basis of the exercise. One should cover diagnosis, one initial therapy, one transition to insulin, and one such co-morbidities as hypertension and dyslipidemia. The case studies serve to test the SDM principles against actual situations. An outline of how to organize the cases, some model cases, and some typical problems is found in Appendix A.26.

Step 8: Discuss implementation

Before adjourning this meeting, an implementation plan needs to be developed. Additional meetings to finalize the plan may be necessary, but at least make a start now. There are several options for moving the community toward full implementation and much will depend on the make-up of the community. Over the past decade numerous medical organizations have implemented SDM. Many have published their experience (a reference list is provided at the end of this chapter).

Once the group has reached consensus on Practice Guidelines and Master DecisionPaths, a timeline for implementing SDM needs to be developed. The timeline should establish when SDM materials will be distributed to the community and when and how patients will be switched to SDM. For most communities the timeline begins almost immediately following participation in the consensus building process. Decisions to start all newly detected cases and to include the Practice Guidelines or a flow sheet in each chart are common. Some other decisions, such as making changes to charting, scheduling patients, and setting up procedures for diabetes education and nutrition may take a little time. At this meeting a priority list of steps that need to be taken and assignment for responsibility to undertake the steps by team members should be made.

Evaluation of Staged Diabetes Management

Once SDM is underway, assess progress periodically, specifically in the areas of patient care, quality of care, and cost of care. This evaluation provides information needed to make changes and improvements and is crucial to the program's success.

Measuring quality

The issue of measuring quality can be broken down into three types of evaluation measure: structural, process, and outcome. Structural measures refer to those program elements that are throughputs: personnel, equipment, facilities, and financing. For nearly half a century, structural measures were predominant in medicine. Physician education, availability of highly technical instruments, the hospital–medical school association, and money spent on these structural elements were believed to be reflected in care. Thus, the more spent the better the outcome. By the mid-1950s, it became clear that structural measures did not necessarily explain differences in outcome. Perhaps the most striking information came from studies comparing surgery rates when patients sought one opinion versus two. A second opinion led to 50 per cent fewer surgeries and lower costs—and medical outcome was not compromised.[3]

The shortcomings of structural measures led to process measures, which focused on the policies, programs, and procedures of health care delivery. Considered part of throughputs, process measures tracked patients through the system and examined whether consistent, documented practices were in place. Practice Guidelines developed because of attention to issues of process.

Process measures became widespread, and in some clinics the belief emerged that the mere existence of standards of care could ensure quality. Federally funded patients were the first to benefit from process measures; that is, professional service review organizations measured physician performance against Practice Guidelines. A typical process measure included the presence or absence of diagnostic criteria for type 2 diabetes in the patient's chart as well as the documentation of patient education and evaluation of complications.

Process measures assumed that beneficial medical outcomes resulted from systematic processes. Research, however, did not entirely support this assumption. Standardized care should have improved outcome, but too often Practice Guidelines were not used. One reason for a lack of implementation of guidelines was that they did not account for the unique resources each community brings to a medical problem. A second reason often cited was that Practice Guidelines tended to be written by "experts" who were not involved in community-based primary care.

Defects in structural and process measures led to outcome measures. By focusing on the end product (medical condition of the patient after the treatment), providers could determine whether a medical intervention led to beneficial results. Since outcomes were so important, many argued, outcome measures alone would suffice. Thus, in the 1980s several medical centers advertised the number of successful heart transplants, the number of patients receiving laser therapy, the five year survival rate for individuals with breast cancer, and so forth. This may have been an excellent way to promote particular health care delivery systems, but it also showed tremendous variations in practice. Concern for these variations, rising costs, renewed focus on quality, and a cost–benefit approach to outcome measurement has led to the current outlook on quality of care. According to this outlook each element of the systems approach to quality assessment has merit. Thus, the key to assessing the impact of SDM is to incorporate structural, process, and outcome measures from the outset.

Process and structural measures

If the SDM Diabetes System Review was completed as part of the needs assessment, note that it was divided according to inputs, throughput, and outputs. This will serve as a baseline measure. If the review was not done for the needs assessment, familiarize the diabetes teams with it now. By creating a team of health professionals and assigning resources to SDM this will result in changing the structure of diabetes care in the community. Note these structural changes in items one to seven of the throughputs. Identifying process measures for SDM is straightforward. The Practice Guidelines and Master DecisionPaths adopted by the community are process measures and the basis for assessing SDM. To assess the process measures, conduct a patient chart audit using the Patient Chart Audit Form found in the Appendix, Figure A.2.

In addition to auditing the patient's charts, answer the following process measure questions.

1. Has the community of health care professionals agreed on the Master DecisionPaths for type 1, type 2, and gestational diabetes?

2. Has a policy been established to include the Practice Guidelines and DecisionPath in each patient's chart or in every exam room?

3. Has a system been devised to track patients using the Master DecisionPath?

4. Has a system been adopted to record and aggregate data according to type of diabetes, stage, and phase?

Outcome measures

Incorporate intermediate and long-term outcome measures into the SDM program. Here are several intermediate outcome measures for consideration:

- HbA_{1c}
- blood glucose (SMBG)
- blood pressure
- microalbuminuria
- lipid profile
- treatment for diabetes
- treatment for hypertension
- treatment for dyslipidemia
- body mass index (BMI)
- medical nutrition plan
- foot examination
- eye examination
- aspirin use
- referral for diabetes education
- referral for medical nutrition therapy

For diabetes in pregnancy, use the following measures:

- miscarriage (type 1 and type 2 diabetes only)
- fetal anomalies (type 1 and type 2 diabetes only)
- large for gestational age (LGA)
- small for gestational age (SGA)
- neonatal hypoglycemia

Long-term measures for type 1 and type 2 diabetes are listed below. The number of intervening variables affecting these outcomes cannot be easily identified. For that reason, monitor these outcomes, but also record possible intervening variables:

- retinal changes
- renal changes
- neurological changes
- cardiovascular disease
- peripheral vascular disease
- foot problems (ulcers, deformities, infections)
- other related complications

Evaluate the long-term measures in light of specific steps taken to alter them. Improved metabolic control should prevent or delay microvascular complications. However, the level of control and how well it is sustained are critical. Unless these factors are taken into account, false conclusions may be made about the relationship between SDM and outcomes. Therefore, be realistic in selecting outcome measures. Minimally, the outcomes should meet the criteria for NCQA Physician Recognition as outlined in Chapter 1.

Ongoing monitoring

Developing a system of ongoing monitoring is fundamental to promoting change while ensuring quality. In 1950, Dr. Deming, the famed developer of the quality movement, proposed the PDSA cycle.[4] He argued that for a program to change and maintain quality, the environment needed planning (P), doing (D), studying (S), and acting (A). Applied to medicine in general and SDM in particular, PDSA promotes ongoing reassessment of medical practices. Recently, such quality assurance movements as Six Sigma have emerged to reinforce the whole movement towards improved quality and reduced error.[5] Arguing that the rate of error in medicine is too high, resulting in significant human and financial costs, the Six Sigma movement attempts to apply mathematical principles to problem identification and resolution. An underlying principle is to assure both effectiveness and efficiency while reducing error. Six Sigma's goal is to reduce error to three mistakes for each one million medical encounters. As an example, it argues that currently there are more than 500 surgical errors each week. Using an approach similar to that of Dr. Deming, instead of the PDSA paradigm, it uses a define–

measure–analyze–improve–control (DMAIC) model. Its key is to measure the scope of the problem first, understand the factors that contribute to error, bring together all involved personnel to find a way to correct the error, implement the change, and measure the outcome. It recognizes that critical to its success are a committed leadership, a management process that incorporates measurement, and the careful selection of change agents who are among the best professionals in the organization.

Whether the Deming approach, Six Sigma, or any of another dozen quality improvement processes, the principles remain the same. Identification and acceptance of a problem must come first. Measurement is key to this. Through measurement both the scope of the problem and possible solutions become known. Selection of an intervention needs to be founded in science. The importance of an evidence based approach cannot not be emphasized enough. Too often the solution is selected based on too little evidence. For years the belief that patients required individual education to learn about diabetes went untested. Only when rising costs made such education prohibitive was there a willingness to understand the role of patient education in the treatment of diabetes and to measure its cost effectiveness. Out of this came an understanding that while education was beneficial, its costs were too high. The question was whether a more cost effective approach could be created. Teaching patients in group classes was proposed. However, unlike individual education, this intervention was thoroughly tested and subjected to statistical analysis. It was shown that individuals had the same amount of improvement in glycemic control when taught in groups as patients taught individually, but at a lower cost.[6]

As illustrated in the discussion of patient education, assessment eventually gets to the question "What does it cost?". Increasingly, cost is important in determining a program's usefulness. Can SDM lead to a better way to determine cost? Staged Diabetes Management reduces variation and generates significant data from short-term, long-term, and ongoing monitoring. A series of studies in a variety of clinical setting have shown cost savings with improved glycemic control.[7–9]

References

1. Institute of Medicine. *Clinical Practice Guidelines.* Field MJ, Lohr KN, eds. Washington, DC: National Academy Press, 1990.
2. Mazze RS, Etzwiler DD, Strock ES, *et al.* Staged Diabetes Management: toward an integrated model of diabetes care. *Diabetes Care* 1994; 17: 56–66.
3. Barr JK, Schachter M, Rosenberg SN, *et al.* Procedure-specific costs and savings in a mandatory program for second opinion on surgery. *Qual Rev Bull* 1990; 16: 25–32.
4. Deming WE. *Out of the Crisis.* Massachusetts Institute of Technology, 1986.
5. Barney M and McCarty T. *The New Six Sigma.* Minneapolis: Pearson Higher Education. 2002.
6. Rickheim PL, Weaver TW, Flader JL and Kendall DM. Assessment of group versus individual diabetes education: a randomized study. *Diabetes Care* 2002; 25(2): 269–274.
7. Mazze R and Simonson G. Staged Diabetes Management: a systematic evidence-based approach to the prevention and treatment of diabetes and its co-morbidities. *Pract Diabetes Int* 2001; 18(7) (Supplement).
8. Sidorov J, Shull R, Tomcavage J, Girolami S, Lawton N and Harris R. Does diabetes disease management save money and improve outcomes? A report of simultaneous short-term savings and quality improvement associated with a health maintenance organization-sponsored disease management program among patients fulfilling health employer data and information set criteria. *Diabetes Care* 2002; **25**(4): 684–689.
9. Benjamin E and Bradley R. Systematic Implementation of Customized Guidelines: The Staged Diabetes Management Approach. *Journal of Clinical Outcomes Management* 2002; **9**: 81–86.

3 Therapeutic Principles for the Treatment of Diabetes

This chapter provides an overview of current diabetes therapies, including medical nutrition therapy (food plan and activity), oral agents, and insulin. The role of each with regard to the treatment of all types of diabetes is discussed. A discussion on evaluating blood glucose control is also included.

Medical Nutrition Therapy Stage

Medical nutrition therapy (MNT) utilizes the selection of healthy food choices and increased physical activity to benefit the treatment of diabetes, hypertension, and associated metabolic derangements. The specific functions of this therapy as a stand-alone intervention or applied in conjunction with a pharmacologic therapy are:

1. blood glucose control
2. weight management
3. blood pressure control
4. lipid control
3. synchronization with pharmacological therapies

MNT is used alone, as treatment for hyperglycemia and/or obesity in type 2 diabetes and gestational diabetes. Its purpose is to moderate caloric intake combined with increased total energy output. Alteration in both the proportion and amount of carbohydrate, protein, and fat can have a profound effect upon blood glucose levels. Specifically, in the non-pregnant person, hypo-caloric diets with even modest weight loss can significantly lower blood glucose levels by an average of 30–60 mg/dL (1.6–3.3 mmol/L).[1] An increase in activity level combined with these measures has the most beneficial effect on lowering blood glucose levels. Increased activity fosters a more rapid and efficient uptake of glucose, which in turn lowers blood glucose levels. Nevertheless, success of MNT is generally short lived. Most individuals are unable to maintain long-term weight reduction. Increased blood glucose levels accompany any weight gain.[1]

Individuals with type 2 diabetes (and to some extent individuals with gestational diabetes) can benefit from exercise. The primary benefits include:

- improved insulin sensitivity, resulting in more efficient uptake of glucose by muscle and fat
- appropriate weight maintenance

Staged Diabetes Management: A Systematic Approach (2nd Edition) R. S. Mazze, E. S. Strock, G. D. Simonson and R. M. Bergenstal
 ISBN: 0 470 86576 8

- improved serum lipid levels
- reduced risk of cardiovascular disease

Complication management is also enhanced by the appropriate application of medical nutrition therapy recommendations, including

- low-protein diet (0.8 g protein/kg/day or ~10 per cent of calories) for overt nephropathy
- reduced sodium consumption (< 2400 mg/day) for hypertension
- reduction in saturated fat (< 10 per cent of total calories) for dyslipidemia

While useful in type 2 diabetes to control blood glucose levels, the benefits of weight reduction in pregnancy, even amongst those who are obese, have to be balanced against the adverse impact on fetal growth and development. In general, weight management in pregnancy is meant to assure caloric levels that allow the developing fetus to grow without adding any further glucose challenge to the mother.

A major role for medical nutrition therapy is in individuals treated with pharmacological agents (such as people with type 1 diabetes treated with insulin, or individuals with type 2 diabetes or gestational diabetes treated either with oral agents or insulin). Food plans are designed to work with and balance the therapeutic effects of pharmacologic agents. In diabetes, a food plan with a moderate amount of carbohydrate (50 per cent of total calories), protein (20 per cent of total calories), and fat (30 per cent of total calories) aids in reducing post-prandial glucose excursions, which enhances the action of the pharmacologic agent. Similarly, by increasing activity level and thereby improving glucose utilization, this enhances the glucose lowering effect of the agent. By incorporating foods high in fiber, thus slowing absorption, the glycemic challenge of the meal can be significantly reduced.

Self-monitored blood glucose and medical nutrition therapy

While most patients treated with pharmacological therapy (whether type 1, type 2, or gestational diabetes) are asked to monitor their blood glucose, individuals with type 2 and gestational diabetes treated by MNT alone often fail to understand the nature of their metabolic derangement. Much of this is due to the lack of emphasis on SMBG. Blood glucose data provide immediate information regarding the effect of the current food and activity plan. Since the food and activity plan are individualized, testing at different times during the day will help pinpoint their effectiveness. Both fasting and post-prandial (2 hours after each meal) data are needed for a proper assessment. During the start and adjust phases, when changes in medical nutrition therapy are likely, SMBG should be performed two to four times per day, varying the time each day until a full picture of the range of blood glucose levels can be created. In the maintain phase, when the target blood glucose goal has been reached and only minor adjustments are needed to stay in target, testing can be decreased. In pregnancy, SMBG needs to be increased to seven times per day to ensure rapid detection and immediate treatment of hyperglycemia.

Oral Agent Stage

The term oral agent was originally synonymous with sulfonylureas. For more than 40 years they were the dominant oral hypoglycemic agent. Now, the oral agents incorporate five general classifications, each with a different action:

- sulfonylureas (glyburide [glibenclamide], glimepiride, gliclazide, and glipizide) stimulate insulin secretion
- meglitinides (repaglinide and nateglinide)

stimulate insulin secretion in a glucose dependent manner

- biguanides (metformin) suppress excess hepatic glucose output and may improve insulin sensitivity at target tissues (muscle and fat)

- thiazolidinediones (pioglitazone and rosiglitazone) are insulin sensitizers; improve glucose uptake in insulin-sensitive target tissue and suppress hepatic glucose output

- alpha-glucosidase inhibitors (acarbose, miglitol) inhibit alpha-glucosidase enzymes in the small intestine that are responsible for breaking down carbohydrate into simple sugars, resulting in a delay in glucose absorption

Oral agents are currently used only in the management of type 2 diabetes and the sulfonylurea glyburide in the management of gestational diabetes. All oral agents have a limited effect on blood glucose control, lowering HbA_{1c} by one to two percentage points. However, these agents present an important opportunity to target the specific defects in type 2 diabetes and gestational diabetes that contribute to hyperglycemia. Because one or more underlying defects may contribute to hyperglycemia it is common to treat diabetes with a combination of oral agents. The major defects targeted by oral agents include:

- excessive hepatic glucose output (metformin and thiazolidinediones)

- decreased insulin sensitivity (metformin and thiazolidinediones)

- insufficient basal insulin (metformin and thiazolidinediones)

- insufficient post-prandial insulin secretion (sulfonylureas and meglitinides)

- excessive carbohydrate intake (alpha-glucosidase inhibitors)

See Chapter 4 for more information about the defects (how they relate to the natural history of diabetes and how these defects are detected). The following is a discussion of the specific mechanism of action of each oral agent class.

Sulfonylureas

The commonly available second- and third-generation sulfonylureas in the United States include glyburide, glipizide, and glimepiride. Sulfonylureas were the first oral agents widely used in the treatment of type 2 diabetes. Sulfonylureas, along with the meglitinides, are considered part of the broad category of compounds called insulin secretagogues. They stimulate insulin secretion from pancreatic β-cells by binding to a plasma membrane protein known as the ATP-sensitive potassium channel.[2] The interaction serves to depolarize the cell by blocking the efflux of potassium. This membrane depolarization opens voltage-gated Ca^{2+} channels, allowing an influx of Ca^{2+} into the β-cell. Insulin containing vesicles bind to the cell membrane in response to the rise in Ca^{2+}, resulting in secretion of insulin into the bloodstream.

Sulfonylureas have an average glucose lowering effect of 50–60 mg/dL (2.8–3.3 mmol/L). The majority of those treated with sulfonylureas experience improved glycemic control measured as a reduction in HbA_{1c} of up to two percentage points. Initial treatment with sulfonylureas is most successful in patients who are lean, have a short duration of diabetes, and follow dietary recommendations. While all sulfonylureas can cause hypoglycemia, some clinicians have noted that the second- and third-generation agents may result in less hypoglycemia and better glycemic control than the first-generation agents. Sulfonylureas, like many glucose lowering agents, tend to contribute to weight gain. Weight gain is due to the increased insulin level in the bloodstream that induces the active uptake and conversion of glucose into triglyceride in adipose tissue. Moreover, insulin induces the uptake and storage of free fatty acids, resulting in weight gain. Weight gain can be minimized by referral to a dietitian, who will provide patients with an appropriate food plan and activity/exercise schedule.

Most sulfonylureas are given once or twice each day. Dose changes are particular to each, with up to five steps needed to reach maximum dose. Sulfonylureas should be used with caution in patients with allergies to sulfa drugs and are contraindicated in the presence of severe renal disease (serum creatinine > 2.0 mg/dL [180 μmol/L]) or hepatic dysfunction. All sulfonylureas except glyburide pass the placental barrier. Thus, with the exception of glyburide (glibenclamide), sulfonylureas should not be used in pregnancy (see Chapter 6).

Meglitinides

Both repaglinide (a benzoic acid derivative) and nateglinide (a D-phenylalanine derivative) are in the meglitinide classification of insulinotropic oral agents. Like sulfonylureas, they are insulin secretagogues that stimulate β-cells to secrete insulin in a glucose-dependent manner.[5] Meglitinides close ATP-dependent potassium channels in the β-cell plasma membrane, inhibiting efflux of potassium and resulting in a membrane depolarization. This causes voltage gated calcium channels to open, allowing an influx of Ca^{2+} into the cells, which in turn stimulates the secretion of insulin from the cell. The key difference between sulfonylureas and meglitinides is that the latter reach peak plasma levels much faster. Meglitinide elimination half-life is more rapid, allowing insulin secretion to coincide more closely with meal related blood glucose excursions. Since meglitinides and sulfonylureas share the same mode of action, they should never be used in combination.

Meglitinides are taken before each meal. When taken as a monotherapy they reduce fasting plasma glucose by up to 60 mg/dL (3.3 mmol/L) and HbA_{1c} by approximately one to two percentage points. When used in combination therapy, HbA_{1c} is decreased by approximately 1.5 percentage points when repaglinide is added to patients treated with metformin.[11] The incidence of hypoglycemia with meglitinides is comparable to that with second-generation sulfonylureas. However, since meglitinides are taken just before a meal they become a more flexible alternative for patients who frequently skip meals or eat at different times throughout the day. Meglitinides can be used in patients with impaired renal function and/or impaired liver function (with a recommendation to titrate more slowly) and becomes an alternative to sulfonylureas for patients with severe sulfa allergies. Meglitinides should not be used in pregnancy.

Biguanides

Metformin, a bignanide, belongs to the category of insulin sensitizers. Based on numerous studies several pharmacologic mechanisms of action have been proposed for the biguanide metformin. These include suppression of excess hepatic glucose production (by the process of glycogenolysis and gluconeogenesis), increase in glucose uptake and utilization in peripheral insulin-sensitive tissues, and reduced glucose uptake in the small intestine.[3] While the precise contributions of each of these potential modes of action are not known, the primary effect of metformin appears to inhibit gluconeogenesis, thereby decreasing hepatic glucose output. Clinical trials have reported a glucose lowering effect of 40–80 mg/dL (2.2–4.4 mmol/L) with decrease in HbA_{1c} of up to 2 per cent.[4] Unlike the insulin secretagogues, metformin does not stimulate the pancreas to secrete insulin, thus it does not cause hypoglycemia when used alone. However, it can lead to hypoglycemia when used in combination with a secretagogue or insulin. Finally, metformin appears to maintain or lower weight, which may be the result of an anorexic effect. Perhaps because of this anorexic effect, metformin appears to enhance the lowering of LDL. Unlike sulfonylureas, metformin does not appear to result in weight gain. Because of a potential for gastrointestinal side effects, metformin is started at a low dose (500 mg or 850 mg) and slowly increased. The clinically effective dose is 2000 mg/day, with a maximum dose of 2550 mg/day. An extended release formulation of metformin has shown similar reduction in glucose levels, but reduced levels of gastro-intestinal side effects, compared with the standard preparation of metformin. The starting dose of extended release metformin is 500 mg with the evening meal that can be titrated to a clinically effective dose of 1500–2000 mg/day based on level of glycemic control and tolerability.

Metformin is in the same drug classification as phenformin. Phenformin was removed from use in the United States by the Food and Drug Administration (FDA) in 1977 because it was linked to an increased risk of lactic acidosis. Lactic acidosis, defined as plasma lactate levels > 5 mmol/L is a very serious metabolic complication because it is fatal in approximately 50 per cent of cases. Metformin appears to be a much safer biguanide, but the risk of lactic acidosis is still present and special precautions for its use are advised. The risk of developing lactic acidosis increases if the metformin level builds up in the bloodstream. Since metformin is cleared primarily by the kidneys, patients with impaired kidney function (serum creatinine > 1.4 mg/dL [120 μmol/L] in women and > 1.5 mg/dL [130 μmol/L] in men should not be treated with metformin. Patients undergoing radiographic studies using iodinated contrast materials should temporarily discontinue metformin therapy prior to or at the time of the procedure since they may lead to an acute decrease in renal function. Therapy can be resumed two days after the procedure once normal renal function has been established. Metformin should be used with caution in elderly patients, especially those over 80 years of age, because kidney function tends to decline with age. Elderly patients should be treated with the lowest dose needed to achieve glycemic targets and the highest doses of metformin should be avoided. Renal function should be monitored periodically in these patients. The risk of lactic acidosis also increases in patients who cannot deliver sufficient oxygen to peripheral tissues. Thus, metformin is contraindicated in patients with congestive heart failure (CHF) who require pharmacologic treatment. Additional precautions for use include patients with pulmonary disease, hepatic impairment, or acute or chronic alcohol consumption.

Because metformin passes the placental barrier, it is not approved for use in pregnancy and during lactation. It is important to note that women with Polycystic Ovary Syndrome (PCOS) is a insulin resistance conditioned associated with PCOS is often treated with metformin for infertility. While the drug has proven beneficial, its effect on the developing fetus is unknown. However, recent reports have shown that women treated with metformin for PCOS have a reduced risk of spontaneous abortion during the first trimester and fewer fetal anomalies; and they appear to have a dramatically reduced risk of developing GDM.[12]

Thiazolidinediones

The thiazolidinedione class of compounds currently consists of pioglitazone and rosiglitazone. Troglitazone was the first compound to be introduced in the thiazolidinedione class and was withdrawn from the market in 2000 due to idiosyncratic hepatotoxicity. Unlike troglitazone, pioglitazone and rosiglitazone do not appear to induce hepatotoxicity. Thiazolidinediones act by improving insulin sensitivity (hence are called insulin sensitizers) and have been shown to improve insulin action in a variety of animal and human studies. While the complete mechanism of action of the thiazolidinedione class of compounds remains unclear, overall this class of compounds elicits their effect by binding to nuclear peroxisome proliferator activated receptors (PPARs). Transcription of numerous genes controlling carbohydrate and lipid metabolism are regulated by PPARs. Several isoforms of PPARs exist and are most abundant in adipose tissue with a low level of expression in liver and muscle. Activation of PPAR-gamma isoforms are responsible for improved carbohydrate uptake and metabolism and PPAR-alpha is involved with alteration of lipid metabolism.[13] Rosiglitazone and pioglitazone have the highest specificity for the PPAR-gamma isoforms with some cross-reactivity with PPAR-alpha isoforms.

While the thiazolidinedione class of compounds has been used clinically since the introduction of troglitazone in 1997, they continue to be one of the most widely studied compounds in the area of diabetes research. Since they improve insulin resistance, the effect of thiazolidinediones is much broader than improving glycemic control;

they have also been shown to improve lipid profiles, reduce hypertension, and lower other cardiovascular risk factors such as decreasing plasminogen activator inhibitor-1 (PAI-1) and fibrinogen levels.[14] The non-hypoglycemic effects of thiazolidinediones on cardiovascular risk factors will be reviewed in Chapter 7. Table 3.1 outlines the action of thiazolidinediones on various tissues or organs that may lead to improved glycemic control.

Taken once daily, the glucose lowering effect of thiazolidinediones has been reported to be approximately 50 mg/dL (2.8 mmol/L) or 1.5 per cent HbA_{1c}.[6] Although not a hypoglycemic agent, when used in combination with insulin it can lead to hypoglycemia and should be used with caution in patients who do not monitor blood glucose. Because rare reports of hepatitis and elevated ALTs, caution should be used when starting thiazolidinedione therapy if ALT levels are mildly elevated (1–2.5 times the upper limit of normal) and therapy should not be initiated for ALT levels > 2.5 times the upper limit of normal. For rosiglitazone and pioglitazone therapy ALT levels should be determined every other month for the first year of therapy and periodically thereafter. Increased ALT monitoring may be required if ALT levels increase during treatment with thiazolidinedione. Discontinue thiazolidinedione therapy if ALT levels exceed three times the upper limit of normal.

Unlike metformin, the thiazolidinediones are known to be associated with modest weight gain of approximately 1–3 kg. The reasons for this may include increased subcutaneous adipose tissue, increased uptake of glucose into adipose tissue with subsequent conversion into triglyceride, and fluid retention. Thiazolidinedione therapy, alone or in combination with other medications for glycemia management, may lead to moderate to severe edema in approximately 4 per cent of patients. In some cases the edema is quite severe and may exacerbate or cause congestive heart failure. Medication should be withdrawn if severe edema occurs and/or any worsening in cardiac status occurs.

Thiazolidinediones are not approved for use in pregnancy because they pass the placental barrier and affect fetal growth and development. Few studies have been conducted with thiazolidinediones to demonstrate their safety and efficacy to treat polycystic ovary syndrome. Since rosiglitazone and pioglitazone are FDA category C drugs they should be used with caution in treating patients with PCOS. Metformin, a FDA category B drug, has been more widely studied to treat PCOS and should be considered for the treatment of PCOS along with medical nutrition therapy.[18]

Alpha-glucosidase inhibitors

Alpha-glucosidase inhibitors represent another pharmacologic class of agents for the treatment of type 2 diabetes. Their action is in the small intestine to inhibit enzymes (alpha-glucosidases)

Table 3.1 Metabolic effects of thiazolidinediones

Tissue/Organ	Effect
Adipose	• Increase expression of insulin-sensitive glucose transporter 4 (GLUT 4)
	• Stimulate formation of subcutaneous adipocytes
	• Inhibit lipolysis and decrease free fatty acid (FFA) release
	• Reduced release of potential mediators of insulin resistance including tumor necrosis factor alpha (TNF-α), resistin and adiponectin[14]
Muscle	• Improved insulin sensitivity and insulin stimulated glucose disposal[15]
	• Enhanced exercise stimulated glucose uptake[16]
Pancreas	• Improved beta-cell function
	• Improved meal stimulated insulin release[17]
Liver	• Modest, if any suppression of hepatic gluconeogenesis[17]

that break down complex carbohydrate into simple sugars (monosaccharides). The inhibition of these enzymes delays the absorption of monosaccharides, lowering postprandial blood glucose levels.

Acarbose and miglitol are alpha-glucosidase inhibitors used as a monotherapy or in combination with a sulfonylurea, metformin, or insulin. The clinical response of alpha-glucosidase inhibitor therapy is a lowering of average blood glucose by approximately 30 mg/dL (1.7 mmol/L) and a decrease in HbA_{1c} of up to one percentage point.[7] The predominant side effects include abdominal pain, diarrhea, and flatulence. Because of the potential for gastrointestinal discomfort, alpha-glucosidase inhibitors should be started at the lowest dose before the largest meal of the day and titrated up gradually. Contraindications include pregnancy and lactation, severe renal disease, chronic intestinal disease, and liver disease (acarbose only).

Combination oral agents

Combinations of sulfonylureas and metformin, repaglinide and metformin, or thiazolidinediones and sulfonylurea can be used to gain the advantage of each drug's unique action. As noted earlier, type 2 diabetes is a disease of both insulin resistance and insulin deficiency. Insulin resistance related drugs, such as the biguanides and thiazolidinediones and be used in combination with the insulin deficiency oral agents – the sulfonylureas and the meglitinides. When used in combination, the addition of a second agent generally occurs after reaching the maximum effective dose of the first agent. The second agent may be increased to maximum dose as well. Combinations of agents that enhance glucose uptake and improve insulin secretion can be started at the same time. This is the case in patients with long-standing type 2 diabetes with fasting and postprandial blood glucose levels averaging 200 mg/dL (11.1 mmol/L) and 270 mg/dL (15 mmol/L) respectively. Additionally, acarbose may be used in combination with a sulfonylurea or metformin, if a primary goal is the correction of postprandial hyperglycemia. Three oral agents, such as rosiglitazone, metformin, and sulfonylurea, can be used in combination as well. However, the same precautions for each agent must be considered. In general this will mean LFT, renal, and cardiovascular evaluations.

Combination oral agent and insulin

The combination of insulin in the evening and metformin, thiazolidinediones, or sulfonylurea in the morning is an alternative to directly initiating insulin therapy alone as well as a means to supplement the effectiveness of insulin. Generally sulfonylurea, thiazolidinedione, or metformin is given with the first meal of the day and intermediate- or long-acting insulin is administered at bedtime. Thiazolidinediones and metformin may also be used in combination with multi-injection insulin regimens. It is recommended that the patient first reach a total daily insulin dose of 0.7 U/kg before adding an insulin sensitizer (see Table 3.2).

Table 3.2 Approximate glucose lowering potential of type 2 diabetes therapies

Treatment	FPG reduction	HbA_{1c} reduction
Sulfonylurea	50–60 mg/dL (2.8–3.3 mmol/L)	1–2%
Metformin	50–60 mg/dL (2.8–3.3 mmol/L)	1–2%
Meglitinide	~60 mg/dL (~3.3 mmol/L)	1–2%
Thiazolidinedione	50–60 mg/dL (2.8–3.3 mmol/L)	1–2%
Alpha-glucosidase inhibitor	15–30 mg/dL (~1.5 mmol/L)	0.5–1%
Combination	100–120 mg/dL (~5.6–6.7 mmol/L)	3–4%

SMBG and oral agents

The use of SMBG is critical for any patient treated with an oral agent, since the resulting data provide an indication of the effect of the medication dose. Since oral agents work throughout the day, testing before each meal and at bedtime is important. Postprandial testing should be performed 2 hours after a meal. In general, at the onset of treatment and during the adjust phase, testing should be performed two to four times per day. During the maintenance phase, testing may be decreased to one or two times per day.

Insulin stage

Insulin, in one form or another, has been available since 1922. There are currently five classes of insulin named according to their length of action: rapid, short (regular), intermediate, prolonged intermediate, and long acting. Since the early 1990s insulin produced by recombinant DNA has been available. In 1996 the first insulin analog, lispro, was introduced in an effort to more precisely control the starting time, peak action, and duration of short-acting insulin.[8] Two amino acids in regular human insulin were transposed to generate an insulin (lispro) with a faster subcutaneous absorption rate compared with regular insulin. A second rapid-acting insulin, aspart, was introduced recently. Both lispro and aspart insulin analogs have comparable (with slight variations) in their action curves. Because of this, Staged Diabetes Management does not differentiate between these two analogs and groups them into a single class called rapid-acting insulins with the designation of "RA". In 2001 the first truly long-acting insulin analog, glargine, was introduced. During the same year, clinical research trials began several different versions of inhaled insulin. Inhaled insulin provides only bolus insulin and requires background or basal insulin to be administered once or twice a daily via injection. It is very likely that in the near future there will be several Food and Drug Administration approved alternatives to subcutaneous (injected) delivery of insulin.

Insulin action

Currently, insulin can be delivered by two mechanisms: injection or infusion pump. Injected insulin is available in all five classes of insulin, while pump therapy uses only rapid or short-acting insulins. Pump therapy provides both continuous infusion and boluses of insulin (to cover meals). For all forms of insulin and all delivery means the action curve is determined by several factors: type of insulin, source of the insulin (animal versus human), buffering compounds, site of injection, and exercise. Thus the absorption rate is not as predictable as the action curves might suggest. Table 3.3 summarizes the time of insulin action including onset, peak effect, and duration.

Some general rules will minimize the variation caused by many of these factors. Since each patient's response to insulin is slightly different, standardizing the general site of injection (arm

Table 3.3 Insulin action times

Insulin	Begins to work	Peak effect	Duration
Rapid Acting (RA)	5–15 minutes	1–2 hours	3–4 hours
Regular (R)	30–45 minutes	2–3 hours	4–8 hours
NPH (N)/Lente	2–4 hours	4–8 hours	10–16 hours
Ultralente (UL)	3–5 hours	8–14 hours	18–20 hours
Glargine (G)	2 hours	None	24 hours

versus abdomen) and the time and duration of exercise is helpful. Determining the insulin action curve of any individual requires SMBG data. Although the regimens prescribed are based on typical insulin action curves, variation between patients prevents absolute certainty in determining when the insulin peak action will occur. Thus, SMBG testing should be used to "map" the insulin action curve. For each insulin regimen Staged Diabetes Management provides a guide to SMBG that identifies the times to test in order to obtain adequate data to map the insulin action curve.

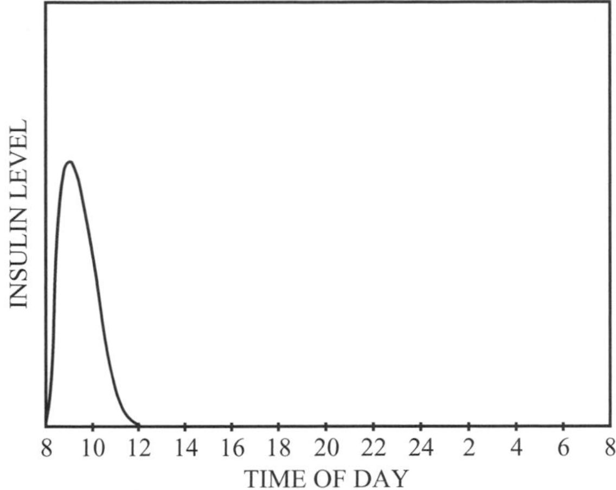

Figure 3.1 Rapid-acting insulin analog action curve

Rapid-acting insulin analogs and inhaled insulin

Lispro (RA) is a human insulin analog first discovered through computer modeling that permits the computational chemist to develop numerous "intramolecular relationships" to predict the action of insulin analogs under various conditions.[9] In this particular case, investigators developed an analog to insulin by reversing amino acids at positions 28 and 29 of the B-chain of human insulin. The resulting human insulin analog has lysine at position 28 and proline at position 29, hence the name lispro. Lispro does not form typical insulin hexamers (like regular insulin) in solution. Therefore, it is absorbed much faster and has a shorter time to peak effect (1–2 hours) and a shorter duration (approximately 3 hours) of action than regular insulin. In a similar manner, aspart, the second rapid-acting insulin to be introduced, is absorbed quickly after subcutaneous injection, peaks within 1–2 hours and is cleared within 4 hours. Thus, their rapid action may enhance glycemic control by enabling injection of insulin at the time of meals when food is ready to be eaten. This makes the timing more precise and estimates of total carbohydrate intake more realistic. Importantly, the action profiles of lispro and aspart have no significant "tail," which reduces the need for additional between-meal carbohydrate (snacks) and the risk of hypoglycemia (see Figure 3.1 compared with Figure 3.2). Premixed insulin formulations are available that combine rapid-acting insulin and intermediate-acting insulin. While these premixed insulins are convenient for patients, dose adjustments are not as easily accomplished. Another rapid-acting insulin analog (currently under review) is glulisine.

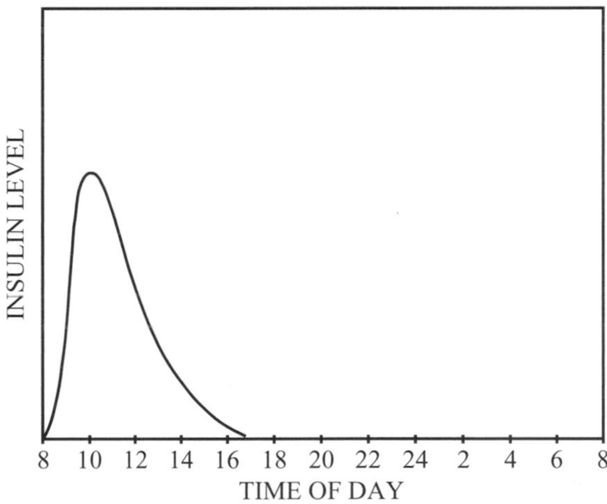

Figure 3.2 Short-acting regular insulin action curve

Inhaled insulin is meant to replace the rapid-acting pre-meal insulins which are generally delivered by either injection or infusion pump. Inhaled insulins are rapid-acting insulins, which are suspended in either powder or liquid. They use an aerosol delivery device designed for intrapulmonary insulin delivery in one or two inhalations. Relatively large amounts of insulin are required in part due to the bioequivalence between inhaled and subcutaneous insulin. Two to three times the amount of inhaled insulin is required to obtain the same insulin kinetics and glucose uptake as subcutaneous short-acting insulin. While it has been reported that inhaled insulin has a shorter overall duration of action and time to peak action (1 hour versus $1\frac{1}{2}$ to 2 hours for short-acting insulin), the pharmacokinetics and pharmcodynamics of inhaled insulin remain uncertain. The incidence of hypoglycemia is similar to that of subcutaneous insulin. The only reported adverse reaction has been a cough which effects as many as 10 per cent of the patients. Underlying lung disorders and smoking do not appear to be a significant contraindication. One precaution is that smokers appear to inhale insulin much more rapidly and reach peak insulin levels in half the time of nonsmokers.

Short-acting insulin

Regular insulin (R) is used before meals (Figure 3.1), and when injected 30–40 minutes before meals should match the breakdown of carbohydrate from the meal and the post-prandial rise in blood glucose. To evaluate the effectiveness of regular insulin, patients should obtain a blood glucose value before the next meal. If a subsequent pre-meal blood glucose level is high, this suggests the previous dose of regular insulin was insufficient for the amount of food consumed at the previous meal. In contrast, if the blood glucose is low, it suggests that too much insulin was taken, too little food was consumed, or the level of activity (such as strenuous exercise) was high. SMBG should be performed immediately before regular insulin is administered.

The generalized action curve for human regular insulin depicted in Figure 3.2 may not be as predictable as is shown. Based on injection site, absorption rate, prandial state, and level of exercise, the onset, peak, and duration of insulin may vary dramatically. Note that regular insulin has an onset of action of 30–45 minutes after the injection, but could be delayed by as much as an additional 30 minutes. The curve to peak effect is steep, reaching its highest point between 2 and 3 hours after the injection. As a general rule, the later the onset of action, the later the time of peak action. The duration of regular is from 4 to 6 hours. Note that the descending curve is slower and has a "tail" or "hangover." Thus, while most of the insulin has been utilized by noon in the illustration above, residual insulin is still available up to as late as 4 pm. Additionally, the overall action curve for regular can be affected by the introduction of a second insulin such as intermediate- or long-acting insulin. In both cases the second insulin may raise the level and duration of peak action.

Intermediate-acting insulin

The duration of intermediate-acting insulin (N) is normally 10–16 hours, but may extend to as much as 20 hours with a peak between 4 and 8 hours. The action profile is shown in Figure 3.3.

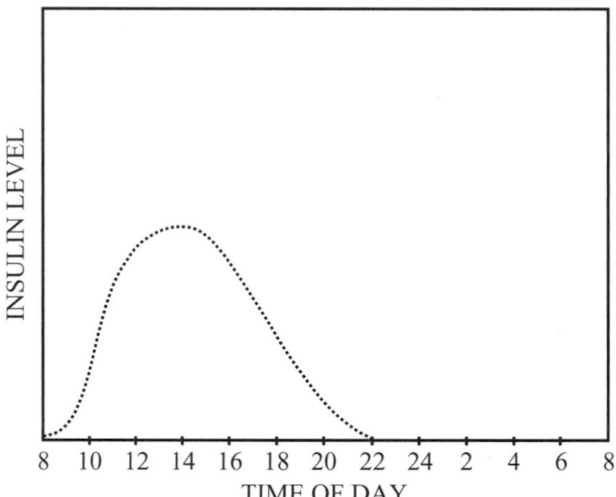

Figure 3.3 Intermediate-acting insulin action curve

Intermediate-acting insulin is often mixed with rapid or short-acting insulins in a "split mixed" regimen. Mixing insulins may affect the absorption rate. When mixed with regular insulin, N may slow the absorption rate by up to 15 minutes, although this effect is not usually of clinical significance. A similarly negligible slowing of the absorption rate occurs when N is mixed with RA. While this has led some physicians to recommend that regular or lispro be given separate from other insulin, the overall effect is minimal and should be considered only if difficulty is noted.

Premixed concentrations of 70/30 (70 per cent N and 30 per cent R), 50/50 (50 per cent N and 50 per cent R), Mix 75/25 (75 per cent NPL and 25 per cent lispro), and Mix 70/30 (70 per cent NPA and 30 per cent aspart) insulin are also available. Premixed insulins are recommended for the elderly and in others who have problems calculating the appropriate ratio. For most patients, however, customized mixing of insulins will be more beneficial for improving glycemic control.

To evaluate the peak effect of intermediate-acting insulin, SMBG should occur between 8 and 14 hours after administration. Testing just before the evening meal will determine whether the morning dose of N was effective. If intermediate-acting insulin is given at the evening meal, its effectiveness can be evaluated by checking fasting blood glucose levels the next morning. It is also suggested that mid-afternoon and 3 AM blood glucose levels be determined if the patient is experiencing symptoms of hypoglycemia at these times. If hypoglycemia is corroborated at mid-afternoon, consider lowering the morning dose of N. If corroborated at 3 AM, consider either lowering the afternoon intermediate-acting insulin or changing the time of administration. If snacks are added, subtract an equal amount of calories at the usual meal times so that the total caloric intake does not increase.

Prolonged intermediate-acting insulin

Figure 3.4 shows the action curve of prolonged intermediate-acting (ultralente) human insulin. The action curve for this human insulin is symmetric. It has both a slow onset and slow dissipation. This can be affected by injection site, exercise, and absorption rate, but less so than regular- or intermediate-acting insulins. The onset occurs over a period of approximately 3 hours. The curve at this point continues to rise at the same rate (slope) until it peaks at between 8 and 14 hours after the injection. The descending slope is the same as the ascending slope with remaining duration of approximately 10 hours. Ultralente is often used in combination with short-acting insulin to provide the basal insulin requirements for the individual who cannot be sure about the timing of each meal. In such a regimen, regular or lispro insulin is used to cover each meal. Adjustment of insulin doses when R or RA and UL are mixed is generally limited to the amount and timing of the short-acting insulin (once basal requirements have been established). Patients can eat and exercise when they like. As long as they have the basal dose of insulin to cover the fasting state, they can adjust their regular insulin requirements by testing before the next meal as well as before and after exercise.

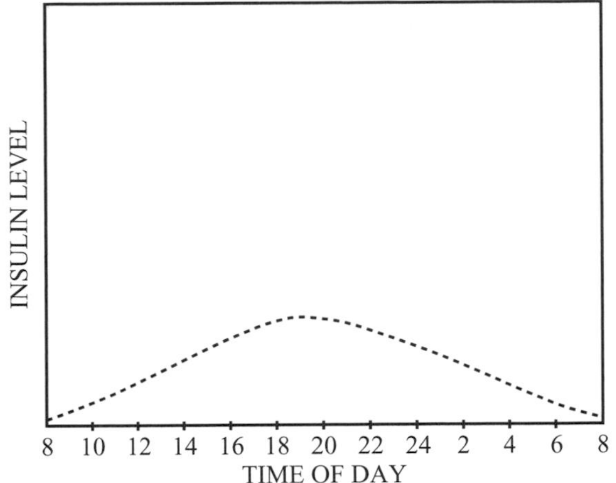

Figure 3.4 Prolonged intermediate-acting insulin (UL) action curve

SMBG for prolonged intermediate-acting insulin is more complex since this form of insulin is meant to improve glycemic control in the fasting state (between meals and overnight). Tests during fasting period should demonstrate normal blood glucose levels. Additionally, if the patient skips a meal, the blood glucose at the time the meal would have been consumed and until the next meal should be near normal. SMBG, therefore, cannot be prescheduled. Rather, it should be done any time the patient feels hypoglycemic, any time a meal is skipped, occasionally overnight (3 AM), and at random times.

When used as basal insulin, especially in type 1 diabetes, two injections of ultralente are normally required to maintain a constant level of background insulin. In such a case, the curves overlap to produce a nearly straight line with no peaks and valleys. Short-acting insulin, as mentioned earlier, is used to respond to each meal. Human ultralente insulin may also be used in place of intermediate-acting insulin (especially in type 2 diabetes) to provide for basal needs and to suppress overnight hepatic glucose output. Administered at 5–6 PM, its peak will occur at approximately 3–4 AM, consistent with intermediate-acting insulin given at bedtime. Because the peak is relatively low when compared to intermediate-acting insulin, the chance of hypoglycemia is much less than with intermediate-acting insulin. The duration of action of long-acting insulin must be carefully monitored when used overnight, since its action can continue well into the next day.

Long-acting insulin analog (Glargine)

Glargine is a long-acting insulin analog that has no peak action, which will provide for basal insulin needs in a multi-injection or inhaled insulin regimens (in the future). Human insulin was modified to create an insulin that is soluble at moderately acidic pH (4.2) and insoluble at neutral pH. When glargine is injected into subcutaneous tissue it forms a micro-precipitate that slowly dissolves and enters the blood stream at a very steady rate (see Figure 3.5). This results in the continuous delivery of insulin for a period of approximately 24 hours at a relatively low dose similar to pancreatic insulin secretion during a fasting state. One significant benefit of glargine over intermediate-acting insulins is a reduction in the risk of nocturnal hypoglycemia and generally improved fasting blood glucose control.[19] Because glargine is supplied at a moderately acidic pH, it should not be mixed with other insulins (which are supplied at neutral pH). Glargine recently received approval by the Food and Drug Administration to allow flexible administration at any time of the day.

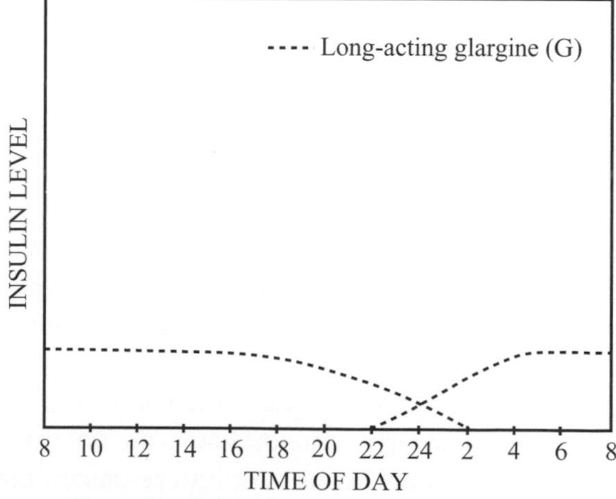

Figure 3.5 Long-acting insulin glargine

Insulin action and stages of therapy

This section graphically displays the integrated action profiles for various insulin regimens. For consistency, rapid-acting insulin is represented as a dotted line, short-acting insulin by short dashes, intermediate-acting insulin by long dashes, and long-acting insulin by solid lines. A simple notation represents insulin regimens. For example, a four-injection regimen of three pre-meal injections of rapid-acting insulin (RA) and one bedtime injection of long-acting insulin glargine (G) is depicted as RA–RA–RA–G. The time periods correspond to pre-breakfast, pre-lunch, pre-dinner, and pre-bedtime.

There are several different ways to administer insulin. It is preferable that the most physiological method to closely mimic normal insulin requirements be employed. This necessitates a balancing basal and bolus requirements, generally resulting in multi-injection regimens. Insulin utilization does not differ in any substantial way based on type of diabetes. Chapters 4–6 will provide details for the use of insulin in type 2, type 1, and gestational diabetes, respectively. Here, the principles related to different regimens are detailed along with their predicted action curves. Note that the Insulin Stage number corresponds with the number of injections. Insulin infusion pump therapy is discussed separately.

Insulin Stage 1
R/N–0–0–0

Insulin Stage 1 (see Figure 3.6) consists of two insulins mixed (or premixed 70/30) at the time of

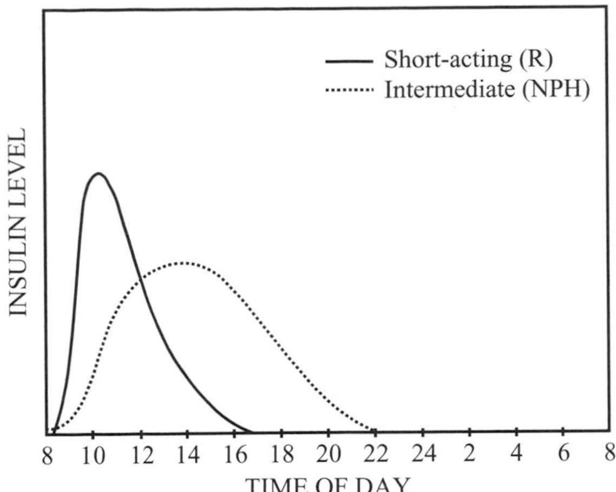

Figure 3.5 Insulin Stage 1 action curve using R/N–0–0–0

injection. Note that between the peak action of regular- and intermediate-acting insulin little exogenous insulin is available. Because this regimen does not mimic normal physiologic patterns of endogenous insulin action, it is not generally recommended. Variations of this regimen may be found in individuals with type 1 diabetes in the "honeymoon" phase. The two peak actions are primarily meant to cover the breakfast, and midday meals. A large evening meal or excessive hepatic glucose output would require additional injections of insulin. Additionally, because this regimen is meant to cover both breakfast and the midday meal with sufficient residual insulin for the evening meal, it often requires a large single dose. This will raise the chance of hypoglycemia, especially in the late afternoon. Thus it is very important that, at the minimum, SMBG be done at the time of the injection, 2 hours after breakfast, and 2 hours after the midday meal. This will ensure that the action of insulin will be accurately measured.

Another alternative to Insulin Stage 1 is a single injection of intermediate- or long-acting insulin at bedtime. This is specifically meant to cover basal insulin needs throughout the night and the following day. Thus, this regimen is especially useful in type 2 diabetes with glargine. There is no peak action of this insulin, thus the risk of overnight hyperglycemia, is substantially reduced. Its initial effect should be to reduce the fasting hyperglycemia, thereby impacting on the daytime blood glucose levels. If fasting glucose levels are normalized, it may result in no additional daytime insulin being needed. More likely is the use of this regimen as a starting point for the introduction of insulin in type 2 diabetes. SMBG should be done immediately prior to the time of the injection, at fasting and one to two times throughout the day. When this regimen is used as a starting point for multiple injections, the first step is to use the bedtime glargine to resolve the fasting hyperglycemia. Once this is accomplished, rapid-acting insulin can be added judiciously before each meal, starting with the meal that consistently leads to the highest daytime blood glucose levels. The results may be as many as three additional injections of RA. By using this approach, however, the total daily insulin requirement will be as much as 20 per cent lower than when fewer injections are used. The addition of RA before meals allows pinpointing of insulin to cover only those meals that produce high blood glucose levels. It is also possible following such a regimen to reduce the number of injections when meals are skipped or if the patient is successful in using medical nutrition therapy to reduce reliance on exogenous insulin. Few patients with type 2 diabetes can be sustained on a single-injection regimen, and it is rarely successful for those with type 1 diabetes.

Insulin Stage 2
R/N–0–R/N–0 or RA/N–0–RA/N–0

This is perhaps the most popular insulin therapy. It consists of two injections of intermediate-acting (N) insulin mixed with short- (R) or rapid-acting (RA) insulin given before the first meal and the evening meal each day (see Figure 3.7).

It comes in two forms: premixed and mixed at the time of injection. There are premixed versions of N with short- and rapid-acting insulins. These premixed versions are not always at the same ratio. There are, for example, 70/30 and 50/50 premixed versions of N and R; there is a mix 70/30 version of N and aspart and a mix 75/25

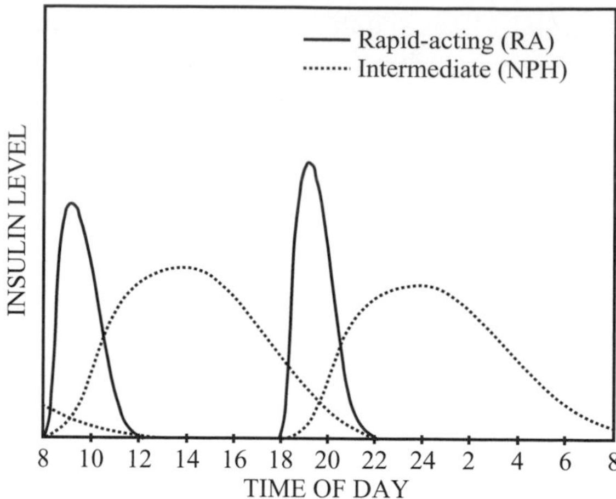

Figure 3.7 Insulin Stage 2 action curve using RA/N–0–RA/N–0

Consistent meals, exercise, and sleep patterns are necessary. Patients on two-injection regimens cannot skip meals, nor should they exercise at varying times without making anticipatory changes in the insulin dose and timing. The peak action of intermediate-acting insulin must be consistent with postprandial periods. Too often this regimen results in overinsulinization by attempting to use high doses of N to cover between- and after-meal periods. To avoid this, consider moving to bedtime G or N (Insulin Stage 3 or 4). SMBG should be done at least four times per day on this regimen: before each meal and at bedtime. Because mid-afternoon hypoglycemia is a possibility, testing 2 hours after the midday meal should also be considered.

version of N and lispro. What they have in common is that a change in the dose does not change the proportion of intermediate to short- or rapid-acting insulin. Thus, when the dose is increased both N and R or RA increase at the same rate. Thus 10 units of premixed 70N/30R insulin contains 7 units of N and 3 units of R. At 20 units of 70N/30R insulin the ratio remains the same (14N and 6R). This significantly limits insulin adjustments and often results in overinsulinization, which occurs when there is too much insulin during basal periods. For instance, if the premixed insulin does not resolve hyperglycemia following breakfast, then an increase in premixed insulin to provide more R would result in more N. This might result in mid-afternoon hypoglycemia, as there is a greater amount of intermediate-acting insulin available. In contrast, the mixture of N and R just before breakfast and dinner allows for any ratio of the two insulins. While in general the starting insulin distribution is two-thirds morning and one-third evening with the ratio 1:2 R:N in the morning and 1:1 R:N in the evening, it is likely that these ratios will be changed in order to optimize the peak actions and duration curves to synchronize with meals. Using the example above, an increase in morning R would not necessitate an increase in morning N when the insulins are dosed separately.

Insulin Stage 3
R/N–0–R–N or RA/N–0–RA–N

Three injections are given each day. N, or intermediate-acting insulin, mixed with short- (R) or rapid-acting (RA) insulin is given before the first meal, R or RA is given before the evening meal, and N is given near bedtime (at least 2 hours after the evening meal), shown in Figure 3.8. A variant of Stage 2, when N is moved to bedtime, more directly impacts morning hyperglycemia. In such a case, use of premixed insulins should cease. Note that this moves the peak action of intermediate-acting insulin to between 5 and 7 am. By more accurately targeting the morning blood glucose levels, this may also impact daytime blood glucose. Often the morning R or RA and N will be lowered if the evening N is effective. At the same time, since the N has been moved to bedtime, the valley between the action of evening R or RA and N is greater. Note that R may be substituted by RA at the same dose. Consult Figure 3.2 for the insulin action curve. Because RA acts more quickly and has a shorter duration, make certain that the patient is advised to eat immediately following administration of RA. Careful meal planning by reducing the caloric content of the evening meal and moving some calories to bedtime will help reduce the postprandial glucose challenge. A variation of Insulin Stage 3 is R or

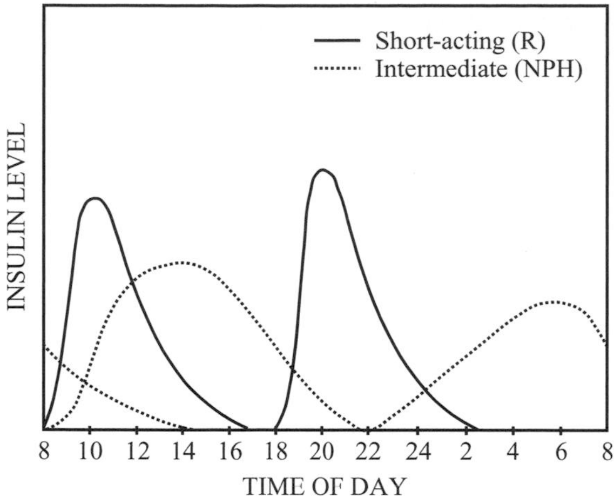

Figure 3.8 Insulin Stage 3 action curve using R/N–0–R–N

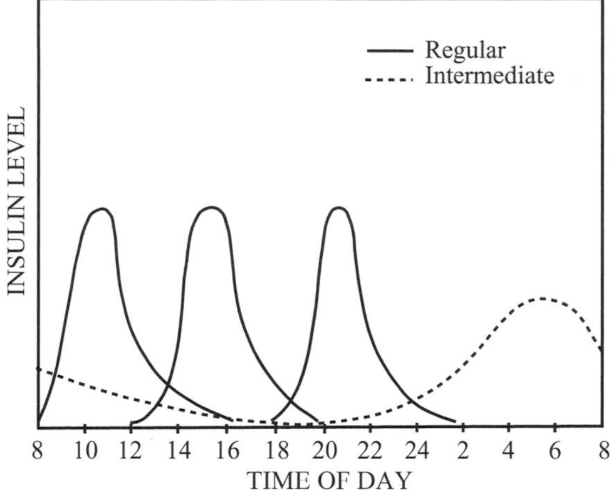

Figure 3.9 Physiologic Insulin Stage 4 action curve using R–R–R–N

RA administered before the midday meal and N given before the evening meal. SMBG should be done at least before each meal and at bedtime. Additional tests may be required if the blood glucose does not respond. Often this regimen results in improved blood glucose, but if it does not, consider replacing the morning N with midday R or RA, especially if the problem is mid-afternoon hypoglycemia.

Physiologic Insulin Stage 4
R–R–R–N or G, or RA–RA–RA–N or G

Four injections are given each day. R or RA is given before each major meal, while intermediate- (N) or long-acting glargine (G) insulin is given at least 2 hours after the evening meal. The major difference between N and G is that N will maintain glucose control overnight and before breakfast (see Figure 3.9) while G will provide basal insulin requirements for a full 24 hour period (see Figure 3.10). Physiologic Insulin Stage 4 may be initiated at diagnosis; alternatively, it may be the next step after Stage 3 has failed to adequately improve blood glucose levels. Physiologic Insulin Stage 4 has many appealing features. It closely mimics normal insulin secretion by targeting the postprandial rise in blood glucose as well as the overnight and fasting hepatic glucose output. It generally results in as much as a 20 per cent reduction in overall insulin requirements. If meals are missed, insulin need not be administered in patients with type 2 diabetes or with gestational diabetes. If unplanned events occur, the insulin dose can easily be adjusted. The negative features include the need for four injections and a greater number of SMBG tests. Weighing the two, the likelihood of improved glycemic control argues in favor of Insulin Stage 4. Because it targets each meal, patients and providers and patients can easily adjust insulin doses.

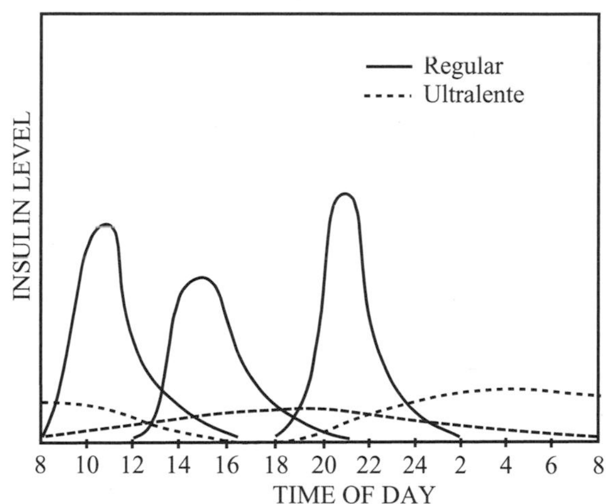

Figure 3.10 Physiologic Insulin Stage 4 action curve using RA–RA–RA–G

With added experience with glargine and other long-acting insulin analogs the timing of the single daily dose may be switched to the morning. In some cases this has been found to improve glycemic control over the single evening injection. Each case will be different. Another variant on Stage 4 is the use of RA as needed with regard to the number of injections. Similar to infusion pump therapy, the patient provides a bolus of RA based on carbohydrate intake and SMBG testing. This permits the greatest flexibility while assuring adequate insulin coverage. Carbohydrate counting and insulin administration are fully detailed in the chapters related to each type of diabetes.

Insulin infusion pump

Insulin infusion pump therapy provides continuous subcutaneous infusion of regular insulin as well as pre-meal boluses as needed. Supplied by an electronic pump approximately the size of a pager and worn externally, the device is programmed to supply adequate insulin to cover overnight and fasting insulin requirements. Prior to each meal or snacks, the patient can instruct the pump to deliver a bolus of regular insulin. Thus, the overall effect has been similar to the insulin action curve for Stage 4.

Combination therapies

Combination insulin and thiazolidinedione

When patients with type 2 diabetes are taking between 1 and 1.5 U/kg insulin per day, it is appropriate to consider either moving to more injections or adding an insulin sensitizer such as a thiazolidinedione. In type 2 diabetes one primary defect is the inadequate expression of GLUT 4, an important glucose transporter in insulin-sensitive cells. Adding a thiazolidinedione to an insulin regimen should enhance the utilization of both the endogenous and exogenous supply of insulin. Since individuals with type 1 diabetes generally are not insulin resistant in insulin-sensitive tissues, this combination therapy is not recommended.

Combination insulin and metformin

The use of metformin in combination with insulin may be beneficial. In this case metformin would suppress hepatic glucose output and improve the uptake of glucose by enhancing insulin sensitivity. Metformin is added to the current insulin stage, with increases in the dose of metformin in accordance with the adjustment guide. Lowering the insulin dose may be necessary, especially overnight insulin (both N and G), to accommodate the effect of metformin on excessive hepatic glucose output. Close SMBG with adjustments to insulin therapy when persistent hypoglycemia occurs is necessary. Follow the insulin adjustment guide for the particular stage and path of insulin therapy.

Evaluating blood glucose control

Five ways to assess glycemic control are self-monitored blood glucose (SMBG), glycosylated hemoglobin (HbA_{1c}), fructosamine assay, plasma glucose assay, and ketone monitoring.

Use of HbA_{1c} and SMBG

Use both HbA_{1c} and SMBG when undertaking intensive therapies and for verification of SMBG.

Since SDM relies on sound SMBG data, confirm the SMBG values with a periodic HbA_{1c} (quarterly). Since HbA_{1c} is a retrospective measure covering an extended time, it is generally not used in women with gestational diabetes. The exception is when diagnosis is based on casual blood glucose > 200 mg/dL (11.1 mmol/L) or when there is concern the patient has underlying type 1 or type 2 diabetes. Under such circumstance, a baseline HbA_{1c} is advisable.

Self-monitored blood glucose

SMBG is a necessary part of treatment for all types of diabetes. The typical testing pattern should have two purposes: (1) to provide data for clinical decision-making and (2) to determine the effectiveness of therapy. For clinical decision-making, SMBG detects glucose patterns to determine the most appropriate timing for food intake, pharmacologic agents, and exercise. The number of tests required varies throughout the Adjust and Maintain Phases. In general, four tests per day are the minimum when clinical decisions are being made. This may be increased during the adjust phase when treatment is being changed frequently. In the Maintain Phase the patient has reached the glucose target and requires monitoring for confirmation and for any further fine adjustments. It may be possible to reduce the number of tests during this phase if the SMBG data are corroborated by HbA_{1c} values. In all cases SMBG must have a defined purpose, and the data must be acted on. Patients will soon abandon SMBG if health care professionals ignore the results.

A general rule with SMBG is that the data should be obtained from a memory based reflectance meter. This reduces the likelihood of error in reporting the test results. SMBG should occur at the decision-making points in the day. This is generally before each meal and near bedtime (2–3 hours after the end of the evening meal). For special circumstances, such as overnight hypoglycemia, mid-afternoon hypoglycemia, and postprandial hyperglycemia, SMBG tests can be added at the appropriate times.

Table 3.4 summarizes the SMBG testing schedule for insulin based therapies. As a general rule testing should always occur prior to administration of insulin so that the correct dose can be calculated. This is a guide; SMBG may have to be individualized to uncover specific problems in each patient.

Table 3.4 SMBG testing schedule for patients treated with insulin

Insulin test time (test immediately prior to insulin administration plus . . .)	
Rapid-acting (RA)	2 hour post meal
Regular (R)	Before next meal
NPH administered AM	Before evening meal
NPH administered PM	Fasting blood glucose
Ultralente	Fasting blood glucose
Glargine (G) at bedtime	Fasting blood glucose

Frequency of SMBG testing

During the initial selection of treatment and when actively adjusting therapy, at least four SMBG tests per day are needed to evaluate treatment. If therapy is failing, more testing is needed until the underlying problem is discovered. Once the patient is in the Maintain Phase, the optimum number of tests is still four times per day. This can be reduced to fewer tests if the blood glucose remains stable for at least 1–3 months and the HbA_{1c} corroborates the SMBG values. Table 3.5 summarizes the testing frequency for each type of diabetes. This overall guide can be shared with all team members and patients as well.

If the circumstances permit reduction of SMBG, one of the following alternative patterns shown in Table 3.6 will provide sufficient data. Many other options exist, but keep in mind that the purpose is to accurately assess overall glycemic control, make decisions about current therapy, and guide selection of alternative therapies.

Table 3.5 Recommended SMBG testing frequency/day

Stage	SMBG in Adjust Phase			SMBG in Maintain Phase		
	Type 1	Type 2	Gestational	Type 1	Type 2	Gestational
MNT	na	2–4+	6–7	na	1–2	6–7
Oral agent	na	2–4+	na	na	1–2	na
Combination	na	2–4+	na	na	1–2	na
Insulin Stage 2	4+	4+	6–7	2–4	2–4	6–7
Insulin Stage 3	4+	4+	6–7	3–4	2–4	6–7
Physiologic Insulin Stage 4 and Pump	4+	4+	6–7	4	2–4	6–7

Table 3.6 Alternate SMBG schedule

3–4 times/day	Skipping every other day
1–2 times/day	Varying time of day
2 times/day	AM and evening snack
4 times/day	1 weekday, 1 weekend day

Data analysis

Numerous automated computer based programs are available for the rapid analysis of blood glucose data stored in memory based reflectance meters. Virtually all programs follow a similar format, associating each blood glucose test with the corresponding time and date. This enables the programs to use a variety of display formats to assist in the process of review and clinical decision-making. The most common formats are:

- list of each blood glucose value with corresponding date and time of test
- summary (mean and standard deviation) of all glucose values within a specified period of time
- display of glucose values in a graphic format
- identification of glucose values above and below preset targets

Each of these computer generated outputs can be saved in print form and attached to the patient's permanent record. Figure 3.11 contains a typical summary report of data collected over a 30 day period. The 26 readings (one per day) resulted in an average SMBG of 110 ± 37 mg/dL (6.1 ± 2 mmol/L). Forty-six per cent of the readings were within the target range (90 to 160 mg/dL [5 to 8.9 mmol/L]). Figure 3.12 shows a more concentrated period of 7 days, during which time 22 SMBG readings were recorded. The horizontal lines show the target range. All of the glucose data were aggregated as if they occurred on one (modal) day. Examining blood glu-

Average of Readings:	110 mg/dL (6.1 mmol/L)
Number of Readings:	26
Maximum Reading:	228 mg/dL (12.7 mmol/L)
Minimum Reading:	74 mg/dL (4.1 mmol/L)
Standard Deviation:	37 mg/dL (2.1 mmol/L)
Number of Days:	9
% Above Target Range:	15
% Within Target Range:	46
% Below Target Range:	38

Figure 3.11 SMBG meter results

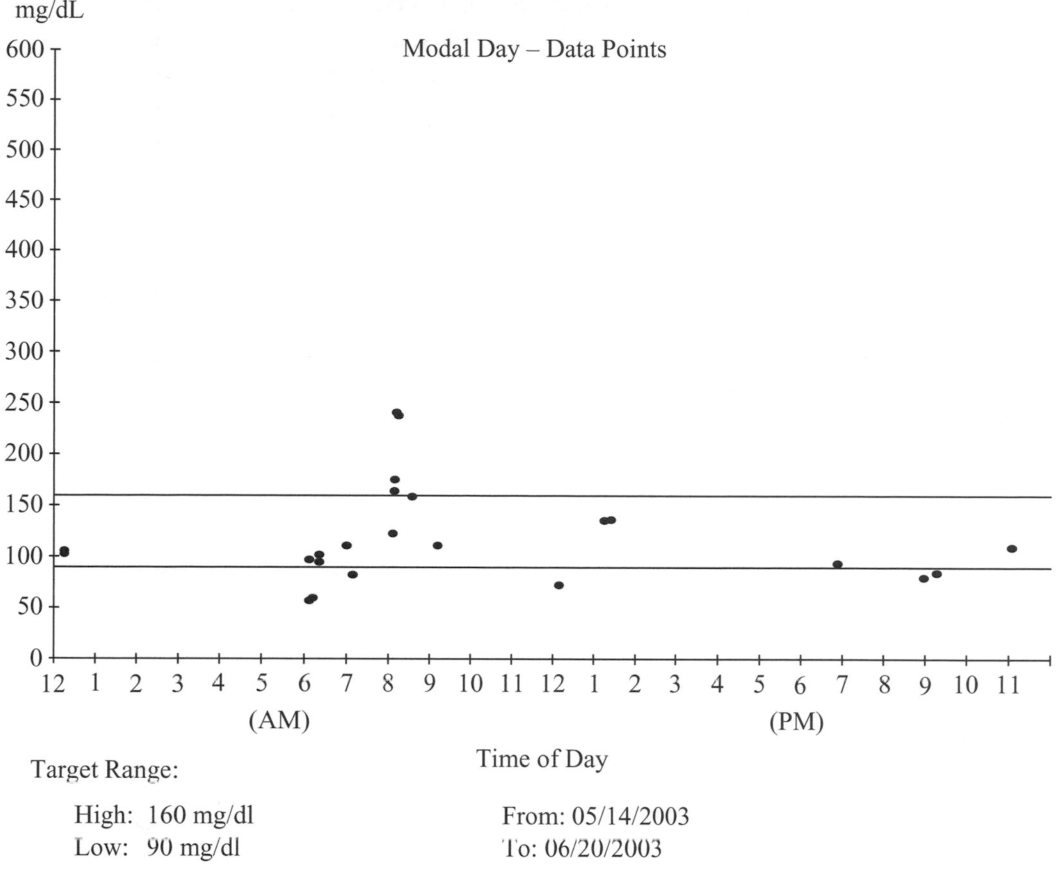

Figure 3.12 SMBG modal day

cose values from this vantage point makes it apparent that morning (6–9 am) blood glucose ranges from 50 to 250 mg/dL (2.7 to 13.9 mmol/L). This helps to identify the variability in control throughout the modal day period. Figure 3.13 illustrates 276 readings taken during 6 months collapsed into a single day. Here a clear pattern emerges, showing significant hyperglycemia between noon and 2 pm. The illustration also shows substantial variation at the same time of day over the 30 days. This plot is typical of type 1 diabetes.

SMBG and verified data

With the advent of SMBG and the use of a variety of reflectance meters, it is natural to question the accuracy and reliability of these devices versus laboratory measurements. Because SMBG is a vital part of diabetes management, SDM has addressed these issues with two major recommendations: (1) use of meters with onboard memories to verify the test value, time, and date and (2) periodic evaluation of the meter against laboratory determinations.

Once the patient understands SMBG and has used the meter for a period of time, re-evaluate the technique (see Figure 3.14). On at least an annual basis, subject the meter to accuracy testing as described in Figures 3.15 and 3.16. Note the changes for the whole-blood method in Figure 3.16.

Ambulatory glucose profiles and continuous glucose monitoring

It has long been hoped that a means of continuous glucose monitoring by non-invasive technology for SMBG would be developed. Several attempts

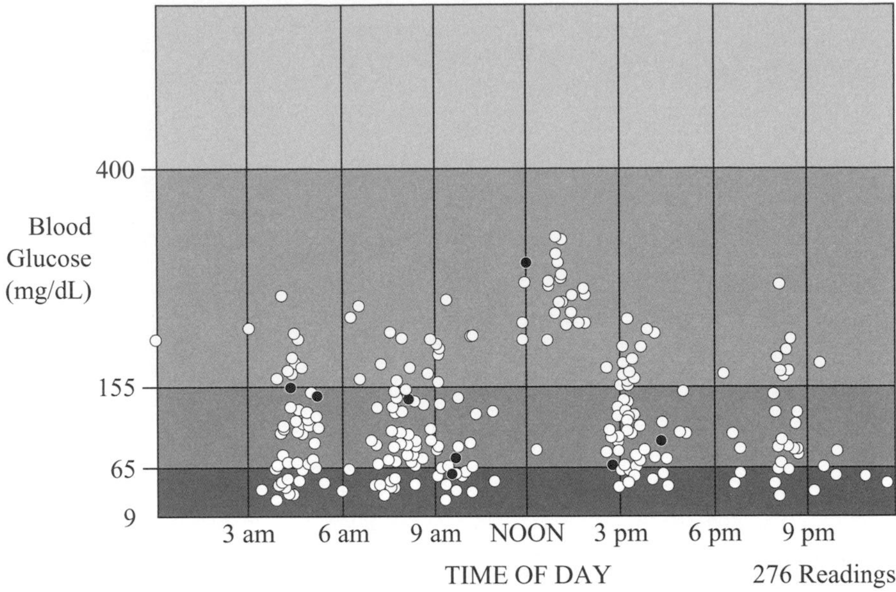

Figure 3.13 Modal day based on six-month SMBG data

using such technologies as near-infrared and mid-infrared spectroscopy of and electrochemical measurement of interstitial fluid glucose have been tried with varying success. When such technology is available, glucose data will be supplied in a much greater quantity, necessitating new ways of describing blood glucose patterns. One new and innovative approach combines the ability of the meter to store glucose data with the time and date with the computer's ability to present and analyze glucose data. The ambulatory glucose profile (AGP) collapses glucose values from several days into a single or modal day.[10] This enables the quick recognition of patterns of hyperglycemia and hypoglycemia and the effect of caloric intake and exercise, as well as overnight hepatic glucose output. Several features of the AGP are helpful in clinical decision-making. First, the AGP is typically different when type 1, type 2, and gestational diabetes are compared. Second, patterns of hypoglycemia and hyperglycemia can be readily discerned (see Figure 3.17). Third, comparisons of serial AGP can be used to measure the efficacy of different regimens.

While the use of SMBG and the production of AGPs provide an approximate representation of glucose excursions throughout the day, they do not provide the information that would be available if glucose were continuously monitored. Currently there are two general categories of continuous monitoring based on sampling technique: non-invasive and invasive. Non-invasive methods use optical scanners, which direct a beam of light through the skin surface. While most light waves are absorbed by the skin surface, waves in the near-infrared region pass through the upper layers of the skin to the deeper portion of the skin that is perfused with blood.[20] The amount of disruption in the light wave caused by varying glucose concentrations is then measured. The first systems using near-infrared spectroscopy (NIRS) were only successful at relatively high blood glucose concentrations and thus not considered clinically acceptable. However, newer, dual-beam technology is sensitive in the low and normal glucose ranges (50–115 mg/dL).[21] Such systems may be the first to provide continuous monitoring without invasive techniques.

Invasive glucose monitoring methods employ transdermal or glucose electrode technologies. The transdermal approach uses reverse iontophoresis by applying low-voltage current to the skin surface thereby causing interstitial fluid, which contains glucose, to pass through the skin.[22] Glu-

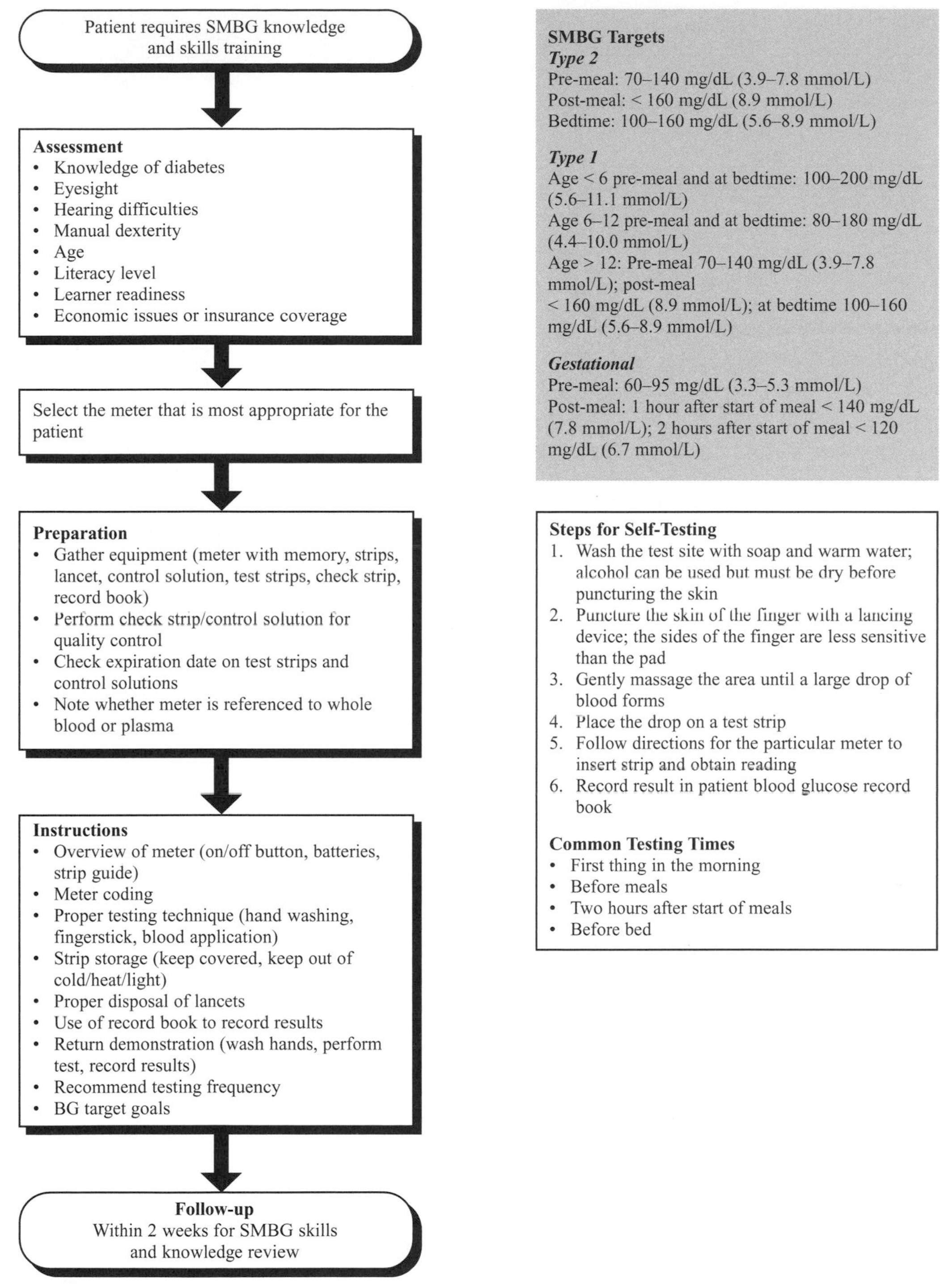

Figure 3.14 SMBG Initial Visit Education

cose in the interstitial fluid is measured by an oxidase reaction. These data are combined with information about skin temperature and sweat (which contains glucose) and factored in during the calculation process. The data are subjected to interpolation based on calibration of the patient's whole blood, which requires that the patient obtain a capillary blood sample every 12 hours.

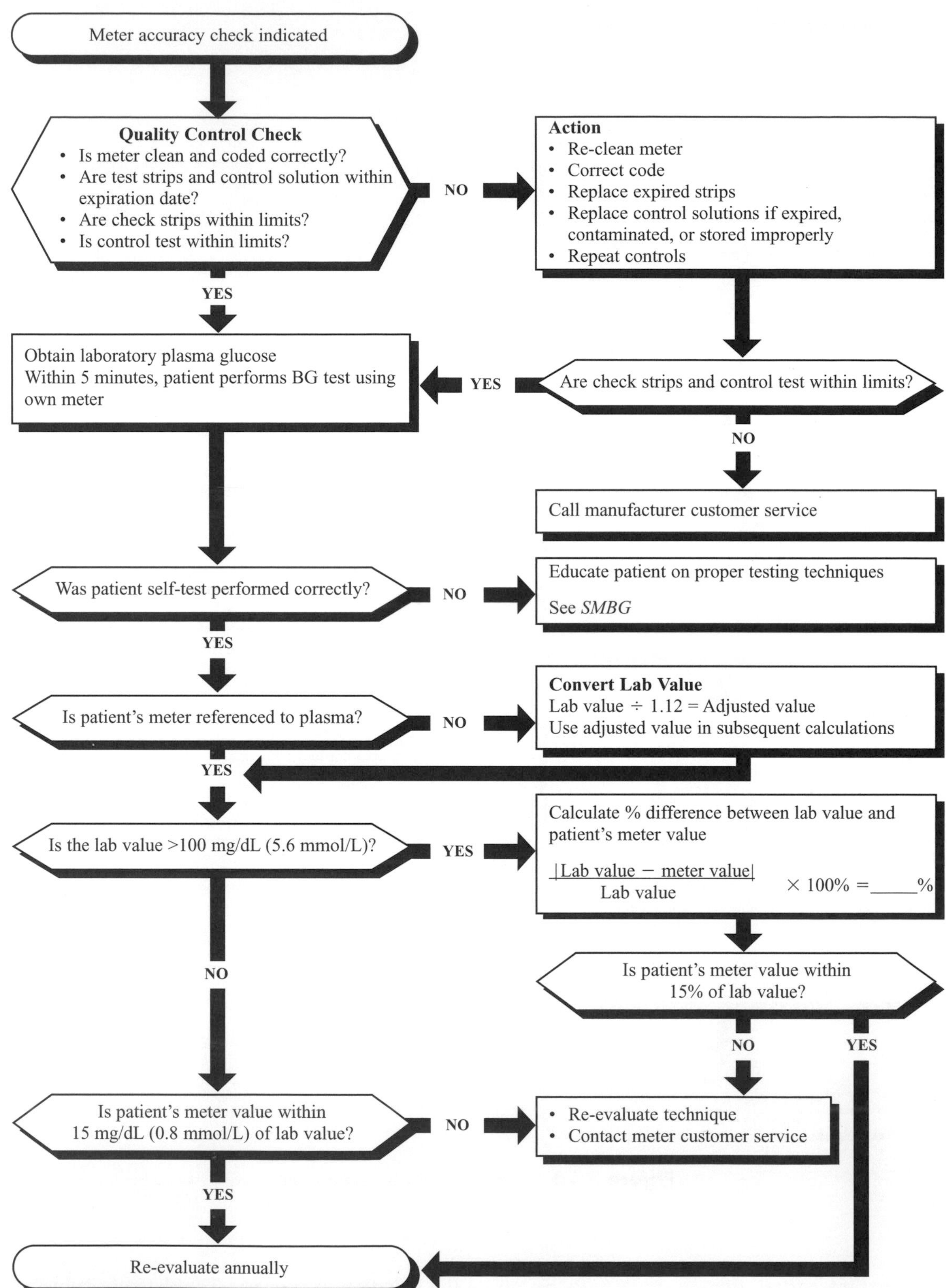

Figure 3.15 Plasma Method

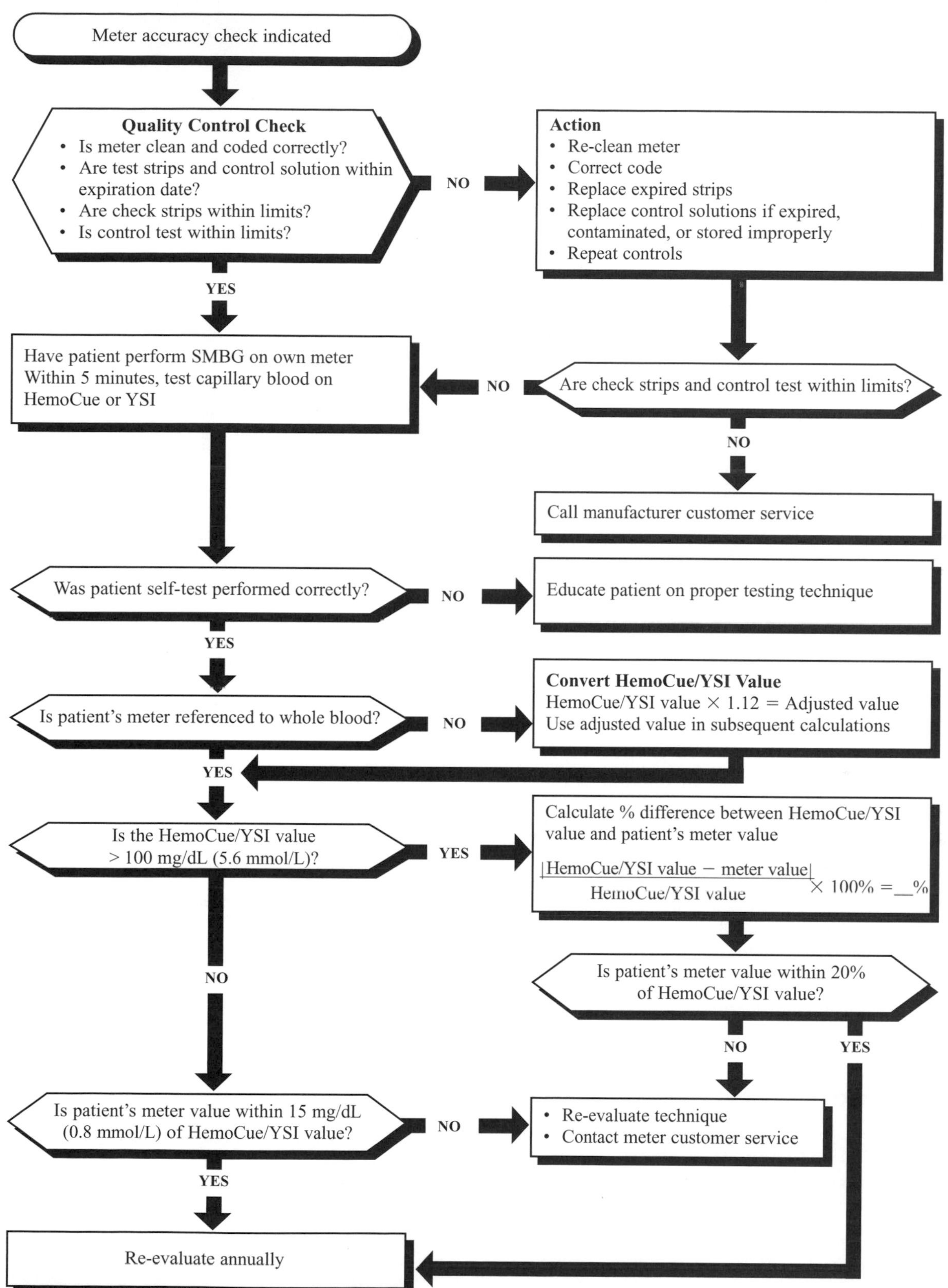

Figure 3.16 Whole Blood Method

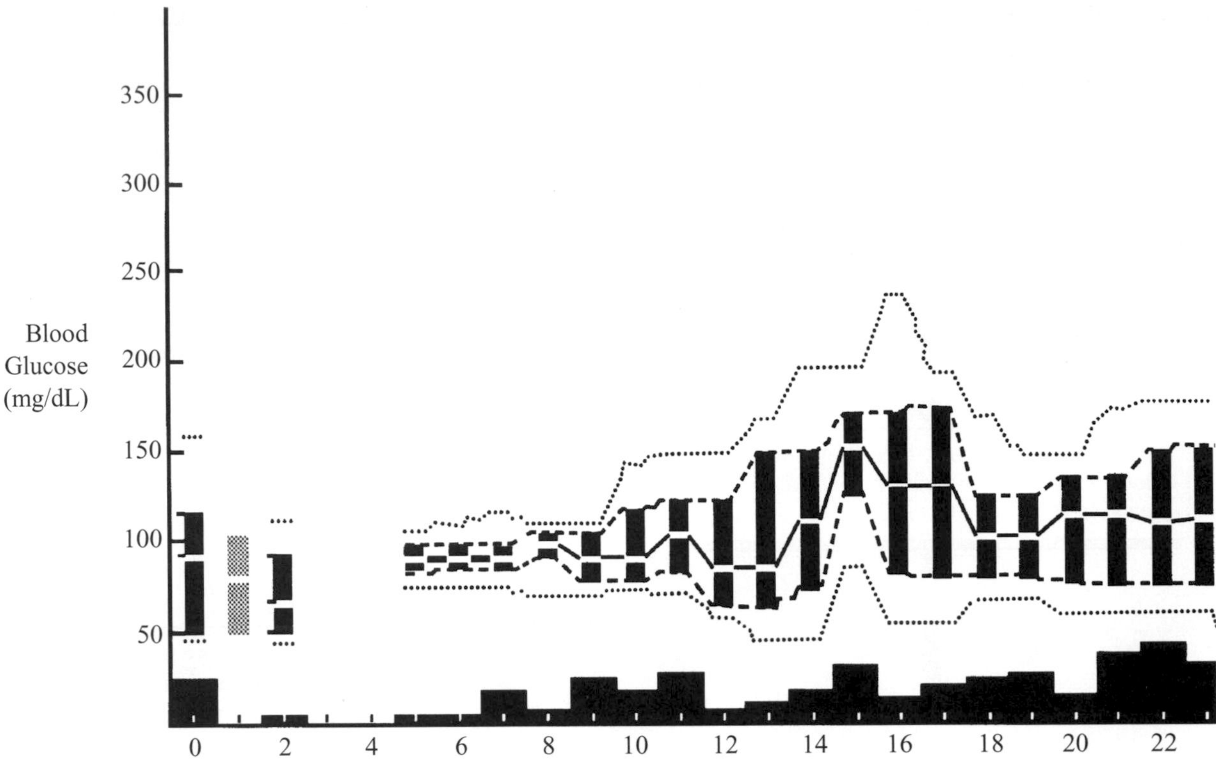

Figure 3.17 Ambulatory Glucose Profile (AGP)

The glucose electrode method differs substantially from transdermal approach. Far more invasive, a thin sensor is inserted into the abdomin, where it measures glucose in interstitial fluid by glucose oxidase reaction every 10 seconds.[23] Glucose data are transmitted to an external monitor (the size of a pager) worn by the patient near the sensor. Like the transdermal method, it requires conventional capillary blood samples obtained by reflectance meters (four times each day) for calibration. The final values are averaged every five minutes and stored in the device.

Glycosylated hemoglobin

Glycosylated hemoglobin, or HbA_{1c}, is used in clinical decision making to corroborate the metabolic control reflected in SMBG values. HbA_{1c} is a relative measure reflecting the average blood glucose level for the previous 8–10 weeks. It should change in the same direction as SMBG values. Correlation between SMBG and HbA_{1c} values is shown in Figure 3.18. Unsuspected

If HbA_{1c} is:	HbA_{1c}*	Average SMBG is:
1 percentage point above normal	7%	~150 mg/dL (8.3 mmol/L)
2 percentage points above normal	8%	~180 mg/dL (10.0 mmol/L)
3 percentage points above normal	9%	~210 mg/dL (11.7 mmol/L)
4 percentage points above normal	10%	~245 mg/dL (13.6 mmol/L)
5 percentage points above normal	11%	~280 mg/dL (15.6 mmol/L)
6 percentage points above normal	12%	~310 mg/dL (17.2 mmol/L)
7 percentage points above normal	13%	~345 mg/dL (19.2 mmol/L)
8 percentage points above normal	14%	~380 mg/dL (21.1 mmol/L)

* assumes normal range of 4–6%
Nathan, DM, et al: *N Engl J Med* 310: 341–346, 1984

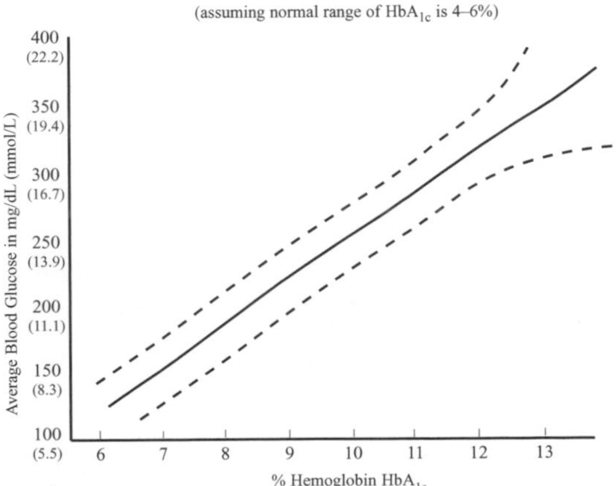

Figure 3.18 Relationship between glycosylated hemoglobin (HbA_{1c}) and blood glucose levels

hyperglycemia, such as that occurring between meals, may also be detected.

For some clinicians the use of glycosylated hemoglobin in place of SMBG has become routine practice. While it may be used to corroborate SMBG values, it should never be substituted. Importantly, specific adjustment of insulin or other therapies requires the day-to-day values provided by SMBG data. Without SMBG (i.e., using only HbA_{1c}), specific times of hyperglycemia, such as morning fasting, are not identified. HbA_{1c} measures glycosylation of hemoglobin in red blood cells that occur over their lifetime (120 days). It is believed that as blood glucose concentrations rise glycosylation increases. It is also cumulative. The older red blood cells will have accumulated more glycosylated hemoglobin, while the newly produced red blood cells will have substantially less. HbA_{1c} is interpreted as an average of all hemoglobin glycosylation. It is used to estimate control over the previous six weeks. Measuring this fraction makes it possible to estimate the overall blood glucose control of the person with diabetes. Note that some laboratories report total glycosylated hemoglobin (HbA_{1a}, HbA_{1b}, and HbA_{1c}). This equates to HbA_{1c} by measuring the difference between the upper limit of normal and the patient value. The delta or difference should be approximately the same as the difference between the upper limit of normal and the patient's value for HbA_{1c}. For clinical purposes the question is whether a particular level of blood glucose can be directly interpolated from HbA_{1c}. It can, but to a limited degree, as depicted in Figure 3.18. Note that the confidence interval (dashed line) in the graph widens as HbA_{1c} increases. When HbA_{1c} is at 12 per cent, the confidence interval reaches approximately 100 mg/dL (5.6 mmol/L). Therefore, HbA_{1c} should be considered a relative measure. As overall blood glucose control deteriorates or improves, eventually this will be reflected in the direction of change in HbA_{1c} value. Correlation between HbA_{1c} and SMBG values ranges from 0.12 to 0.50. This is due to the frequency of SMBG, which permits random and often sporadic testing. Hypothetically, if continuously monitored, the correlation between HbA_{1c} and plasma blood glucose would approach unity. Where HbA_{1c} does contribute information is when the patient is new to the office and no history of individual blood glucose values has been collected, and also in pregnancy when, again, no history of blood glucose values is available.

The second purpose of measuring HbA_{1c} and SMBG is to assess whether a therapy is achieving its goal. Too often patients are maintained on unproductive therapies. HbA_{1c} is an excellent measure of the overall efficacy of a therapy. If HbA_{1c} rises, the therapy is not working and modification or change is necessary. Similarly, if SMBG values remain high, the current therapy is failing. As a general rule, a drop of between 0.5 and 1 percentage point HbA_{1c} every month (consistent with an average decrease of from 15 to 30 mg/dL or 0.8 to 1.7 mmol/L) should be expected if the therapy is working. Thus, the goal for a patient who starts therapy with a HbA_{1c} level 6 per cent above the upper limit of normal should reach near-normal levels within 6–9 months of the onset of treatment. If the current therapy is not progressing toward this goal at an adequate pace, then moving to the next stage or therapy is appropriate.

Frequency of HbA_{1c}

Frequency of HbA_{1c} depends on the phase of therapy and the usefulness of SMBG data. At diagnosis or during the adjustment phase, obtaining an HbA_{1c} at 8 to 12 week intervals provides a measure from baseline as to the effectiveness of the therapy. If the patient cannot provide SMBG data, HbA_{1c} may need to be continued at 8 to 12 week intervals until the patient reaches the maintenance phase. If SMBG is reliable, quarterly measures of HbA_{1c} are adequate. Once in maintenance, measurement of HbA_{1c} every 3–4 months is reasonable. Optimally, HbA_{1c} results should be available before seeing the patient. Too often the SMBG data (especially if erratic) do not provide sufficient information to confirm how well the current therapy is working. If the HbA_{1c} is available before the patient is seen, these data can be compared and control can be more accurately assessed. If this is not possible, if there is a discrepancy between HbA_{1c} and SMBG, the patient should be contacted. If HbA_{1c} is not available, a fasting plasma glucose should be obtained, which provides the best alternative overall assessment (in the office) of glycemic control. This test should be compared to the SMBG results.

Fructosamine

The fructosamine assay can be used to determine the overall level of blood glucose control during the previous 2–3 weeks. This colorimetric assay measures the number of fructosamine linkages formed between glucose and serum proteins (primarily albumin). Fructosamine may be used to complement, but not replace, quarterly HbA_{1c} determinations for monitoring overall glycemic control.

Casual (random) and fasting plasma glucose

With the introduction in 1997 of new diagnostic criteria for diabetes has come a change in terminology. "Random plasma glucose" has been renamed "casual plasma glucose" to indicate that this measure is done without regard to prandial state and with fewer than 8 hours of fasting. Although generally used for diagnosing diabetes, both the casual plasma glucose (CPG) and the fasting plasma glucose (FPG) are rarely used to evaluate overall glycemic control. Once treatment is underway, in the absence of other data FPG may be used to assess the body's ability in a steady state to respond to hepatic glucose output. Thus, it reflects the least glucose stimulated state. Measured sequentially over a period of several months, the FPG should provide data that indicate whether glycemic control is improving. It does not, however, reflect the glucose challenge that occurs after each meal. In this manner it cannot be used as a replacement for SMBG or HbA_{1c}. In contrast, the CPG is a very weak measure since it reflects either a pre-prandial or post-prandial state, depending on when the last meal was taken. Therefore, the CPG should not be used alone to assess overall glycemic control. It can be used with the FPG, but would be a very inaccurate assessment.

Ketone monitoring

All patients with type 1 diabetes and women with diabetes in pregnancy should monitor their ketones regularly. Ketones are also useful in type 2 diabetes at the time of diagnosis to help differentiate between diabetes classifications. For individuals with type 1 diabetes ketones should be checked whenever there is blood glucose > 240 mg/dL (13.3 mmol/L) or an illness or infection. For gestational diabetes and type 2 diabetes in pregnancy, the purpose of monitoring ketones is to assure that the patient is not starving in order to lower blood glucose. Starving ketosis is a common problem in pregnancy complicated by hyperglycemia and should not be dismissed. These women should initially test on a daily basis until starvation can be ruled out. After confirming no ketones, testing can be reduced to one to two times per week.

References

1. Franz MJ, Monk A, Barry B, *et al*. Effectiveness of medical nutrition therapy provided by dietitians in the management of non-insulin dependent diabetes mellitus: a randomized, controlled clinical trial. *J Am Diet Assoc* 1995; **95**: 1009–1017.
2. Beck-Nielsen H, Hother-Nielsen O and Pedersen O. Mechanism of action of sulphonylureas with special reference to the extrapancreatic effect: an overview. *Diabetes Med* 1988; **5**: 613–620.
3. Bailey CJ. Biguanides and NIDDM. *Diabetes Care* 1992; **15**: 755–772.
4. Herman LS, Schersten B, Bitzen PO, Kjellstrom T, Lindgarde F and Melander A. Therapeutic comparison of metformin and sulfonylurea, alone and in

various combinations. *Diabetes Care* 1995; **17**(2): 1100–1108.

5. Fuhlendorff J, Rorsman P, Kofod H, *et al.* Stimulation of insulin release by repaglinide and glibenclamide involves both common and distinct processes. *Diabetes* 1998; **47**: 345–351.
6. Inzucchi SE, Maggs DG, Spollett GR, *et al.* Efficacy and metabolic effects of metformin and troglitazone in type 2 diabetes mellitus. *N Engl J Med* 1998; **338**(13): 908–909.
7. Coniff R and Krol A. Acarbose: a review of US clinical experience. *Clin Ther* 1997; **19**(1): 16–26.
8. Howey DC, Bowsher RR, Brunelle RL and Woodworth JR. [Lys(B28), Pro (B290]-human insulin: a rapidly absorbed analogue of human insulin. *Diabetes* 1994; **43**: 396–402.
9. DiMarchi RD, Chance RE, Long HB, Shields JE and Slieker LJ. Preparation of an insulin with improved pharmacokinetics relative to human insulin through consideration of structural homology with insulin-like growth factor I. *Horm Metab Res (Suppl. 2)* 1994; **41**: 93–6.
10. Mazze RS, Lucido D, Langer O, Hartmann K and Rodbard D. Ambulatory glucose profile: representation of verified self-monitored blood glucose data. *Diabetes Care* 1987; **10**: 111–117.
11. Moses R, Slobodniuk R, Boyager S, *et al.* Effect of repaglinide addition to metformin monotherapy on glycemic control in patients with Type 2 diabetes. *Diabetes Care* 1999; **22**: 119–124.
12. Glueck CJ, Wang P, Goldenberg N and Sieve-Smith L. Pregnancy outcomes among women with polycystic ovary syndrome treated with metformin. *Hum Reprod* 2002; **17**: 2858–2864.
13. Smith U. Pioglitazone: mechanism of action. *Int J Clin Pract* 2001; **121**: 13–18.
14. Stumvoll M and Haring HU. Glitazones: clinical effects and molecular mechanisms. *Ann Med* 2002; **34**: 217–224.
15. Inzucchi SE *et al.* Efficacy and metabolic effects of metformin and troglitazone in type 2 diabetes mellitus. *N Engl. J Med* **338**: 867–872.
16. Hallsten K, Virtanen KA, Lonnqvist F, *et al.* Rosiglitazone but not metformin enhances insulin- and exercise stimulated skeletal muscle glucose uptake in patients with newly diagnosed type 2 diabetes. *Diabetes* 2002; **51**: 3479–3485.
17. Ovalle F and Bell DS. Clinical evidence of thiazolidinedione-induced improvement in pancreatic beta-cell function in patients with types diabetes mellitus. *Diabetes Obes Metab* 2002; **4**: 56–59.
18. Iuorno MJ and Nestler JE. Insulin lowering drugs in polycystic ovary syndrome. *Obstet Gynecol Clin North Am* 2001; **28**: 153–164.
19. Home PD and Ashwell SG. An overview of insulin glargine. *Diabetes Metab Res Rev* 2002; Suppl 3: S57–S63.
20. Koschinsky T and Heinemann L. Sensors for glucose monitoring: technical and clinical aspects. *Diabetes Metab Res Rev* 2001; **17**: 113–123.
21. Gabriely I, Wozniak R, Mevorach M, *et al.* Transcutaneous glucose measurement using near infrared spectroscopy during hypoglycemia. *Diabetes Care* 1999; **22**: 2026–2032.
22. Garg SK, Potts RO, Ackerman NR, *et al.* Correlation of finger stick blood glucose measurements with Glucowatch Biographer glucose results in young subjects with type 1 diabetes. *Diab Care* 1999; **22**: 1708–1714.
23. Bode BW, Gross TM, Thorton KR, *et al.* Continuous glucose monitoring used to adjust diabetes therapy improves glycosylated hemoglobin: a pilot study. *Diab Res Clin Pract* 1999; **46**: 183–190.

PART TWO
THE TREATMENT OF DIABETES

4 Type 2 Diabetes

Statistics from the Centers for Disease Control National Center for Chronic Disease Prevention and Health Promotion report that in the year 2003 there were approximately 17.0 million Americans with diabetes.[1] The majority (~95 per cent) of these individuals have type 2 diabetes. Moreover, 5.9 million of the 17 million people have undiagnosed type 2 diabetes.[2] Aggregating both the detected and undetected cases, more than 10 per cent of the adult population currently has type 2 diabetes. Annually, as many as 800 000 new cases are detected and about half that number die with type 2 diabetes as an underlying or contributing factor. Thus the number of people with type 2 diabetes is growing by nearly 500 000 each year. If the population is segmented into high-risk groups, these proportions change significantly. Among those over the age of 65, the percent of people with diabetes doubles to 20 per cent. For those who are in high-risk racial or ethnic groups, the numbers can be up to fivefold greater. Even among children and adolescents the incidence and prevalence of type 2 diabetes is rising. This phenomenon is worldwide. It has been estimated that 300 million people will have diabetes by the year 2025.

Whether in the United States or elsewhere the common factors associated with this substantial increase in the number of people with diabetes are: (1) better surveillance; (2) aging population; (3) increased prevalence of obesity in children and adults; (4) poor nutrition; and (5) reduction in activity.

Etiology

In simplest terms, type 2 diabetes is both a genetically and environmentally mediated disease characterized by a combination of insulin resistance in peripheral tissues (muscle, liver, and adipose) coupled with relative insulin deficiency. It is unclear which factor occurs first, insulin resistance or insulin deficiency. In most cases individuals with type 2 diabetes have both conditions in varying degrees, perhaps reflecting the multifactorial nature of the pathogenesis of the disease. It is important to note that both insulin resistance and insulin deficiency are progressive in nature. Staged Diabetes Management relies on at least a basic understanding of the biochemical and molecular derangements leading to insulin resistance and relative insulin deficiency in order to make informed clinical decisions regarding the prevention and treatment of the disease. This is especially true with the dramatic proliferation in therapeutic options for managing type 2 diabetes

Staged Diabetes Management: A Systematic Approach (2nd Edition) R. S. Mazze, E. S. Strock, G. D. Simonson and R. M. Bergenstal
 ISBN: 0 470 86576 8

mellitus, targeting insulin resistance (thiazolidinediones, biguanides) and insulin deficiency (sulfonylureas, meglitinides, insulin, and insulin analogs).

Deficiency in β-cell function

Individuals destined to develop type 2 diabetes may have two defects related to insulin secretion. First, they may fail to secrete adequate insulin at the start of a meal. This first-phase insulin is needed to overcome the initial glucose challenge of a meal and to signal the liver to reduce its production of endogenous glucose. After some (unknown) duration of disease, the β-cells are unable to adequately respond to the post-prandial rise in glucose. The defects in the biphasic β-cell response eventually contribute to a net decrease in available insulin. This defect in insulin secretion appears to be found in normoglycemic relatives of individuals with type 2 diabetes, suggesting that reduced production of insulin may be an early defect in the progression to type 2 diabetes.

In the years prior to and early in the progression of type 2 diabetes, individuals are often hyperinsulinemic due to the β-cell response to increasing insulin resistance in peripheral tissues. Interestingly, individuals may be both hyperinsulinemic and hyperglycemic at the same time because there is a *relative insulin deficiency* that develops. That is, the hyperinsulinemia may not be sufficient to overcome insulin resistance, altering glucose metabolism to the point where hyperglycemia develops. Moreover, early during this hyperinsulinemic state there appears to be β-cell dysfunction manifested as diminished first-phase insulin secretion and reduced response to glucose challenges. With time the natural history of diabetes dictates that β-cell dysfunction continues to worsen, resulting in even further declines in insulin secretion. A vicious cycle develops as glucose levels rise in the blood stream, creating a glucose toxic environment, further weakening the β-cell and allowing glucose levels to rise higher.

Why the β-cell dysfunction? While this remains an area of intense scientific research, it appears that many factors combine to cause β-cell dysfunction. These include:

- alterations in β-cell sensitivity to insulin secretagogues
- glucose toxicity
- lipid deposition in the β-cell (lipotoxicity)
- increased demands of insulin secretion due to insulin resistance

Insulin deficiency may occur relatively early in the natural history of type 2 diabetes in certain populations. It has been suggested that if the traditional diet of a population were relatively low in carbohydrates, then the average amount of insulin produced by individuals in this population would be low relative to populations accustomed to diets high in carbohydrate. It has been reported that such individuals generally produce less insulin than weight matched populations accustomed to high-carbohydrate diets. Thus, the change to a Western style diet for Asian-Americans might explain the significant increase in the incidence of type 2 diabetes in this population. Their insulin deficiency makes them unable to produce adequate amounts of insulin to maintain normal blood glucose levels. Such individuals are not to be confused with other groups who also have experienced a significant alteration in diet. It has been postulated that certain ethnic groups, including American Indians and Polynesians, have a genetic predisposition for survival which favors the storage of energy (fat) when food is plentiful coupled with conservation of energy stores during times of famine. As access to consistent food supplies becomes possible, the very same "thrifty genes" that were advantageous during cycles of feast and famine become deleterious when food is always plentiful, as they tend to gain weight and become severely insulin resistant.

Insulin resistance

Research is emerging on the molecular mechanisms of insulin resistance leading to type 2 diabetes, but the entire picture is far from complete. One thing is clear, the development of insulin resistance in peripheral tissues is multifactorial and is not caused by a single defect; rather, a combination of defects in several signaling pathways leading to reduced insulin mediated glucose uptake. The following section briefly highlights the current understanding of this complex and multifaceted metabolic disorder.

Insulin resistance appears to start at the level of the insulin receptor. These receptors are located on the surface insulin sensitive cells and set off a cascade of events leading to glucose uptake and metabolism. The first step in this cascade is the activation of the receptor via the autophosphorylation of key tyrosine residues. The activated receptor contains intrinsic tyrosine kinase activity, resulting in the phosphorylation of key signaling proteins called insulin receptor substrates (IRS-1, IRS-2, and IRS-3). Insulin resistance at the receptor level is thought to occur primarily by the inhibition of receptor tyrosine kinase activity[3] and secondarily to a minor reduction in the number of insulin receptor in individuals with type 2 diabetes.[4] Stimulation of phosphotyrosine phosphatase (PTPase), an enzyme that inactivates the insulin receptor by cleavage of the phosphate groups from phosphotyrosine residues, has been shown to result in increased insulin resistance.[5]

Relationship between obesity and insulin resistance

A positive correlation between excess weight gain (obesity) and insulin resistance has been established for decades, but the precise cause and effect relationship has yet to be clearly delineated. One of the mysteries to unravel is how increased storage of triglyceride (fat) in adipose tissue can result in insulin resistance in muscle and liver tissue. One explanation is the rise in free fatty acid (FFA) levels associated with obesity. Obese individuals tend to have elevated FFA levels due to suppressed lipogenesis and increased lipolysis coupled with a diet high in fat. Elevated FFA levels have been shown to decrease insulin mediated glucose uptake in skeletal muscle,[6] and increase hepatic glucose output,[7] resulting in hyperglycemia. Thus, obesity related increases in FFA level provide a direct linkage between fat deposition excess (weight gain) and insulin resistance in other insulin-sensitive tissues.

Another intriguing connection between obesity and insulin resistance has been the identification of tumor necrosis factor α (TNFα). This cytokine is secreted from adipose tissue and skeletal muscle and has been shown to have a multitude of effects including induction of tumor cell lysis, modulation of lipid metabolism, and septic shock. TNFα has been implicated in causing insulin resistance and type 2 diabetes.[8] Data supporting this are quite compelling. For example, TNFα levels have been shown to positively correlate with body mass index (BMI) in individuals with type 2 diabetes[9] and to impair insulin stimulated glucose uptake in muscle.[10] The mechanism of action is thought to occur by a TNFα induced reduction in insulin receptor mediated phosphotyrosine kinase activity and direct inactivation of IRS-1. TNFα is not the only factor that contributes to obesity related insulin resistance. Additional research is needed to fully understand insulin resistance in peripheral tissues.

Influence of body fat distribution on insulin resistance

The influence of body fat distribution plays a critical role in the development of insulin resistance. For example, individuals with central or truncal fat distribution (waist to hip circumference ratio > 1) have higher levels of insulin resistance compared to those with lower body fat distribution in the gluteofemoral region.[11] The classic morphological categorizations of "apple" versus "pear" shape are easy to distinguish clinically and provide a basis for identification those patients with highest levels of insulin resistance.

Why does fat stored at one location in the body differ from others in contributing towards insulin resistance? Current research has demonstrated that the answer is linked to differences in metabolic activity of the various fat stores. Central or truncal fat stores are more metabolically active than lower body fat stores. Metabolically active means that the fat tissue can effectively store triglyceride by the action of lipoprotein lipase and quickly break down triglyceride by the action of lipases, releasing free fatty acids into the bloodstream. It is the flux of free fatty acids into the bloodstream that is thought to lead to increased insulin resistance in the liver and skeletal muscle.

Insulin has a direct and indirect effect on hepatic glucose production. High levels of circulating insulin normally act to suppress hepatic glucose output, inhibit lipolysis, and regulate central nervous system control of hepatic glucose production and appetite. In persons with insulin resistance, these high levels of circulating insulin appear to be ignored by the liver, fat cells, and CNS, resulting in excessive hepatic glucose output in the presence of both hyperglycemia and hyperinsulinemia.

Pre-diabetes

Figure 4.1 shows the three variables that depict the natural history of undiagnosed or poorly treated type 2 diabetes. By understanding the natural history, it is possible to find clues as to the underlying defects that contribute to hyperglycemia. Before the onset of overt type 2 diabetes, blood glucose levels rise above the normal range, resulting in a state of impaired glucose homeostasis (pre-diabetes). Impaired glucose homeostasis includes two categories, impaired fasting glucose (IFG) and impaired glucose tolerance (IGT).

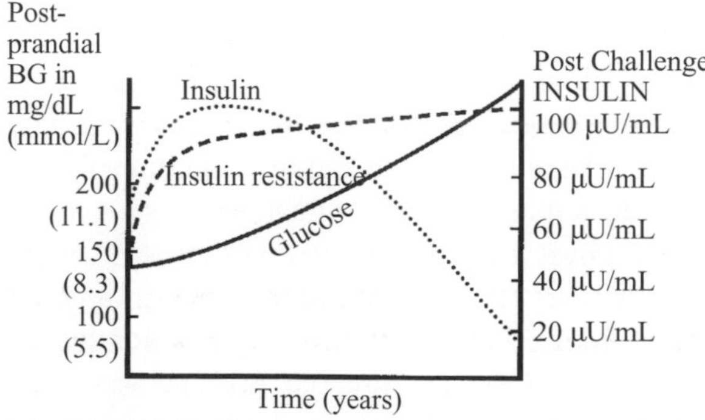

Figure 4.1 The natural history and underlying defects of type 2 diabetes

Diagnosis of IFG is made if the fasting plasma glucose is between 100 and 125 mg/dL (5.6 and 6.9 mmol/L) and diagnosis of IGT is made if the 75 g oral glucose tolerance test two hour value is between 140 and 199 mg/dL (7.8 and 11 mmol/L).

As previously mentioned, individuals with either pre-diabetes or type 2 diabetes often have elevated plasma insulin levels (hyperinsulinemia). Pancreatic β-cells attempt to maintain normal insulin production in response to increasing insulin resistance by synthesizing and secreting insulin in an attempt to maintain euglycemia. This can be indirectly measured by determining the amount of insulin in the blood using an insulin radioimmunoassay (RIA). As the patient moves from pre-diabetes to diabetes, first phase insulin secretion, characterized by a sudden burst of insulin released in response to a post-prandial rise in blood glucose, is gradually lost. The β-cells are not able to sustain the demands of synthesis and secretion of insulin and, over the course of years, gradually lose the ability to secrete adequate amounts of insulin. This decline in β-cell function is called β-cell exhaustion. One factor implicated in causing β-cell exhaustion is glucose toxicity resulting from persistent hyperglycemia.[12] The length of time from excessive insulin production to the exhaustion of pancreatic cells is related in part to the persistence and level of hyperglycemia. This process generally occurs over several years and is modulated by such factors as diet, activity, and weight gain. Eventually, if near-normal glycemia is not restored, it is possible for the patient to reach a state in which insulin production is so compromised (insulin deficiency) as to limit the only viable therapeutic option to exogenous insulin.

Confounding these factors is that some individuals with type 2 diabetes produce excessive hepatic glucose. One of insulin's functions is to suppress hepatic glucose production and increase the formation of glycogen during the fed state. Hepatic insulin resistance (characterized by the inability of basal levels of insulin found during the fasting state to adequately suppress the formation of excess glucose by the liver via the process of gluconeogenesis) results in elevated fasting blood glucose levels.

Throughout, the progression toward diabetes is a concomitant process linked to increasing insulin resistance. Known as part of the metabolic syndrome, it was previously called Reaven's syndrome, syndrome X, dysmetabolic syndrome, and insulin resistance syndrome. Thought to be the effect of both cellular and vascular insulin resistance, it is characterized by obesity, hypertension, dyslipidemia, and renal disease (see Chapter 7 for a complete discussion).[5]

No method to predict the onset of impaired glucose homeostasis or subsequent type 2 diabetes currently exists. These events are compounded by genetic predisposition to insulin resistance and obesity along with environmental factors such as diet composition and activity levels. Because the genetic component is so important, certain ethnic and racial groups are at higher risk for developing type 2 diabetes. Table 4.1 shows the approximate risk of developing type 2 diabetes in different populations.

Table 4.1 Approximate risk of developing type 2 diabetes

Factor	Risk Range
Age > 65 years old	15–25%
American Indian	30–50%
Hispanic	20–30%
African-American	15–20%
Asian	10–12%
Caucasian	5–8%
Previous gestational diabetes	20–80%

Overview of treatment options for type 2 diabetes

There are five regimens currently available for treating type 2 diabetes:

1. medical nutrition therapy
2. oral agent monotherapy
3. combination of different classes of oral agents
4. combination of oral agent(s) and insulin
5. insulin

All pharmacologic therapies are supplemented by appropriate medical nutrition therapy.

The need for appropriate medical nutrition therapy and exercise/activity has long been recognized as a cornerstone in the treatment of type 2 diabetes. An appropriate food plan helps to achieve glycemic targets, promote appropriate lipid levels, control blood pressure, and maintain reasonable weight while meeting the nutritional needs of the individual. In conjunction with exercise, medical nutrition therapy aims at improved glycemic control through modifications in daily carbohydrate intake and total number of calories. As a consequence of reducing caloric intake, some modest weight reduction is expected. Studies have shown that even modest weight loss can dramatically improve glycemic control due to an increase in insulin sensitivity, thus reducing insulin resistance, which results in improved glucose utilization.[6] If an increase in exercise/activity is included, glucose disposal is enhanced in the muscle in order to meet the enlarged energy demands. The combined effect results in reduced insulin resistance, lower plasma insulin levels, and improved glycemic control. When medical nutrition therapy fails to improve glycemic control or when blood glucose levels are moderately high at diagnosis (fasting plasma glucose 200–300 mg/dL (11.1–16.6 mmol/L), an oral agent combined with medical nutrition therapy is required.

The five classes of oral agents can be divided into hypoglycemic agents, which include sulfonylureas (first, second, and third generation) and meglitinides, both of which are considered secretagogues. The meglitinide family of compounds, like sulfonylureas, stimulate insulin secretion from β-cells in response to a glucose challenge. The non-hypoglycemic agents include biguanides, alpha-glucosidase inhibitors, and thiazolidinediones. Both the hypoglycemic and non-hypoglycemic drugs are described in detail in Chapter 3.

The most commonly used oral agents are the sulfonylureas and biguanides. Recently these two drugs were combined in one compound, making it possible to treat both the insulin resistance and insulin deficiency associated with type 2 diabetes with one agent. Of the remaining oral agents, alpha-glucosidase inhibitors work by inhibiting glucosidase enzymes in the small intestine that are responsible for the break down of carbohydrate into monosaccharide. This principally targets post-prandial blood glucose levels. Thiazolidinediones act as insulin sensitizers by reducing insulin resistance at the cellular level. The oral agents described above work in conjunction with an appropriate food and exercise/activity plan.

If medical nutrition therapy and exercise interventions plus oral agent monotherapy are inadequate in their ability to achieve target blood glucose levels (fasting plasma glucose of between 80 and 140 mg/dL or 4.4 and 7.7 mmol/L), a combination of oral agents or combination oral agent and insulin may be used. If these fail to restore normal blood glucose levels, or if blood glucose levels are beyond the effective range of oral agents, insulin alone may be indicated.

In insulin based therapies, a food plan helps by reducing or maintaining weight (improving insulin sensitivity) and assures that there is an appropriate amount of carbohydrate at each meal to prevent hypoglycemia and hyperglycemia. Exogenous insulin therapies work by augmenting the individual's own endogenous production of insulin. Since current therapy relies on short-, intermediate-, and long-acting insulin, meals, snacks, and exercise/activity must be synchronized with the pharmacokinetics of insulin action. Exogenous insulin in its two short-acting forms, regular and rapid-acting, is used to cover post-meal rises in blood glucose or to correct currently elevated glucose levels. Intermediate-acting NPH or long-acting ultralente and glargine insulins provide basal insulin requirements. Because of variation in action patterns, hypoglycemia may occur if too much insulin is administered, insufficient carbohydrate is ingested, or the timing of meals, insulin, and exercise is not synchronized. Referral for medical nutrition therapy is highly recommended when initiating insulin therapy.

The impact of the DCCT, UKPDS, and other major studies

The Diabetes Control and Complications Trial (DCCT) in 1993 was the first major study to demonstrate that tight glycemic control prevents the microvascular complications of type 1 diabetes.[17] Subsequent smaller studies in type 2 diabetes confirmed the importance of overall metabolic control in preventing, or slowing the progression of microvascular and macrovascular disease.[14–17] It was however, not until 1998 with the completion of the United Kingdom Prospective Diabetes Study (UKPDS) that there was a significant change in the management of type 2 diabetes. Results of the 20 year UKPDS demonstrated that poor metabolic control adds to the risk of both microvascular and cardiovascular disease.[18,19] The epidemiologic data from the UKPDS showed that for each percentage point decrease in HbA_{1c}, there was a 23 per cent reduction in the risk of retinopathy and a marginal reduction in risk of myocardial infarction. More importantly, the study confirmed two previous observations: (1) maintenance of near-normal blood glucose for an extended time will require multi-drug therapies often leading to reliance on insulin, and (2) attention to intensive blood pressure control provides an added benefit in terms of cardiovascular risk reduction. Since its publication, numerous studies have confirmed and expanded the UKPDS findings. Type 2 diabetes appears to be part of a larger syndrome with consequences for almost every major organ system. Attention to each of the associated diseases is more urgent than previously thought. This has consequences for both the early detection and intensive treatment of those at risk for and with type 2 diabetes. Type 2 diabetes is often detected

7–10 years after it actually develops.[20] This explains why so many individuals with type 2 diabetes present at diagnosis with associated comorbidities, such as retinopathy, nephropathy, neuropathy, hypertension, and/or dyslipidemia. Under such circumstances, the issue of glycemic control for those diagnosed late may seem less important than in type 1 diabetes.

One question often put forward is: why treat hyperglycemia vigorously if the microvascular and macrovascular complications have already developed? The findings from the UKPDS suggest that reduction in HbA_{1c} may also reduce the risk of progression of microvascular disease.[19,21,22] This has led to an overriding question: what means should be used to improve glycemic control in type 2 diabetes. Few would argue that if medical nutrition therapy were selected as the solo therapy and successfully reduced blood glucose, this regimen would be beneficial at very low risk. On the other hand, some would argue that reliance on oral agents and/or insulin may present a greater risk of adverse events, such as hypoglycemia, weight gain, liver damage, and lactic acidosis. Such risks, some argue, outweigh the benefits of reduced microvascular and macrovascular disease.

Because of the overwhelming evidence supporting the benefits of tight glycemic control in type 2 diabetes, the principle followed in Staged Diabetes Management is to optimize glycemic control without relying on pharmacologic agents when possible, but to use oral agents and/or insulin when blood glucose levels at diagnosis are greater than 200 mg/dL (11.1 mmol/L) fasting or 250 mg/dL (13.9 mmol/L) casual or when medical nutrition therapy alone fails to reach the target blood glucose goals. This is founded on our current understanding of the natural history of type 2 diabetes and the therapeutic benefits of each of the treatment modalities.

Prevention of type 2 diabetes

Can type 2 diabetes be prevented? The previous discussion suggested several pathways to the development of type 2 diabetes. The concept of genetic predisposition to type 2 diabetes has received significant attention. Supporting this theory is the high prevalence of type 2 diabetes among such genetically homogeneous populations as American Indians, Samoans, and Hispanics. Additional evidence comes from the high concordance rate for type 2 diabetes among identical twins. For these groups it has been hypothesized that their high prevalence is due to "thrifty genes."[23] The idea of a thrifty gene that favors storing energy over expending energy is supported by a high preponderance of obesity in these high-prevalence groups. This suggests not only a genetic, but also a morphologic explanation linking hyperglycemia to obesity through insulin resistance.

A genetic explanation of type 2 diabetes is by the high prevalence of early type 2 diabetes among women with previous gestational diabetes. Is it possible to prevent type 2 diabetes in these women, or are they inevitably likely to develop this disease due to a genetic predisposition? Recent evidence suggests that the increased risk of developing type 2 diabetes in women with GDM may be an artifact. These women may already have type 2 diabetes which, went undiscovered until their pregnancy. GDM, may indeed be an early sign of type 2 diabetes. Supporting this view are two factors: (1) the high incidence of subsequent type 2 diabetes; and (2) an increasing reliance on pharmacological interventions to control blood glucose in pregnancy. Contradicting this view is the wide variation (20 to 80 per cent) in the incidence of subsequent type 2 diabetes. In fact, the risk is altered if there is no family history of diabetes, the pregnancy was uncomplicated by obesity, and where there are no subsequent pregnancies.

Do genetic, morphologic, and physiologic factors combine to cause type 2 diabetes, or do they act independently? Evidence supports all three positions. Most likely, the risk of type 2 diabetes will be highest among women who have a family history of type 2 diabetes, are significantly obese, and have experienced gestational diabetes. In contrast, the lowest risk would be in lean Caucasian males with no family history of diabetes. The need to clarify the impact of these three factors is based on the question as to what could be done to prevent the inevitability of developing type 2 diabetes. For example, if genetic factors were the key, then insulin-sensitizing agents would be beneficial well in advance of overt hyperglycemia. If, on the other hand, obesity were the principal factor, medical nutrition therapy as well as increased exercise/activity would be beneficial to prevent type 2 diabetes. If, however, pancreatic β-cell exhaustion is the root cause, early use of insulin combined with drugs that block rapid absorption of carbohydrates may be the solution. If a combination of factors leads to diabetes, perhaps prevention will require a combination of interventions. This has been demonstrated in a series of studies completed in Europe and the United States. Collectively they support the notion that a careful assessment of risk factors, interventions in lifestyle that may modify these factors, and ultimately consideration of pharmacologic agents may be the best means of preventing the onset of type 2 diabetes. The US multi-center Diabetes Prevention Program (DPP) and The Finnish Diabetes Prevention Study have shown that intensive interventions aimed at significant changes in life style (reduction in caloric intake and increased consistent activity) lower weight, which, in turn, reduces the risk of developing overt type 2 diabetes.[24,25] In the presence of such data it is necessary to – at the very least – promote appropriate nutrition and activity level combined with very close surveillance so that those at the highest risk (impaired glucose homeostasis) could be offered treatment. When these intensive steps fail to arrest the deterioration in glycemic control, then non-hypoglycemic pharmacological agents, such as metformin and thiazolidinediones, might be used. In the DPP, metformin was able to reduce the incidence of type 2 diabetes by 31 per cent compared with placebo. The reduction in risk was even more dramatic in obese patients with body mass index greater than 35 kg/m^2.

Note: Before continuing, it might be helpful to review the structure of Staged Diabetes Management for type 2 diabetes. The SDM DecisionPaths and Practice Guidelines present the stages and phases of diabetes diagnosis and treatment. Phases refer to three specific periods in diabetes management – start treatment (diagnosis and initial therapy), adjust treatment (modifying therapy in order to achieve glycemic targets), and maintain treatment (reaching the therapeutic goal). Stages are the treatment options. This information should be shared with the patient and family members.

Type 2 diabetes detection and treatment

(The following guidelines are for non-pregnancy. Type 2 diabetes complicated by pregnancy is discussed in Chapter 6.)

This discussion provides the basis for screening, diagnosis, and treatment of type 2 diabetes. It begins with the Type 2 Diabetes Practice Guidelines, followed by the Master DecisionPath. The latter lays out an orderly sequence of therapeutic stages shown to improve glycemic control. Specific DecisionPaths for each stage (treatment options) as well as Diabetes Management Assessment DecisionPaths (medical visit, education, nutrition, adherence assessment) along with a complete description of each item and the rationale for decisions are also presented.

As this section is reviewed, note the following:

- Diagnosis of diabetes should be documented in the chart and meet criteria set by the American Diabetes Association or other similar national organizations and the World Health Organization.[20]

- All individuals with diabetes should be treated with medical nutrition therapy, either as a primary therapy or in combination with pharmacologic agents.

- At diagnosis, oral agents need careful consideration since some factors such as underlying liver and kidney disease, pregnancy, and age may preclude the use of some or all of these agents.
- If oral agent therapy fails to improve and eventually restore glycemia to within target goals, combinations of oral agents from different classifications, or combination oral agent–insulin regimens, may be required.
- Combination therapies using insulin sensitizers may be initiated as either a transition to insulin (oral agent and insulin) or after insulin doses reach 0.7 U/kg.
- Severe hyperglycemia (BG > 300 mg/dL or 16.9 mmol/L) requires immediate initiation of insulin therapy.
- Reversing direction in the Master DecisionPath is possible. Patients started on insulin can, with appropriate lifestyle modifications, stop insulin and start oral agent therapy or medical nutrition therapy alone to control blood glucose levels.
- Diabetes should be treated from a multidisciplinary approach. The Diabetes Management Assessment DecisionPaths review the practices of dietitians, nurse educators, and psychologists.
- Type 2 diabetes is part of metabolic syndrome; such patients are at high risk for hypertension, dyslipidemia, and renal disease and as such should therefore be carefully evaluated and closely monitored thereafter.

Type 2 Diabetes Practice Guidelines

Type 2 Diabetes Practice Guidelines are divided into seven sections: screening, diagnosis, treatment options, targets, monitoring, follow-up, and complications surveillance (see Figure 4.2).

Screening

Identifying the person with type 2 diabetes begins with surveillance for risk factors.

Symptoms

Many patients present with no symptoms of type 2 diabetes. This may be because the symptoms themselves are subtle or because the patient has become used to the symptoms over several years and does not associate them with any particular illness. Frequently, fatigue, urinary tract infections, yeast infections, skin irritations, and other vague complaints accompany type 2 diabetes. As glucose control deteriorates, blurred vision and mild neuropathy may be reported. When hyperglycemia is severe, some patients develop the classical symptoms of diabetes: weight loss, dehydration, polyuria, polyphagia, and polydipsia. Unfortunately, many of these symptoms are often attributed to aging and not necessarily to diabetes.

Urine ketones

Type 2 diabetes is generally distinguished by the absence of ketonuria. On rare occasions when patients are under stress (sepsis or myocardial infarction), accompanied by high blood glucose levels or during periods of starvation or with high protein/fast diets, ketones may be detected.

Medical Emergencies

Some patients with undetected cases of type 2 diabetes may present in coma due to extremely high levels of blood glucose. Although very rare,

Screening	Screen all patients every 3 years starting at age 45; if risk factors present, start earlier and screen annually
Risk Factors	• BMI > 25 kg/m² (especially waist-to-hip ratio > 1) • Family history of type 2 diabetes (especially first-degree relatives) • Age (risk increases with age) • Hypertension (⩾ 140/90 mm Hg) • Dyslipidemia (HDL ⩽ 35 mg/dL [0.90 mmol/L] and/or triglyceride ⩾ 250 mg/dL [2.8 mmol/L]) • Previous impaired fasting glucose (IFG) with fasting plasma glucose 100–125 mg/dL (5.6–6.9 mmol/L) • Previous impaired glucose tolerance (IGT) with oral glucose tolerance test (OGTT) 2 hour glucose value 140–199 mg/dL (7.8–11 mmol/L) • Previous gestational diabetes: macrosomic or large-for-gestational age infant • Polycystic ovary syndrome • Acanthosis Nigricans • American Indian or Alaska Native; African-American; Asian; Native Hawaiian or Other Pacific Islander; Hispanic
Diagnosis	
Plasma Glucose	Casual ⩾ 200 mg/dL (11.1 mmol/L) plus symptoms, fasting ⩾ 126 mg/dL (7.0 mmol/L), or 75 gram oral glucose tolerance test (OGTT) 2 hour glucose value ⩾ 200 mg/dL (11.1 mmol/L); if positive, confirm diagnosis within 7 days unless evidence of metabolic decompensation (ketones)
Symptoms	Often none Common: blurred vision; urinary tract infection; yeast infection; dry, itchy skin; numbness or tingling in extremities; fatigue Occasional: increased urination, thirst, and appetite; nocturia; weight loss
Urine Ketones	Usually negative
Treatment Options	Medical nutrition therapy; oral agent (α-glucosidase inhibitor, metformin, repaglinide, nateglinide, sulfonylurea, thiazolidinedione); combination therapy (oral agents, oral agent–insulin); Insulin: Stages 2, 3, 4
Targets	
Self-Monitored Blood Glucose (SMBG)	• More than 50% of SMBG values within target range • Pre-meal; 70–140 mg/dL (3.9–7.8 mmol/L) • Post-meal (2 hours after start of meal): < 160 mg/dL (8.9 mmol/L) • Bedtime: 100–160 mg/dL (5.6–8.9 mmol/L) • No severe (assisted) or nocturnal hypoglycemia Adjusted pre-meal target upwards if decreased life expectancy; frail elderly; cognitive disorders; or other medical concerns (cardiac disease, stroke, hypoglycemia unawareness, end-stage renal disease)
Hemoglobin HbA_{1c}	Within 1.0 percentage point of upper limit of normal (e.g., normal 6.0%; target < 7.0%) • Frequency: 3–4 times per year • Use HbA_{1c} to verify SMBG data
Monitoring	
SMBG	2–4 times per day (e.g., before meals, 2 hours after start of meal, bedtime); may be modified due to cost, technical ability, availability of meters; if on insulin, check 3 AM SMBG as needed
Method	Meter with memory and log book
Follow-up	
Monthly	Office visit during adjust phase (weekly phone contact may be necessary)
Every 3 Months	Hypoglycemia; medications; weight or BMI; medical nutrition therapy; BP; SMBG data (download meter); HbA_{1c}; eye screen; foot screen; diabetes/nutrition continuing education; smoking cessation counseling, aspirin therapy
Yearly	In addition to the 3 month follow-up, complete the following: history and physical; fasting lipid profile; albuminuria screen; dilated eye examination; dental examination; neurologic assessment; complete foot examination (pulses, nerves, ABI and inspection); immunizations
Complications Surveillance	Cardiovascular, renal, retinal, neurological, foot, oral, and dermatological See *Chronic Complications MasterDecisionPath*

Figure 4.2 Type 2 Diabetes Practice Guidelines

this is a medical emergency requiring appropriate treatment. See "Hospitalization for Diabetic Ketoacidosis and Hyperglycemic Hyperosmolar Syndrome" in Chapter 9 for further discussion and treatment DecisionPaths.

Screening for Diabetes

Screening for type 2 diabetes is based on the presence of risk factors (see Table 4.2). The American Diabetes Association (ADA) recommends that all individuals be tested for diabetes beginning at age 45. Other national organizations throughout the world vary on the notion of age-related universal screening due to the variation in when each risk groups develop diabetes. Some groups develop diabetes well in advance of 45 years old and may indeed present with significant complications if they are first detected at age 45. Screening for diabetes should be based on epidemiologic data concerning the risk of developing diabetes and its complications in particular groups. American Indians, Alaska Natives, African-Americans, Asians, Native Hawaiians and other Pacific Islanders, and Hispanics develop diabetes more frequently and at an earlier age. Additional risk factors include obesity, family history of diabetes, hypertension, dyslipidemia, previous impaired glucose homeostasis, and women with previous gestational diabetes. While each clinician must decide when it is best to screen, it is clear that individuals with any of these risk factors require special attention.

There are two different screening approaches (see Figure 4.3). The most economical screening method is to use capillary blood measured by a reflectance meter. This is not a replacement for a laboratory measurement, but is sufficiently accurate to justify diagnostic testing. A casual capillary value of > 140 mg/dL (7.8 mmol/L) or a

Table 4.2 Risk factors for type 2 diabetes

Factor	Comment
Overweight/obesity	The majority of people with type 2 diabetes are more than 20% above ideal body weight with a body mass index (BMI) > 25 kg/m^2.
Family history	There is a strong genetic predisposition—individuals with siblings with type 2 diabetes are at especially high risk; identical twins have an 80–95% concordance rate.
Age	Incidence increases with age—at age 40 expect 3–5%, at age 50 expect 5–8%, between ages 60 and 75 expect an increase to 15%, and by age 80 to 25%. For high-risk ethnic groups such as American Indians and Hispanics, the age of onset lowers to as early as 7 years of age.
Hypertension, hypertriglyceridemia, and low HDL cholesterol	Metabolic syndrome (insulin resistance syndrome).
Impaired fasting glucose (IFG) and/or impaired glucose tolerance (IGT)	Expect 5–10% of patients with IFG and/or IGT to develop type 2 diabetes each year. For ethnic groups at highest risk, expect as high as 15–20% to develop type 2 diabetes each year.
Gestational diabetes mellitus (GDM)	20–80% of those with gestational diabetes will develop type 2 diabetes as early as 5 years after initial diagnosis of gestational diabetes. GDM is considered an "unmasking" of type 2 diabetes during pregnancy.
Race or ethnic background	American Indians, Alaska Natives, African-Americans, Hispanics, Asians, and Native Hawaiians and other Pacific Islanders have between three and ten times greater risk of developing type 2 diabetes.

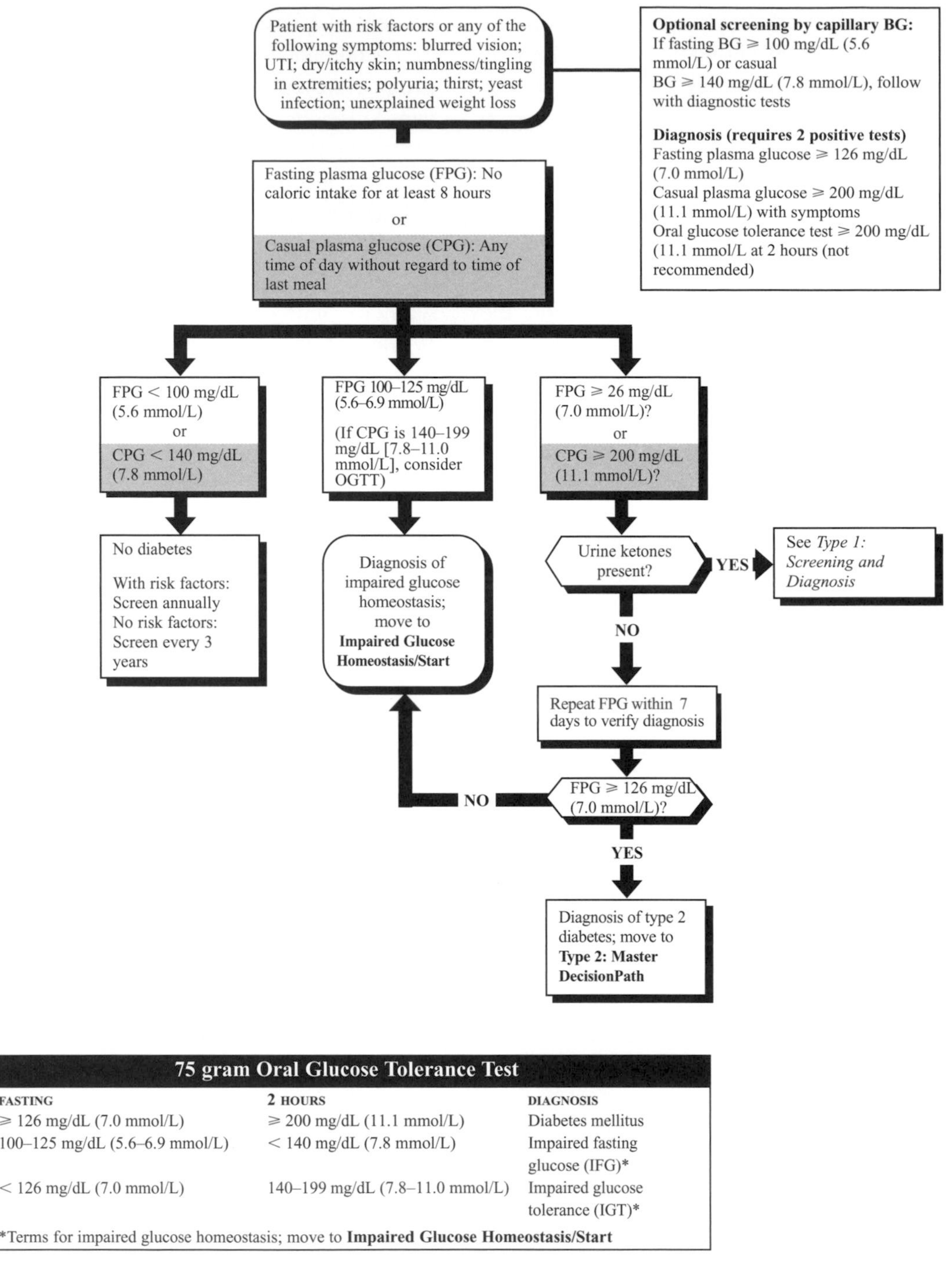

75 gram Oral Glucose Tolerance Test

FASTING	2 HOURS	DIAGNOSIS
⩾ 126 mg/dL (7.0 mmol/L)	⩾ 200 mg/dL (11.1 mmol/L)	Diabetes mellitus
100–125 mg/dL (5.6–6.9 mmol/L)	< 140 mg/dL (7.8 mmol/L)	Impaired fasting glucose (IFG)*
< 126 mg/dL (7.0 mmol/L)	140–199 mg/dL (7.8–11.0 mmol/L)	Impaired glucose tolerance (IGT)*

*Terms for impaired glucose homeostasis; move to **Impaired Glucose Homeostasis/Start**

Figure 4.3 Type 2 Diabetes Screening and Diagnosis DecisionPath

fasting > 100 mg/dL (5.6 mmol/L) would be sufficient evidence to require follow-up with a laboratory plasma glucose test. The alternative is to use the more costly, but more accurate, laboratory fasting or casual plasma glucose value as the screening test.

Diagnosis

The diagnostic criteria for type 2 diabetes accepted by the American Diabetes Association[26] and the World Health Organization are summarized in Table 4.3.

Table 4.3 Diagnostic criteria for diabetes and impaired glucose homeostasis (pre-diabetes). In the absence of metabolic decompensation, repeat diagnostic test on a subsequent day.

	Fasting Plasma Glucose (at least 8 hours after last caloric intake)	Casual Plasma Glucose (without regard to time of last meal)	75 Oral Glucose Tolerance Test
Diabetes	Fasting plasma glucose $\geqslant$ 126 mg/dL (7.0 mmol/L)	Casual plasma glucose $\geqslant$ 200 mg/dL (11.1 mmol/L) plus symptoms (polyuria, polydipsia, or unexplained weight loss)	2 hour plasma glucose $\geqslant$ 200 mg/dL (11.1 mmol/L)
Impaired Glucose Homeostasis (Pre-diabetes)	Impaired fasting glucose Fasting plasma glucose 100–125 mg/dL (5.6–6.9 mmol/L)		Impaired glucose tolerance 2 hour plasma glucose 140–199 mg/dL (7.8–11.0 mmol/L)
Normal	Fasting plasma glucose $<$ 100 mg/dL (5.6 mmol/L)		2 hour plasma glucose $<$ 140 mg/dL (7.8 mmol/L)

The diagnosis of diabetes can be made on the basis of either a fasting plasma glucose or casual plasma glucose (with symptoms) that has been confirmed on a different day by any one of these. Alternatively an oral glucose tolerance test can be used. The fasting plasma glucose test is recommended. However, since many patients initially present having recently eaten, SDM suggests that the first test be completed on that day using the casual plasma glucose criteria. Because patients do not readily identify or even recognize polyuria, polydipsia, or weight loss, it may not be possible to obtain an accurate history. Consider recurrent infections (urinary tract and yeast), fatigue, and changes in vision as important symptoms. In the absence of any symptoms, use the casual plasma glucose as a screening test. If positive, follow with a fasting plasma glucose test. A fasting state is characterized by at least 8 hours without caloric intake. Use of the oral glucose tolerance test (OGTT) should not be routine. It is reserved for those patients for whom the casual plasma glucose is between 140 and 199 mg/dL (7.8 and 11.0 mmol/L) and type 2 diabetes is suspected. If the fasting plasma glucose value is $\geqslant$ 100 and $<$ 126 mg/dL (5.6 and 7 mmol/L), the patient has impaired fasting glucose.

HbA_{1c} and the detection of type 2 diabetes

Glycosylated hemoglobin HbA_{1c}, or simply HbA_{1c}, is not used in the diagnosis of diabetes. HbA_{1c} can be measured by several different methods and as such has not been sufficiently standardized. Some laboratories report total glycosylated hemoglobin (HbA_{1a}, HbA_{1b}, and HbA_{1c}), while others report only the "c" fraction. One method is equated to the other by measuring the difference between the upper limit of normal and the reported value. The delta for total glycosylated hemoglobin and HbA_{1c} is approximately equivalent. In general, any delta above the upper limit of normal or any value reported above the upper limit of normal suggests the presence of hyperglycemia. The opposite is not necessarily the case. When there is a rapid onset of type 1 diabetes, the HbA_{1c} may initially appear normal. In rare instances the abnormally high or low HbA_{1c} may be due to a hemoglobinopathy (such as sickle-cell trait).

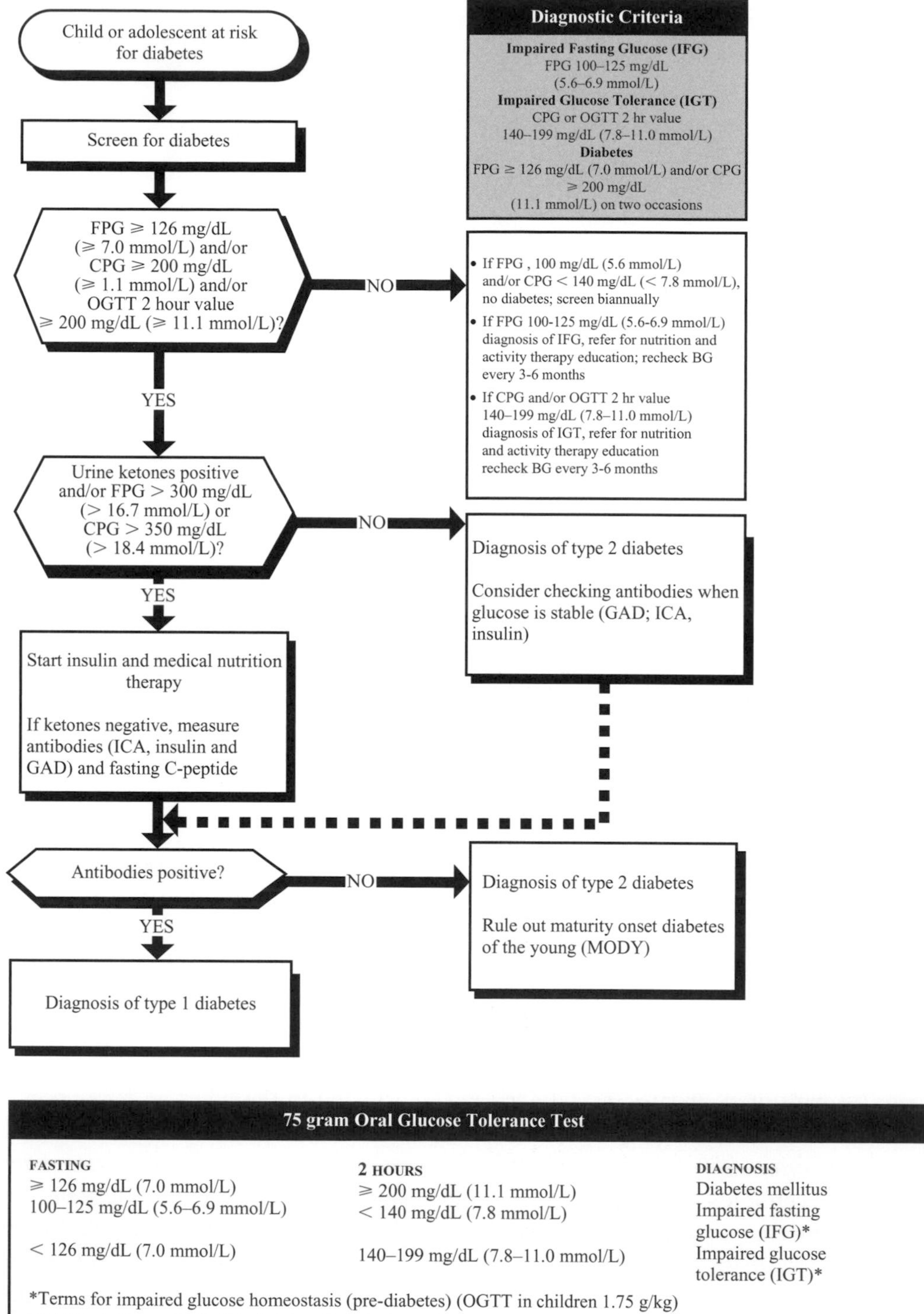

75 gram Oral Glucose Tolerance Test

FASTING	2 HOURS	DIAGNOSIS
⩾ 126 mg/dL (7.0 mmol/L)	⩾ 200 mg/dL (11.1 mmol/L)	Diabetes mellitus
100–125 mg/dL (5.6–6.9 mmol/L)	< 140 mg/dL (7.8 mmol/L)	Impaired fasting glucose (IFG)*
< 126 mg/dL (7.0 mmol/L)	140–199 mg/dL (7.8–11.0 mmol/L)	Impaired glucose tolerance (IGT)*

*Terms for impaired glucose homeostasis (pre-diabetes) (OGTT in children 1.75 g/kg)

Figure 4.4 Screening and Differential Diagnosis of Diabetes in Children and Adolescents DecisionPath

Insulin levels, C-peptide, and the detection of type 2 diabetes

Insulin in blood is measured by either insulin levels or C-peptide representing the amount of insulin in the blood. Both measures are increasingly in use for the differentiation between type 1 and type 2 diabetes, and to determine the extent of insulin deficiency. Insulin levels represent the total amount of both endogenous and exogenous insulin in the blood. In contrast, C-peptide measures only endogenous insulin. For individuals who are currently not treated with insulin, the measures are interchangeable. However, for the individual currently treated with exogenous insulin, in order to determine whether any endogenous insulin is being produced the C-peptide assay is used. This assay measures the connecting peptide "C" portion of the insulin peptide chain that is cleaved when proinsulin is processed into mature biologically active insulin. Because it is produced as part of the insulin peptide, it is equivalent to the amount of insulin secreted. Since it is not found in "vial" insulin, it can be used as a basis for differentiation between endogenously secreted and exogenous insulin. In type 2 diabetes, depending upon the duration of disease, endogenous insulin levels can be high, normal, or low, thus they are not used for the diagnosis of type 2 diabetes.

Screening and diagnosis for children and adolescents

In recent years the number of individuals under the age of 18 with type 2 diabetes has increased dramatically. Chapter 5 provides the details for screening, diagnosis, and classification as well as management of children and adolescents with type 2 diabetes. Here, some of the key principles for screening and detection in this group are reviewed. While there are no requirements regarding the screening of children and adolescents suspected or at risk for type 2 diabetes, SDM has taken the position that screening should be considered in any high-risk child or adolescent. The first principle is that screening and diagnosis in children do not differentiate between type 1 and type 2 diabetes. Since the incidence of type 1 diabetes is as high as or higher than the incidence of type 2 diabetes in adolescents and since incidence is a factor of risk group membership, the first step is to understand the risk group membership of the individual. In general, Caucasian children are at a higher risk of developing type 1 diabetes, while children of minority groups are at higher risk of type 2 diabetes. Lean children are more likely to have type 1 and obese children are at greater risk of type 2 diabetes. Despite these trends, exceptions are more often the rule. Thus, an underlying principle is to rule out type 1 diabetes first and, in the absence of a clear distinction between types of diabetes, treat the child or adolescent with insulin for any apparent persistent hyperglycemia. Surveillance for urine ketones should be considered paramount in this process as moderate to high ketones invariably suggest type 1 diabetes.

Impaired glucose homeostasis (pre-diabetes)

Many scientists and clinicians believe that treating individuals with elevated plasma glucose levels that are lower than diagnostic criteria can prevent type 2 diabetes. Individuals with fasting plasma glucose levels between 100 and 125 mg/dL (5.6 and 6.9 mmol/L) or two hour OGTT values between 140 and 199 mg/dL (7.8 and 11.0 mmol/L) are considered to have impaired glucose homeostasis (IGH). Studies using non-hypoglycemic oral agents as well as changes in diet and activity have shown that these measures can significantly reduce the risk of developing overt diabetes.[27] Annually, 5–10 per cent of the individuals with impaired glucose homeostasis will develop diabetes if no intervention is undertaken.[20]

Staged Diabetes Management provides DecisionPaths to guide the start (see Figure 4.5) and follow-up of treatment for IGH. As with type 2 diabetes a complete history and physical should be done and a baseline HbA_{1c} measured. The HbA_{1c} should be within the normal range for the laboratory. To establish a medical nutrition therapy, begin by obtaining a food and physical

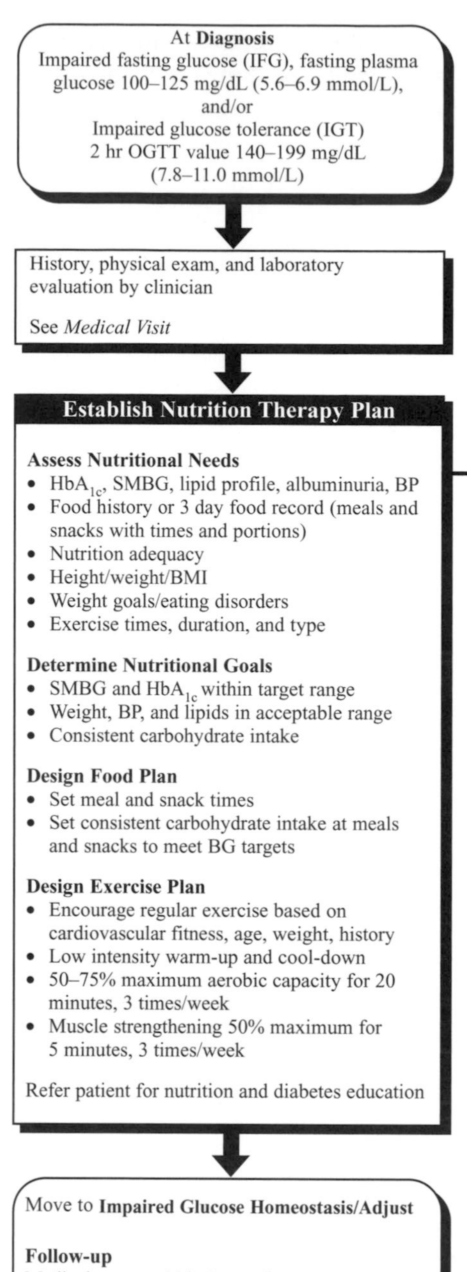

Targets
- HbA_{1c}: within normal range
- Lipid profile: within normal range
- Blood pressure: < 130/80 mmHg

Management Guidelines
- Lipids: serum cholesterol < 200 mg/dL (5.2 mmol/L); LDL< 100 mg/dL (2.6 mmol/L); triglycerides < 150 mg/dL (1.7 mmol/L)
- Nutrition: saturated fats < 10% total calories (< 7% with elevated LDL); total fat 30% of total calories (< 30% if obese with elevated LDL); cholesterol < 300 mg/day
- Weight: BMI < 25 kg/m^2 (see *BMI Chart*); determine reasonable body weight; if BMI > 25 kg/m^2, decrease calories by 10–20% and add exercise
- Hypertension: BP < 130/80 mmHg; if BP ⩾ 130/80 mmHg, reduce sodium to < 2400 mg/day
- Albuminuria: < 30 mg/24 hour or < 30 mg/g creatinine; if > 300 mg/24 hour or > 300 mg/g creatinine (macroalbuminuria), reduce protein intake to 0.8 gm/kg/day or ~10% total calories

Sample Food Plan

MEAL	CHO	MEAT/SUB	ADDED FAT
Breakfast	3–4	0–1	0–1
Snack	1–2	0	0–1
Lunch	3–4	2–3	1–2
Snack	1–2	0	0–1
Dinner	3–4	2–3	1–2
Snack	1–2	0	0–1

- **1 CHO** = 1 carbohydrate serving = 15 g carbohydrate; 60–90 calories
- **1 Meat/Sub** = 1 oz serving (28 gm) = 7 g protein; 5 g fat; 50–100 calories
- **1 Added Fat** = 1 serving = 5 g fat; 45 calories
- **Vegetables** = 1–2 servings/meal; not counted in plan

See *Carbohydrate Counting* and *Food Choices*

Figure 4.5 Impaired Glucose Homeostasis/Start

activity history. This may require asking the patient to maintain a diary for 3–4 days. On the basis of this information, a food and exercise/activity plan can be recommended. A sample food plan providing approximately 50 per cent of total calories from carbohydrate, 30 per cent from fat, and 20 per cent from protein is provided in the DecisionPath in Figure 4.5. Note that along with the appropriate food plan is an exercise regimen designed to increase aerobic capacity and muscle strengthening. Follow-up is at three month intervals until the blood glucose level is normalized. These measures should help prevent the onset of type 2 diabetes and most likely reduce the risk of associated microvascular and macrovascular complications. If the patient is unable or unwilling to follow the prescribed food and exercise plan, refer to the discussion in the "Adherence Assessment" section at the end of this chapter.

Because some groups, most notably American Indians, are at such an increased risk of developing type 2 diabetes (up to 50 per cent prevalence) and often develop diabetes early in life, the question is whether there are other earlier markers of type 2 diabetes besides IGH. Numerous studies have shown that well in advance of hyperglycemia there is an elevation in serum insulin levels. Measuring serum insulin levels or other more precise measures of insulin resistance (clamp studies), while currently not routinely used, may become a more useful predictor of type 2 diabetes and may identify those for whom early pharmacologic interventions (with insulin-sensitizing agents) and lifestyle modifications would be beneficial to prevent the disease.

Treatment options

Treatment of type 2 diabetes may require both behavioral and pharmacological interventions. Independent of the final therapy, medical nutrition therapy and exercise are considered integral to successful outcomes. Generally, treatment for type 2 diabetes has been divided into three periods: (1) medical nutrition alone; (2) oral pharmacological agents; (3) insulin. Both the provider and patient often see each period as a major milestone in the progression of diabetes. This is an error. The means of treatment does not necessarily reflect the degree of severity. Two measures, hyperglycemia and complications, are truer reflections of severity of disease.

The overall purpose of medical nutrition therapy is to improve glucose and lipid levels by reducing the glycemic effect of excessive carbohydrate intake and decreased energy expenditure. Thus, for medical nutrition therapy to be effective, alterations in food and increase in activity are required. Both steps improve insulin sensitivity and thus lower blood glucose levels. Current food and exercise plans seek to alter the composition and quantity of calories to (1) gradually lower glycemia; (2) maintain or reduce weight; (3) increase physical activity; and (4) promote healthful eating for optimal nutrition.

Five classifications of oral agents are currently available for managing type 2 diabetes: sulfonylureas, biguanides (metformin), alpha-glucosidase inhibitors (acarbose, miglitol), thiazolidinediones (pioglitazone, rosiglitazone), and meglitinides (repaglinide, nateglinide). The secretagogues (sulfonylureas and meglitinides) stimulate insulin secretion. The sensitizers, metformin (reduces hepatic glucose) and thiazolidinediones (increase insulin utilization at target tissue) improve insulin sensitivity. Alpha-glucosidase inhibitors suppress the alpha-glucosidase enzyme in the small intestine, which breaks down carbohydrate into monosaccharides, resulting in lower post-prandial glucose levels.

Oral agents may be given alone or in combination with other oral agents. Generally, oral agents from one classification are combined with another from a different classification. Thus common combinations are sulfonylureas with metformin or thiazolidinediones. In this case, the combination is designed to overcome insulin deficiency and insulin resistance. An exception is that the combination of metformin and thiazolidinediones is used to overcome both excessive hepatic glucose output and improve insulin sensitivity. Oral agents may also be given in combination with insulin. Such regimens often use the insulin to supplement basal insulin and the oral agent, such as a secretagogues, to improve bolus insulin requirements by improving β-cell function.

Insulin therapies include rapid-acting analogs (RA), short-acting regular (R), intermediate-acting NPH, prolonged intermediate-acting ultralente (U), and long-acting glargine (G) insulin (see Chapter 3 for further details). Designed to replace or supplement endogenous insulin, they overcome both insulin resistance and insulin deficiency.

Targets

Numerous studies have demonstrated that while any improvement in glycemic control is beneficial, near-normal levels of blood glucose (HbA_{1c} < 7 per cent) afford the best protection against the development and progression of microvascular disease in type 2 diabetes.[18,28] To achieve this goal, more than 50 per cent of self-monitored blood glucose values should be between 70 and 140 mg/dL (4.0 and 7.8 mmol/L) pre-meal, < 160 mg/dL (8.9 mmol/L) 2 hours after the start of the meal, and between 100 and 160 mg/dL (5.6 and 8.9 mmol/L) at bedtime. Achieving these SMBG targets normally correlates with an HbA_{1c} target of within 1 percentage point of the upper limit of normal (see Table 4.4). However, these goals may not be readily achievable, or safe, in some patients (e.g. elderly or people with cognitive disorders) and may have to be adjusted upward.

Monitoring

Appropriate management of type 2 diabetes always includes SMBG. Three different patterns of SMBG correspond to starting, adjusting, and maintaining the treatment goal.

During the *start phase*, independent of the type of therapy, data gathering is an essential early step in ensuring that the blood glucose levels are responding to the prescribed regimen. SMBG should be performed at defined times throughout the day to collect data on fasting, pre-meal, 2 hours post-meal, and overnight blood glucose levels.

During the *adjust phase*, SMBG should be synchronized to the action of the principal therapy – medical nutrition therapy, oral agent, or insulin action curves – to determine where hyperglycemia or hypoglycemia occur. SMBG should be performed at least three times each day to ensure continued improvement in blood glucose levels until targets are achieved. Patients should perform SMBG at different times throughout the day, including fasting, before meals, 2 hours after the start of meals, bedtime, and 3 AM as needed. The goal is to adjust therapy based on blood glucose patterns.

During the *maintain phase*, SMBG can be reduced to correspond with the patient's desire to have feedback and the therapeutic needs. For example, if the patient is maintained on the same dose of sulfonylurea, testing might be limited to three times per day, 2 days per week. If circumstances change, such as increased activity, alteration in food plan, or sudden alterations in therapy during inter-current events, increased testing is recommended to enhance clinical decision-making.

Because many studies have shown that patients may falsify or fail to record their SMBG results, meters with a memory should be used.[29,30] These meters directly record the blood glucose value with the corresponding time and date of test. Some devices can provide a running average the blood glucose data. More importantly, they can be connected to a computer, which will display the data in several formats that can facilitate clinical decision-making. Whether used routinely or more frequently for special situations, SMBG data provide patients with direct feedback on how well their individual therapy is working and assist

Table 4.4 HbA_{1c} and average SMBG correlation[23]

If HbA_{1c} is	Average SMBG is
1 percentage point above normal	150 mg/dL (8.3 mmol/L)
2 percentage points above normal	180 mg/dL (10.0 mmol/L)
3 percentage points above normal	210 mg/dL (11.7 mmol/L)
4 percentage points above normal	245 mg/dL (13.6 mmol/L)
5 percentage points above normal	280 mg/dL (15.5 mmol/L)
6 percentage points above normal	310 mg/dL (17.2 mmol/L)

clinicians with information needed to make appropriate decisions about therapy. The absence of SMBG data makes clinical decision-making almost impossible for both the patient and the clinician. Determining appropriate diet, exercise, oral agent, or insulin dose requires a source of constant, accurate feedback. Currently only SMBG can provide such feedback.

Follow-up

When starting or adjusting therapy, follow-up should be scheduled bi-weekly or monthly. An important element of SDM is that treatment options that are ineffective should be detected early and changes made rapidly. More frequent phone contact may be required, especially when adjusting insulin doses. The overall expectation is an average monthly decrease in average blood glucose of 15–30 mg/dL (0.8–1.7 mmol/L), which would translate into a drop in HbA_{1c} of 0.5–1.0 percentage points, until targets are reached. However, not until the end of the second month will the impact of the initial therapy be fully reflected in the HbA_{1c} levels. This is a safe rate of decline and generally does not place the patient at risk of either absolute or relative hypoglycemia. During the maintain phase, quarterly visits should be scheduled where weight, glycemic control (HbA_{1c}), and adherence to medical nutrition therapy can be assessed.

Annually, a fasting lipid profile, albuminuria screen, complete foot examination (pulses, nerves, and inspection), dental examination, and dilated eye examination are recommended. Additionally, nutrition and diabetes skills review and evaluation of other risk factors (smoking, alcohol intake, and weight management) are beneficial. Completing this evaluation (with appropriate referral) is necessary to meet national standards for diabetes management.

Insulin resistance and complication surveillance

Additionally, surveillance for disorders associated with insulin resistance (such as hypertension and dyslipidemia) as well as microvascular and macrovascular complications of diabetes should occur (see Chapters 8 and 9). For example, a foot check with a 10 g, 5.07 monofilament for sensation and an examination for pressure points, injuries, and ulcers is a necessity. As many as 80 per cent of those with type 2 diabetes have a serious co-morbidity. In many cases the complication can be managed and its progression slowed if found early. Staged Diabetes Management provides explicit protocols for the detection and treatment of the major microvascular and macrovascular complications. Periodic screening, rapid intervention, and close follow-up can significantly reduce the consequences of these complications.

Type 2 Diabetes Master DecisionPath

Note: Type 2 diabetes complicated by pregnancy is reviewed in Chapter 7.

Once the diagnosis has been confirmed, the next step is to choose the appropriate treatment modality. Staged Diabetes Management provides a Master DecisionPath for type 2 diabetes to facilitate rapid selection of the starting therapy and to lay out the options if the therapy fails to improve glycemic control. Staged Diabetes Management stresses the need to reach an agreed-upon therapeutic goal, which may entail moving the patient from simple to more complex regimens. It also allows for movement from more complex to less complex regimens as long as glycemic targets are maintained. A principle of SDM is to share the Master DecisionPath and the therapeutic goals with the patient. Through this process, the patient knows the options and the therapeutic goal.

The Type 2 Diabetes Master DecisionPath is shown in Figure 4.6. Four general treatment alternatives (medical nutrition therapy, oral agent, combination of oral agents, and insulin) are avail-

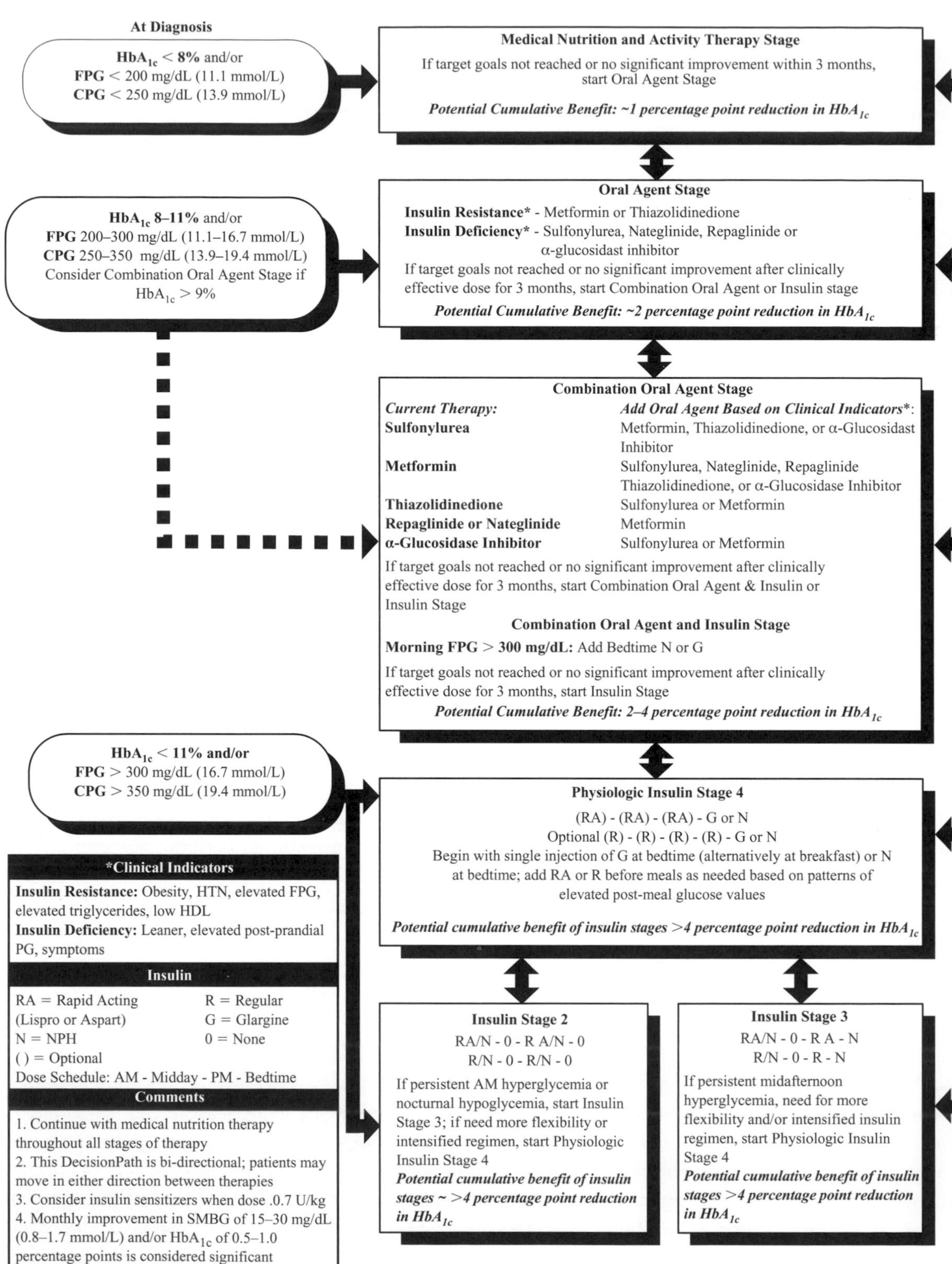

Figure 4.6 Master DecisionPath for Type 2 Diabetes

able at diagnosis. Selection should be based on both a realistic assessment of the patient's willingness to follow the regimen and scientific rationale. Patient acceptance is most related to understanding the regimen, cost, comfort, and specific fears related to certain types of treatment. This contrasts with the medical view, which seeks the most effective treatment from a scientific and clinical perspective. Balancing the two views is important.

While SDM is designed to be customized by the community, it is important to note that there is a scientific basis for selecting a starting therapy. It is recognized that limited resources, patient willingness, or ability to follow a specific regimen may not enable the clinician to initiate the most efficacious therapy. Staged Diabetes Management has a built-in mechanism in the Specific DecisionPath that evaluates a therapy against specific goals. If the therapy does not meet the goals, it is adjusted until maximum effectiveness is obtained. If targets are not achieved, a new therapy is initiated. The sequential movement to new therapies has timelines to assure that no patient remains on a therapy that is ineffective.

From a scientific perspective, if at diagnosis the fasting plasma glucose is < 200 mg/dL (11.1 mmol/L) or the casual plasma glucose is < 250 mg/dL (13.9 mmol/L), medical nutrition therapy should be initiated. Numerous studies provide evidence that most nutritional interventions have a maximum effective lowering of 100 mg/dL (5.6 mmol/L) in blood glucose. On average, the benefits of nutritional intervention are a reduction in blood glucose of 50 mg/dL (2.8 mmol/L) or approximately 1.0–1.5 percentage points in HbA_{1c}. Thus, this therapy is reserved for those who have recently developed type 2 diabetes in whom mild insulin resistance is the principal underlying defect.

The primary goal of medical nutrition therapy for diabetes is to achieve glycemic targets by a combination of moderating carbohydrate intake coupled with increased exercise/activity. Modest weight reduction of 5–10 pounds may be sufficient to restore near euglycemia when plasma glucose is relatively low, but is considered to be a secondary goal of medical nutrition therapy.[31] Blood glucose levels may not improve due to weight loss in those patients with profound insulin deficiency. Dietary interventions combined with increased activity tend to increase insulin sensitivity and utilization, resulting in improved glucose uptake.

Glycemic control in patients with moderate hyperglycemia (casual plasma glucose 250–350 mg/dL [13.9–19.4 mmol/L] and fasting plasma glucose 200–300 mg/dL [11.1–16.7 mmol/L]) may be treated effectively by oral agents. The selection of the most appropriate oral agent is based on such factors as obesity, insulin resistance, and insulin deficiency as well as pregnancy, and liver and kidney disease. In general, insulin sensitizing agents should be reserved for those with insulin resistance (obese patients) and insulin secretagogues should be used in those with insulin deficiency. Oral agents, except glyburide (a glibenclamide), pass the placental barrier and are, therefore, contraindicated in pregnancy. Additionally, since many oral agents are *metabolized* in the liver, patients with severe liver disease should not be given these drugs. For individuals with significant kidney disease (serum creatinine > 2.0 mg/dL or 180 μmol/L), only thiazolidinediones and meglitinides (repaglinide or nateglinide) may be used. In patients with serum creatinine between 1.4 and 2.0 mg/dL (120 and 180 μmol/L), alpha-glucosidase inhibitors, meglitinides, sulfonylureas, or thiazolidinediones may be used. Any oral agent can be used in the absence of kidney disease (serum creatinine < 1.4 mg/dL or 120 μmol/L) if there are no other contraindications for use.

Recently, a combination of an insulin sensitizing agent and an insulin secretagogue have been used in patients with an $HbA_{1c} > 9$ per cent. When blood glucose reaches this level usually both insulin resistance and insulin deficiency are significantly involved, resulting in significantly elevated blood glucose levels. The combined effect of the two classifications is to lower HbA_{1c} by as much as four percentage points. In general, monotherapies lower HbA_{1c} by no more than two percentage points. Thus, if the patient is at HbA_{1c} of 10 per cent, a combination of oral agents with appropriate medical nutrition intervention should be able to reach the goal of $HbA_{1c} < 7$ per cent. These values are research-based averages and will differ among individuals.

When casual plasma glucose is > 350 mg/dL (19.4 mmol/L) or fasting plasma glucose is > 300 mg/dL (16.7 mmol/L), single oral agents or a combination of oral agents with appropriate medical nutrition therapy are generally not sufficient to lower blood glucose into the target range. Under such circumstances, insulin should be considered as the starting therapy. Additionally, during a pregnancy complicated by type 2 diabetes (pre-gestational diabetes) when blood glucose levels > 200 mg/dL (11.1 mmol/L) insulin should be the initial therapy. In all of these cases, the risk of glucose toxicity is very high. Should this occur, the pancreatic β-cells will weaken, thereby producing less insulin. This may start a cascade effect in which the β-cells weaken even more in the presence of rising blood glucose levels. The net result raises the risk of hyperosmolar hyperglycemic syndrome. The underlying cause of significant hyperglycemia (fasting blood glucose is > 300 mg/dL (16.7 mmol/L)) is usually advanced type 2 diabetes in which there is severe insulin deficiency and insulin resistance. While in some cases, the insulin deficiency may be reversed with weight reduction and improved insulin sensitivity, the majority of these patients will permanently require exogenous insulin.

Fundamental principles

1. *Acute illness at diagnosis.* Insulin should be initiated in the presence of any ketonuria beyond small (see Insulin Stage 2, 3, or 4). Once the patient has been stabilized and blood glucose levels are consistently below 300 mg/dL (16.7 mmol/L) in non-pregnant patients, reliance on exogenous insulin may be reconsidered (especially when the patient's HbA_{1c} is within two percentage points of the upper limit of normal).

2. *Moving between therapies.* Effective management requires a goal and a reasonable time to meet that goal. Unfortunately, many patients with type 2 diabetes remain in the adjust phase for prolonged periods of time without reaching glycemic targets. Often, no change in therapy is made, even when it is obvious glycemic control is not improving. To avoid this problem, SDM provides guidelines for deciding when a therapy has reached its maximum effectiveness and, therefore, should be added to or changed. Table 4.5 summarizes these guidelines. They are based on a slow and steady adjustment in therapeutic dose to the optimum dose before changing the stage. These times have been studied and they present little danger of hypoglycemia, reduce the risk of prolonged hyperglycemia, and restore patient confidence that goals are achievable.

Table 4.5 Suggested timelines to reach target

Stage	Time
Medical nutrition therapy	2–3 months
Oral agent	3 months
Insulin stages	6–12 months

3. *Therapies, not patients, fail.* It is recognized that both patients and physicians are reluctant to start insulin therapies, even when blood glucose is high, before fully exhausting simpler treatment stages (oral agents). Typically, the patient is started on an oral agent, which cannot achieve the goal of near-normal blood glucose. The patient interprets this as a failure, as does the physician. But whose failure? Perhaps the patient had already mentioned a reluctance to use insulin. Perhaps the physician wanted to give the patient an opportunity to exhaust the oral agents before turning to insulin. In either case, the scientific evidence suggests that the therapy will fail.

4. *Treat to target.* SDM is based on the notion that the patient and physician have agreed upon a reasonable target and that the therapy has been selected to reach that target. With this in mind, SDM has set the criteria for changing the therapy: HbA_{1c} should decrease by at least one percentage point per month. If, after reaching the maximum effective dose, the current therapy cannot achieve this, then the next therapy should be initiated. Thus, even if the patient is started on oral agents when insulin is indicated, with appropriate adjustments at 2–4 week intervals, it would require 8–12 weeks to achieve maximum dose of one oral agent and another 8–12 weeks to maximize the dose of combination oral agent therapy. Thus, 16–24 weeks, or 4–6 months, would pass before insulin is considered. Allowing for further adjustments, delays in contacting patients, re-education, and other factors, within a year of the start of treatment a patient's therapy should include insulin if glycemic targets have not been achieved. If by then initiating insulin therapy is still not possible, seeking the assistance of a specialist would be appropriate.

Medical Nutrition Therapy Stage

Medical nutrition therapy (MNT) can be used alone or in combination with pharmacologic interventions. Although considered a cornerstone of all medical interventions in diabetes, its role and scope of effectiveness is often misunderstood. As a stand-alone therapy it is most effective when fasting plasma glucose is < 200 mg/dL (11.1 mmol/L) or casual plasma glucose is < 250 mg/dL (13.9 mmol/L) at diagnosis. The DecisionPath for starting medical nutrition therapy is shown in Figure 4.7. For exercise, see "Exercise Assessment."

Medical Nutrition Therapy/Start

In general, the principles of starting MNT are the same whether the therapy is stand-alone or in combination with a pharmacologic agent. It is well established that the vast majority of individuals with type 2 diabetes are obese and thus insulin resistant. For these individuals, weight and activity management (see Exercise Assessment) are important tools in the quest to re-establish normal glycemic levels. Food planning attempts to achieve sufficient dietary management to improve glycemic control and to improve such other physiological parameters as lipids, blood pressure, and albuminuria. Activity management (or exercise) attempts to increase energy utilization in a manner that is sensitive to the patient's age, fitness, and lifestyle. *If individuals should require a pharmacologic agent, they should continue to be treated with a food and exercise plan that may require some modifications (i.e., timing of meals) in order to prevent hypoglycemia and hyperglycemia.*

The first step in determining the appropriate food plan is to complete a physical examination. The variables that determine the appropriate food plan and eventual dietary compliance go well beyond the current physical well-being of the individual. Psychosocial issues and economics must be considered. A thorough assessment of the patient's readiness and ability to follow a food plan to re-establish a balance between caloric input and energy output is necessary. Sharing the Master DecisionPath with the patient, providing food choices, and clearly establishing the metabolic goals are necessary steps in this process.

At the initial nutrition visit, obtain the following information:

- Medical history
- Assessment of nutritional needs by food history and/or three day food record
- Medications that affect diet prescription such as hypertension medications, lipid-lowering medications, and diabetes medications that impact on the gastrointestinal systems (such as alpha-glucosidase inhibitors and metformin)
- Laboratory data: HbA_{1c}, plasma glucose

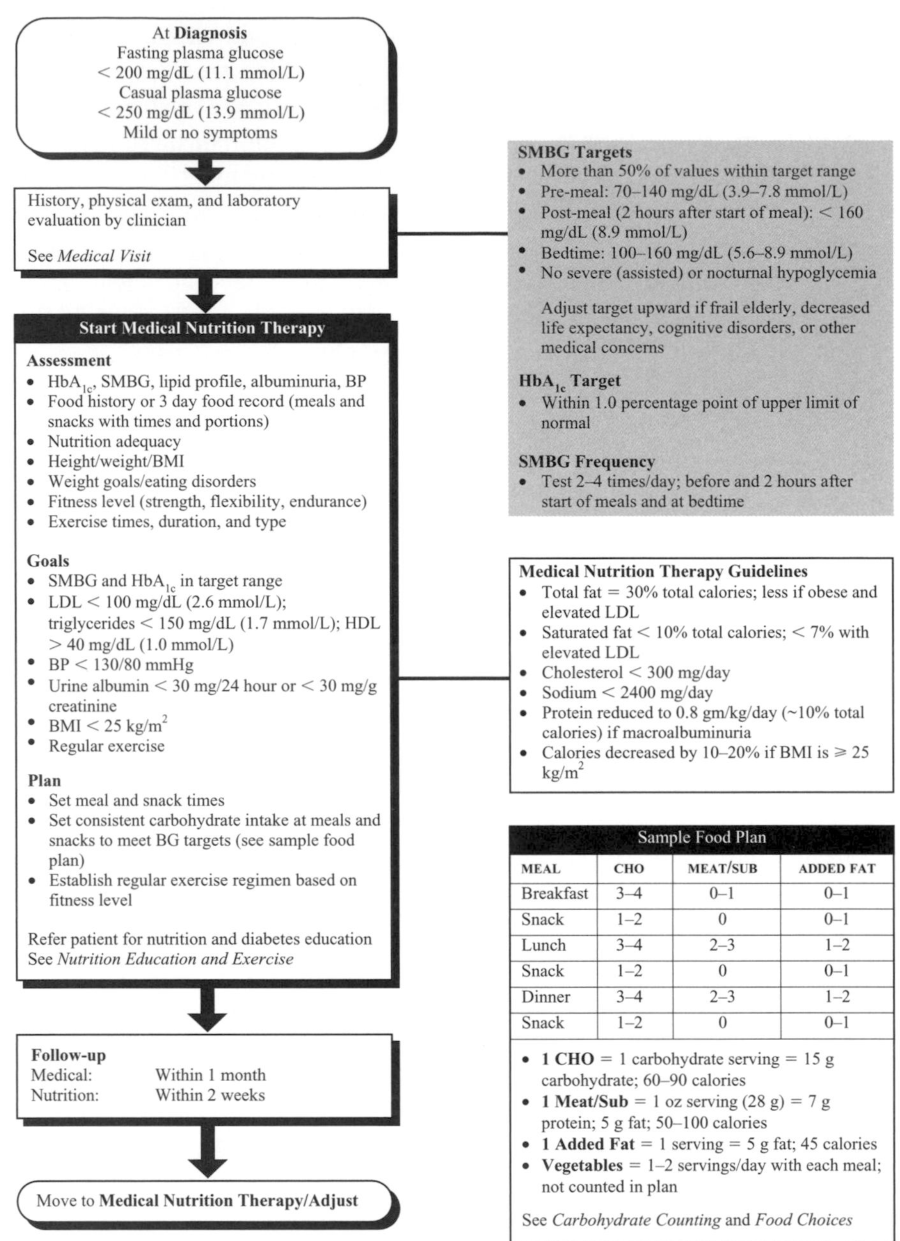

MEAL	CHO	MEAT/SUB	ADDED FAT
Breakfast	3–4	0–1	0–1
Snack	1–2	0	0–1
Lunch	3–4	2–3	1–2
Snack	1–2	0	0–1
Dinner	3–4	2–3	1–2
Snack	1–2	0	0–1

Figure 4.7 Medical Nutrition Therapy/Start

level, fasting lipid profile, blood pressure, renal function and liver function tests (ALT)

- Goals for patient care: target blood glucose, target HbA_{1c}, method and frequency of blood glucose monitoring and weight management
- Medical clearance for patient to exercise and/or other pertinent information related to daily activities

Assess obesity. To determine the appropriate nutrition intervention, include an assessment of body mass index (BMI – divide weight measured in kilograms by the square of the height measured in meters – kg/m^2). Recently, the National Heart, Lung, and Blood Institute identified overweight as a BMI of 25–29.9 kg/m^2 and obesity as $\geqslant 30\ kg/m^2$. See the BMI chart in the Appendix (Figure A.5) to calculate the BMI. Body mass index correlates well with body fat as a clinical measure of obesity. A loss of two units of BMI corresponds to a decrease in body weight of about 5–6 kg (11 to 13.2 lb).

Once the BMI has been determined, obtain this additional information:

- Thorough diet history including past experience with meal planning
- Dietary restrictions due to allergies, religion, culture, finances, and preferences
- Weight history including any significant loss or gain in weight over the past five years
- Weight goals
- Current appetite, recent loss of appetite
- Eating or digestion problems
- Eating schedule
- Meal preparation practices
- Typical day's food intake (to be evaluated for approximate calories and nutrient composition, other nutritional concerns, frequency, and timing of meals)
- Frequency and choices in restaurant meals
- Alcohol intake
- Use of vitamins or nutritional supplements

Obtain data related to physical activity and exercise:

1. What type of activity does the patient currently do?
2. Does the patient exercise regularly?
3. What limitation does the patient have that would hinder or prevent exercise?
4. Is the patient willing or interested in becoming more physically active?

Assess psychosocial/economic issues (see the "Behavioral Issues and Assessment" section). During the visit, include a review of the living situation, cooking facilities, finances, educational background, employment, ethnicity, religious background, and belief considerations. Next, develop a plan that includes a combination of patient and healthcare team goals related to diabetes management, such as target HbA_{1c}. The food plan prescription should be individualized to the patient based on diet history, food patterns and preferences, and other collected data, as well as socioeconomic issues, ethnic/cultural issues, religious practices, and lifestyle.

Medical nutritional interventions are behavioral in their approach. Begin by establishing a blood glucose target and the period of time it should take to reach this goal. This decision needs to be made by the patient and the physician. Next, determine the degree to which the individual is ready to alter caloric intake as part of a strategy for controlling blood glucose. Sometimes readiness to change is a function of knowledge. Individuals with diabetes must first understand the disease, treatment options, and long-term prognosis before they are ready to accept a therapeutic choice. The SDM section on patient education addresses this point and provides details regarding the approach to education. SDM uses three principles in the development of a food plan: replace, reduce, and restrict.

The first step in designing an effective food plan is to replace high caloric and high carbohydrate foods and drinks with substitutes that are similar in volume and taste. *Replacing* regular soda pop with diet soda is one example: the same size portion and a similar taste. Replacing full fat ice cream with a low fat, low sugar substitute is another example. In general, patients are willing to do this as it causes the least inconvenience and is easy to fit into their current lifestyle. If this fails to adequately lower blood glucose (expect a drop of 20–30 mg/dL (1.2–1.7 mmol/L) within the first week, consider more aggressive caloric reductions and restrictions. If, over a period of two

Table 4.6 Estimation of calorie requirements for adults

	kcal per lb DBW	kcal per kg DBW
Men and physically active women	~15	~30
Most women, sedentary men, adults over age 55	~13	~28
Sedentary women, obese adults, sedentary adults over age 55	~10	~20

to three weeks, the trend does not continue, then move to the second principle. *Reduction* of caloric intake is accomplished by reducing the portion size of key foods and drinks. Begin with a total reduction of approximately 10 per cent. The easiest way to accomplish this is to reduce all caloric intake during meals and snacks. Keep slowly reducing total calories (5 per cent/week) until total caloric intake reaches 75 per cent of the original intake or a reduction by 500 kcal/day. This should result in a weight reduction of approximately 1 pound weekly. Blood glucose should continue to improve. If this fails, significant *restrictions* need to be placed on intake of certain food or drinks, for example, total omission of regular soda pop, high-fat milk, cheese, butter, ice cream, salad dressing, and sweetened syrups may be required.

The replace, reduce, restrict approach is one strategy. A far more comprehensive approach is usually needed. If medical nutrition therapy is to work for a long period of time, then the plan must target blood glucose and weight maintenance or reduction simultaneously. Begin with a calculation of target weight (assuming that the blood glucose has already been agreed upon). The target weight can be determined by finding the upper limit of the normal range of the BMI for the patient. Next, plan to move towards this goal in increments of 1 to 2 points. For example, if the current BMI of a 5 ft. 8 in. male patient is 32 kg/m^2 his long term goal would be a BMI of 24 kg/m^2, requiring a weight loss of at least 50 lb (23 kg). The initial target would be a weight loss of 5 lb. (2 kg). This could be accomplished by a net reduction in daily caloric intake of 500 kcal/day for a period of five weeks. To reach the long-term goal, the patient would continue on the new dietary regimen for approximately one year. Although this seems to be a long period of time, it has been found that the changes in lifestyle, that lead to the weight loss will be more likely to be sustained.

The regimen can be modified for both daily activity level and age. Persons with a sedentary lifestyle generally need fewer calories to maintain their metabolic rate. Typically, an obese and sedentary individual requires one-third fewer calories to maintain the same body weight than an active leaner person. See Table 4.6.

Harris–Benedict equation. The Harris–Benedict equation is another way to determine caloric requirements.[32] It is a close estimation of basal energy expenditure (BEE), shown in Table 4.7.

Table 4.7 Basal energy expenditure (BEE)

Female BEE

$655 + (9.6 \times W) + (1.8 \times H) - (4.7 \times A)$

Male BEE

$66 + (13.7 \times W) + (5 \times H) - (6.8 \times A)$

W = actual weight in kg; H = height in cm; A = age in years

BEE × activity factor = total caloric requirement

Activity Factors

- very sedentary = 1.1
- sedentary/most people = 1.2
- aerobic exercise 3 times/week = 1.3
- aerobic exercise 5 times/week = 1.5
- daily aerobic exercise = 1.6

Adjustment in body weight for obese patients. The BEE should be modified for obese individuals, since it assumes a certain metabolic rate for all tissues. An obese person has a greater percentage of body fat, which is much less metabolically active. Thus, caloric needs calculated on the basis of an obese person's actual body weight would be skewed very high. Obese persons do, however, have an increased caloric expenditure required for walking and moving excess weight or the increase in body protein for structural support of extra fat tissue. Because of these concerns, the following formula is suggested for obese patients. This formula is based on physiologic theory, rather than direct clinical research. Use the adjusted body weight obtained through this calculation in place of actual weight in the formula for BEE.

Adjusted weight (kg) $= (\text{ABW} - \text{DBW}) \times 0.25 + \text{DBW}$

ABW = actual body weight

DBW = desirable body weight

0.25 = percentage of metabolically active body fat tissue

Macronutrient composition. Although reduction in total caloric intake is effective, yet another approach evaluates the macronutrient composition of the food plan. Staged Diabetes Management recommends plans are individualized according to a person's lifestyle, eating habits, and concurrent medical conditions. For example, if weight is a concern, total fat should be reduced; if elevated cholesterol is a concern, saturated fat should be reduced to less than 10 per cent of total fat; and if hypertension is a concern, sodium intake should be reduced to < 2400 mg/day.

Educating individuals about food planning involves teaching basic concepts of nutrition, diabetes nutrition guidelines, and discussing ideas for altering current food plans to meet these guidelines. Points of focus include the following.

1. *When and how much to eat.* Space food throughout the day to avoid long times between meals and snacks. Choose smaller portions. Eat smaller meals and snacks. Avoid skipping meals and snacks (if part of food plan).

2. *What to eat.* Choose a variety of foods each day. Choose foods lower in fat. Avoid foods high in added sweeteners such as soda pop, syrup, candy, and desserts.

3. *How to make food choices.* Include a simple definition of carbohydrate, protein, and fat, with examples of food sources of each; discuss nutrition guidelines, such as eating less fat and carbohydrates, using less added sweetener, eating more fiber, and reducing total caloric (fat) intake for weight loss if appropriate; and suggest grocery shopping tips for making these changes in their current eating pattern.

4. *Changes in food plan when taking medications.* Since patients may eventually be placed on oral agent or insulin therapy, it is appropriate to indicate that some changes in the food plan may take place when these therapies are initiated. Additional attention to food and eating awareness is recommended for obese individuals. This can be achieved by discussing the connection between portion size and carbohydrates; the calorie and fat content of foods; and the importance of self-monitoring behaviors, such as food records designed to increase awareness of total food consumption and stimuli that promote overeating.

Carbohydrate counting and the exchange lists. Carbohydrates are quickly broken down to glucose in the digestive track and thus have the greatest immediate impact on blood glucose levels. Therefore, accounting for the amount of carbohydrate intake is of particular concern when generating a food plan for the individual with diabetes. One approach, called carbohydrate counting, has patients consume a specific number of carbohydrate choices (15 g carbohydrate/choice) at each meal or snack. Carbohydrate counting allows for synchronization of pharmacologic therapy to the glucose patterns that emerge from following an established food plan (see the Appendix, Figure A.14). Patients using pre-meal rapid-acting insulin or rapid-acting meglitinides can be taught to adjust the pre-meal dose based on the number of carbohydrates they plan to ingest at the next meal. After experimentation, many patients can become adept at these adjustments (often with excellent results). This approach is best when packaged foods are used with the nutritional labels that contain the amount of calories coming from carbohydrates. The approach is least effective when portion sizes are hard to estimate and the composition of the food or drink is unknown.

Foods are divided into three categories: carbohydrates, meats and meat substitutes, and added fat. For each category, each unit contains a relatively fixed range of calories (see Table 4.8). The exchange lists, which group foods into six lists with all foods on any one list containing approximately the same proportion of carbohydrate, fat, and protein, can be used to select foods from the three categories. The six lists are starch, meat and meat substitutes, vegetables, fruit, milk, and fat. Because foods can be exchanged within one list it allows greater variety in food choices while maintaining consistency in nutrient content. A food plan would include choices in the three categories for each meal and snack. For example, a typical breakfast might include three carbohydrate choices (banana, milk, and toast), one meat choice (ham), and one fat choice (butter). The total calories would be 270 (CHO) + 100 (meat) + 45 (fat) = 415 kcal.

Reinforcement, doctor/patient relationship. In order to support and sustain medical nutrition interventions there are many areas that need to be addressed by the patient and the health care provider. Some of these are listed here.

- *Agreement on short-term goals.* Short-term goals should be specific, "reasonable and realistic," and achievable in 1–2 weeks. Goals should address eating, exercise, and blood glucose monitoring behaviors. The focus should be to change one or two specific behaviors at a time in each area, e.g. eat breakfast and use less margarine, walk for 15 minutes twice a week, test blood glucose before and after the main meal three times a week.

- *Collection of important clinical data.* Provide instructions on how to record food intake (actual food eaten and quantities, times of meals), exercise habits (type, frequency, and duration), and blood testing results.

- *Documentation.* Include in the patient's permanent record the assessment and intervention. The report should include a summary of assessment information, long-term goals, education intervention, short-term goals, specific actions recommended, and plans for further follow-up, including additional education topics to be reviewed.

Coordinated exercise/activity plan. Medical nutrition therapy incorporates a food plan with exercise or activity designed to optimize glucose uptake and insulin utilization. The approach to exercise and activity is detailed in this chapter.

Table 4.8 Calories and food exchanges

Type of Food	Calories (kcal/kg)	Exchange List
Carbohydrates	60–90	Starch, fruit, milk
Meat and meat substitutes	50–100	Meat
Added fat	45	Fat

Glucose monitoring. Although the patient may be started on a regimen based solely on MNT to improve glycemic control, it is especially important not to omit SMBG. In general, SMBG is used too infrequently with such patients. This places the patient and health care professional at an enormous disadvantage. Lacking SMBG data, it is almost impossible for the patient or professional to have adequate data to determine how well the nutrition therapy is working. Patient knowledge of target blood glucose ranges and blood glucose testing technique need to be assessed. During the start treatment phase, when data are being collected to determine whether medical nutrition therapy and increased exercise are reasonable choices, SMBG must occur at least 2–4 times each day. The testing schedule of fasting, before meals, 2 hours after the start of the meal, and before bedtime should be used in order to develop patterns of blood glucose levels throughout the day. This should be combined with testing before and after exercise (at least twice during the initial treatment phase). Testing using an SMBG meter with memory is the only certain way to ensure accurate data. Do not employ SMBG as a punitive measure. Patients are likely to fabricate results to please the healthcare team if SMBG is used punitively.

HbA_{1c} should be used in association with SMBG, but not as a replacement (see Table 4.4). Since several assays for glycosylated hemoglobin exist, one way to standardize the HbA_{1c} is to report the difference between the reported value and the upper limit of normal. Thus, when the upper limit of normal is 6 per cent, an HbA_{1c} of 10.5 per cent is 4.5 per cent above normal. The average SMBG value for a period of at least 1 month with two to four tests per day should correlate with the HbA_{1c} level. Minimally, the SMBG values and HbA_{1c} should move in the same direction. If this is not the case, suspect error in SMBG.

During the start phase (1–2 weeks), all SMBG data should be reviewed weekly. Examine blood glucose records for the incidence of hyperglycemia, hypoglycemia, and number of blood glucose values in target range. If several values exceed 300 mg/dL (16.7 mmol/L), consider initiating an oral agent (see the oral agent section that follows). A follow-up contact within 2 weeks of the initial visit should be made. At that time, review baseline data (SMBG). A 5 per cent reduction in mean blood glucose should have been possible by this time. If this level is reached, a second appointment 2 weeks later should show continued reduction. If, after the second follow-up, blood glucose levels (based on verified data) do not show at least 15 mg/dL (0.8 mmol/L) improvement, adjust the food plan, reassess the exercise prescription, and consider starting an oral agent.

Medical Nutrition Therapy/Adjust

Evaluate progress. Optimally, patients should be seen two weeks after the start of MNT to review their progress. At this visit, weigh the patient and determine whether there have been changes in diet, alterations in medication, and changes in exercise habits. Review SMBG records for frequency of testing, time of testing, and results. Assess blood pressure and obtain any pertinent laboratory data. As it is too early to uncover a change in HbA_{1c}, measure blood glucose by reflectance meter during the visit. Obtain the patient's food records completed since initial visit or take a 24 hour food recall (see Figure 4.8).

To determine whether the therapy is effective, examine the SMBG records for patterns of reduced blood glucose levels. Patterns are three consecutive days in which there is little change in blood glucose at a particular time of the day (within 1–2 hour intervals). To corroborate the blood glucose values check the reflectance meter's memory. This can be accomplished by either downloading the stored glucose data or scrolling though the device. If there is a pattern of higher blood glucose, then alterations in the food plan are necessary. If it is lower blood glucose, the regimen is working. However, these values must be corroborated by HbA_{1c}. Since only two weeks have passed, the HbA_{1c} will not change to any appreciable degree. In this case wait another 2–4 weeks before a second HbA_{1c} assay is performed.

If there have been episodes of hypoglycemia, they are related to exercise or skipped meals. If

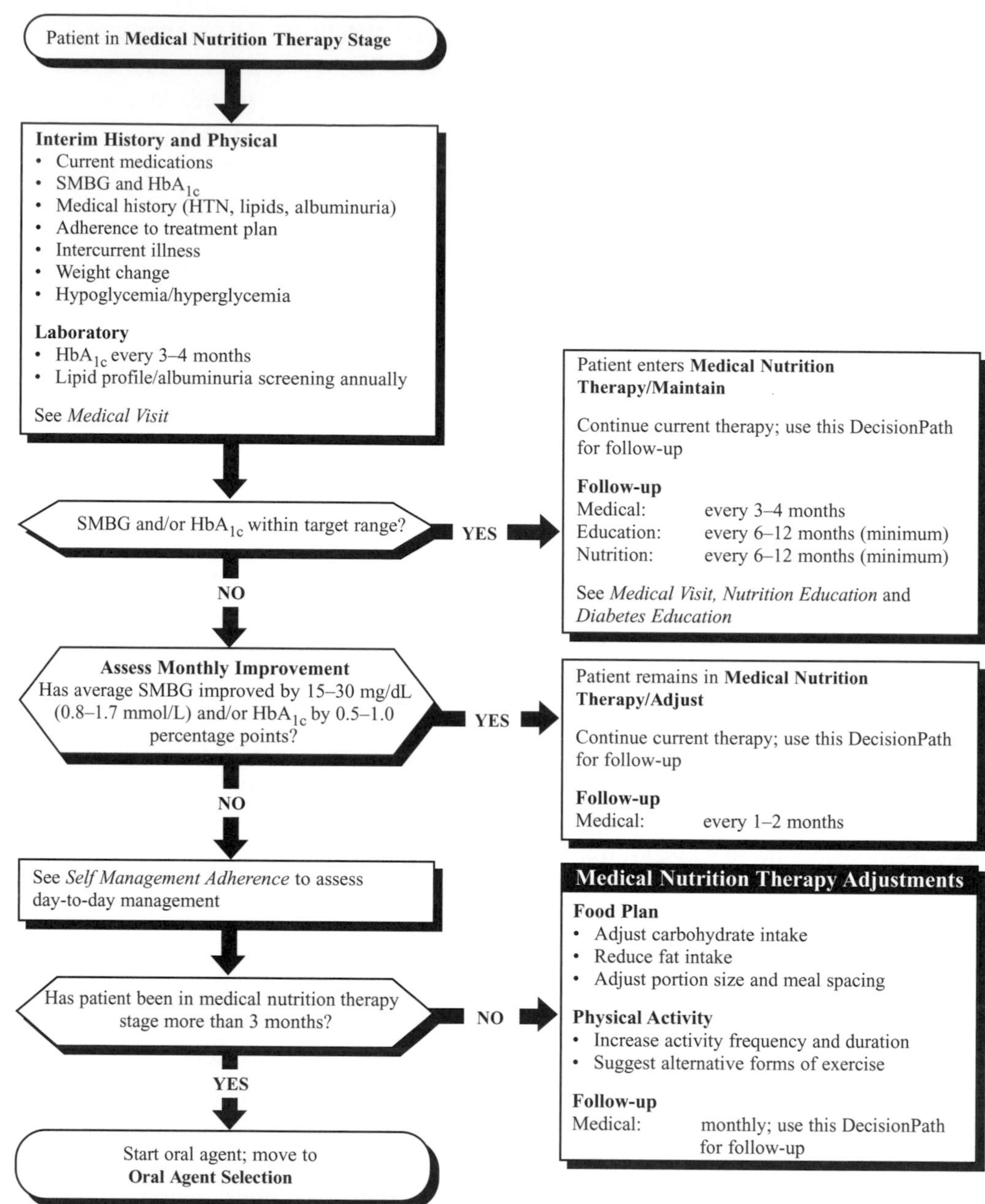

Figure 4.8 Type 2 diabetes Medical Nutrition Therapy/Adjust

there is a pattern of hyperglycemia, generally it will appear as post-prandial blood glucose values > 160 mg/dL (8.9 mmol/L). Alterations in food plan should continue for up to three months. Staged Diabetes Management provides the general guideline of between 0.5 and 1 percentage point improvement in HbA_{1c} and a parallel lowering of average blood glucose of 15–30 mg/dL (0.8–1.7 mmol/L) monthly. If this target has not been achieved in at most three months, then the food plan should be supplemented by oral medications.

Corrective measures.

- *Changes in exercise and/or activity levels.* Patient should have gradually increased physical activity with a minimum goal of 10–15 minutes of physical activity three to four times a week. Is the patient willing or able to do more?

- *Change in food habits*. Patient eats meals and snacks on a regular basis and makes appropriate food choices in reasonable portions. If caloric intake has been excessive, can the patient reduce calorie intake by moderate amounts (approximately 250–500 calories per day)? Can the patient make further improvements in the overall quality of the diet?

- *Change in weight*. Weight maintenance or modest weight loss would be an appropriate outcome. If the patient's weight increases, have positive changes in food selection and/or exercise been made? Or is weight gain related to rehydration as a result of improved glycemic control?

- *Achievement of short-term goals*. Determine whether the patient has achieved short-term goals established in previous visits and whether they are willing to set new goals.

- *Intervention*. Identify and recommend the changes in food and exercise that can improve the outcome, such as meal spacing; appropriate portions and choices; meal and snack schedule; and exercise frequency/duration/type/timing, including exercise after meals to reduce post-prandial hyperglycemia. Adjust food plan if necessary based on patient feedback. Reset short-term goals based on recommendations.

Self-management skill review. Do any survival self-management skills need to be reviewed (e.g. hypoglycemia prevention, illness management)? Are continuing self-management skills needed (e.g. use of alcohol, restaurant food choices, label reading, handling special occasions, and other information to promote self-care and flexibility)?

Set follow-up plans. A second follow-up visit is recommended if:

1. patient is newly diagnosed
2. patient is having difficulty making lifestyle changes
3. additional support and encouragement is required
4. major goal is weight loss

If no immediate follow-up is needed, schedule the next appointment within 3–4 months.

Communication/summary to referral source. A written documentation of the nutrition assessment and intervention should be completed and placed in the patient's medical record. This documentation should include summary of assessment information, education intervention, short-term goals, specific actions recommended, and plans for further follow-up, including additional education topics to be reviewed.

Follow-up visits. All follow-up visits should include weight in light clothing without shoes; changes in medication; and changes in exercise habits. Review SMBG records, including frequency of testing, time of testing and results. Exam current blood pressure level and HbA_{1c} value. Complete a 24 hour food recall, and check for food plan problems and/or concerns.

Again, evaluate whether therapy is working or if change is needed, based on the following:

- Improvement in HbA_{1c} or at target.

- Changes in blood glucose values – is there a downward trend in blood glucose values? Have there been episodes of hypoglycemia? Is it related to exercise or skipped meals? Is there a pattern of hyperglycemia? Are post-prandial blood glucose values less than 160 mg/dL (8.9 mmol/L)? What percent of blood glucose values are within the target range? An overall decrease in blood glucose values of 15–30 mg/dL (0.8 to 1.7 mmol/L) per month should be obtained.

- Changes in exercise and/or activity levels – patient has gradually increased physical activity with a minimum goal of 15–20 minutes of physical activity three to four times a week. Is the patient willing or able to do more?

- Change in food habits – patient eats meals and snacks on a regular basis and makes appropriate food choices in reasonable portions. If calorie intake has been excessive, can patient reduce calorie intake by moderate amounts (approximately 250–500 calories per day)? Can the patient make further improvements in the overall quality of the diet?

- Weight maintenance or modest weight loss would be an appropriate outcome. If patient's weight has increased, have positive changes in food selection and/or exercise been made?

- Determine whether patient has achieved short- and long-term goals. Do these goals remain appropriate for the patient, or should new ones be established?

- During the adjust phase, therapy is modified to accelerate reaching the target blood glucose level. Increase in exercise levels, decrease in caloric intake, and other strategies may be enlisted to ensure further glucose reduction at an accelerated rate. The period of experimentation with steps to reduce blood glucose requires SMBG four times per day and monthly visits. HbA_{1c} levels should begin to respond to the overall lower blood glucose during the first month. However, not until the end of the second month will the impact of the initial therapy be fully reflected in the HbA_{1c} levels. From there on, reduction by at least 0.5 percentage points in HbA_{1c} per month should continue until targets (HbA_{1c} within 1.0 percentage point of the upper limit of normal) are achieved.

Follow-up intervention. Too often members of the healthcare team other than the physician are reluctant to recommend changes in therapy. This leads to both reduced efficiency and needless error in treatment. If any of the following are uncovered by any team member (especially dietitian or nurse), consider contacting provider for immediate alteration in therapy:

- blood glucose levels (average SMBG) have not shown a downward trend

- blood glucose levels (average SMBG) have not reached the target range by 3–6 months

- HbA_{1c} has not shown a downward trend

- HbA_{1c} has not reached target range by 3–6 months

- Hypertension (blood pressure $> 130/80$ mm Hg) has not responded to dietary changes, weight loss, and/or exercise changes

- Lipids outside target range after 4–6 months of nutrition intervention (see Chapter 8)

Note: If laboratory data show no improvement and/or the patient is not willing to make food and exercise behavior changes, a change in therapy will be required. If the patient is treated with an oral agent, consider a combination of oral agents, combination oral agent-insulin, or insulin therapy. Otherwise, consider referral to a specialty team. If medical nutrition therapy fails, be certain that long-term goals, ongoing care, weight maintenance or loss, and overall glucose and lipid control are discussed. Reset short-term goals and review self-management skills. Determine whether any survival or continuing level self-management skills need to be addressed or reviewed. Additional follow-up visits are recommended if the patient needs and/or desires assistance with additional lifestyle changes, weight loss, and/or further self-management skill training. Written documentation of the intervention should include a summary of outcomes of nutrition intervention (medical outcomes, food and exercise behavior changes), self-management skill instruction/review provided, recommendations based upon outcomes, and plans for follow-up.

Medical Nutrition Therapy/Maintain

This may prove to be the most difficult phase to sustain. During this phase, blood glucose and HbA_{1c} target levels have been achieved. Patients often reduce SMBG testing and abandon their food and exercise plans. If at any time the patient exceeds the SMBG or HbA_{1c} levels, return the patient to the adjust treatment phase. Consider referral for diabetes and nutrition education every 6–12 months. Ongoing education that reinforces the importance of a food and exercise/activity plan is a critical factor in helping patients maintain glycemic control.

Exercise assessment

The importance of exercise in restoring a balance between food intake and energy expenditure is paramount in diabetes management. Increased activity level improves insulin sensitivity, which has a direct impact on glycemic control. Some studies have been able to quantify this relationship by showing that 6 weeks of regular exercise will result in an average drop in mean blood glucose of between 30 and 45 mg/dL (1.7–2.5 mmol/L).[33] This is equivalent to a drop of 1–1.5 percentage points HbA_{1c}.

Developing an exercise prescription begins with assessing the patient's cardiovascular fitness and making appropriate adjustments based on age, weight, and medical history. (see Figure 4.9). As shown in Photo 4.1, one option for assessing a patient's overall fitness level is to measure the amount of oxygen that can be delivered to the body (VO_2 max). Often a registered dietitian or exercise specialist can be very helpful. In his or her absence, common sense plays a major role. Exercises should be comfortable, frequent, consistent, and reasonable. They should be based on the patient's ability and motivation. Fitting exercise into the lifestyle of most patients requires some innovative thinking. Some exercises can be done sitting, standing, and even lying down. Most are not stressful and are designed for the older patient. Aerobic (walking, swimming) and anaerobic (lifting) exercises are both important. Setting the long-term goal between 50 and 75 per cent maximal heart capacity adjusted for age is a safe and efficacious plan.

Exercise may need to vary with the seasons. While walking outdoors is fine in good weather, walking indoors in shopping centers is best for inclement weather. Exercise must be combined with lower caloric intake. (Walking to the bakery is not good exercise if it results in increased caloric intake.) Start the exercise prescription with intermediate goals using low-intensity warm-up and cool-down exercises. Begin with walking and lifting exercises using the daily routine as the guide (e.g. walking instead of driving, carrying items). During the start period, maintain weekly contact until a pattern has been achieved. The use of exercise to reduce blood glucose level is less likely to occur initially unless the food plan has changed as well.

See Appendix A.16 through A.18 for a detailed outline of exercise plan goals, follow-up and education topics.

If the exercise prescription is ineffective, consider resetting the goals. Determine the patient's readiness to do exercise, re-educate as to the relationship between exercise and glucose control, and consider referral to an exercise specialist.

Oral Agent Stage

Oral agent therapy should be considered under three circumstances. First, consider oral agents for the newly diagnosed patient with type 2 diabetes with a fasting plasma glucose between 200 and 300 mg/dL (11.1 and 16.7 mmol/L) or a casual plasma glucose between 250 and 350 mg/dL (13.9 and 19.4 mmol/L). When plasma glucose reaches these levels, insulin resistance, excess hepatic glucose output, and insufficient insulin secretion are likely causes of persistent hyperglycemia. Since medical nutrition therapy alone usually will lower glucose by no more than

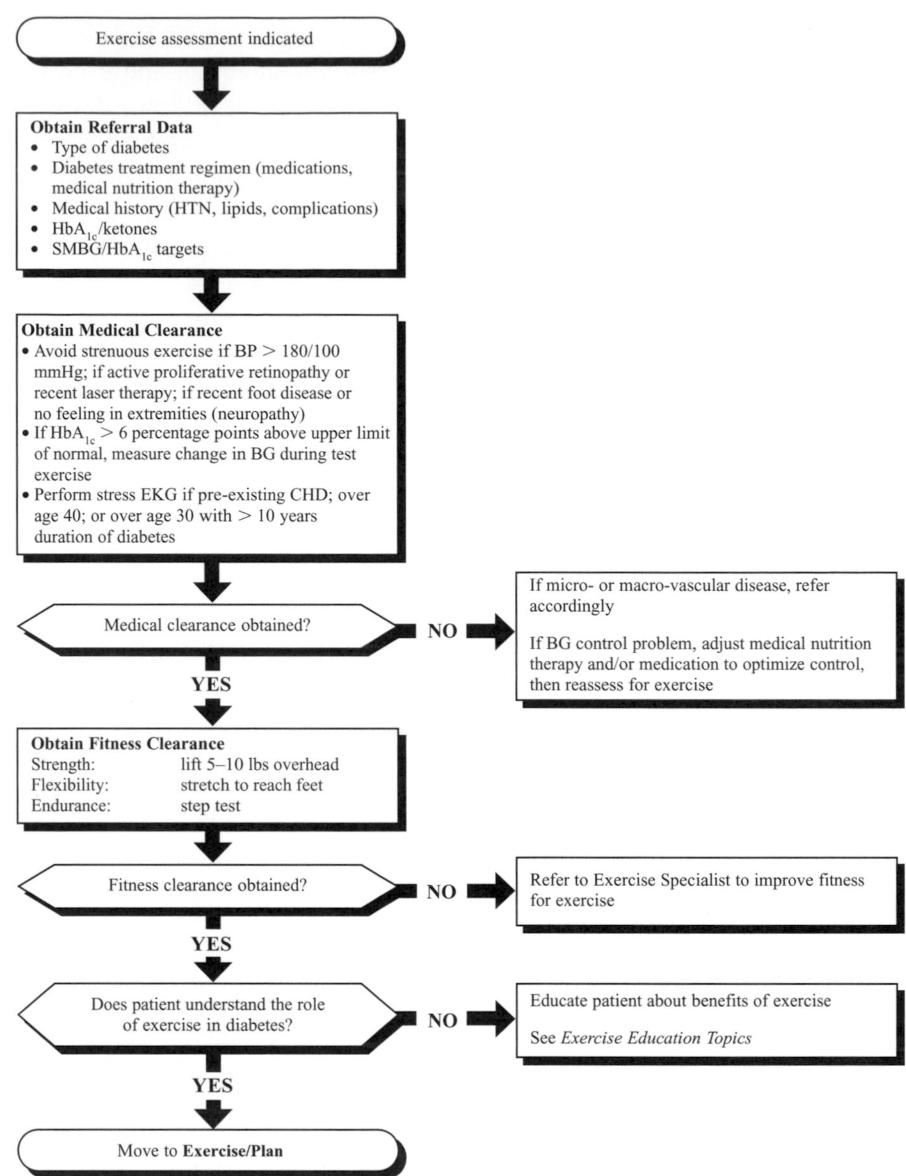

Figure 4.9 Exercise Assessment DecisionPath

50–75 mg/dL (2.8–4.2 mmol/L), a pharmacologic agent is needed. Second, consider an oral agent when medical nutrition therapy fails to improve glycemic control by at least 0.5 percentage point HbA_{1c} monthly. Third, consider an oral agent as a therapy to replace low-dose insulin (< 0.2 U/kg) if the patient has achieved glycemic targets.

Five classifications of oral agents are currently available for managing type 2 diabetes: sulfonylureas (glyburide, glipizide, and glimepiride), biguanides (metformin), alpha-glucosidase inhibitors (acarbose, miglitol), thiazolidinediones (pioglitazone, rosiglitazone), and meglitinides (repaglinide, nateglinide). Selecting the appropriate oral agent has become a very critical part of good diabetes management.

Oral agent selection and contraindications

Before considering initiation of an oral agent, certain factors must be addressed.

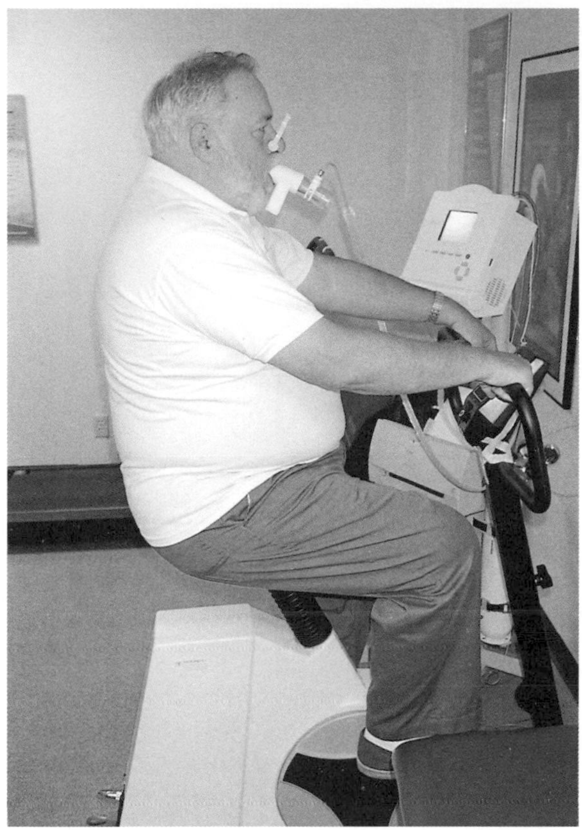

Photo 4.1 Exercise assessment: Determining VO_2 max

Step 1. The first step should be a review of the contraindications, regulations and other factors that might remove an agent for consideration. In the United States, the Food and Drug Administration (FDA) regulates the use of pharmacological agents. In general, the regulations are applicable to other countries. However, each country may have its own regulations, which need to be considered.

- Currently, metformin is the only oral agent that has been approved by the FDA for use in non-pregnant individuals with type 2 diabetes or insulin resistance (polycystic ovary syndrome) under the age of 18. For these individuals see Chapter 5.
- Only one oral agent, glyburide, has been reported effective in controlling hyperglycemia in pregnancy and not to pass the placental barrier (see Chapter 7).
- Since oral agents are either metabolized in, or cleared by, the liver, they are not recommended for patients with severe liver disease (see Figure 4.10). Thiazolidinediones, in particular, may cause liver damage. Therefore, serum transaminase levels must be monitored before the initiation of and during thiazolidinedione therapy.
- The next factor to consider is serum creatinine since some oral agents are cleared by, the kidney. Thiazolidinediones and meglitinides may be used with underlying kidney disease (serum creatinine > 2.0 mg/dL or 180 μmol/L). When serum creatinine is between 1.4 and 2.0 mg/dL (120 and 180 μmol/L), all current oral agents except metformin may be used. Only when serum creatinine is below 1.4 mg/dL (120 μmol/L) can metformin be initiated.
- Some patients may have allergies to sulfa containing medications (sulfonylureas).
- The gastro-intestinal side effects of alpha-glucosidase inhibitors and metformin can be severe and should be explained in detail before initiation

Step 2. The second step is to determine whether one or a combination of oral agents is needed. Generally, when HbA_{1c} is below 9 per cent monotherapy is used. Between 9 and 11 per cent a combination of agents from two different classifications can be used, such as sulfonlyurea and metformin.

Step 3. The third step is to determine whether the underlying defect is primarily insulin resistance or insulin deficiency. At diagnosis most individuals with insulin resistance are overweight or obese – BMI > 27 kg/m^2 – and therefore would be started on either metformin or a thiazolidinedione. The choice between the two is not

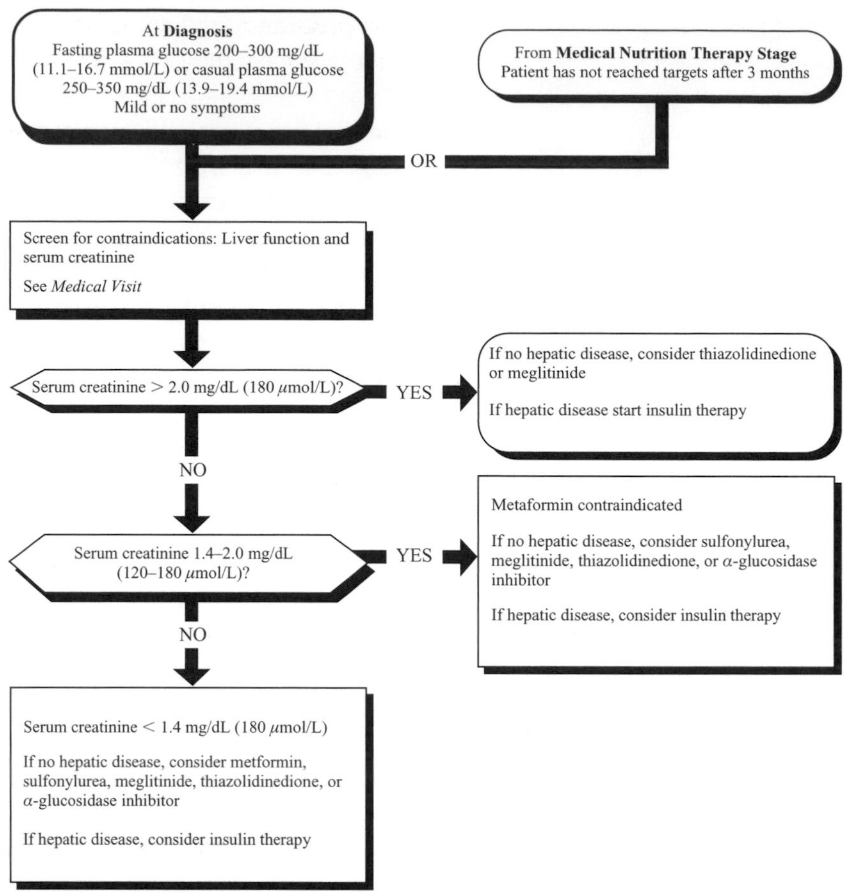

Indicators for Use of Oral Agents

	METFORMIN	SULFONYLUREA	α-GLUCOSIDASE INHIBITOR	THIAZOLIDINEDIONE	MEGLITINIDES
Positive	Obesity Dyslipidemia Insulin resistance	FPG > 250 mg/dL (13.9 mmol/L) CPG > 300 mg/dL (16.7 mmol/L)	Post-meal hyperglycemia (with failure on metformin)	Obesity Dyslipidemia Insulin resistance	Flexible meal schedule Renal insufficiency Post-meal hyperglycemia
Negative	Lactic acidosis Hypoxia > 80 years old CHF	Hypoglycemia Weight gain Sulfa allergy (rarely)	Gastro-intestinal disturbances	Edema Liver disease Altered metabolism of oral contraceptives Weight gain	Hypoglycemia Weight gain

Note: Oral agents are not approved for use in pregnancy.

Figure 4.10 Oral agent selection for individuals 18 years and older

clear. Because metformin suppresses hepatic glucose output, it is often targeted at fasting plasma glucose, whereas the thiazolidinedione is better suited to post-prandial blood glucose abnormalities. Since both drugs are non-hypoglycemic, there is little concern for low blood glucose levels. Both drugs have some cardiovascular benefit by improving the lipid profile. Secretagogues should be considered in lean patients with relative insulin deficiency.

Oral Agent/Start

OA–(OA)–(OA)–0

Initiation of any oral agent should begin with the minimum dose, independent of the patient's weight. Oral agents are generally given before breakfast and/or the evening meal. The meglitinides are rapid acting and meant to be given before each meal. The code for all oral agent administration is provided above. The first OA (without parenthesis) denotes the most popular time (pre-breakfast) for OA administration. The OA in parenthesis denotes optional or alternate times. Two factors should be considered when using sulfonylureas: (1) risk of hypoglycemia and (2) allergic reaction (rare). Generally, oral hypoglycemic agents (sulfonylureas, repaglinide and nateglinide) are safe, in terms of the risk of hypoglycemia, at this low dosage level. Use caution in patients with a history of allergies to sulfa drugs. Since metformin, thiazolidinedione, and alpha-glucosidase inhibitors do not stimulate pancreatic insulin secretion, they are not considered hypoglycemic drugs. However, since they may be used in the future with other hypoglycemic agents or insulin, precautions should be taken to monitor blood glucose frequently when starting any of these drugs. Additionally, these drugs have other contraindications (see Chapter 3 for details). Metformin can have acute gastrointestinal side effects, and, because it is a biguanide like phenformin, patients with pre-existing pulmonary, kidney, liver, or cardiovascular disease should not be given this drug because of the increased risk of lactic acidosis. Alpha-glucosidase inhibitors, too, have side effects, particularly gastric distress (abdominal pain, diarrhea, and flatulence).

Thiazolidinediones have been associated with idiosyncratic liver damage requiring serum transaminase levels to be monitored before starting therapy and throughout the course of treatment. See Chapter 3 for details on serum transaminase monitoring for the different thiazolidinediones.

It is no longer necessary to avoid all oral agents in pregnant women or women with child-bearing potential. One agent, glyburide, has been used very successfully to control hyperglycemia throughout pregnancy. As it does not pass the placental barrier, it should have no deleterious effect on the developing fetus. Recently, metformin has been successfully used for women with type 2 diabetes and PCOS who are seeking to ovulate.

It is important to confirm the defect(s) before selecting one of the oral agents. The identification of the principal underlying defect(s) relies on more data than often are available at diagnosis. Ideally, three forms of information would be helpful at the point of diagnosis: fasting plasma glucose, HbA_{1c}, and plasma insulin level. Generally, only a casual or fasting plasma glucose is available. In that case, follow the Type 2 Diabetes Master DecisionPath using the glucose criteria from the diagnostic tests. If at diagnosis a baseline HbA_{1c} and fasting plasma glucose are available, then consider the information in Table 4.9 to guide selection of the appropriate therapy. If insulin level is available, refer to the discussion "Insulin Level."

Combinations of oral agents can be given immediately following diagnosis. When the fasting plasma glucose is between 250 and 300 mg/dL (13.8 and 16.7 mmol/L), if HbA_{1c} is greater than three percentage points above normal at diagnosis, consider starting a secretagogue and sensitizer. For extremely insulin resistant patients, a combination of metformin and thiazolidinedione should be considered. If a less optimal therapy is selected because of a lack of sufficient data at diagnosis, once in treatment use the SMBG, HbA_{1c} (and, if feasible, insulin levels) to detect the underlying defect and to adjust the treatment appropriately.

Insulin level. Use these modifications to Table 4.9. In most individuals at diagnosis there are morphological signs of insulin resistance. The patient has central body obesity, with a waist to hip ratio greater than one. Corroborating insulin resistance would be the finding of higher than normal plasma insulin levels. As mentioned previously, insulin resistance is treated with insulin sensitizing agents. If, alternatively, plasma insulin levels are substantially below the lower limit of the normal range, consider initiating insulin therapy. In this case, exogenous insulin will be required to overcome absolute insulin deficiency and any residual insulin resistance.

For patients with no pre-existing contraindications (especially no liver or kidney disease), the choice of alpha-glucosidase inhibitor, metformin, thiazolidinediones, sulfonylurea, or meglitinide should be based on the degree of obesity, risk of hypoglycemia, and known allergies to certain

Table 4.9 Therapy selection at diagnosis using HbA_{1c} and fasting plasma glucose

	HbA_{1c} within < 1.5 percentage points above upper limit of normal	**HbA_{1c} 1.5–3 percentage points above upper limit of normal**	**HbA_{1c} > 3–5 percentage points above upper limit of normal**	**HbA_{1c} > 5 percentage points above upper limit of normal**
Fasting plasma glucose 126–199 mg/dL (7.0–11.0 mmol/L)	Start Medical Nutrition Therapy Stage	Start Medical Nutrition Therapy Stage; consider Oral Agent Stage (thiazolidinedione, sulfonylurea, or alpha-glucosidase inhibitor)	Start Oral Agent Stage (sulfonylurea, repaglinide, nateglinide, metformin, or thiazolidinedione)	Start Physiologic Insulin Stage 4
Fasting plasma glucose 200–300 mg/dL (11.1–16.7 mmol/L)	Start Medical Nutrition Therapy stage; consider oral agent stage (metformin thiazolidinedione, or alpha-glucosidase inhibitor)	Start Oral Agent Stage (metformin, sulfonylurea, repaglinide, nateglinide or thiazolidinedione)	Start Oral Agent Stage; consider starting Insulin: Stage 2, 3, or 4* (metformin, thiazolidinedione, sulfonylurea, repaglinide or nateglinide)	Start Physiologic Insulin Stage 4
Fasting plasma glucose 301–400 mg/dL (16.7–22.2 mmol/L)	Start Oral Agent Stage (metformin, thiazolidinedione, sulfonylurea, or repaglinide)	Start Oral Agent Stage; consider starting Insulin: Stage 2, 3, or 4*	Start Insulin: Stage 3 or 4*	Start Physiologic Insulin Stage 4
Fasting plasma glucose > 400 mg/dL (> 22.2 mmol/L)	Start Insulin Stage 3	Start Insulin: Stage 3 or 4*	Start Physiologic Insulin Stage 4	Start Physiologic Insulin Stage 4

*Same as Physiologic Insulin Stage 4

drugs. In general, European, Latin American, and Canadian experience with metformin promote its use in obese patients over use of sulfonylureas. This is especially true if the patient is at risk of hypoglycemia. If, however, the patient has a history of gastrointestinal problems, metformin may exacerbate this condition and should either be avoided or used cautiously. Scientifically, alpha-glucosidase inhibitors make the most sense if the defect can be isolated to an elevated post-prandial rise in blood glucose levels.[34] Since each of these is a starting therapy at diagnosis, patients should be told that it is likely to be changed once additional information from SMBG and serial HbA_{1c} is available.

The food plan and exercise program for an individual starting at diagnosis on an oral agent follows the same principles as for the patient on medical nutrition therapy alone (see Figures 4.8, 4.9, and 4.10). Special attention should be paid, however, to patients on sulfonylureas, repaglinide, alpha-glucosidase inhibitors, and metformin. Because sulfonylureas and meglitinides can cause hypoglycemia, it is important to emphasize that the patient must maintain a consistent food plan and avoid skipping meals. Gastric distress from either alpha-glucosidase inhibitors or metformin cannot easily be overcome by altering the diet. The oral agents available as monotherapies or combination therapies are summarized in Table 4.10.

Follow-up. During the first week the patient should do SMBG four times each day, preferably at varying times in order to produce a complete picture of metabolic response to the oral agent. At the end of 1 week's testing, review SMBG data to determine whether the blood glucose has been altered and if any hypoglycemic episodes have occurred. If average blood glucose decreases by more than 10 per cent continue with the minimum dose. Schedule the next visit for 2 weeks following initiation of the oral agent.

Oral Agent/Adjust
OA–(OA)–(OA)–0

If the SMBG has not been lowered significantly (approximately 20 per cent) after 2–4 weeks, increase the dose of oral agent. Depending upon the specific agent, the increased dose may be

Table 4.10 Oral agents

	Size (mg)	Dose (mg)	Duration	Per Day
First-generation Sulfonylureas				
Tolbutamide	500	500–3000	6–12 hours	2–3
Acetohexamide	250, 500	250–1500	12–24 hours	1–2
Tolazamide	100, 250, 500	100–1000	12–24 hours	1–2
Chlorpropamide	100, 250	100–500	up to 60 hours	1
Second-generation Sulfonylureas				
Glyburide (Glibenclamide)	1.25, 2.5, 5.0	1.25–20	24 hours	1–2
Glyburide (micronized)	1.5, 3	0.075–12	24 hours	1–2
Glipizide	5, 10	5–40	10–24 hours	1–2
GlipizideXL (extended release)	5, 10	5–20	24 hours	1
Third-generation Sulfonylureas				
Glimepiride	1.0, 2.0, 3.0, 4.0, 8.0	1–8	24 hours	1
Alpha-glucosidase Inhibitors				
Acarbose	25, 50, 100	25–300	3–5 hours	1–3 (before meals)
Miglitol	25, 50, 100	25–300	3–5 hours	1–3 (before meals)
Biguanides				
Metformin	500, 850, 1000	500–2550	10+	1–3
Meglitinides				
Repaglinide	0.5, 1, 2	0.5–4	4–6 hours	1–4 (before each meal)
Nateglinide	60, 120	120–480	4–6 hours	1–4 (before each meal)
Thiazolidinediones				
Pioglitazone	15, 30, 45	15–45	24 hours	1
Rosiglitazone	2, 4, 8	4–8	12–24 hours	1–2

given at a different time, as shown in Table 4.10. Be sure to confirm that the original medical nutrition therapy is being followed. Continue this therapy for 1–2 weeks using SMBG data to determine impact. Most oral agents can be adjusted weekly. At most no more than two weeks should elapse without adjustment in oral agents if blood glucose does not respond. Only the thiazolidinediones require a longer period (1–2 months) before blood glucose change occurs. Staged Diabetes Management is designed to permit up to four dosage increases (depending upon the oral agent) before the maximum dose is reached. Note, that the clinically effective dose is not necessarily the maximum dose. For example, the clinically effective dose of sulfonylureas is approximately two-thirds maximum dose and the clinically effective dose of metformin is 2000 mg/day, not the maximum dose of 2550 mg/day. Because individual differences to dose response exist, close monitoring with verified SMBG data is essential during this phase. For patients on sulfonylurea or repaglinide, episodes of hypoglycemia may occur as the dose is increased.

Glycosylated hemoglobin values should begin to decrease due to lowered blood glucose levels within 4–8 weeks following initiation of treatment. If HbA_{1c} level shows no improvement, consider the following.

- Hemoglobinopathy, such as sickle cell trait
- Increase daily testing
- Patient not adhering to diabetes regimen

The long-term HbA_{1c} target should be set to within one percentage point of the upper limit of normal with at least a 0.5 percentage point reduction each month. If the current average SMBG is $>$ 250 mg/dL (13.9 mmol/L), expect a 30 mg/dL (1.7 mmol/L) decrease in blood glucose over the next month and a one percentage point decline in HbA_{1c}. If this is not accomplished, increase the dose of the oral agent according to the guide. If the maximum dose is reached, consider combination therapy or insulin therapy.

Oral Agent/Maintain
OA–(OA)–(OA)–0

If the patient has reached the therapeutic goal on the oral agent, treatment now turns to maintenance. During this phase, attempt to maintain glycemic control within target range without making significant demands on the patient. SMBG testing schedules and frequency of contact with the health care professional are individualized. Insufficient contact (especially for the elderly) may cause the patient to lose interest in the intensified treatment and become less likely to follow the therapeutic regimen, thereby worsening glycemic control. For some patients close contact, frequent visits, and careful assessment of behaviors related to the treatment regimen are the cornerstones of good care. Minimally, all patients should be seen every 3–4 months. Assessment for complications (Chapters 8 and 9) and evaluation of the overall impact of the therapy on glycemic control should be continued.

During both the adjust and maintain phases, patients may experience transient weight gain (3–5 pounds) with sulfonylurea, meglitinide, or thiazolidinedione therapy due to improved uptake of glucose as glycemic control improves. This is expected and can be reversed once near-normal levels of glucose are achieved. If the patient reports symptoms of hypoglycemia, consider moving some meal related carbohydrate to snacks, or add a carbohydrate choice to snacks.

Alternate mono and combination oral agent therapy

Table 4.11 provides a general guide as to whether to change the oral agent, add a second agent, or move to insulin therapies. SMBG and HbA_{1c} data are necessary to detect the principal defect and to then select the appropriate change in the current therapy. Always consider the principal defect first. Since each class of oral agents works differently, they may be combined if one or the other has failed to improve control. In general, maintain the maximum or clinically effective dose of the current oral agent and slowly add the second oral

Table 4.11

Current Therapy	Add one of these pharmacological agents: SULFONYLUREA	METFORMIN	THIAZOLIDINE-DIONE	REPAGLINIDE OR NATEGLINIDE	α-GLUCOSIDASE INHIBITOR	BEDTIME NPH OR GLARGINE INSULIN*
SULFONYLUREA		✓ **Positive:** obesity, dyslipidemia, AM FPG >200 mg/dL **Negative:** CHF, renal disease, lactic acidosis, GI disturbances	✓ **Positive:** Insulin resistance, AM FPG >200 mg/dL **Negative:** liver disease, peripheral edema	**Not Indicated**	**Positive:** Elevated post-prandial glucose **Negative:** Limited glucose lowering, GI disturbances	**Positive:** Transition therapy to multi-dose insulin, AM FPG >300 mg/dL **Negative:** Minimal clinical benefit
METFORMIN	✓ **Positive:** FPG >250 mg/dL, CPG >300 mg/dL, consider in lean patients, **Negative:** weight gain, hypoglycemia, sulfa allergy		✓ **Positive:** severe insulin resistance, obesity, persistent dyslipidemia **Negative:** liver disease, peripheral edema	✓ **Positive:** Consider in lean patients, elevated post-prandial glucose, variable meal schedule **Negative:** hypoglycemia, weight gain	**Positive:** elevated post-prandial glucose **Negative:** Limited glucose lowering, GI disturbances	✓ **Positive:** Best with bedtime NPH, limited weight gain **Negative:** may not lower post-meal glucose
THIAZOLIDINE-DIONE	✓ **Positive:** FPG >250 mg/dL, CPG >300 mg/dL, consider in lean patients, **Negative:** weight gain, hypoglycemia, sulfa allergy	✓ **Positive:** obesity, dyslipidemia, severe insulin resistance **Negative:** CHF, renal disease, lactic acidosis, GI disturbances		**Not Indicated**	**Not Indicated**	**Positive:** AM FPG >300 mg/dL **Negative:** may not lower post-meal glucose
REPAGLINIDE OR NATEGLINIDE	**Not Indicated**	✓ **Positive:** obesity, dyslipidemia **Negative:** CHF, renal disease, lactic acidosis, GI disturbances	**Not Indicated**		**Not Indicated**	**Not Indicated**
α-GLUCOSIDASE INHIBITOR	**Positive:** Consider in lean patients, FPG >250 mg/dL, CPG >300 mg/dL **Negative:** weight gain, hypoglycemia, sulfa allergy	**Positive:** obesity, dyslipidemia **Negative:** CHF, renal disease, lactic acidosis, GI disturbances	**Not Indicated**	**Not Indicated**		**Positive:** AM FPG >300 mg/dL **Negative:** minimal clinical benefit
INSULIN STAGE 2, 3, 4	**Not Indicated**	✓ **Positive:** limited weight gain, insulin dose >0.7 U/kg **Negative:** CHF, renal disease, lactic acidosis, GI disturbances	✓ **Positive:** Dyslipidemia, insulin dose >0.7 U/kg **Negative:** liver disease, peripheral edema	**Not Indicated**	**Positive:** No systemic side-effects **Negative:** Limited glucose lowering, GI disturbances	

*Most patients using only bedtime insulin will benefit most from multi-dose insulin therapy

✓ = preferred combination

agent, starting with its minimum dose. Increase the dose of the second oral agent if glycemic targets are not being achieved until maximum dose is reached.

Starting with combination oral agent therapy

For some individuals a combination of substantial insulin resistance and insulin deficiency are present at diagnosis. These individuals are usually obese with HbA_{1c} between 9 and 11 per cent. In most cases this is due to the discovery of diabetes late in its natural history. A combination of an insulin sensitizer and secretagogues at the initiation of therapy targets both the insulin resistance and the insulin deficiency. Both agents should be started at minimum dose and slowly increased until the target blood glucose is reached. Combinations of drug categories that exist in one tablet, such as metformin and glyburide or metformin and rosiglitazone may also be used at the start of treatment.

Failure of all oral agent therapies

If oral agent therapy fails to bring the patient into glycemic control, initiation of combination oral agent–insulin therapy or Insulin Stage 2, 3, or 4 will be required. The Type 2 Diabetes Master DecisionPath should have already been shown to the patient, and insulin therapy should have been explained as an option. If this is not the case, it is important to reiterate the need to consider alternative therapies since it is unlikely that continuing with oral agents at their maximum dose will improve control any further. Indeed, if insulin therapy is not initiated, any persistent hyperglycemia places the patient in acute risk of glucose toxicity and at a greater risk of developing macrovascular and microvascular complications (see Chapters 8 and 9). Under such circumstances, exogenous insulin is required since β-cell production of insulin has been severely and perhaps permanently affected. If hyperglycemia is allowed to continue, the sequence of glucose toxicity and β-cell weakening will worsen to a point where production of insulin is seriously compromised.

The next section details the use of insulin combined with an oral agent. The selection requires a careful evaluation to individualize the therapy.

The addition of insulin to an oral agent

In patients previously treated by oral agents, insulin may be introduced as an adjunct to oral agent therapy. This is preferable for those patients who were started on an oral agent, reached the maximum effective dose, and were given a second oral agent, but still were not able to achieve glycemic targets. For most other patients, especially those in whom mean fasting SMBG exceeds 300 mg/dL (16.7 mmol/L), starting insulin as the monotherapy is more appropriate than trying other oral agents. For the latter circumstance, skip this step and follow the DecisionPaths for insulin therapy. In the section following insulin therapies, rationale and methods for the addition of insulin sensitizers to the current insulin therapy are reviewed.

Combination Oral Agent–Insulin Therapy/Start OA–(OA)–(OA)–N or G

For some time researchers and clinicians have been examining the efficacy of bedtime insulin and daytime oral agents.

While virtually every oral agent has undergone some evaluation with insulin, the most frequently tested are metformin and the sulfonylureas. The purpose of sulfonylurea and insulin is to optimize the benefits of both. A meta-analysis of controlled studies using sulfonylurea and insulin in combination demonstrated improvements in glycemic control when compared with insulin monotherapy.[35] Since insulin is an effective means of lowering blood glucose levels, other oral agents that target insulin resistance by increasing insulin sensitivity (metformin and thiazolidinedione) can be used in combination with insulin. Acarbose has also been approved for use with insulin. In this case the purpose of acarbose is to reduce the post-prandial blood glucose rise after a meal while primarily relying on insulin to provide for basal insulin requirements.

When oral agents alone or in combination fail to restore near euglycemia, combination therapies that include bedtime intermediate (N) or long-acting (glargine) insulin are often considered. It is well recognized that insulin, when used properly, will significantly improve glycemic control at virtually any level of hyperglycemia. However, this is at the risk of hypoglycemia, especially when high doses of insulin are required or when the patient chooses to skip a meal. It is for this reason that bedtime low-dose insulin is combined with an oral agent to lower blood glucose overnight while reducing the risk of hypoglycemia. It is also well known that multiple defects are at work in type 2 diabetes.

While mild insulin deficiency and insulin resistance may be addressed by oral agents, often these are insufficient to overcome an absolute reduction in endogenous insulin secretion. In such cases, addition of bedtime low-dose insulin will supplement endogenous insulin. The current bedtime insulins have substantial differences that need to be considered before they are used. N is an intermediate-acting insulin with a peak action at between 4 and 8 hours after administration. Taken overnight, it may lead to early morning hypoglycemia. Glargine (G) is a long acting analog which lasts up to 24 hours and has no peak action. The latter, therefore, acts more like basal insulin and may be used as such. Use of either insulin places more responsibility with the patient. It is, for example, necessary to monitor blood glucose before each insulin injection. With N it may be necessary to measure blood glucose at 3 AM (or whenever hypoglycemic symptoms appear). Because the insulins may be added to non-hypoglycemic oral agents (such as metformin and thiazolidinediones), monitoring of blood glucose for hypoglycemia must be increased.

Adding insulin to sulfonylurea therapy. Begin by reducing the current dose of sulfonylurea by one-half. Give this amount in the morning. Next, introduce one injection of N or G insulin at bedtime, or approximately 2–3 hours after the evening meal. The amount of insulin should be low (0.1 U/kg) at the start. Since there is always a risk of hypoglycemia (less nocturnal hypoglycemia with G) with the introduction of insulin, move a carbohydrate choice from the evening meal to bedtime. Do not add to the total caloric intake as this will eventually be the cause of weight gain and thus may discourage further reliance on insulin. Make certain that SMBG is measured before each meal, before the bedtime insulin is administered, and, if using N insulin, at 3 AM at least once during the first week to evaluate the impact on overnight blood glucose levels. If nocturnal hypoglycemia is discovered, consider changing from N to G. Adjust insulin dose based on patterns of fasting blood glucose.

Adding insulin to acarbose, metformin, or thiazolidindione therapy. Continue the current dose of oral agent and add bedtime N or G insulin at 0.1 U/kg. Since there is a risk of hypoglycemia with the introduction of insulin, move a carbohydrate choice to the time the bedtime insulin is given. Do not supplement the food plan with additional calories. Make certain that SMBG is performed before meals, before the bedtime insulin is administered, and at 3 AM at least once during the first week to evaluate the impact on overnight blood glucose levels.

Combination Oral Agent–Insulin Therapy/Adjust OA–(OA)–(OA)–N or G

If fasting blood glucose fails to decrease during the first week of therapy, increase N or G in increments of 2–4 units based on patterns of blood glucose until fasting glycemic targets are achieved or 0.4 U/kg is reached. Note, that often significant amounts of bedtime insulin are required due to the combination of insulin resistance and excess hepatic glucose output. Regular or rapid-acting insulin may be added to the evening meal if the 2 to 3 AM blood glucose continues to remain high. Reducing carbohydrate intake at the evening meal may also assist in lowering fasting blood glucose.

Throughout the oral agent–insulin therapy period, be prepared to reduce or increase the insulin as dictated by blood glucose levels and to maintain the current dose of the oral agent. If the intent is to transition the patient to insulin only therapy, slowly reduce the oral agent and replace with pre-meal R or RA insulin. If G insulin is used as the basal insulin, then use the RA insulin analogs for pre-meal insulin. Within 1 month both daily blood glucose and HbA_{1c} should show improvement. If the overall blood glucose has improved marginally but fasting blood glucose has remained high, increase N or G insulin at bedtime up to 0.4 U/kg. If no improvement in fasting blood glucose has been noted, insulin-only therapies should be considered (see guidelines for initiating insulin therapy found in the next section).

Combination Oral Agent–Insulin Therapy/ Maintain

OA–(OA)–(OA)–N or G

Because oral agent–insulin therapy is generally not used as a "final" treatment, the long-term impact on the patient is unknown. Theoretically, it should help the patient in two ways: exogenous insulin should rest the pancreas while ensuring improved glycemic control; the insulin sensitizing agent (metformin and thiazolidinedione) should reduce insulin resistance. If the combination is with an insulin secretagogue, the benefits are less clear, except to reduce reliance on multiple injections of insulin. Lacking controlled studies, it remains to be determined whether combined therapy is better than insulin alone. An important point to keep in mind is to not eliminate SMBG during the maintain phase and to monitor for weight gain.

Failure of all combination therapies

When combination therapies fail, the next stage is insulin. The Type 2 Diabetes Master DecisionPath should have already been shown to the patient, and insulin therapy should have been discussed as an option if combination therapy failed to bring the patient into glycemic control. If this is not the case, it is important to reiterate the need to consider alternative therapies since it is unlikely that continuing with combination therapy will improve control. Staged Diabetes Management does not recommend treating a patient with type 2 diabetes with more than two oral agents in combination because these individuals are likely to be both insulin resistant and significantly insulin deficient with insufficient endogenous insulin production. No combination of oral agents will be able to overcome the insulin deficiency at this stage. Should oral agents be continued and hyperglycemia result, there is an added danger of severe glucose toxicity and thus a "temporary weakening" of β-cells.

Insulin therapy

Because initiation of insulin is a major step in diabetes therapy, it may be helpful to review with the patient some key principles of his or her care and the Type 2 Diabetes Master DecisionPath (see Figure 4.6). It is important to note that patients starting insulin may need a revised food plan and exercise program synchronized to insulin action.

Hyperinsulinemia, hyperglycemia, and weight gain

A major concern about introducing insulin in type 2 diabetes is whether exogenous insulin contributes to hyperinsulinemia-induced atherogenesis. Current evidence supports improved glycemic control to prevent retinal, renal, and neurological complications. Contrary to popular belief among many health professionals, there is little evidence to support a direct cause and effect between hyperinsulinemia (from exogenous insulin) and atherosclerosis. Historically, based on results from the 1978 University Group Diabetes Program (UGDP), sulfonylureas and insulin have been implicated in increasing cardiovascular disease and related death via a purported hyperinsulinemic atherogenic profile. The United Kingdom Prospective Diabetes Study provides no evidence for an increase in cardiovascular risk by either sulfonylureas or insulin.[18,36] Thus, avoiding the use of insulin or sulfonylureas in order to improve blood glucose control because of the fear of increasing cardiovascular disease is not justified. In fact, if improved control results from introducing insulin, the net result may be a reduction in lipid levels, which in turn may reduce the risk of cardiovascular disease.[33]

Introducing exogenous insulin to improve glycemic control raises concerns about hypoglycemia and weight gain. While hyperglycemia may indeed be rectified, if insulin is introduced too rapidly at high dose patients may experience symptoms of relative or "true" hypoglycemia. It is not uncommon to lower blood glucose by > 100 mg/dL (5.6 mmol/L) when high dose insulin is used. In SDM, insulin is started at the lowest safe dose and is adjusted slowly so that HbA_{1c} decreases at a rate of 0.5–1 percentage point HbA_{1c} per month (or average SMBG of 15–30 mg/dL [0.8–1.7 mmol/L]). When the patient experiences high blood glucose levels there is probably some weight loss or stabilization (both by volume of fluid loss and glucose excretion). Using insulin to restore near-normal glycemia is likely to be accompanied by a 3–10 lb weight gain. This is normal and can be minimized by modifying diet or increasing exercise at the start of insulin therapy. As part of an intensive regimen, the exogenous insulin may cause some "hunger." There is a tendency to chase the insulin with food, which results in added caloric intake. This can be prevented by maintaining the same caloric (carbohydrate) intake and moving the calories to synchronize with the insulin action curve. (For example, if due to the peak action of intermediate-acting insulin the patient experiences mid-afternoon hypoglycemia, reduce the caloric intake at the midday meal and use some of these calories [carbohydrate] for a mid-afternoon snack. The net effect is to maintain the same caloric intake, but to distribute it more effectively to reduce hypoglycemia.)

Treatment options

Insulin therapy in type 2 diabetes is similar to that for type 1 diabetes because the same insulins and regimens are used (although pump therapy is relatively rare in type 2 diabetes). Where the two differ is how the insulin is used to overcome the underlying defect. In type 1 diabetes the destruction of the pancreatic β-cells results in total reliance on exogenous insulin. This is rarely the case in type 2 diabetes. Depending upon the duration of the disease and the severity of insulin resistance and insulin deficiency, exogenous insulin has varying functions. Most individuals with type 2 diabetes produce some insulin. The defect may be in the amount of insulin (relative insulin deficiency), the timing of insulin secretion (second-wave defect), or insulin activity at the receptors (insulin resistance). Thus the choice of therapy first takes into consideration the underlying defects. If the principal defect is relative insulin deficiency a combination of change in diet and low-dose insulin may resolve the problem. If the defect is related to insulin resistance, the exogenous insulin will have to address both excess hepatic glucose output and resistance at target tissue. This generally calls for higher-dose insulin.

There are several approaches to insulin therapy. SDM divides each insulin regimen into two components: basal or background and bolus or meal related. Combinations of basal and bolus insulin can be used for conventional and intensive management. In conventional insulin therapy, insulin action is matched to carbohydrate intake (see Chapter 3 for insulin action curves). This regimen relies on a consistent schedule of food intake and exercise/activity. Since insulin is given to anticipate when food is ingested, it is important to maintain a consistent eating schedule to optimize the insulin action. Typically, the regimen calls for fewer injections and attempts to optimized mixed dosing. Once the most popular regimen, it is now being replaced by a more physiological insulin delivery regimen: intensive insulin therapy. In this regimen insulin is altered to match energy intake and expenditure. These regimens consist of three or more injections of insulin per day and are coordinated with food intake and activity level. Because it comes closer to mimicking the normal physiologic state, intensive insulin therapy provides a better chance of optimizing blood glucose control. Typical of this approach are frequent changes in insulin dose, more numerous SMBG, and a willingness to alter schedules.

The goal of both approaches is to optimize control without increasing weight or risking hypoglycemia. In general, carbohydrate intake need not increase; rather, the total carbohydrate intake can be distributed differently to synchronize more closely with insulin peak action.

Note: Because it is highly unlikely that an individual treated with a single injection of insulin alone will achieve near-normal glycemic control, no pathway is provided for that circumstance in the Type 2 Diabetes Master DecisionPath.

Generally, for consistency insulin therapies use pre-meal and bedtime as the times to administer insulin. Whether basal or bolus, conventional or intensive, generally insulin may be given at four specific times during a day related to meals, activity, and sleep. The times are before breakfast (fasting), midday meal, evening meal, and at bedtime (3–4 hours after the evening meal). The insulins are denoted as regular (R), rapid acting (RA), intermediate acting (N), and long acting (G). The insulin regimen R/N–0–R–N denotes breakfast regular and intermediate insulin, no insulin before lunch, regular insulin before the evening meal, and intermediate insulin before bedtime. See Chapter 3 for a complete review of insulin action curves.

Medical nutrition therapy is continued if the patient is moving from an oral agent to insulin. In newly diagnosed patients, medical nutrition therapy is instituted along with insulin initiation. Follow the same program discussed in the sections on medical nutrition therapy. Furthermore, if patients prefer to not eat between meal snacks, rapid-acting insulin will also be a better choice than regular insulin.

Short-acting insulin. choosing between regular or rapid acting (lispro or aspart). No clear criteria currently exist for choosing between regular short-acting and rapid-acting insulin for type 2 diabetes. However, in clinical practice, some principles have emerged that may be helpful in choosing between these two forms of insulin. For patients whose lifestyle makes food and activity planning very difficult, RA, which is injected just prior to eating has a more predictable action curve (peak within 1 to $1\frac{1}{2}$ hours, overall action 3 hours). For patients already under treatment for whom regular insulin before each meal has not resulted in improved post-prandial glucose levels, using RA in place of R is recommended. This maintains the patient on the same number of injections. For all other patients, at diagnosis or in treatment, either R or RA could be used at the same dose. R insulin is a good choice for patients that eat many small meals throughout the day. RA is preferred in SDM because it is generally more predictable, is convenient for the patient, and can be more easily adjusted. In the sections on insulin adjustments, additional criteria for switching between these two insulins are discussed.

Starting insulin with a new diagnosis of type 2 diabetes

The benefits of early detection of type 2 diabetes are based on the evidence that the long-term complications of diabetes are directly related to the severity of persistent hyperglycemia. Klein and colleagues[14] showed that on average a person has approximately 10 years of undetected diabetes before the diagnosis is made. Additionally, timely diagnosis avoids further metabolic decompensation and the risks of Hyperglycemic Hyperosmolar Syndrome (HHS) (see Chapter 10). While in the past many patients with type 2 diabetes presented long after complications occurred, this can be avoided through better surveillance. Rarely is there a sudden weight loss at the early onset of type 2 diabetes. The classic signs of polyuria, polydipsia, and polyphagia occur much later. Thus, unless screened often and early enough, the discovery of diabetes may occur late in its natural history. When this occurs and there are classic signs, these serve as an indication for considering insulin at diagnosis, since blood glucose levels must have been relatively high for a long period of time.

At diagnosis of type 2 diabetes, initiation of insulin therapy should occur immediately if fasting plasma glucose is > 300 mg/dL (16.7 mmol/L) or casual plasma glucose is > 350 mg/dL (19.4 mmol/L) without regard to symptoms. At these high plasma glucose levels, medical nutritional therapy alone or in combination with an oral agent normally will not sufficiently lower the blood glucose level into the target range. Furthermore, patients with persistent hyperglycemia at these levels experience glucose toxicity and are at increased risk for HHS. Finally, some individuals may actually be gradual developers of type 1 diabetes (termed latent autoimmune diabetes in adults), for whom insulin therapy will prevent diabetes ketoacidosis.

Determine whether insulin will be initiated on an inpatient or outpatient basis. Many institutions have developed systems that allow for the safe initiation of insulin on an outpatient basis. If resources for education and medical follow-up are not available, the patient should be hospitalized. If the patient is at risk for HHS (see Chapter 10), if there is uncertainty as to type of diabetes, or if the individual cannot care for him or herself, consider hospitalization immediately.

Once it is determined that insulin is required, and the patient is willing to take insulin, the next question is which stage should be started. In general the factors that are taken into consideration are:

- number of injections patient is willing to take
- underlying defect
- transient condition causing metabolic decompensation
- patient lifestyle

If the patient is willing to take insulin multiple times per day, the starting stage should be based mainly on the underlying defect. One defect associated with the need for exogenous insulin is relative insulin deficiency. As the natural history of type 2 diabetes progresses, if persistent hyperglycemia goes unchecked, the β-cells weaken due to glucose toxicity, resulting in insulin deficiency, affecting both basal and meal stimulated insulin secretion. A second determinant may be a transient condition – an underlying infection, MI, or steroid use at diagnosis. This may cause blood glucose to rise above 400 mg/dL (22.2 mmol/L). Refer to Table 4.12 for appropriate insulin stage.

SMBG is not optional with initiation of insulin therapy. Minimally, SMBG should be immediately before each injection and before bedtime. Additionally, 3 AM blood glucoses should be measured intermittently. If using RA insulin, 2 hour post-meal tests are useful to adjust the dose. Elderly patients often forget to eat, thus insulin therapies should be used carefully and thoughtfully. Patients with difficulty in taking insulin, patients who drive long distances, and individuals who operate heavy equipment should be well educated about insulin's use and SMBG before initiating this therapy.

Certain state and federal regulations prohibit individuals using insulin from working at particular jobs. This is especially true in interstate commerce. The necessity to find the therapy that extends life, reduces complications, and improves overall health should take precedence over the desirability to retain employment. Unfortunately, reality requires a balance. The patient should be informed of the necessity for insulin and the relationship between persistent hyperglycemia and, for example, retinopathy. Education often is the key to making a decision as to whether to accept insulin therapy, chance serious eye complications (including blindness), and retain employment. Counseling and other services may be required.

Because type 2 diabetes often affects the middle-aged, working person, managing diabetes in the workplace may become difficult. Multiple

Table 4.12 Selecting Insulin: Stage 2, 3, or 4 (Physiologic)

	Primarily fasting hyperglycemia	Primarily post-prandial hyperglycemia	Fasting and post-prandial hyperglycemia	Cannot detect problem
Stage 2	×			
Stage 3	×			
Stage 4 (Physiologic)		×	×	×

injections offer the most flexibility. Physiologic Insulin Stage 4 permits the patient to skip meals, add more R or RA insulin as needed, and make daily changes in treatment.

Insulin Stage 2 is less forgiving. It requires a schedule that allows for a lunch break at a fixed time. It also requires a consistent activity schedule.

Preparing the patient to use insulin: multiple injections and insulin adjustment

Regimens requiring administration of insulin at multiple times are far more physiologic, generally require less total insulin, and usually result in a more flexible schedule for the patient. Many physicians and patients are concerned with the discomfort of multiple-injection insulin regimens. Studies have repeatedly shown that the newer 31 gauge needles are almost painless if inserted at the correct angle (90 degrees) and if the injection site is rotated within the same general area. Additionally, needleless syringes are available to help patients with needle phobia. Currently studies are underway testing the feasibility, safety, and efficacy of inhaled insulin preparations, which may make multiple insulin administration more acceptable to patients (and health care providers).

Blood glucose monitoring

All patients should be performing SMBG independent of the number of injections they are taking. These data are necessary for meaningful communications between the patient and the healthcare professional. The type of meter to be used for SMBG varies. However, SMBG should have these important attributes. First, the meter should have a memory, making it possible to record and store data for retrieval. This also ensures the accuracy and reliability of the patient's information. Second, the meter should be simple to use and require only a small blood sample. Third, testing should be scheduled to coincide with the meals, activity, and insulin adjustments to optimize collecting data for clinical decision-making. Fourth, testing should take into account the need to adjust insulin dose based on changes in blood glucose.

Unlike the case with oral agent regimens, patients are expected to play a very important role in the daily adjustments in insulin dose. There are two approaches to adjusting treatment using SMBG data – pattern or immediate response. The two are meant to address most situations. When they do not, it is generally necessary to collect more SMBG data and to confirm that the patient's behavior is consistent with the instructions. Pattern response suggests that each individual has a consistent set of blood glucose/insulin relationships. This consistency is characterized by predictable patterns in which specific insulin doses are related to known glycemic levels. For example, increasing the morning intermediate-acting N insulin will consistently result in a decrease in late afternoon (pre-evening meal) blood glucose levels. Therefore, the purpose of initial SMBG is to determine whether such a pattern can be easily identified. When, after trial and error (even within 3 days) such a pattern has been identified, treatment of type 2 diabetes may follow a predictable path. Generally, however, identifying a specific pattern takes substantially longer. Because of changes in food plan, exercise, seasons, and so on, patterns may change. Therefore, the concept of patterned response should be continually reassessed.

Immediate response recognizes that an acute situation has developed requiring an immediate action, such as hypoglycemia (insulin reaction), hyperglycemia, or an anticipated change in food plan or exercise. This occurs whenever blood glucose is below 60 mg/dL (3.3 mmol/L) or greater than 250 mg/dL (13.9 mmol/L). Refer to "Hospitalization for Problems Related to Glycemic Control" in Chapter 10 for additional information.

Insulin Stage 2, 3, or Physiologic Insulin Stage 4?

For newly diagnosed patients starting on insulin, the Type 2 Diabetes Master DecisionPath (see Figure 4.6) indicates three insulin regimens using rapid or short-acting and intermediate- or long-acting insulins. The conventional approach is to begin with Insulin Stage 2 and proceed to the next stages if this two-injection regimen fails to bring the patient into glycemic control. Some clinicians prefer a more physiologic regimen, beginning with Stage 4 and removing insulin as warranted. A third approach which SDM has found very effective, is to begin with bedtime long-acting (G) insulin with subsequent addition of up to three injections of RA before meals as needed for daytime management of post-prandial hyperglycemia (0–0–0–G built up to RA–RA–RA–G). This section discusses each regimen, beginning with Stage 2.

Stage 2 Insulin: conventional approach

Following a thorough history, physical, and laboratory evaluation and after review of the target blood glucose levels, the decision as to whether to hospitalize to start the patient on an insulin regimen should be made. In most cases hospitalization is unnecessary. Assuming that insulin will be started on an ambulatory basis, the time of insulin initiation becomes the next question.

Note: For all insulin therapies the starting dose formula has been carefully selected to meet the immediate metabolic requirements of the individual while reducing the risk of hypoglycemia and severe hyperglycemia.

Insulin Stage 2/Start
R/N–0–R/N–0 or RA/N–0–RA/N–0

Morning insulin start. If the first time the patient starts this therapy is in the morning, the total daily dose is calculated as 0.3 U/kg (see Figure 4.11). The total daily dose is divided into two periods roughly associated with breakfast and the evening meal (approximately 10 hours apart). The pre-breakfast dose is two-thirds of the total daily requirement. This is further divided into one-third R or RA and two-thirds N. The small amount of R or RA is to cover breakfast. The intermediate-acting insulin is to cover lunch and the afternoon period. Review the insulin action curves described in Chapter 3. Note the likely times of peak action. Glucose excursions after lunch will have to be measured (SMBG) to determine whether adequate insulin is available. Also keep in mind that afternoon exercise will affect blood glucose levels. The pre-evening meal insulin is calculated as one-third of the total daily dose equally split between R or RA and intermediate-acting insulin and given as one injection before the evening meal. For example, a patient with a current weight of 200 lb (91 kg) would receive either 27 or 28 total units of insulin. (Here we use 28 since it is more easily divisible.) Of the 28 units, 18 would be given in the AM and 10 in the PM. Of the 18 units in the AM, 12 units would be N and 6 units would be R or RA. The PM dose would be 5 units N and 5 units R or RA. For the frail elderly, or others using 75/25, 70/30 or 50/50 pre-mixed insulins, the doses would be 18 units of premixed insulin in the AM and 10 units of premixed insulin in the PM. The disadvantage of pre-mixed insulin is that the ratio is constant. If the patient on a premixed regimen experienced post-breakfast hyperglycemia, both the N and R or RA would have to be increased at a ratio of 2:1. This may resolve the post-breakfast hyperglycemia, but may cause mid-afternoon hypoglycemia.

Afternoon or evening insulin start. If the therapy is being started in the afternoon or evening, the starting dose is one-third of the normal total daily dose (0.1 U/kg), which is equally divided between N and R or RA insulin. The next day the patient would be on the total daily dose as described above. The patient should be taught both insulin administration technique and how to monitor blood glucose. SMBG should be performed every 4 hours. If blood glucose levels are > 250 mg/dL (13.9 mmol/L), consider additional small doses (1–2 units) of R or RA with SMBG 1–2 hours after the insulin injection. This therapy is temporary. Have the patient return the next morning to initiate daily insulin administration (see previous section).

Immediate follow-up. Self-monitored blood

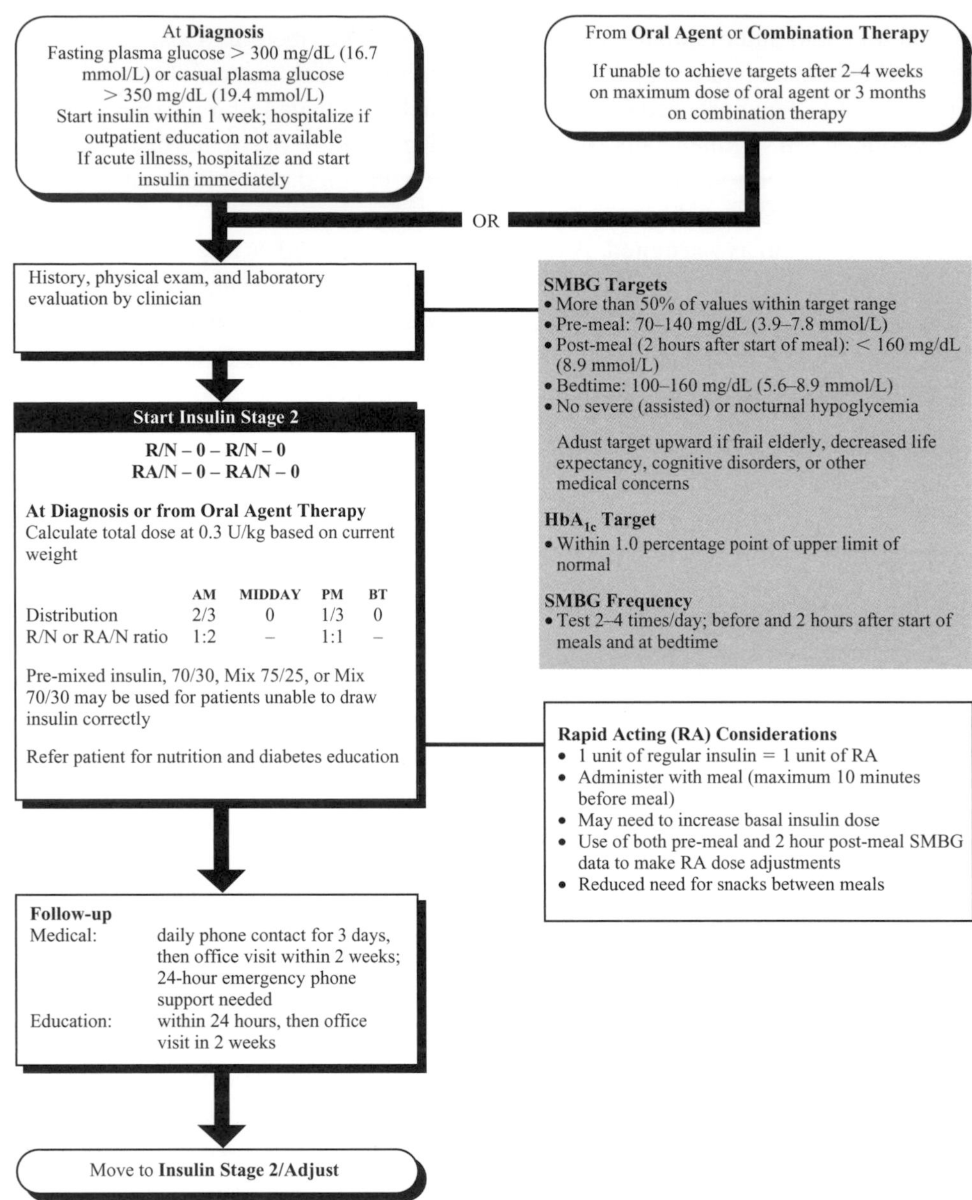

Figure 4.11 Type 2 Insulin Stage 2/Start DecisionPath

glucose is the best way to assess the impact of insulin therapy. The minimum SMBG for this treatment regimen is four times per day (before meals and at bedtime). An evening snack may be necessary to prevent overnight hypoglycemia. One or two carbohydrate choices taken from earlier in the day and moved to bedtime can be provided as a snack. To avoid nocturnal hypoglycemia, consider SMBG at 3 AM at least once per week (or whenever symptoms occur).

During the first several days it is imperative to maintain glucose levels at a point that will avoid both hypoglycemia and hyperglycemia. Additionally, co-management with the various health professionals who will be involved in diabetes care must be established. The nurse educator and dietitian are vital components of the healthcare team and should be incorporated into care as soon as feasible. This is especially important in ambulatory management. The guidelines for insulin adjustments begin immediately. Along with making arrangements for both nurse and dietitian follow-up, establish target blood glucose levels.

Although near euglycemia is the overall goal of

treatment to prevent microvascular and macrovascular complications (see Chapters 8 and 9), any improvement from baseline benefits individuals with type 2 diabetes. Setting the initial goal at fasting < 200 mg/dL (11.1 mmol/L) and post meal < 250 mg/dL (13.9 mmol/L) is the first step in ensuring eventual near-normal levels of blood glucose. This interim target was established to promote the overall goal of gradual (safe) reduction in blood glucose. While any improvement in blood glucose is acceptable, the overall long-term goal is to achieve near-normal glycemic control. Thus, it is appropriate to react to consistent patterns of high blood glucose with increased insulin.

Medical nutrition therapy. As with all pharmacologic therapies, medical nutrition therapy is part of the overall treatment approach. Start as if the person was treated solely by nutrition therapy (see Medical Nutrition Therapy/Start). Modifying the nutrition therapy to avoid hypoglycemia may be necessary. To do this, consider altering the timing of both food intake and exercise to synchronize with the insulin action curve. Some initial weight gain (3–5 lb) may occur with the introduction of insulin. This is due to the uptake and metabolism of glucose as glycemic targets are being reached or as a result of rehydration. Subsequent weight gain, however, is due to chasing insulin with food. In SDM, alterations in the timing of meals, snacks, and exercise are the principal tools by which hyperglycemia and hypoglycemia are prevented. If hyperglycemia or hypoglycemia do occur, immediately consider changing the insulin regimen.

Insulin Stage 2/Adjust
R/N–0–R/N–0 or RA/N–0–RA/N–0

Adjustments to Insulin Stage 2 are based on patterns of SMBG values (see Table 4.13).
Follow these general principles:

- Look for a pattern – at least 3 days of similar blood glucose values.

Table 4.13 Insulin Stage 2, pattern adjustment guidelines (see Figure 4.12 for letter designations)

Time	< 70 mg/dL (< 3.9 mmol/L)	140–250 mg/dL (7.8–13.9 mmol/L)	> 250 mg/dL (> 13.9 mmol/L)
AM or 3 AM	↓PM N 1–2 U (a,b)	↑PM N 1–2 U (a)	↑PM N 2–4 U (a)
MIDDAY (MID)	↓AM R or RA 1–2 U (c,e)	↑AM R or RA 1–2 U (f,g)	↑AM R or RA 2–4 U (f,g)
PM	↓AM N 1–2 U (d,e)	↑AM N 1–2 U (f,h)	↑AM N 2–4 U (f,h)
	< 100 mg/dL (< 5.6 mmol/L)	160–250 mg/dL (8.9–13.9 mmol/L)	> 250 mg/dL (> 13.9 mmol/L)
BEDTIME (BT)	↓PM R or RA 1–2 U (e)	↑PM R or RA 1–2 U (f)	↑PM R or RA 2–4 U (f)

Notes

a. Evaluate nocturnal hypoglycemia; check 3 AM BG
b. Consider adjusting bedtime snack
c. Consider adding or adjusting mid-morning snack
d. Consider adding or adjusting afternoon snack
e. Evaluate whether previous exercise is causing hypoglycemia
f. Consider adding exercise
g. Consider decreasing mid-morning snack
h. Consider decreasing afternoon snack
i. No mid-morning snack usually needed with RA
j. No afternoon snack usually needed with RA
k. Consider adding AM N if long interval betweeen midday and evening meal or afternoon hyperglycemia

AM N: 50% MIDDAY R dose
MIDDAY R: ↓ 50%
AM and PM R: No change

Figure 4.12 Type 2 diabetes insulin adjustment considerations

- Make initial adjustments to target the consistently low blood glucose first. Follow this by targeting patterns of high blood glucose.
- Normally, target only one insulin at a time and at one time point (AM or PM).
- Change dose by 1–4 units depending on the level of hyperglycemia or hypoglycemia.
- Become familiar with insulin action curve principles (see Chapter 3).

- Avoid adding calories to total food intake to prevent hypoglycemia.

Instead, move carbohydrate choices (e.g., save dessert for bedtime snack).

Target blood glucose and insulin adjustments. During the first several months of insulin therapy, the patient should demonstrate improved glycemic control. HbA_{1c} should drop approximately 0.5–1 percentage point per month and mean SMBG 15–30 mg/dL (0.8–1.7 mmol/L) per month (see Figure 4.13). If these rates are met, the same insulin doses are kept. If the rates are not met, increase the insulin doses following the adjustment guidelines.

Insulin Stage 2/Maintain
R/N–0–R/N–0 or RA/N–0–RA/N–0

When SMBG and HbA_{1c} targets are met, alterations to the insulin, food plan, and exercise

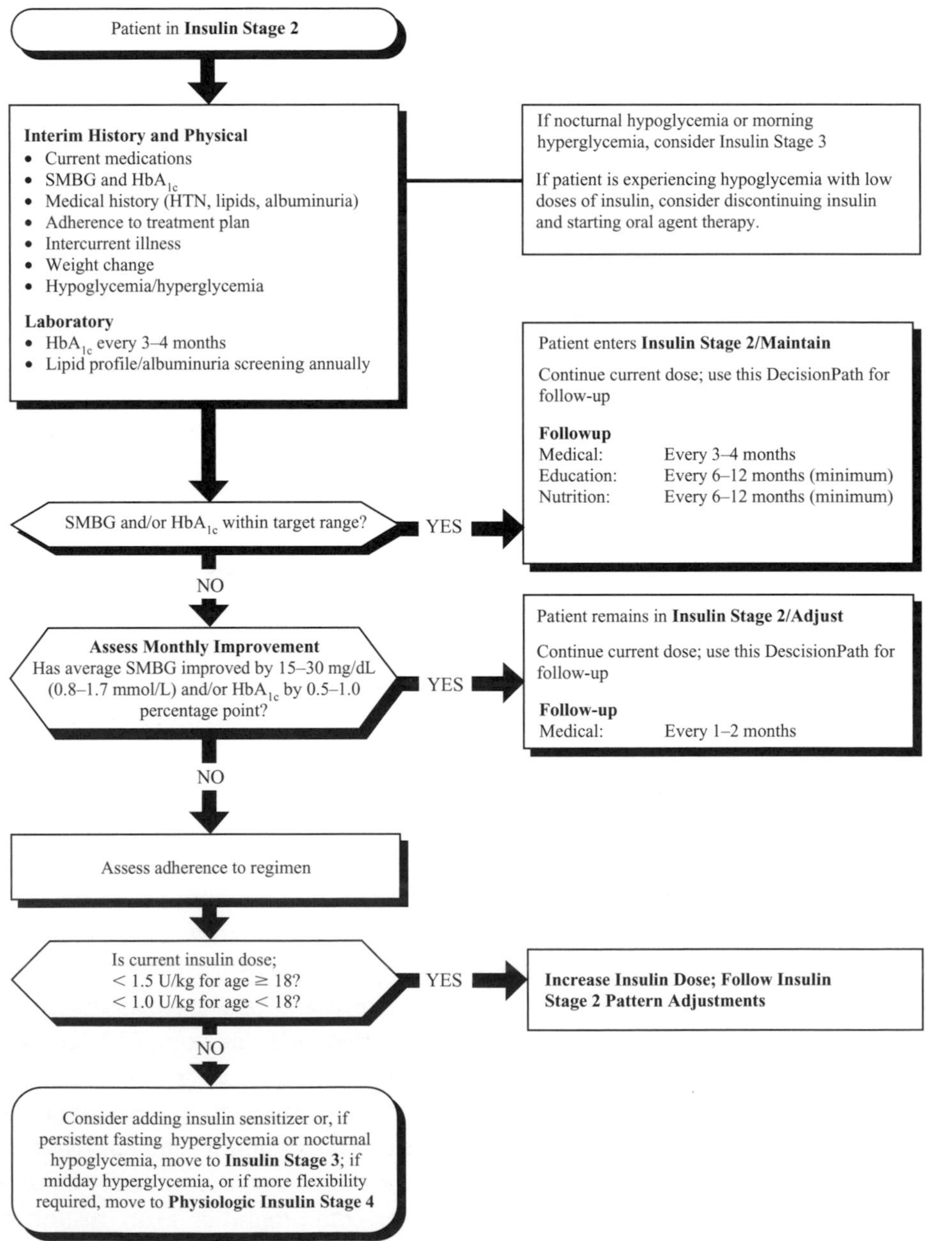

Figure 4.13 Type 2 diabetes Insulin Stage 2/Adjust DecisionPath

regimens are likely to be required to maintain glycemic targets. To prevent both hyperglycemia and weight gain, encourage a schedule of blood glucose and weight monitoring. While neither need be as regimented as during start and adjust phases, both are required to detect either increasing blood glucose or weight. At a minimum SMBG should occur prior to each insulin injection, with at least one daily two hour post-prandial (at varying meals each day). Weight should be monitored weekly. Some changes in insulin dose and timing should be expected. The patient might be provided with some general rules for making insulin adjustments based on consistent patterns of blood glucose.

Choosing a three-injection regimen

If Insulin Stage 2 has failed to allow the patient to achieve glycemic targets (reach maintain phase) after 6 months of adjustment, or if a pattern of persistent fasting hyperglycemia or nocturnal hypoglycemia occurs at any time, consider a three-injection regimen. In addition, consider moving to a three-injection regimen if patients require more flexibility to fit their lifestyle. The patient should have already seen the Type 2 Diabetes Master DecisionPath and (hopefully) will have already agreed to considering alternate therapies requiring an increased number of injections if the current therapy has failed to reach the overall goals.

A common pathway for individuals with type 2 diabetes is Insulin Stage 3, which is a slight modification of Insulin Stage 2 where the evening meal intermediate-acting insulin (N) is moved to bedtime. This should improve the fasting blood glucose level and reduce the likelihood of nocturnal hypoglycemia.

Insulin Stage 3

Most newly diagnosed patients do not start with three injections because historically these are used in patients who were started on Insulin Stage 2 and ultimately required bedtime intermediate-acting insulin. There is no reason that the three-injection regimen could not be used at diagnosis (this is often the case in gestational diabetes). If Insulin Stage 3 is used at diagnosis, make certain that a thorough history, physical, and laboratory evaluation are completed and that the target blood glucose levels are reviewed.

Note: For all insulin therapies the starting dose formula has been carefully selected to meet the immediate needs of the individual while reducing the risk of hypoglycemia as well as hyperglycemia.

Insulin Stage 3/Start: at diagnosis
R/N–0–R–N or RA/N–0–RA–N

Morning insulin start. If the patient starts this therapy in the morning, the total daily dose is calculated as 0.3 U/kg (see Figure 4.13). The total daily dose is divided into three periods associated with breakfast, the evening meal (approximately 10 hours apart) and bedtime (at least 3 hours after dinner). The pre-breakfast dose is two-thirds of the total daily requirement. This is further divided into one-third R or RA and two-thirds N. The R or RA insulin will lower post-breakfast glucose and the intermediate-acting insulin N is for lunch and the afternoon period. The evening dose is calculated as one-third of the total daily requirement and evenly split between R or RA at dinner and intermediate-acting insulin N at bedtime. By placing N insulin at bedtime, its principal action is moved closer to the morning.

Afternoon or evening insulin start. If the therapy is being started in the afternoon or evening, the starting dose is one-third the normal starting dose (0.1 U/kg) equally split between N and R or RA. The short-acting insulin is given before dinner and the intermediate-acting insulin before bedtime. The next day the patient would be on the total daily dose as described above for starting Insulin Stage 3 in the morning. The patient should be taught both insulin administration technique and how to monitor blood glucose. The patient should self-monitor blood glucose every 4 hours. If blood glucose levels are $>$ 250 mg/dL (13.9 mmol/L), consider additional small doses (1–2 units) of R or RA with SMBG an hour after the insulin. This therapy is temporary. Have the patient return the next morning to initiate daily insulin administration (see previous section).

During the first several days it is imperative to maintain glucose levels at a point that will avoid both hypoglycemia and hyperglycemia. Have the patient SMBG at least four times per day (before meals and at bedtime). Additionally, co-management with the various health professionals who will be involved in diabetes care must be established. The nurse educator and dietitian are vital components of the healthcare team and should be incorporated into care as soon as feasible. This is especially important in ambulatory management. The guidelines for insulin adjustments begin immediately. Along with making arrangements for both nurse and dietitian follow-up, establish target blood glucose levels.

Insulin Stage 3/Start: from Insulin Stage 2 R/N–0–R–N or RA/N–0–RA–N

Three conditions can be addressed by Insulin Stage 3 that may have been encountered in Insulin Stage 2:

- morning fasting blood glucose consistently above target range
- nocturnal hypoglycemia
- varying time of evening meal

Morning fasting blood glucose may be high for several reasons. The principal causes relate to a high bedtime glucose, early AM excessive glucose output (dawn phenomenon), Somogyi effect, and insufficient exogenous basal insulin. One consequence of relative insulin deficiency may be excess hepatic glucose production (gluconeogenesis). The second factor, high evening blood glucose, is usually the result of a larger meal or proportionately higher carbohydrates at the evening meal and at bedtime. The third cause for high fasting plasma glucose, dyschronized insulin peak action, may result in low blood glucose from 2 to 4 AM and a rebound to hyperglycemia (Somogyi effect) by morning. The latter is often the cause of nocturnal hypoglycemia. Alternatively, nocturnal hypoglycemia may result from too much intermediate-acting insulin at dinner coupled with insufficient bedtime snack. If adjustments to the Insulin Stage 2 regimen have failed to overcome these problems, moving the intermediate-acting insulin to at least 3 hours after the evening meal (this bedtime injection is shown as BT in figures and tables) should provide some resolution. Before doing this, however, be certain that overinsulinization has not occurred (>1.5 U/kg). If this is suspected, consider reducing the total daily insulin dose to 1 U/kg and redistributing it according to Insulin Stage 3 (see Figure 4.14).

To start Insulin Stage 3, move the current dose of evening meal N insulin to bedtime. Make certain SMBG occurs at this time. One or two carbohydrate choices from earlier in the day can be moved as a bedtime snack. Readjust both the evening R or RA and the morning R or RA after 3 days on this regimen. Most probably the morning R or RA will be reduced and the evening R or RA will be increased. The total daily dose should still follow the pattern of a maximum of 1.5 U/kg.

Before beginning pattern adjustment, determine which insulin is responsible for the glucose pattern. Intermediate-acting insulin (N) is meant to reach its peak near the morning to lower the fasting blood glucose value. The overlap of R and N between midnight and 2 AM may require adjusting the evening snack. This should not be the case in individuals using RA because of its shorter action curve. In addition, residual bedtime N may be present when the morning R or RA is administered. Measurement of blood glucose post-breakfast thus becomes important when starting Stage 3.

Insulin Stage 3/Adjust R/N–0–R–N or RA/N–0–RA–N

The patient should realize that it will be necessary to frequently adjust the morning short-acting insulin. The first sign of too much morning R or RA will be post-breakfast or midday hypoglycemia. Reduction in morning R or RA (see Table 4.14) will resolve this problem. An additional adjust-

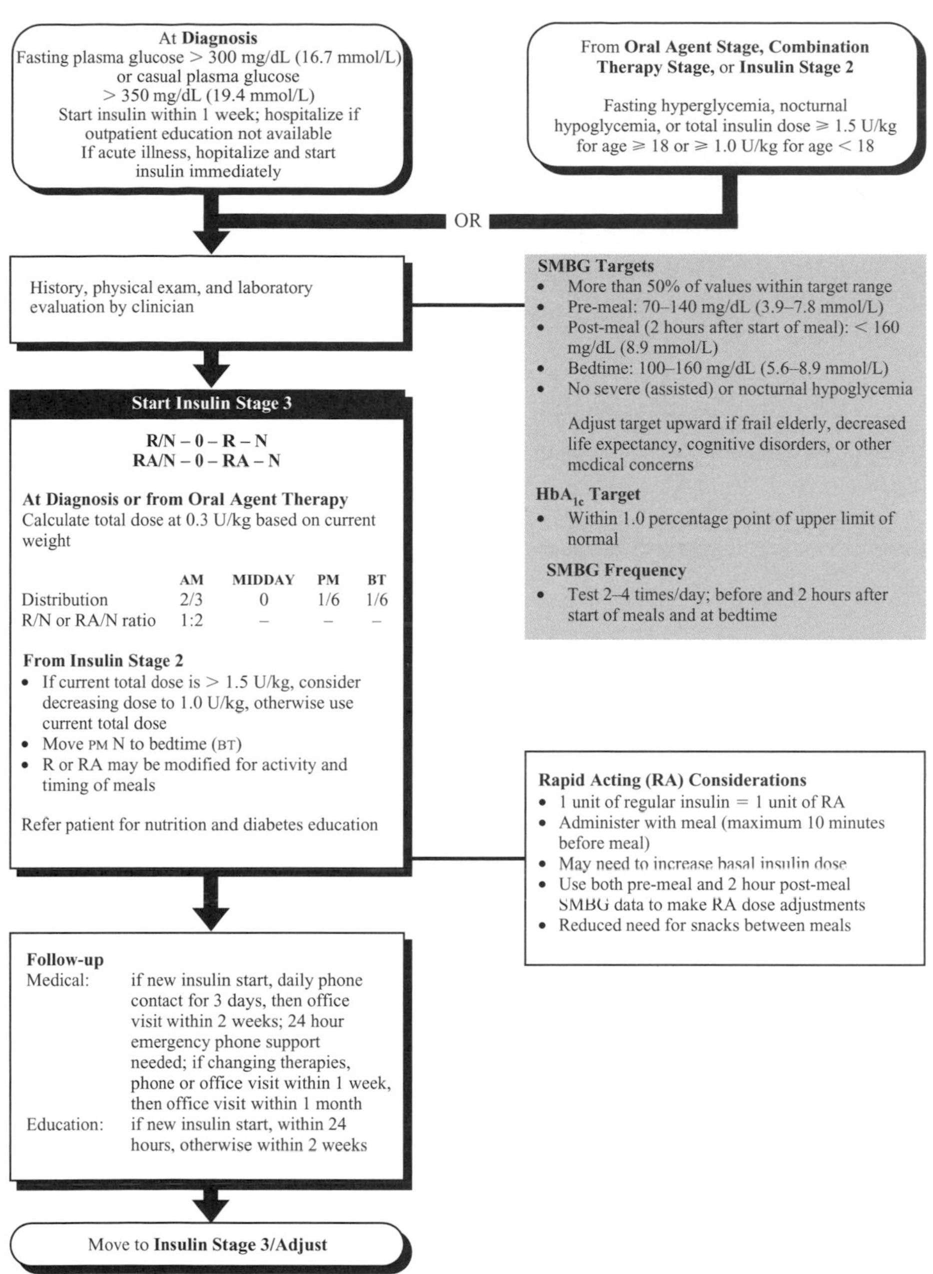

Figure 4.14 Type 2 diabetes Insulin Stage 3/Start

ment in breakfast carbohydrate intake or mid-morning snack may be needed. If the pre-evening meal glucose goes up, use the same formula as before, i.e., raise the morning N. This will increase the amount of insulin available to cover carbohydrate intake at lunch. Alternatively, if the bedtime N lowers the fasting blood glucose, the intermediate-acting insulin requirements during the daytime may need to be reduced. If the pre-dinner blood glucose is < 80 mg/dL (4.4 mmol/L) for three consecutive days, consider lowering the morning N. Keep in mind the impact of exercise on both when there is too much or too little insulin. Exercise in the mid-afternoon should be closely followed by SMBG before and after the exercise period. If possible, avoid adding additional calories in order to prevent weight gain.

The third adjustments are related to the bedtime blood glucose levels. These are affected most by food intake at dinner and by the amount of short-

Table 4.14 Insulin stage 3 pattern adjustment guidelines (see Figure 4.12 for letter designations)

Time	< 70 mg/dL (< 3.9 mmol/L)	140–250 mg/dL (7.8–13.9 mmol/L)	> 250 mg/dL (> 13.9 mmol/L)
AM or 3 AM	↓PM N 1–2 U (a,b)	↑PM N 1–2 U (a)	↑PM N 2–4 U (a)
MIDDAY (MID)	↓AM R or RA 1–2 U (c,e)	↑AM R or RA 1–2 U (f,g)	↑AM R or RA 2–4 U (f,g,i)
PM	↓AM N 1–2 U (d,e)	↑AM N 1–2 U (f,h)	↑AM N 2–4 U (f,h)
	< 100 mg/dL (< 5.6 mmol/L)	160–250 mg/dL (8.9–13.9 mmol/L)	> 250 mg/dL (> 13.9 mmol/L)
BEDTIME (BT)	↓PM R or RA 1–2 U (e)	↑PM R or RA 1–2 U (f)	↑PM R or RA 2–4 U (f)

acting insulin used. In addition, many people snack throughout the evening without having a discrete evening meal. This may influence the type of short-acting insulin selected and/or the dose administered. Blood glucose at bedtime should not exceed 160 mg/dL (8.9 mmol/L). Consider increasing R or RA before dinner or changing the meal content. Hyperglycemia at bedtime will often result in a high fasting blood glucose (see Insulin Stage 2 for general principles).

Insulin Stage 3/Maintain
R/N–0–R–N or RA/N–0–RA–N

When patients reach their metabolic targets using Insulin Stage 3, they enter the maintain treatment phase. In this phase changes in insulin, food plan, and exercise regimens are likely to be less frequent. Despite this reduction in changes to therapy, surveillance with SMBG is necessary. Because of the addition of a third injection and perhaps fear of hypoglycemia overnight, some patients may add too many calories as part of the evening snack. A schedule of consistent weight monitoring should be encouraged. While neither SMBG nor weight monitoring need be as regimented as during start and adjust phases, both are required to detect trends of either increasing blood glucose or weight. At minimum, SMBG should occur prior to each insulin injection with at least one post-prandial (at varying meals each day). Because this would mean no fewer than four tests a day, for patients who have maintained their metabolic goal for at least 1 month, consider alternate day testing or reducing the number of tests to two a day at different times each day. Some changes in insulin dose and timing should be expected. Food plan should consider further alterations in timing and size; carbohydrate and/or caloric intake should not increase by an appreciable amount. The patient should be reminded of the general rules, such as relying on 3 day patterns before changing insulin dose.

Physiologic Insulin Stage 4: mimicking normal insulin secretion

Multiple-injection regimens are far more adjustable and will most likely result in a more flexible schedule for the patient. Dividing the insulin into smaller doses reduces the chance of local discomfort and likely provides a more consistent time action profile. Additionally, regimens with more injections generally require less insulin overall.

If Insulin Stage 3 has failed to move the patient into the maintain phase of therapy after 6 months of experimentation, or if the patient at diagnosis is willing to try a more intensive regimen, then a four-injection regimen should be considered. The patient should already have been introduced to the Type 2 Diabetes Master DecisionPath, and alternate therapies, requiring an increased number of injections, should have been discussed. Stage 4 is the most physiologic regimen and offers the patient more flexibility regarding timing of meals. Staged Diabetes Management encourages providers to discuss the advantages of Stage 4 with their patients, especially those starting insulin at diagnosis or after oral agents have failed.

Physiologic Insulin Stage 4/Start: at diagnosis
R–R–R–N or G or RA–RA–RA–N or G

If starting Stage 4 at diagnosis, ask the patient to do SMBG four times/day (before each meal and at bedtime (plus overnight one to two times during the first week). Two approaches can be used to initiate this therapy: formula or experiential. For the formula method calculate the total daily dose at 0.3 U/kg. If using N insulin, calculate the amount as 30 per cent of the total daily dose (of all insulins). Divide the remaining 70 per cent equally and administer as either R or RA before each meal. Thus, for a 200 lb. (90 kg) adult, 28 total units of insulin would be given. Eight units (rounded from 8.4) of N would be given at bedtime and 6 units (rounded) of R or RA would be given before each meal. If using G insulin, 50 per cent of the total dose (14 units) would be given at bedtime as G and 4 units (rounded) of R or RA would be given before each meal, resulting in a total of 26 units. Adjustments to this regimen may be made after 3 days of a consistent pattern.

An alternative method is to start with N or G at bedtime calculated at 0.1 U/kg (0–0–0–G). During the next seven to ten days make 1–2 unit adjustments in the dose until 0.3 U/kg has been reached or fasting plasma glucose (without any hypoglycemia is reduced by at least 60 mg/dL (3.2 mmol/L)). Next, review all blood glucose values to identify the pattern of blood glucose that consistently is highest over more than 3 days (e.g. midday, PM, or bedtime). Add an injection of RA or R insulin (0.1 U/kg) to the preceding meal. Thus if the pre-evening meal BG is consistently the highest add RA or R insulin prior to the mid-day meal. The new regimen would be 0–RA–0–G. Adjust this insulin every 3 days by 1–2 units until 0.2 U/kg or the pre-evening meal BG has reduced by least 60 mg/dL (3.2 mmol/L). Repeat this for the next highest blood glucose pattern. Eventually, the patient will be on a regimen of RA–RA–RA–G at the minimum amount of insulin necessary to physiologically mimic insulin requirements. This gradual introduction of pre-meal insulin based on SMBG data reinforces the experiential aspects of diabetes self-management. The patient quickly learns how small increments of insulin given at the appropriate time affect BG level. By relying on low-dose basal insulin initially to improve fasting plasma glucose, an added benefit is that the patient begins the day with improved glucose levels. Meal related BG excursions become less dramatic. By identifying the most serious pattern of hyperglycemia first, the insulin can be targeted and thereby used more sparingly. The result is generally a total insulin dose of < 1 U/kg.

Physiologic Insulin Stage 4/Start (moving from Stage 3)
R–R–R–N or G or RA–RA–RA–N or G

The Stage 4 regimen makes insulin adjustments very easy. Each blood glucose determination has a direct relationship to the previous insulin dose. For example, if the bedtime blood glucose level is high, increase the PM R or RA insulin. Similarly, if the fasting blood glucose is high, increase the bedtime N or G.

Before initiating this regimen from Stage 3, make certain the total daily insulin dose has not reached > 1.5 U/kg, if so, reduce to 1.0 U/kg. For patients continuing with N, seventy per cent of the insulin is given in the form of R or RA distributed before meals and 30% as N at bedtime. In this case R or RA is used for all meal-related increases in blood glucose, while bedtime N is used to provide for basal insulin needs. If the patient is starting G, reduce the total insulin dose by 20%. Next, calculate the R or RA insulin at 50% of the new total daily dose distributed before meals and G at 50 per cent of the new total daily dose administered at bedtime.

Physiologic Insulin Stage 4/Adjust
R–R–R–N or G or RA–RA–RA–N or G

Because this regimen allows for targeting the insulin action to particular post-prandial blood glucose excursions, make certain that SMBG occurs before each insulin administration. The blood glucose value determined at that point will help decide how well the insulin given before the last meal worked and will help calculate the insulin to be given at the current meal. Start by identifying the highest blood glucose. Increase by 1–4 units the insulin prior to the high blood glucose (see Table 4.15). Continue until this blood glucose is lowered to within target. Now find the next highest blood glucose. Repeat until all blood glucoses are within target. For example, if the highest blood glucose is fasting, then increase N or G by 1–4 units. Once the fasting has been resolved, turn to the next blood glucose that is persistently highest. Assume it is the pre-evening meal blood glucose. Increase the midday R or RA by 1–4 units.

Table 4.15 Physiologic Insulin Stage 4 pattern adjustment guidelines (see Figure 4.12 for letter designations)

Time	< 70 mg/dL (< 3.9 mmol/L)	140–250 mg/dL (7.8–13.9 mmol/L)	> 250 mg/dL (> 13.9 mmol/L)
AM or 3 AM	↓BT N or G 1–2 U (a,b)	↑BT N or G 1–2 U (a)	↑BT N or G 2–4 U (a)
MIDDAY (MID)	Stop or ↓AM R or RA 1–2 U (c,e)	Start or ↑AM R or RA 1–2 U (f,g)	Start or ↑AM R or RA 2–4 U (f,g,i)
PM	Stop or ↓MID R or RA 1–2 U (d,e)	Start or ↑MID R 1–2 U (f,h)	Start or ↑MID R or RA 2–4 U (f,h,j,k)
	< 100 mg/dL (< 5.6 mmol/L)	160–250 mg/dL (8.9–13.9 mmol/L)	> 250 mg/dL (> 13.9 mmol/L)
BEDTIME (BT)	Stop or ↓PM R or RA 1–2 U (e)	Start or ↑PM R or RA 1–2 U (f)	Start or ↑PM R or RA 2–4 U (f)

Physiologic Insulin Stage 4/Maintain
R–R–R–N or G or RA–RA–RA–N or G

Upon reaching their glycemic targets, patients enter the maintain treatment goal phase. Normally, fewer alterations to the insulin, food plan, and exercise regimens will be required. However, surveillance with SMBG is necessary. To prevent both hyperglycemia and weight gain, encourage a schedule of blood glucose and weight monitoring. At a minimum, SMBG should be done prior to each insulin injection with at least one post-prandial (at varying meals each day). Because this would mean no fewer than four tests a day, for patients who have maintained their metabolic goal for at least 1 month, consider alternate-day testing or reducing the number of tests to two a day at different times each day. Some changes in insulin dose and timing should be expected. Monitor weight at least weekly. Food plan should consider further alterations in timing and portion size, keeping in mind that the total caloric intake should not increase appreciably. The patient should be reminded of the general rules for changing insulin doses – a minimum of 3 days of the same pattern. Patients should be reminded to contact their health care provider if blood glucose levels begin to rise. HbA_{1c} should continue to be determined every 3–4 months.

New treatment alternatives

Several new treatment regimens based on non-hypoglycemic oral agents have been developed, which may help optimize insulin therapies. Among these are drugs that decrease hepatic glucose output, increase glucose uptake in muscle, reduce total insulin dose, or inhibit the break down and rapid absorption of carbohydrates.

Adding a thiazolidinedione to insulin therapies

Individuals with type 2 diabetes may have several metabolic defects. Patients treated with insulin usually have both fasting and post-prandial hyperglycemia, suggesting that along with insulin resistance they have reduced insulin secretion. The exogenous insulin is generally meant to compensate for the weakened pancreatic β-cells. Thus, the insulin resistance is not directly affected. Thiazolidinediones represent a distinct classification of oral agents in diabetes, the primary action of which is based on increasing insulin sensitivity. Rosiglitazone and pioglitazone were studied in combination with insulin in type 2 diabetes. When used in combination with insulin, they lower blood glucose by approximately 40–50 mg/dL

(2.2–2.8 mmol/L). Although not hypoglycemic *per se*, when used in combination with insulin they can lead to hypoglycemia and therefore patients should closely monitor blood glucose. Patients who are or may become pregnant, or those with moderate to severe heart failure, with liver disease, or at risk for liver disease, should not be prescribed thiazolidinedione (see Chapter 3).

Combination Thiazolidinedione–Insulin/Start and Adjust

Generally, the insulin sensitizers are added when the total daily insulin dose reaches 1 U/kg. The first step is to maintain the current insulin regimen. The second step is to prescribe thiazolidinedione at the minimum dose taken with the first meal of the day. Make certain the SMBG continues at least four times per day and expect to alter the current insulin dose within 1–3 weeks. The patient should be instructed to report blood glucose levels below 70 mg/dL (3.9 mmol/L). When adjusting insulin see the specific insulin stage guidelines. If there is no change in blood glucose, increase thiazolidinedione every 8 weeks until the maximum dose is reached. If adjustments in thiazolidinedione fail to improve control, consider halting the thiazolidinedione and moving to the next insulin stage (3 or 4). If the thiazolidinedione was introduced in Stage 4, consider referral to an endocrinologist if glycemic targets are not achieved.

Adding metformin to insulin therapies

The addition of metformin, a biguanide, to insulin is primarily to suppress hepatic glucose output.[34] While the exact mechanism is not clearly established, in the liver metformin appears to inhibit gluconeogenesis, thereby decreasing hepatic glucose output. Although by itself it is not hypoglycemic, it can lead to hypoglycemia when used in combination with insulin. Metformin has also been reported to cause a modest reduction in weight. Thus its use is generally to target fasting plasma glucose as well as weight gain.

Its principal side-effect is gastrointestinal discomfort; therefore, it should be started at a low dose (500 or 850 mg) and slowly increased. Its dose–response curve shows steady increase in improvement in effectiveness at each dose level up to a maximum blood glucose lowering potential at ~2000 mg/day. Special precautions for its use are required because of the possible side-effect of lactic acidosis (see Chapter 3). Patients with heart, liver, kidney, or pulmonary disease may be at an increased risk of lactic acidosis and, therefore, should not use this drug. Additionally, it is not approved for use in pregnancy.

Combination Metformin–Insulin/Start and Adjust

Patients in Insulin Stage 2 or 3 with persistent fasting hyperglycemia who refuse to move to the next insulin stage and patients in Physiologic Insulin Stage 4 with a total insulin daily dose of > 1 U/kg of insulin may benefit from the addition of metformin. In addition, patients with risks for cardiovascular disease may benefit from addition of metformin. Starting the combination therapy is simple. Follow the metformin start and adjust guidelines presented in the section on oral agents in type 2 diabetes while also following the insulin stage-specific adjustment guidelines. Start with the lowest dose (500 or 850 mg) and increase the dose every 1 to 2 weeks if control does not improve. The clinically effective dose of metformin is 2000 mg per day. Make certain to continue SMBG and be prepared to lower the insulin dose if needed.

Adding alpha-glucosidase inhibitors to insulin therapies

Acarbose and miglitol are alpha-glucosidase inhibitors that slow the breakdown of carbohydrate in the small intestine, resulting in lower post-prandial blood glucose excursions. They are effective drugs for those patients treated with insulin for whom elevated post-prandial blood glucose levels is still a significant problem. When used in combination with insulin they tend to lower HbA_{1c} by up to 1 percentage point.

Combination Alpha-Glucosidase Inhibitor–Insulin/Start and Adjust

Patients in any insulin stage with persistent postprandial hyperglycemia who are having difficulty lowering their carbohydrate intake may benefit from the addition of alpha-glucosidase inhibitor. Initiating the combination therapy is simple. Start with 25 mg of alpha-glucosidase inhibitor before the largest meal of the day and slowly add 25 mg of alpha-glucosidase inhibitor before the other meals over the course of the next few weeks. Continue to increase dose of alpha-glucosidase inhibitor based on tolerability and glycemic control until the normally clinically effective dose of 50–100 mg three times a day is achieved. Continue following the insulin-stage-specific adjustment guidelines. Make certain to continue SMBG and be prepared to lower the insulin dose if needed.

Back to baseline

When insulin alone or in combination with an oral agent fails, it may be appropriate to halt progression through the stages of SDM and to consider a short period of back to baseline. This means that the patient's insulin should be reduced to minimum level to maintain blood glucose values between 120 and 250 mg/dL (6.7–13.9 mmol/L) without experimentation and to reduce the number of injections to minimum (start with the 0–0–0–N or G regimen, if possible) to determine the physiologic needs of the patient.

Back to baseline is necessary when there is constant change in therapy along with weight gain. Holding the patient at baseline may allow detection of the patient's metabolic needs without interference from intervening variables. At this point reinforce medical nutrition therapy. Increased SMBG is necessary to detect the problem areas. Use a 2 week period for this review, making certain that blood glucose levels do not exceed 250 mg/dL (13.9 mmol/L). At the end of the period, if insulin needs to be added the stage of therapy often becomes a variation of Stage 4. This is not surprising since it is the most physiologic use of insulin. *If this back to baseline is not successful, consider co-management with a diabetes specialist.*

Co-management option

Staged Diabetes Management DecisionPaths emphasize the option of co-managing the patient by seeking advice and assistance from nurse educators, dietitians, and diabetes specialists. A diabetes specialist should not only be expert in diabetes management, but should also have a fully qualified team assisting in the patient assessment. The specialist and team should follow the accepted practice guidelines, and the patient should be briefed on the specialist's approach before the referral. Expect a complete report with the new regimen and with new goals for treatment. These expectations should be preset as if in a contract.

Adjusting and maintaining insulin treatment: a special note

The goal throughout the adjusting phase is to identify problem areas and provide interventions to address them. To accomplish this, general guidelines are needed. During this phase the target blood glucose level has been narrowed to a range of 70–140 mg/dL (3.9–7.8 mmol/L) pre-meal. If this target has been reached and verified by SMBG data from a memory-based meter, continue with pattern response. If the attempt to achieve glycemic control within the narrow range fails by resulting in either lower or higher blood glucose values, immediate response is required until near euglycemia is restored. Low blood glucose or hypoglycemia is generally the result of lack of synchronization between insulin administration and food intake. To counter the rapid decrease in blood glucose, have the patient ingest carbohydrates sufficient to respond to the decrease in blood glucose level. In general, patients with type 2 diabetes will not become hypoglycemic rapidly. Obesity and insulin resistance generally preclude this condition. Remember that glucose level is a constantly changing velocity measure as opposed to a static physiologic measure. To rapidly reach a steady state, the individual must counteract the effect of insulin with food. Injectable glucagon may be used to counter severe hypoglycemia when the person is unable to self-treat, is unconscious, or has not responded to repeated treatment with food. Persistent hypoglycemia should be treated vigorously in consultation with a diabetes specialist.

Maintain treatment goal phase

Regardless of the type of therapy, the maintain phase refers to a period during which both provider and patient agree that no further changes in therapy are forthcoming. This decision should be based on achieving optimized control for the individual patient. It should be understood that during stabilization, while minor adjustments are likely, significant changes in treatment should not be necessary.

Management of acute complications

While striving for glycemic control, several acute situations may occur that require immediate attention. This section contains guidelines for managing the acute complications associated with type 2 diabetes.

Managing severe hyperglycemia

Severe hyperglycemia occurs when blood glucose is $>$ 400 mg/dL (22.2 mmol/L). When the individual with confirmed type 2 diabetes presents with severe hyperglycemia, the first step is to rule out risk of going into hyperglycemic hyperosmolar syndrome (HHS). This is based on clinical symptoms (polyuria, polydipsia, and/or polyphagia), physical examination (dehydration), and laboratory data (serum glucose $>$ 400 mg/dL or 22.2 mmol/L) and/or plasma osmolarity $>$ 300 mOsm/L; lactic acidosis, small to moderate ketones). If the risk of HHS is high, hospitalization may be necessary (see Chapter 10).

Managing hypoglycemia

Low blood glucose ($<$ 70 mg/dL (3.9 mmol/L) with symptoms and $<$ 60 mg/dL (3.3 mmol/L) with no symptoms) often results from skipped meals while on a sulfonylurea, repaglinide, nateglinide or insulin. In addition, using too much insulin (overinsulinization) may result in hypoglycemia. The first step is to determine whether the patient is having a seizure or is unconscious (see Figure 4.15). If either condition occurs, immediate medical attention is necessary. If SMBG is available, measure the blood glucose first to make certain the level is low. If not immediately available, administer glucagon and follow by obtaining a blood glucose value. Thereafter monitor blood glucose closely. When the reaction is controlled, investigate the cause of hypoglycemia. In general, for patients treated with a sulfonylurea, repaglinide on nateglinide, too little food will cause such a severe reaction. Additionally, patients treated with insulin alone or in combination with oral agents that suppress hepatic glucose output or improve insulin sensitivity are at high risk for hypoglycemia at lower doses of insulin.

If the patient is conscious, the next question is whether the patient requires assistance to overcome the hypoglycemia. Again, measure blood glucose to confirm hypoglycemia. Some patients will experience relative hypoglycemia when the blood glucose drops rapidly from 200 mg/dL to 100 mg/dL (11.1 mmol/L to 5.6 mmol/L). If the patient is truly hypoglycemic and needs assistance but is conscious and not having a seizure, administer fruit juice, regular soda pop, or a commercial glucose gel. Once stabilized, investigate the cause of the hypoglycemic episode. Consider re-educat-

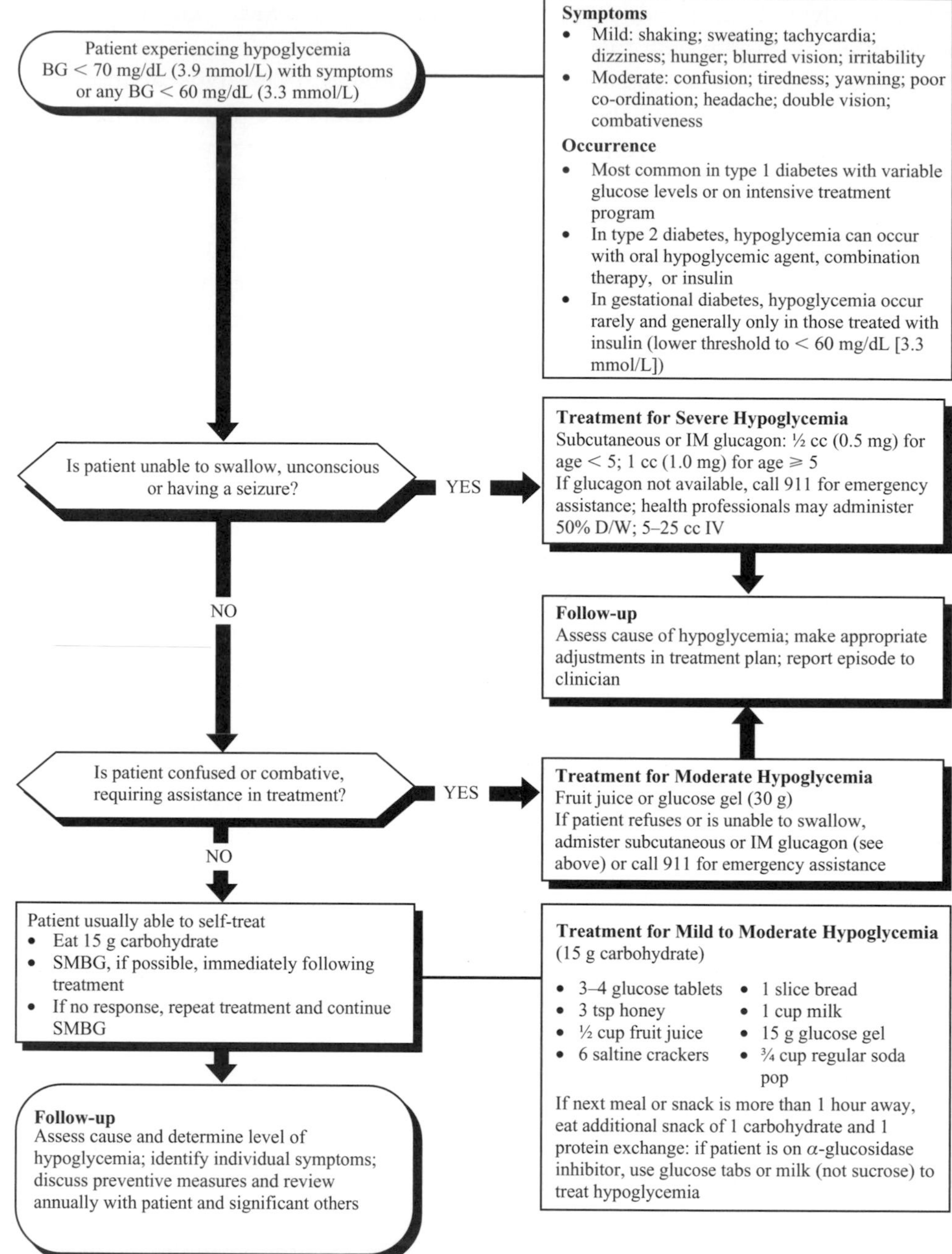

Figure 4.15 Hypoglycemia Treatment DecisionPath

ing the patient and re-evaluating the food plan, exercise, and insulin dosage and timing.

If the patient is having mild to moderate hypoglycemia with symptoms but is able to self-manage, SMBG should be used to document the blood glucose levels during hypoglycemic episodes. It is also important to determine the cognitive state of the individual during such episodes. A person should be able to report the symptoms and the action taken to overcome the hypoglycemia.

Treatment of mild to moderate hypoglycemia generally includes ingesting 15 grams of carbohydrate and retesting blood glucose. When the blood glucose reaches 100 mg/dL (5.6 mmol/L), it is safe to cease treatment and monitor every 2 hours until the next meal. SMBG is the best way to ascertain the response to counter hypoglycemia. It is also a good learning tool for future episodes. Remember that glucose level is a velocity measure, constantly changing, as opposed to a static physiologic measure. To rapidly reach a steady state, the individual must counteract the effect of insulin with glucose. Persistent hypoglycemia should be treated vigorously in consultation with an endocrinologist specializing in diabetes.

Recommend to patients:

- self-monitor blood glucose routinely (two to four times per day)
- follow prescribed food plan
- do not delay meals or snacks
- eat extra carbohydrate or adjust insulin for planned exercise
- be aware of warning signs and treat promptly
- always carry food or glucose tablets to treat hypoglycemia
- anticipate schedule changes – SMBG four times per day may be required
- always consume carbohydrate when consuming alcohol
- make sure friends, coworkers, teachers, and room-mates are aware of symptoms of hypoglycemia and appropriate treatment
- have glucagon available for severe hypoglycemia (review instructions periodically and remind patient and/or family members to check expiration dates)

Review causes/symptoms/treatment with patient, family, friends, coworkers, teachers, and room-mates. Preventing hypoglycemia requires careful reassessment of the possible contributing factors: high-dose hypoglycemic oral agent, over-insulinization (> 1 U/kg in adults), starvation, increased activity, alcohol intake without food, and hypoglycemia unawareness. To prevent the onset of hypoglycemia, SMBG should be required at least two to four times per day. Patients on sulfonylureas may be switched to non-hypoglycemic oral agents. Consider switching patients on single or two injections of insulin to Insulin Stage 3 or 4.

Management during illness

The most appropriate approach to diabetes management during illness is to consider the event from a purely experiential perspective. Blood glucose levels normally increase during illness due to release of stress hormones without regard to prandial state. Patients should be instructed to maintain their usual food plan, oral agent, and/or insulin regimen. Non-caloric fluid intake (water, broth, diet soda pop) may be increased. If patients have nausea or vomiting, initiate their sick day food plan (if available). Increase SMBG and urine ketone testing to every 2–4 hours. If SMBG > 240 mg/dL (13.3 mmol/L) on two consecutive tests, patients may have to supplement their current regimen with R or RA insulin (10 per cent of total daily dose) every 2–4 hours as necessary. Patients should be instructed to contact their provider if SMBG > 240 mg/dL (13.3 mmol/L) and/or they develop moderate to high ketones (rare in type 2 diabetes). Since hyperglycemic hyperosmolar syndrome can occur, frequent telephone contact may be required to prevent the illness from becoming a medical emergency (see Chapter 9). Very ill patients may need to be managed in a medical facility if SMBG is persistently above 400 mg/dL (22.2 mmol/L), if high ketones are present for more than 6 hours, if there is persistent vomiting or diarrhea, or if there is inadequate phone contact.

Type 2 diabetes and pregnancy

For a full discussion of preconception planning and treatment of type 2 diabetes in pregnancy see Chapter 7, Pregestational and Gestational Diabetes. In general the principles outlined in Figure 4.16 should always be followed.

Note: All women actively seeking to become pregnant should be at near-normal blood glucose prior to conception. Women who are not protected from pregnancy and are sexually active should not be given oral agents (exception is the sulfonyurea glyburide) – the main therapy should be medical nutrition therapy alone or with glyburide or insulin.

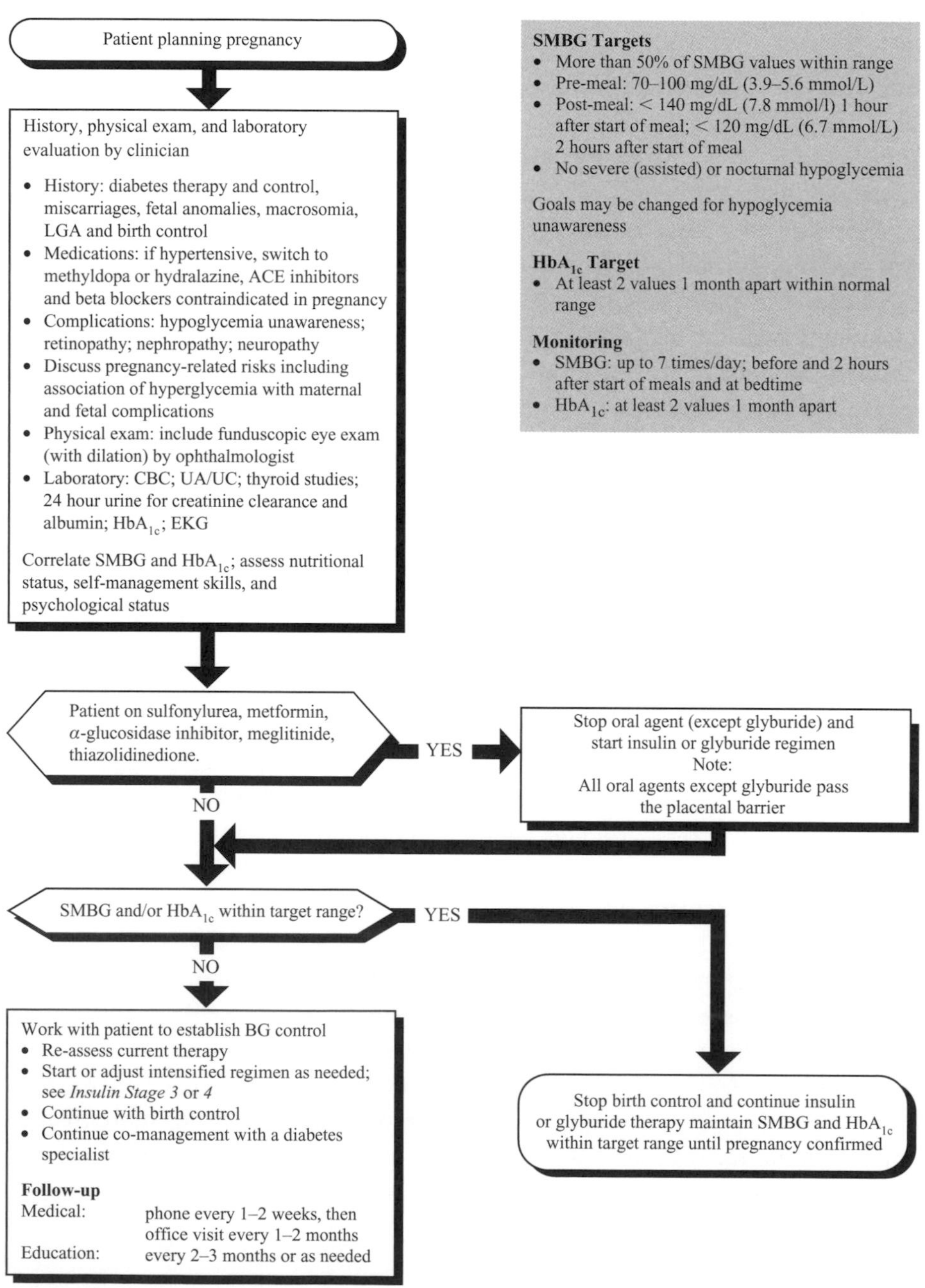

Figure 4.16 Guidelines for Pregestational and Gestational Diabetes

Patient education

All patients require education to understand their diabetes, to learn how to manage it, and to recognize when complications are occurring. This section reviews the principles of education specific to type 2 diabetes. It is preferable to refer patients needing diabetes and nutrition education to nurses and dietitians trained in providing education to individuals with diabetes. This, however, may not be possible. This section provides an overview of the areas covered by patient education in order to acquaint the clinician with what is to be expected if an educator is available, or what is to be addressed if an educator is not available. Where appropriate, the specific education needed for each therapy is also detailed. A complete set of DecisionPaths describing diabetes education, medical nutrition therapy, and exercise assessment can be found in the Appendix.

Diabetes education

Quality diabetes education starts with the establishment of an education plan (see Figure 4.17 and the Appendix, Figures A.8 and A.9). Briefly, the education plan is developed after an extensive physical, psychological, and social assessment of the patient. Based on this assessment, therapeutic (SMBG and HbA_{1c}) and self-management goals are established. The topics to be discussed at the initial diabetes education visit include pathophysiology, medication action and administration, SMBG technique, prevention and treatment of hypoglycemia, and procedures for handling diabetes related medical emergencies. For patients treated with insulin, additional education topics include insulin action, insulin injection technique, site rotation, proper use of glucagon, insulin storage, syringe disposal, and urine ketone monitoring. In order to ensure quality diabetes education, the American Diabetes Association has established a set of 15 diabetes education content areas (see Figure 4.18).

Ideally, patients should have access to specially trained diabetes educators. In the United States,

Establish Education Plan

Assessment
- Height/weight (BMI)/BP/foot exam with monofilament
- Risk factors (family history, obesity, ethnicity, GDM)
- Diabetes knowledge/skills
- Psychosocial issues (denial, anxiety, depression)
- Economic/cultural factors
- Readiness to learn/barriers to learning
- Lifestyle (work, school, food, and exercise habits)
- Tobacco/alcohol use
- Support systems
- Health goals

Goals
- SMBG/HbA_{1c} in target
- Achieve self-management knowledge/skills/ behavior (SMBG, medications, nutrition, exercise)

Plan
- Teach initial education topics
- Establish 3 behavior change goals with patient (exercise, nutrition, medications, monitoring)

Figure 4.17 Guidelines for establishing a diabetes education plan

American Diabetes Association Education Content Areas

1. Pathophysiology of diabetes and treatment options
2. Medical nutrition therapy
3. Physical activity
4. Medications
5. Blood glucose monitoring and use of results
6. Prevention, detection, and treatment of acute complications
7. Prevention, detection, and treatment of chronic complications
8. Goal Setting
9. Psychosocial adjustment
10. Preconception care, pregnancy, and gestational diabetes management

Figure 4.18 Required education content areas for American Diabetes Association recognition

such educators are certified by the National Certification Board of Diabetes Educators. Known as certified diabetes educators (CDEs), they are qualified to provide both basic and advanced diabetes education. Patients have responsibility in terms of self-management and, therefore, must leave the office confident in their skills and understanding. Arrange a follow-up educational visit within 2–4 weeks (or sooner if starting insulin) to review understanding and skills.

Nutrition education

Nutrition education is an integral part of assisting the patient in following a food plan. A registered dietitian with experience in diabetes should counsel the patient as soon as feasible. At the initial nutrition visit, general education about the interrelationship between food and diabetes should be discussed along with a nutritional assessment and the creation of an initial food plan (see Figure 4.19). The food plan should incorporate consistent carbohydrate intake at established meals and, for patients using insulin, integration of the insulin regimen with the food plan. In addition, the food plan should take into account basic medical nutrition therapy guidelines for fat, cholesterol, and sodium intake (see Figure 4.20). For more specific information, see the Appendix (Figures A.8 and A.9) as well as information on carbohydrate counting and food choices (Figures A.14 and A.15). The next visit will be a reassessment combined with an individualized food plan that reflects the ethnic, socio-economic, and special preferences of the patient while addressing the needs of one with diabetes. Here integration of blood glucose results, food plan records, and exercise are discussed. The patient should understand the importance of appropriate food intake, know how to measure caloric intake, and be aware of the effects different nutrients have on blood glucose level.

Establish Nutrition Therapy Plan

Assessment
- Food history or 3 day food record (meals, times, portions)
- Nutrition adequacy
- Height/weight/BMI
- Weight goals/eating disorders
- Psychosocial issues (denial, anxiety, depression)
- Economic/cultural factors
- Nutrition/diabetes knowledge
- Readiness to learn/barriers to learning
- Work/school/sports schedules
- Exercise (times, duration, types)
- Tobacco/alcohol use
- Vitamin/mineral supplements

Goals
- SMBG/HbA$_{1c}$ in target
- Achieve desirable body weight (adults)
- Normal growth and development (children)
- Consistent carbohydrate intake

Plan
- Establish adequate calories for growth and development/reasonable body weight
- Set meal/snack times
- Integrate insulin regimen with medical nutrition therapy (insulin users)
- Set consistent carbohydrate intake
- Encourage regular exercise
- Establish adequate calories for pregnancy/lactation/recovery from illness

Figure 4.19 Guidelines for establishing a nutrition therapy plan

Medical Nutrition Therapy Guidelines
- Total fat = 30% total calories; less if obese and high LDL
- Saturated fat < 10% total calories; < 7% with high LDL
- Cholesterol < 300 mg/day
- Sodium < 2400 mg/day
- Protein reduced to 0.8 g/kg/day (~10% total calories) if macroalbuminuria
- Calories decreased by 10–20% if BMI > 25 kg/m^2

Figure 4.20 Medical nutrition therapy guidelines

Exercise/activity education

Patients are often unaware of the importance of exercise (or increased activity) and its relationship to metabolic control. Exercise education begins with detailing how exercise affects blood glucose levels. Once the patient understands the role of exercise or activity in managing diabetes, the next step is to develop an exercise (activity) plan (see Figure 4.21). Careful evaluation of overall fitness

Establish Exercise Plan

Goals
- Consistent exercise schedule
- Include aerobic (jog, swim, bike) and anaerobic (weight lifting, push-ups) exercises
- Frequency: 3 times/week
- Duration: 30 minutes/session
- Intensity: 50–75% maximum heart capacity (220 − age = 100%)
- If obese, expend 700–2000 calories/week

Plan
- Individualize based on fitness level, age, weight, personal goals, and medical history
- Select type of exercise with patient
- Set exercise schedule with patient
- Measure, record, and review SMBG before and 20 minutes after exercise
- Patient to record type, duration, and intensity
- Patient to note any symptoms, i.e., pain, dizziness, shortness of breath, hypoglycemia

Follow-up
Each week for 2 weeks

Figure 4.21 Guidelines for establishing an exercise plan

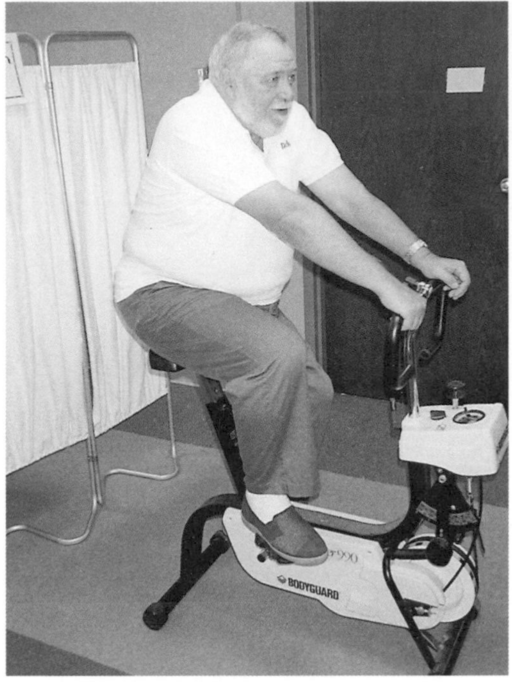

Photo 4.2 Endurance: stationary bike

level is important. Any concerns about cardiovascular disease should be evaluated prior to starting an exercise program. Generally, the patient should be evaluated for fitness on three parameters:

1. endurance (repetitive movements), shown in Photos 4.2 and 4.3
2. strength (lifting weight resistance bands), shown in Photo 4.4
3. flexibility (stretching), shown in Photo 4.5

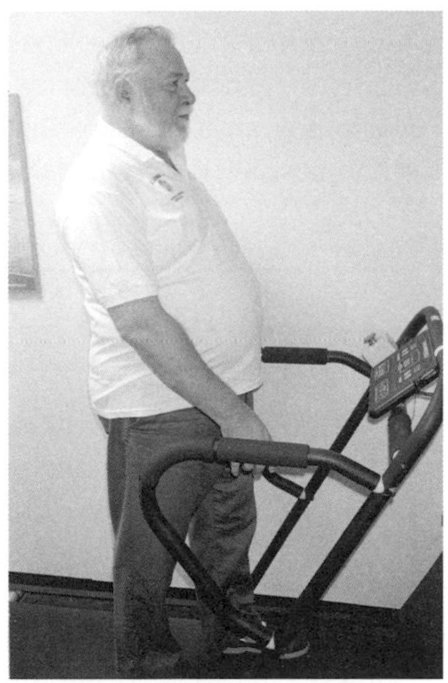

Photo 4.3 Endurance: treadmill

Endurance can be measured by asking the patient to step up and down from a one-step stool continuously for 1 minute. If a stationary exercise bicycle is available, repeated peddling with midrange resistance for 1 minute is another means of assessing endurance. While there are some general standards that are age and gender specific, the patient should be able to perform these activities without any apparent stress. Strength is measured by stretching a standard resistance band or lifting a five pound weight with an outstretched arm. Again, age- and gender-specific tables will provide the average expected strength that would permit eventual repeated exercise. Flexibility can be measured in several ways: simple stretching while standing; touching toes while standing or

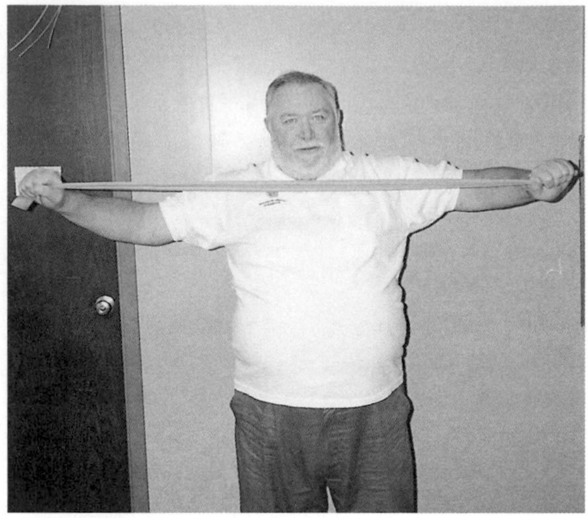

Photo 4.4 Strength: resistance bands

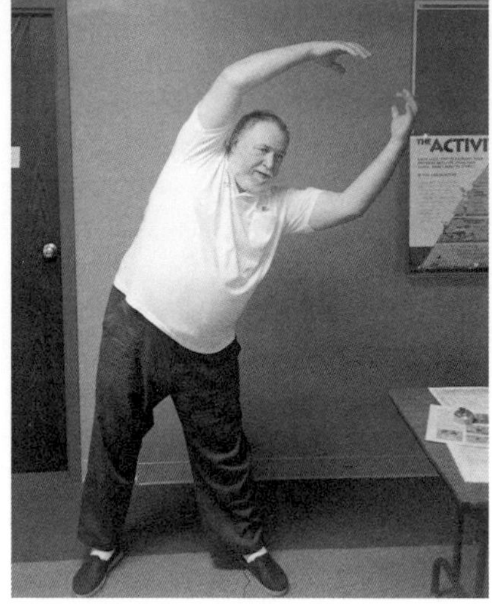

Photo 4.5 Flexibility: stretching

lying; or reaching with both feet flat on the ground. Collectively, these measures are meant to provide an overall rapid assessment of the patient's fitness for exercise.

The level of exercise is determined individually and must answer such questions as when, how often, how long, and at what pace. The Appendix contains Specific DecisionPaths for exercise assessment, developing an exercise plan, and exercise education topics. SMBG testing should occur before and immediately following exercise. For routine exercise, this should be repeated three to five times until a clear pattern emerges. Many patients report significant improvement in blood glucose levels when exercise is included in the overall treatment strategy. While an exercise specialist is desirable, many CDEs are qualified to evaluate fitness and to develop an exercise prescription.

Behavioral issues and assessment

Behavioral issues may be divided into two general categories: adherence to regimen and underlying psychological or social pathology. While nonadherence to a specific regimen may have underlying pathology, it is suggested in a primary care setting to first determine whether the problem is due to other causes. Staged Diabetes Management provides a simple set of pathways to review possible avenues to explore before considering psychological and social causes. Assessment begins with an evaluation of the current level of glycemic control as reported by the patient (SMBG) and the laboratory (fasting plasma or HbA_{1c}). This is because medical intervention is justified when the current therapy is not working. If the correlation between SMBG and HbA_{1c} (see Figure 4.22) is poor, make certain that technique, device, and reporting by the patient are understood. Have patients demonstrate SMBG technique using their meter and draw a simultaneous blood sample for the laboratory. If the correlation between patient and laboratory data is still poor, consider re-education.

Adherence assessment

Four diabetes-related areas of adherence that can be readily assessed in the primary care setting include medical nutrition, medication, SMBG,

If HbA_{1c} is:	HbA_{1c}*	Average SMBG is:
1 percentage point above normal	7%	~150 mg/dL (8.3 mmol/L)
2 percentage points above normal	8%	~180 mg/dL (10.0 mmol/L)
3 percentage points above normal	9%	~210 mg/dL (11.7 mmol/L)
4 percentage points above normal	10%	~245 mg/dL (13.6 mmol/L)
5 percentage points above normal	11%	~280 mg/dL (15.6 mmol/L)
6 percentage points above normal	12%	~310 mg/dL (17.2 mmol/L)
7 percentage points above normal	13%	~345 mg/dL (19.2 mmol/L)
8 percentage points above normal	14%	~380 mg/dL (21.1 mmol/L)

* assumes normal range of 4–6%

Nathan, DM, et al: *N Engl J Med* **310**: 341–346, 1984

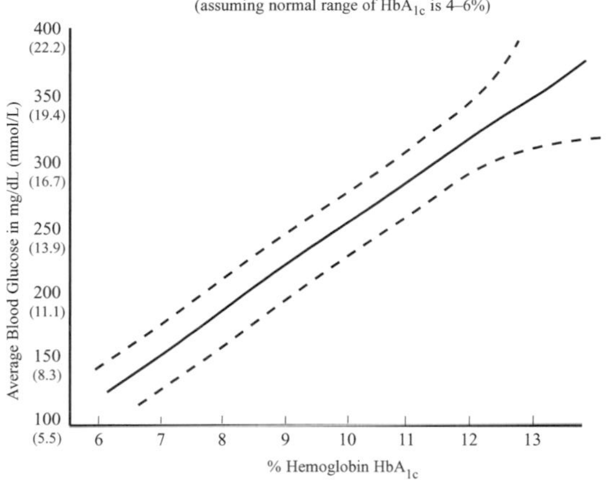

Figure 4.22 Relationship between glycosylated hemoglobin HbA_{1c} and blood glucose levels

and exercise. Each area is approached in a similar manner. First, determine whether the patient understands the relationship between the behavior and diabetes. Second, determine whether the patient is prepared to set explicit short-term behavioral goals. Third, determine why the goals are not met; and fourth, be prepared to return to a previous step along this pathway if the current step is not completed.

The Specific DecisionPath for assessing adherence to nutrition therapy is shown in Figure 4.23. DecisionPaths for assessing adherence to medication, SMBG, and exercise regimens are located in the Appendix. Based on the transtheoretical model of behavior change,[37] all of the adherence DecisionPaths begin with whether the patient understands the connection between the behavior and diabetes. It has been found that changing behavior without understanding why it is important to do so will most likely fail. Thus, providing the patient with specifics as to how food, exercise, medications, or SMBG is related to diabetes management and prevention of complications is critical. Next, determine specifically what the patient is willing to do. In most cases, any misunderstanding as to the importance of adhering to the prescribed regimen can be resolved through this systematic approach. The next step involves setting goals with the patient. Set simple, reasonable, and explicit short-term goals like "replace whole milk with skim milk" or "increase walking by 10 minutes per day." Next, determine whether the patient has met or is attempting to meet the goals. Be prepared to reset the goals and move back a step. As the behavior changes, negotiate new explicit goals. Always ask the patient to help set the new goal. There are, however, those patients for whom this approach will not work. Some patients are not ready to change their behaviors. Continued reinforcement for change, combined with education, will sometimes overcome this reluctance to modify behavior. If this is not effective consider referral to a behavioral expert.

Psychological and social assessment

The diagnosis of type 2 diabetes carries with it the risk of psychological and social dysfunction. Almost half of newly diagnosed cases are uncovered after a complication (such as retinopathy or heart disease) has been discovered. The knowledge that they may havc had undetected diabetes for several years combined with the added burden of diabetes related complications presents a unique dilemma. On the one hand the individual is expected to return to normal life; on the other hand he or she is expected to be responsible for self-management. With the need to restore near euglycemia, this becomes even more problematic. The initiation of a new approach to treatment (such as introducing insulin therapy), may also cause both psychological and social dysfunction. This is often reflected in how the individual adjusts to changes in lifestyle brought about by type 2 diabetes and its treatment.

Patients' ability to acquire the new knowledge and skills is related to their psychological and social adjustment. Such psychological factors as

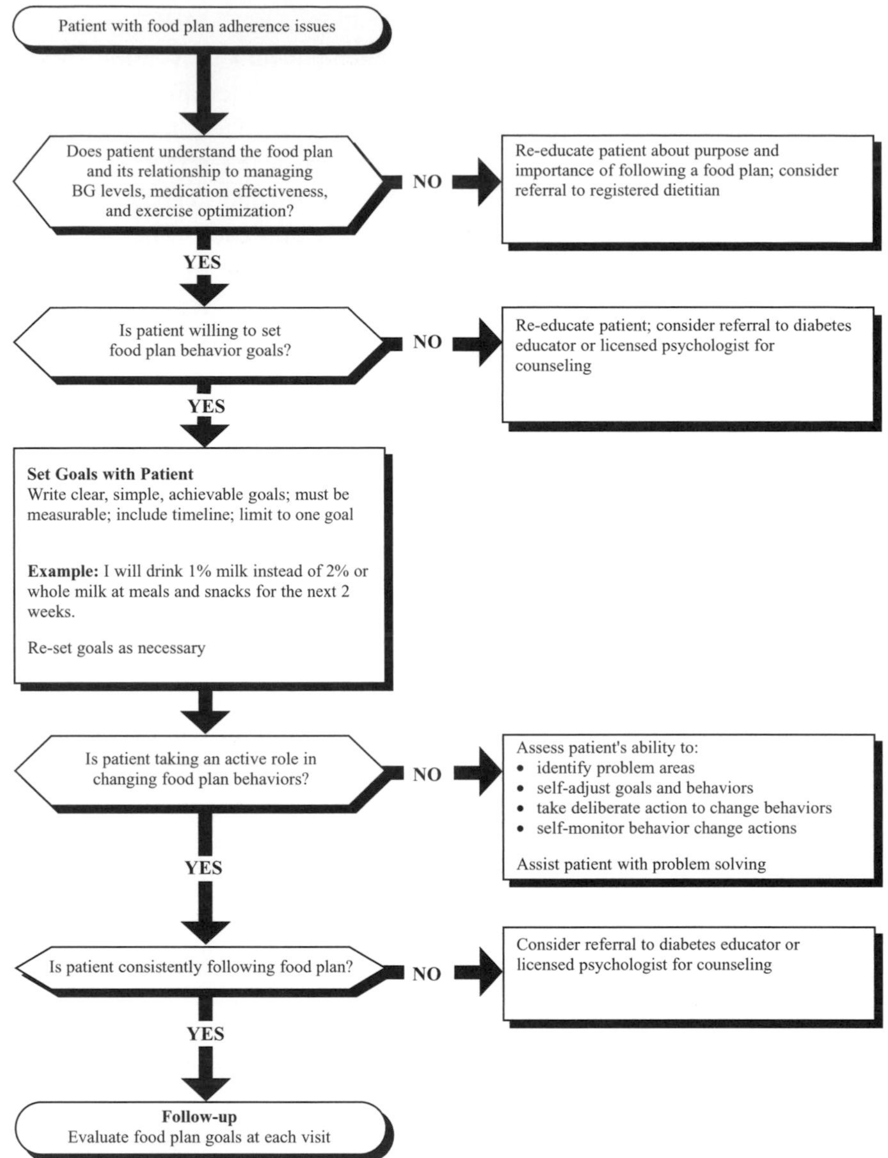

Figure 4.23 Nutrition Therapy Adherence Assessment DecisionPath

depression and anxiety and social factors such as conduct disorders significantly interfere with acquiring self-care skills and with accepting the seriousness of diabetes. Additionally, eating disorders may directly affect the efficacy of treatment and may present serious, long-lasting complications. If the psychological and social adjustment of the individual with diabetes proves to be dysfunctional, it will most likely be reflected in poor glycemic control. This, in turn, raises the risk of acute and chronic complications, which contribute still further to the psychological and social dysfunction. To break this cycle it is necessary to identify the earliest signs of dysfunction and to intervene as soon as possible.

The primary care physician generally initiates psychological and social interventions in diabetes only after symptoms occur. Many of the more common symptoms can be found in the Psychological and Social Assessment DecisionPath (see Figure 4.24). In anticipation of such symptoms, it might be appropriate for primary care physicians

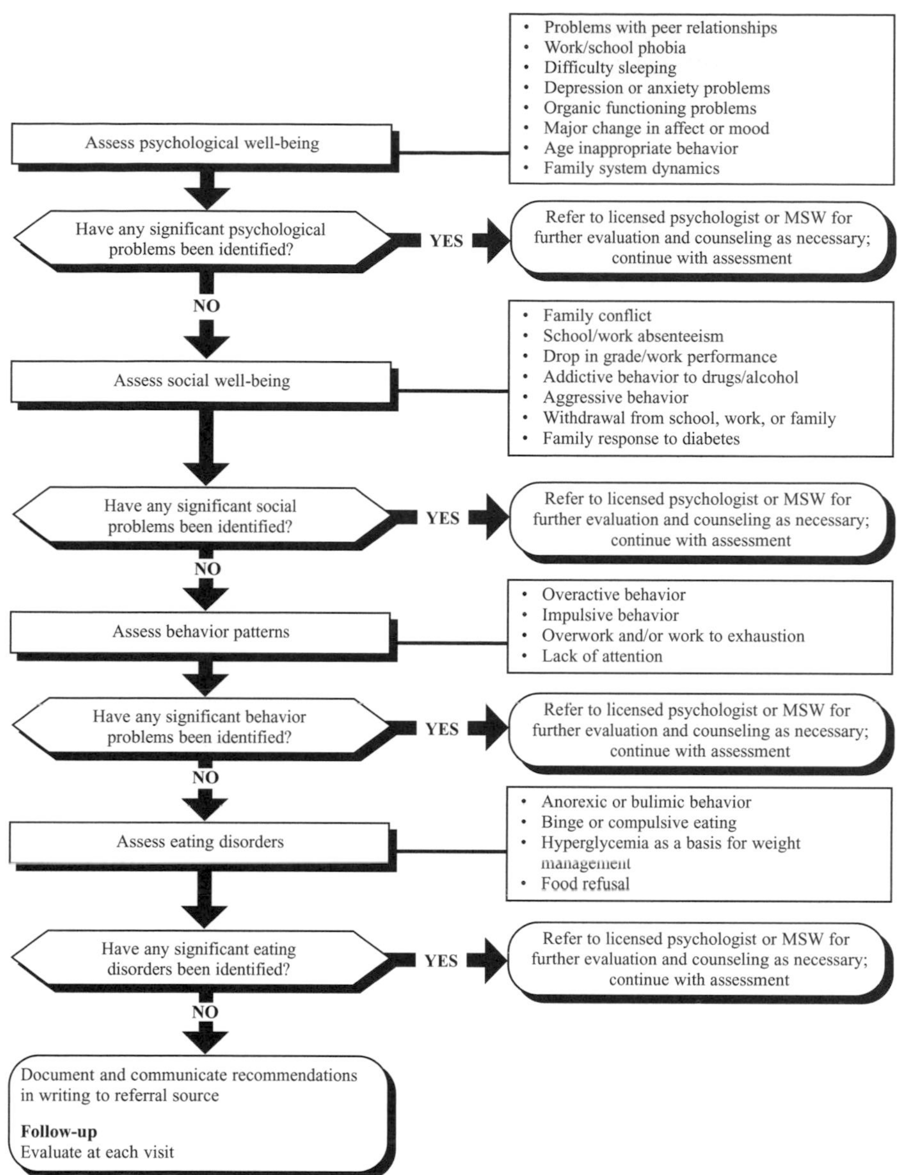

Figure 4.24 Psychological and Social Assessment DecisionPath

to refer newly diagnosed patients, and patients for whom significant changes in therapy are being contemplated, to a psychologist or social worker trained to detect the earliest symptoms of psychological or social dysfunction and to intervene before they result in destructive behaviors. Often one or two counseling sessions are required to detect underlying psychological or social problems and to intervene effectively. Recognizing these early warning signs requires a complete psychological and social profile of the individual. One approach to obtaining this information is to begin the patient encounter with the idea that diabetes will be co-managed by the patient and the physician (and team) and that the patient will be empowered to make decisions. Most patients begin interactions with physicians assuming the power to make all clinical decisions rests with the physician.

For successful diabetes management (where 90

per cent is the responsibility of the patient) co-empowerment of the patient with the health care team effectively brings the patient onto the team and ensures that the patient understands and takes on clinical care responsibilities. Co-empowerment recognizes that the patient and physician may have a different view of the seriousness of the disease, the responsibilities of each health care professional, and the expectations of the patient's performance. The individual with diabetes may feel the physician will make all decisions related to care and the patient should be passive. Alternatively, the physician may feel the patient should make daily decisions about diet, insulin, and exercise.

Co-empowerment is an agreement between the patient and health care team that delineates the responsibilities and expectations of each participant in care and also provides the DecisionPath all team members have agreed to follow. From a psychosocial perspective, it may be seen as a contract in which the patient spells out in detail his or her expectations and in which health care professionals have an opportunity to determine how well those responsibilities and expectations fit with the diabetes management plan. It presents an opportunity to review behaviors that may be dysfunctional to the overall treatment goal. The person who refuses to test, who is hyperactive at work, or who binge eats must be encouraged to share this information with the health team. Similarly, the physician who believes in strict adherence to regimens or the dietitian who expects 100 per cent compliance with a restrictive food plan must be able to state these expectations and have them challenged by the patient. Through this process of negotiation, a consensus as to goals, responsibilities, and expectations can be reached that will benefit the person with diabetes as well as the health care team members.

References

1. Centers for Disease Control National Center for Chronic Disease Prevention and Health Promotion. *National Diabetes Fact Sheet*, 2003.
2. American Diabetes Association. *Diabetes 1996: Vital Statistics.*
3. Youngren JF, Goldfine ID and Prately RE. Decreased muscle insulin receptor kinase correlates with insulin resistance in normoglycemic Pima Indians. *Am J Physiol* 1997; **273**: E276–E283.
4. Sinha MK, Pories WJ, Flickinger EG, Meelheim D and Cara JF. Insulin-receptor kinase activity of adipose tissue from morbidly obese humans with and without NIDDM. *Diabetes* 1987; **36**: 620–625.
5. Kusari J, Kenner KA, Suh KI, Hill DE and Henry RR. Skeletal muscle protein tyrosine phosphatase activity and tyrosine phosphatase 1B protein content are associated with insulin action and resistance. *J Clin Invest* 1994; **93**: 1156–1162.
6. Boden G, Chen X, Ruiz J, White JV and Rossetti L. Mechanisms of fatty acid-induced inhibition of glucose uptake. *J Clin Invest* 1994; **93**: 2438–2446.
7. Foley JE. Rationale and application of fatty acid oxidation inhibitors in treatment of diabetes mellitus. *Diabetes Care* 1992; **15**: 773–784.
8. Moller DE. Potential role of TNF-alpha in the pathogenesis of insulin resistance and type 2 diabetes. *Trend Endocrinol Metab* 2000; **11**: 212–217.
9. Bertin E, Nguyen P, Guenounou M, Durlach V, Potron G and Leutenegger M. Plasma levels of tumor necrosis factor-alpha (TNF-alpha) are essentially dependent of visceral fat amount in type 2 diabetic patients. *Diabetes Metab* 2000; **26**: 178–182.
10. Youd JM, Rattigan S and Clark MG. Acute impairment of insulin-mediated capillary recruitment and glucose uptake in rat skeletal muscle in vivo by TNF-alpha. *Diabetes* 2000; **49**: 1904–1909.
11. Abate N. Insulin resistance and obesity. Role of fat distribution pattern. *Diabetes Care* 1996; **19**: 292–294.
12. Leahy JL, Bonner Weir S and Weir GC. β-cell dysfunction induced by chronic hyperglycemia. Current ideas on mechanism of impaired glucose-induced insulin secretion. *Diabetes Care* 1992; **15**: 442–455.
13. Diabetes Control and Complications Trial Research Group. The effect of intensive treatment of diabetes on the development and progression of long-term complications in insulin-dependent diabetes mellitus. *N Engl J Med* 1993; **329**: 977–986.
14. Kuusisto J, Mykkanen L, Pyorala K and Laakso M. NIDDM and its metabolic control predict coronary

heart disease in elderly subjects. Diabetes 1994; **43**: 960–967.
15. Klein R. Hyperglycemia and microvascular and macrovascular disease in diabetes. *Diabetes Care* 1995: **18**: 258–268.
16. Ohkubo Y, Kishikawa H and Araki E. Intensive insulin therapy prevents the progression of diabetic microvascular complications in Japanese patients with non-insulin-dependent diabetes mellitus: a randomized prospective 6-year study. *Diabetes Res Clin Pract* 1995; **28**: 103–117.
17. Garg A. Treatment of diabetic dyslipidemia. *Am J Cardiol* 1998; **81**(4A): 47B–51B.
18. UK Prospective Diabetes Study Group. Intensive blood-glucose control with sulphonylureas or insulin compared with conventional treatment and risk of complications in patients with type 2 diabetes (UKPDS 33). *Lancet* 1998; **352**: 837–853
19. Turner RC, Millns H, Neil HA, *et al.* Risk factors for coronary artery disease in non-insulin dependent diabetes mellitus: United Kingdom Prospective Diabetes Study (UKPDS: 23). *Br Med J* 1998; **316**: 823–828.
20. Harris MI. Classification, diagnostic criteria, and screening for diabetes. *Diabetes in America* 1995; NIH Publications No. 95-1468(2): 15–36.
21. Meigs JB, Singer DE, Sullivan LM, *et al.* Metabolic control and prevalent cardiovascular disease in non-insulin-dependent diabetes mellitus (NIDDM): the NIDDM patient outcome research team. *Am J Med* 1997; **102**: 38–47.
22. Stern MP and Haffner SM. Dyslipidemia in type II diabetes: implications for therapeutic intervention. *Diabetes Care* 1991; **14**: 1144–1159.
23. Neel, JV. Diabetes mellitus: a "thrifty" geno-type rendered detrimental by "progress?" *Am J Hum Genet* 1962; **14**: 353–62.
24. Knowler WC, Barret-Connor E, Fowler SE, *et al.* Reduction in the incidence of type 2 diabetes with lifestyle intervention or metformin. *N Engl J Med* 2002; **346**: 393–403.
25. Uusitupa M, Louheranta A, Lindstrom J, Valle T, Sundvall J, Eriksson J and Tumomilehto J. The Finnish Diabetes Prevention Study. *Br J Nutr* 2000; Suppl 1: S137–142.
26. American Diabetes Association. Report of the Expert Committee on the Diagnosis and Classification of Diabetes Mellitus. *Diabetes Care* 2003; **26**: S5–S20.
27. Azen SP, Peters RK, Berkowitz K, Kjos S and Xiang A, Buchanan TA. Tripod (troglitazone in the prevention of diabetes): a randomized, placebo-controlled trial of troglitazone in women with prior gestational diabetes mellitus. *Control Clin Trials* 1998; **19**: 217–231.
28. Nathan DM. Inferences and implications: do results from the Diabetes Control and Complications Trial apply in NIDDM? *Diabetes Care* 1995; **18**: 251–257.
29. Mazze RS, Shamoon H, Parmentier R, *et al.* Reliability of blood glucose monitoring by patients with diabetes. *Am J Med* 1984; **77**: 211–217.
30. Mazze RS. Measuring and Managing hyperglycemia in pregnancy: from glycosurin to continuous blood glucose monitoring. *Seminars in Perinatology* 2002; **26**(3): 171–180.
31. Watts NB, Spanheimer RG, DiGirolamo M, *et al.* Prediction of glucose response to weight loss in patients with non-insulin-dependent diabetes mellitus. *Arch Intern Med* 1990; **150**: 803–806.
32. Frankenfield DC, Muth ER and Rowe WA. The Harris–Benedict studies of human basal metabolism: history and limitations. *J Am Diet Assoc* 1998; **98**: 439–445.
33. Devlin JT. Effects of exercise on insulin sensitivity in humans. *Diabetes Care* 1992; **15**: 1690–1693.
34. Chiasson JL, Josse RG, Hunt JA, *et al.* The efficacy of acarbose in the treatment of patient with non-insulin-dependent diabetes mellitus. *Ann. Intern Med* 1994; **12**: 928–935.
35. John JL, Wolf SL and Kabadi UM. Efficacy of insulin and sulfonylurea combination therapy in type II diabetes: a meta-analysis of the randomized placebo-controlled trials. *Arch Intern Med* 1996; **156**: 259–264.
36. UK Prospective Diabetes Study Group. Effect of intensive blood-glucose control with metformin on complications in overweight patients with type 2 diabetes (UKPDS 34). *Lancet* 1998; **352**: 854–865.
37. Prochaska JO, Norcross JC and Diclemente CC. *Changing for Good*. New York: Avon, 1994.

Kahn CR. Causes of insulin resistance. *Nature* 1995; **373**: 384–385.

Reaven GM, Laws A. Insulin resistance, compensatory hyperinsulinemia, and coronary heart disease. *Diabetologia* 1994; **37**: 948–952.

Wing RR, Blair EH, Bononi P, Marcus MD, Watanabe R, Bergman RM. Caloric restriction per se is a significant factor in improvements in glycemic control and insulin sensitivity during weight loss in obese NIDDM patients. *Diabetes Care* 1994; **17**: 30–36.

Klein R, Klein BEK and Moss S. The Wisconsin Epidemiologic Study of Diabetic Retinopathy: a review. *Diabetes Metab Rev* 1989; **5**: 559–570.

Nathan DM, Singer DE, Hurxthal K and Goodson JD. The clinical information value of the glycosylated hemoglobin assay. *N Engl J Med* 1984; **310**: 341–346.

Monk A, Barry B, McClain K, Weaver T, Cooper N and Franz M. Practice guidelines for medical nutrition therapy provided by dietitians for persons with non-insulin dependent diabetes mellitus. *J Am Diet Assoc* 1995; **95**: 999–1006.

Franz, MJ, Monk A, Barry B, *et al.* Effectiveness of medical nutrition therapy provided by dietitians in the management of non-insulin dependent diabetes mellitus; A randomized, controlled clinical trial. *J Am Diet Assoc* 1995; **95**: 1009–1017.

Jensen-Urstad KJ, Reichard PG, Rosfors S and Lindblad LEL, Jensen-Urstad MT. Early atherosclerosis is retarded by improved long-term blood glucose control in patients with DDM. *Diabetes* 1996; **45**: 1253–1258.

Bailey CJ, Path MRC and Turner RC. Metformin. *N Engl J Med* 1996; **334**: 574–579.

5 Type 2 Diabetes and Metabolic Syndrome in Children and Adolescents

The development of insulin resistance or metabolic syndrome and type 2 diabetes in children and adolescents is considered a new epidemic.[1] A rise in childhood obesity, a decline in exercise/activity level, and a realization that not all childhood hyperglycemia results from type 1 diabetes have joined to cause special medical attention to focus on children and adolescents who are at especially high risk for a series of disorders known as metabolic syndrome, insulin resistance syndrome, or syndrome X. All of which reflect the increased realization that obesity, hyperglycemia, hypertension, dyslipidemia, and renal disease may be closely connected.

Currently there are no national data from the United States as to the incidence or prevalence of either insulin resistance or type 2 diabetes in individuals under the age of 18. Neither the Centers for Disease Control and Prevention nor the National Diabetes Data Group of the National Institute of Diabetes and Digestive and Kidney Diseases are able to provide accurate data as to the number of children and adolescents with known type 2 diabetes. Similarly, information related to childhood hypertension and dyslipidemia is scarce. Most epidemiological data regarding type 2 in children and adolescents comes from small population studies limited to specific regions or ethnic groups that may limit their findings, often to just those being studied. However, it is clear that before the early 1990s type 2 diabetes was rarely diagnosed in children and adolescents, but by 1999 the diagnosis increased to 8–45 per cent of all new cases across the United States.[2] The factors contributing to this increasing number are (1) better surveillance; (2) increased prevalence of obesity in children and adolescents; (3) poor nutrition with diets high in fat and carbohydrate; and (4) sedentary lifestyle.

The risk factors associated with type 2 diabetes include:[3]

- overweight – BMI greater than 85th percentile for age and gender
- family history of type 2 diabetes in 1st or 2nd degree relative
- hypertension – BP > 95th percentile for age and gender
- dyslipidemia – HDL < 40 mg/dL (1.1 mmol/L), triglycerides > 250 mg/dL (2.8 mmol/L)
- previous impaired glucose homeostasis – impaired fasting glucose and/or impaired glucose tolerance (prediabetes)
- low (< 2000 g) or high birth weight (> 4000 g)
- high-risk ethnic group (American Indian, Alaska Native, African-American, Mexican-American)

Staged Diabetes Management: A Systematic Approach (2nd Edition) R. S. Mazze, E. S. Strock, G. D. Simonson and R. M. Bergenstal
 ISBN: 0 470 86576 8

- polycystic ovary syndrome
- Acanthosis Nigricans
- sedentary lifestyle
- poor nutrition

Etiology

The etiology of type 2 diabetes in children and adolescents appears to be similar to that of adults. Hyperglycemia is due to a combination of insulin resistance and relative insulin deficiency. This has been reviewed extensively in Chapter 4 and will be reviewed briefly.

Figure 5.1 shows the three variables that depict the natural history of type 2 diabetes in children. Like adults, children pass through three phases: (1) normal glycemia with hyperinsulinemia; (2) prediabetes (impaired fasting glucose (IFG) – fasting plasma glucose between 100 and 125 mg/dL (5.6 and 6.9 mmol/L) – or impaired glucose tolerance (IGT) – 75 g oral glucose tolerance test two hour value between 140 and 199 mg/dL (7.8 and 11 mmol/L); (3) diabetes.

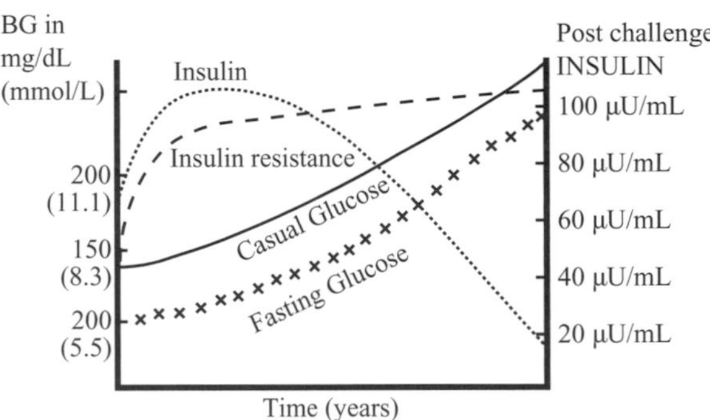

Figure 5.1 The natural history and underlying defects of type 2 diabetes in children and adolescents

A major differentiation between children with type 1 and type 2 diabetes is that children and adolescents with impaired glucose homeostasis or type 2 diabetes may have elevated plasma insulin levels at the time of diagnosis. Pancreatic β-cells respond to increasing insulin resistance by synthesizing and secreting more insulin in an attempt to maintain euglycemia. This can be indirectly measured by determining the amount of insulin in the blood using an insulin radioimmunoassay (RIA). In rare cases, those with long-standing undetected type 2 diabetes, insulin levels are low due to a gradual loss in first-phase insulin secretion. The β-cells are not able to sustain the demands of increased synthesis and secretion of insulin and, over the course of several years, gradually lose the ability to secrete adequate amounts of insulin. This decline in β-cell function has been called 'β-cell exhaustion' and may be triggered by persistent hyperglycemia (glucose toxicity) and well as hyperlipidemia (lipotoxicity).[4] This process is modulated by such factors as diet, activity, and weight gain. Eventually, if near-normal glycemia is restored, insulin production improves.

As mentioned previously, confounding these factors is the fact that some children with type 2 diabetes have a concomitant process linked to increasing insulin resistance (seen as polycystic ovary syndrome in females and/or Acanthosis Nigricans in both females and males from ethnic groups at highest risk for diabetes). Also known as the metabolic syndrome, it is marked by obesity and such conditions as hypertension, dyslipidemia, and renal disease. While there is no method to accurately predict which children will develop insulin resistance or diabetes, genetic factors plus obesity present the highest risks. Hispanics, African-Americans, Native Americans, and Asian-Americans have an incidence rate that varies from two- to tenfold that of Caucasians.

Prevention of type 2 diabetes

Can insulin resistance or type 2 diabetes be prevented in children? The concept of genetic predisposition to insulin resistance and type 2 diabetes has received significant attention. Supporting this theory is the high prevalence of obesity and type 2 diabetes in American Indian, Samoan, and Hispanic children and adolescents. The idea that a thrifty gene favoring storing energy over expending energy is prevalent in these ethnic minorities is supported by a high preponderance of obesity in their children.[5] This suggests both a genetic and a morphologic explanation linking hyperglycemia to obesity through insulin resistance.

Do these factors act independently in children? Evidence suggests that the highest risk of type 2 diabetes among all children would be in obese American Indian children. The lowest risk would be in lean Caucasian children with no family history of diabetes. Can diabetes be prevented in the former group? If obesity is the principal factor, medical nutrition therapy as well as increased exercise/activity will be beneficial to prevent type 2 diabetes. If, however, genetic defects in the pancreatic β-cell of insulin-sensitive tissue is the root cause then early use of either insulin or insulin sensitizers may be the solution. If a combination of factors leads to diabetes, perhaps prevention will require a combination of interventions. Unfortunately, there are no reported studies that have consistently addressed the issues around preventing type 2 diabetes in children. Studies in adults suggest that promotion of appropriate nutrition and activity level combined with very close surveillance, so that those at the highest risk (impaired glucose homeostasis) could be offered treatment, may be the best that can be currently undertaken.

Major studies

The underlying principles in the management of insulin resistance and/or type 2 diabetes in children are based principally on small studies of children plus studies in adults. The major dilemma is whether intensive treatment at the onset of disease is appropriate in children. There is no evidence that allowing blood glucose or blood pressure to worsen is beneficial. As type 2 diabetes is part of a larger syndrome with consequences for almost every major organ system and since these co-morbidities are more prevalent in individuals with long-standing hyperglycemia, it is likely that intensive treatment in children would be beneficial. In adults, type 2 diabetes is often detected 7–10 years after it actually develops.[6] This may be the case in children. If this occurs it would increase the likelihood that adolescents would present at diagnosis with such associated co-morbidities as retinopathy, nephropathy, neuropathy, hypertension, and/or dyslipidemia.

Initiation of intensive treatment in children presents some risks. Few would argue that if medical nutrition therapy were selected as the solo therapy and successfully reduced blood glucose, blood pressure, and lowered weight this regimen would be beneficial at very low risk. On the other hand, some would argue that reliance on metformin and/or insulin may present a greater risk of adverse events. While metformin presents no risk of hypoglycemia or weight gain, its use in children has been limited and whether there are consequences remains unclear. Insulin, which has been used in children since 1922, has its own risks: hypoglycemia and weight gain. Anti-hypertensive drugs also have unknown risks in children. Such risks, some argue, outweigh the benefits of reduced microvascular and macrovascular disease.

The principle followed in Staged Diabetes Management is to optimize metabolic control without relying on pharmacologic agents when possible. Nevertheless, when blood glucose or blood pressure is elevated or when medical nutrition therapy alone fails, SDM supports the careful initiation of pharmacological agents.

Overview of treatment options for children and adolescents with type 2 diabetes

It would be preferable to identify a single treatment option that addresses many of the components of the metabolic syndrome. Among the three options (medical nutrition, metformin, or insulin) for treatment of type 2 diabetes, medical nutrition therapy does just this. In children medical nutrition therapy takes on special significance. An appropriate food plan to assure normal growth and development must be balanced with one that helps to achieve glycemic targets, maintain reasonable weight and not contribute to either hypertension or dyslipidemia. In conjunction with exercise, medical nutrition therapy aims at improved glycemic control through modifications in daily carbohydrate intake and total number of calories. Too few studies exist in children and adolescents related to medical nutrition therapy as treatment for type 2 diabetes. While there are some parallels with adults, such as the effect of weight loss on glycemic control, it is still uncertain as to how much caloric reduction is appropriate in light of the need to assure proper growth and maturation.

Obese children tend to be more sedentary. There are data that suggest that caloric utilization by obese children is less than half that of normal-weight children due to this inactivity. Thus increased activity and weight reduction are needed to reduce insulin resistance, lower plasma insulin levels, and improve glycemic control.

When medical nutrition therapy fails to improve, for example, glycemic control or when blood glucose levels are moderately high at diagnosis (fasting plasma glucose 200–300 mg/dL (11.1–16.6 mmol/L), metformin combined with medical nutrition therapy is required. This non-hypoglycemic agent (a biguanide) has its major effect on suppression of excessive hepatic glucose output. If this fails to restore normal blood glucose levels, or if blood glucose levels are beyond the effective range of metformin at diagnosis, insulin alone may be indicated. Insulin based therapies depend upon a food/activity plan to help by reducing or maintaining weight (improving insulin sensitivity) and assure that there is an appropriate amount of carbohydrate at each meal to prevent both hypoglycemia and hyperglycemia. Exogenous insulin therapies work by augmenting the individual's own endogenous production of insulin. Meals, snacks, and exercise/activity must be synchronized with the pharmacokinetics of insulin action. Current therapy is a combination of short-, intermediate-, and long-acting insulin, Exogenous insulin in its two short-acting forms, regular and rapid acting, are used to cover post-meal rises in blood glucose or to correct currently elevated glucose levels. Intermediate-acting NPH or long-acting ultralente and glargine provide basal insulin requirements. Because of variation in action patterns, hypoglycemia may occur if too much insulin is administered, insufficient carbohydrate is ingested, or the timing of meals, insulin, and exercise is not synchronized. Referral for medical nutrition therapy is highly recommended when initiating insulin therapy to avoid excessive weight gain associated with intiation of this therapy.

The remainder of the chapter is divided into three inter-related sections. The first is related to obesity, the second to the detection and treatment of type 2 diabetes, and the third to the other components of the metabolic syndrome.

Obesity and weight management in children and adolescents

This discussion provides the basis for screening, diagnosis and the treatment of obesity and weight related problems with children. It begins with the Weight Management for Children and Adolescents Practice Guidelines, followed by the Master DecisionPath. The latter lays out an orderly sequence of therapeutic interventions that target specific elements of weight management. Specific DecisionPaths for each treatment options along with a complete rationale for decisions are also presented.

Weight Management Practice Guidelines

Staged Diabetes Management Practice Guidelines are structured to address screening and diagnosis, treatment options, metabolic targets, monitoring, and follow-up. Figure 5.2 shows the Weight Management for Children and Adolescents Practice Guidelines. Specific DecisionPaths provide the means to safely initiate therapy to achieve metabolic targets.

Screening

Unlike adults, the distribution of BMI (weight in kilograms/height in meters^2) in children and adolescents is age related. Standard growth charts for girls and boys are provided by the US National Center for Health Statistics (Figures 5.3 and 5.4). They are meant for an American population and based on a cross-section of individuals from various ethnic and racial groups. For use outside of the U.S. they need to be carefully adjusted based on local data. The child should be placed without shoes and hat, erect with the back against the measuring device. The head should be in the Frankfort plane (an imaginary line from the lower margin of the eye socket to the notch above the tragus of the ear) so that it remains parallel to the horizontal headpiece and perpendicular to the vertical measuring bar. Weight should be measured by a standardized scale without shoes and heavy clothing. It is important to stress that height and weight should be determined at each visit and that the healthcare team continue to discuss appropriate weight for height with the patient.

Risk factors

Some children are born overweight for gestational age. They are often the result of untreated or poorly treated hyperglycemia in pregnancy. In its severest form, it is know as fetal macrosomia. Such children have a birth weight exceeding the 90th percentile for gestational age, they have enlarged organs and are cushingoid in appearance. Most children, however, are born normal weight and become obese due to lifestyle and genetics. The most consistent risk factors for childhood obesity are hereditry, insulin resistance, diet, sedentary lifestyle, and low socioeconomic status. Additionally, it should be noted that the probability of a child being overweight is related to family history of obesity. For example, a child born to parents that are both overweight has an 80 per cent probability of being an overweight child compared with only a 7 per cent probability if both parents are normal weight.[7] This finding highlights the debate of whether it is nature or nurture that leads to childhood and adult obesity. The answer is, both.

Diagnosis

There currently are five categories that children and adolescents may fall in with regards to weight (based on age): underweight $<$ 5th percentile BMI, normal weight 5–85th percentile BMI, overweight 85–95th percentile BMI, clinical obesity 95–97th percentile BMI and severe obesity $>$ 97th percentile BMI. These percentiles must be readjusted for non-U.S. populations and for minorities within the U.S.

Screening

Obtain height and weight on all children > 2 years of age at each visit; using NCHS charts, plot height, weight and BMI

BMI Calculations

- (weight in pounds/height in inches/height in inches) × 703
- metric: weight in kilograms/(height in meters)^2

Risk Factors

- Birth weight > 4000 g or < 2000 g at term
- Child of a mother with GDM in any pregnancy
- Low economic status
- Low self-esteem/self-efficacy
- Single-parent household
- Use of commodity foods
- A diet high in fat/calories/fast foods
- Eating snacks with empty calories
- Drinking sweetened soft drinks or fruit juice
- Sedentary lifestyle, e.g. watching television or using computers/games > 2 hours/day
- Lack of involvement with physical activity or sports, especially family based activities
- Lack of a home based model for physical activity
- Low intake of fruits and vegetables
- Disturbed eating behaviors (no structured meals, excessive dining out of home, binge eating)

Diagnosis

At risk for overweight > 85th percentile BMI*
Clinical obesity > 95th percentile BMI
Severe obesity > 97th percentile BMI

Treatment Options

- If BMI is 85th–95th percentile start weight management program
- If BMI is > 95th percentile; start weight loss program, rule out hypothyroidism, consider referral to pediatric endocrinologist to rule out endocrine abnormality start weight mangement program
- If no contraindication, start or increase activity program
- Avoid numbers-based goals for weight
- Encourage caregiver participation
- Referral for individual or family counseling should be considered
- If available, consider referral to pediatric dietitian

Targets

No weight gain; increased activity; BMI within normal percentile for age and gender; maintain normal growth and development; maintain self-esteem

Monitoring

Maintain normal growth and development; monitor for nutritional adequacy of food intake and daily activity. Recommend monthly follow-up; monitor height, weight, and BMI

Follow-up

Weekly Office visit or counseling as needed; phone contact may be sufficient; positive verbal reinforcement

Every 3 Months Height, weight, and BMI; review activity and nutrition intake; blood pressure; fasting lipid profile as needed; assess development; positive verbal reinforcement

Yearly History and physical; neurologic examination; dental examination; continue nutrition and activity education; positive verbal reinforcement; pediatric depression assessment; assess for other components of metabolic syndrome

Figure 5.2 Weight Management for Children and Adolescents Practice Guidelines

Treatment options

Generally, treatment is designed to provide a long-term solution to weight management problems. Depending upon weight category, the treatment moves from sustaining the current weight (preventing weight gain) to promoting weight loss. Reduction in 'empty calories' such as regular soda, chips, and sweets will often result in a reduction of 250–500 calories/day, which should result in a 0.5–1.0 pound (0.22–0.45 kg)/week reduction in weight. Each treatment is individualized consisting of changes in dietary intake combined with activity level. Pharmacological interventions are not an option. A team approach in which the family, health care provider, and patient work together

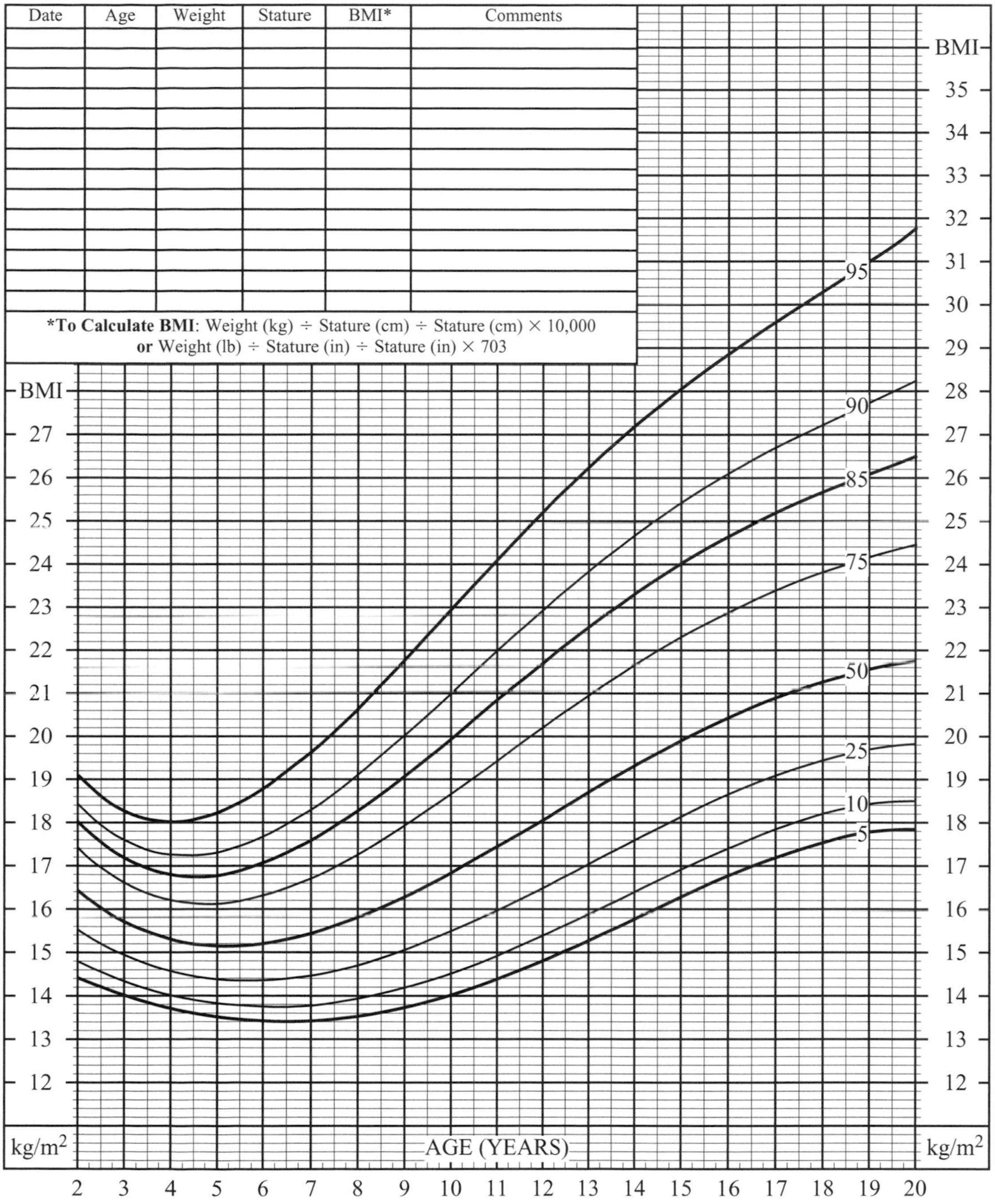

Date	Age	Weight	Stature	BMI*	Comments

***To Calculate BMI**: Weight (kg) ÷ Stature (cm) ÷ Stature (cm) × 10,000
or Weight (lb) ÷ Stature (in) ÷ Stature (in) × 703

BMI
35
34
33
32
31
30
29
28
27
26
25
24
23
22
21
20
19
18
17
16
15
14
13
12
kg/m^2

95
90
85
75
50
25
10
5

AGE (YEARS)
2 3 4 5 6 7 8 9 10 11 12 13 14 15 16 17 18 19 20

SOURCE: Developed by the National Center for Health Statistics in collaboration with the National Center for Chronic Disease Prevention and Health Promotion (2000). http://www.cdc.gov/growthcharts

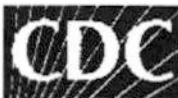

Figure 5.3 Female BMI-for-age chart

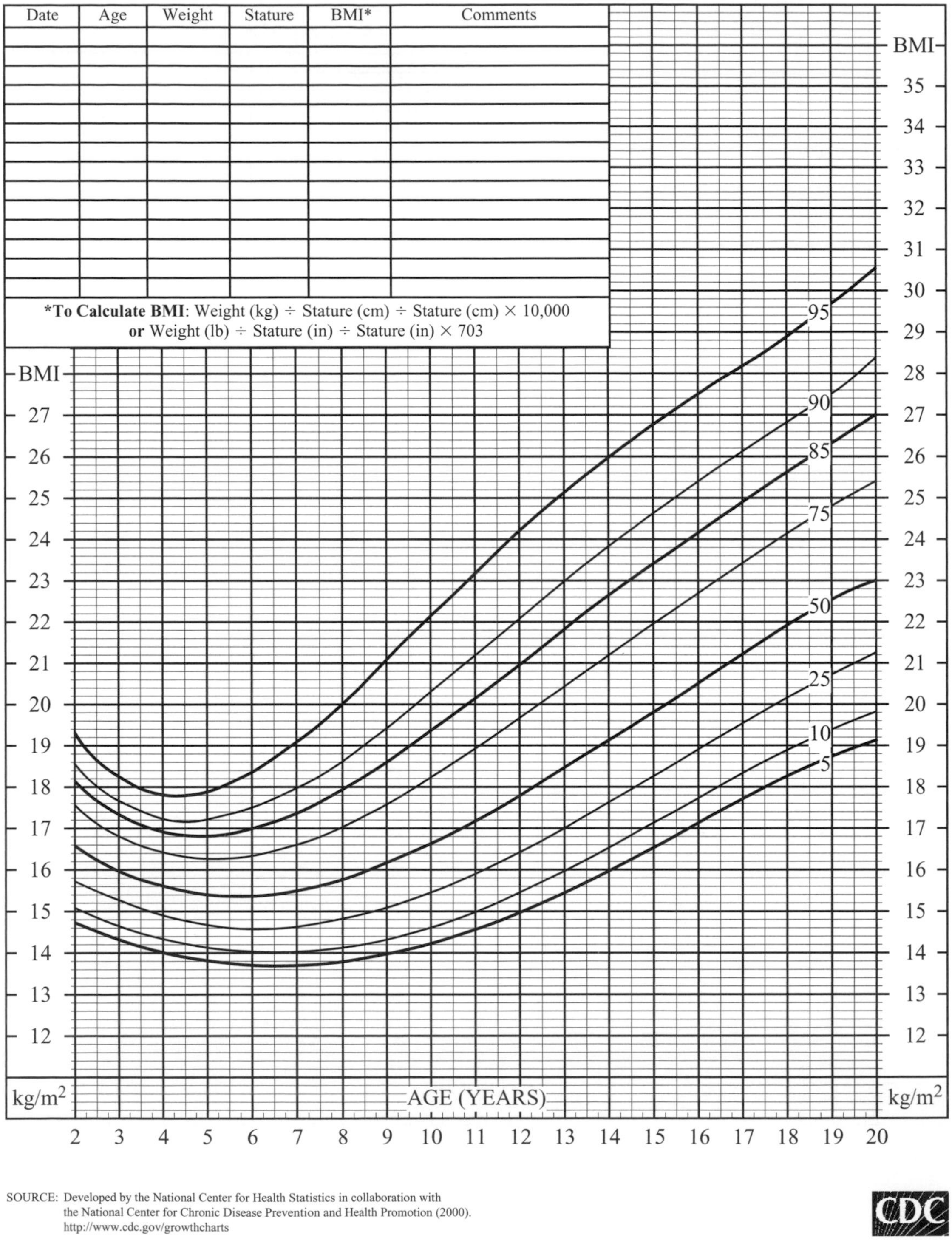

Date	Age	Weight	Stature	BMI*	Comments

***To Calculate BMI**: Weight (kg) ÷ Stature (cm) ÷ Stature (cm) × 10,000
or Weight (lb) ÷ Stature (in) ÷ Stature (in) × 703

BMI

35 34 33 32 31 30 29 28 27 26 25 24 23 22 21 20 19 18 17 16 15 14 13 12

95 90 85 75 50 25 10 5

kg/m²

AGE (YEARS)

2 3 4 5 6 7 8 9 10 11 12 13 14 15 16 17 18 19 20

SOURCE: Developed by the National Center for Health Statistics in collaboration with
the National Center for Chronic Disease Prevention and Health Promotion (2000).
http://www.cdc.gov/growthcharts

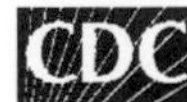

Figure 5.4 Male BMI-for-age chart

with common and clear goals is a necessity. Psychosocial issues related to self-esteem and body image must also be taken into account.

Targets

The short-term goal is to stop weight gain with the long-term goal to re-establish normal BMI. One strategy that works well in children and adolescents that are still growing in height is to work on maintaining current weight and having the patient 'grow' into a more appropriate BMI. Weight loss of approximately 0.5–1.0 pound (0.22–0.45 kg)/week is a reasonable target. The length of time it will take to accomplish weight loss depends upon numerous factors. These factors include the patient's willingness to participate in the weight loss/maintenance process, family support, and ability to participate in activity/exercise. The process is one of behavior change and thus requires several small changes in behavior with achievable goals established along the way. This process must also assure proper growth and development.

Monitoring

It is recommended that the patient keep a daily diary for activity and food intake and that this is reviewed at each office visit at which time height and weight is measured and BMI calculated.

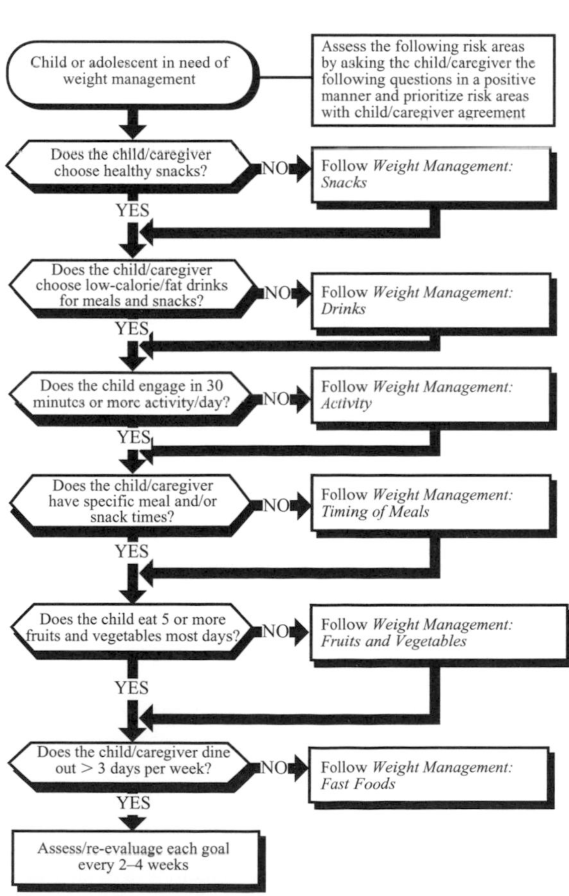

Figure 5.5 Weight Management in Children and Adolescents Master DecisionPath

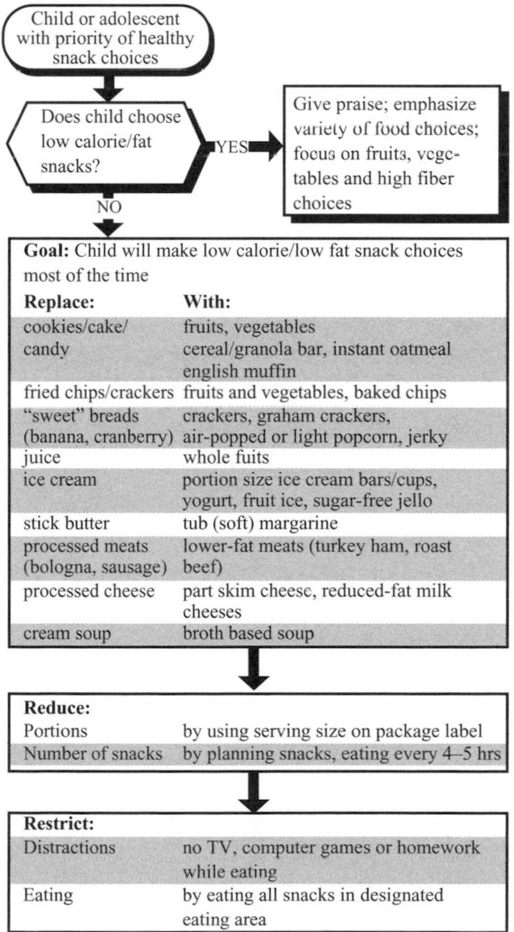

Figure 5.6 Weight Management: Snacks

Follow-up

During the initial intervention, weekly contact with the health care provider and at least monthly office visits to calculate the BMI is recommended. Thereafter, quarterly visits are recommended until weight goals are reached. Because these children are at high risk for any of the comorbidities associated with obesity, it is advisable to evaluate lipid, glucose, and blood pressure and to assess overall growth and development. On an annual basis a complete review for insulin resistance and weight-related disorders should be completed.

Weight management in children and adolescents Master DecisionPath

Weight management is a behavioral issue. The predominant interventions rely on a series of behavioral approaches that target specific actions concerning eating habits and physical activity. The overall approach seeks first to replace high-calorie foods and drinks with lower-calorie substitutes; if this fails, then to reduce energy intake while increasing energy output; and if this fails, to restrict intake to very specific foods and drink. The Weight Management in Children and Adolescents Master DecisionPath (Figure 5.5) stages the

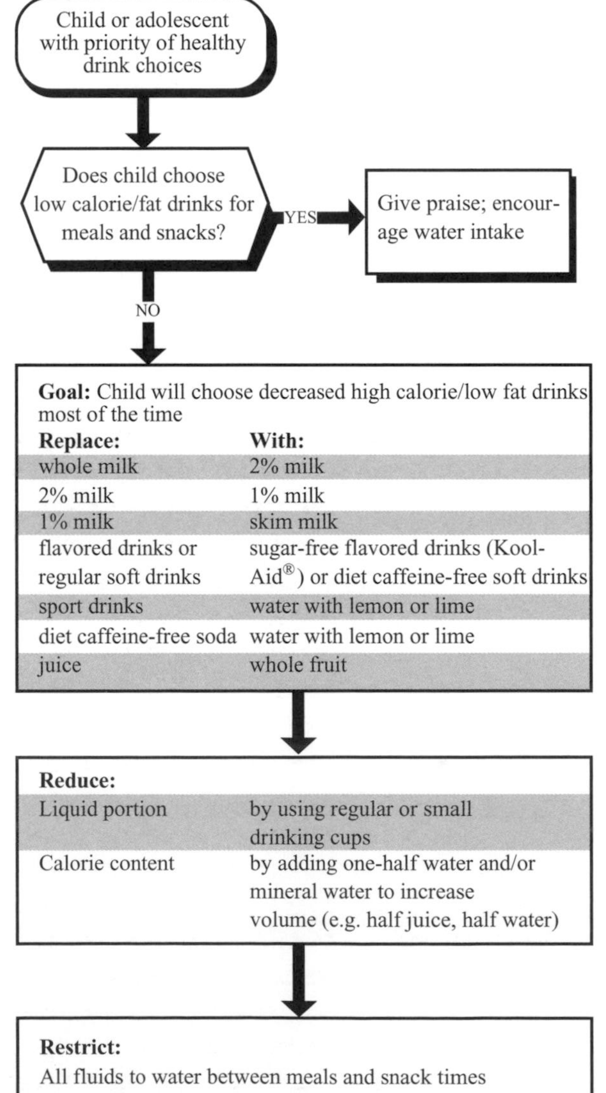

Figure 5.7 Weight Management: Drinks

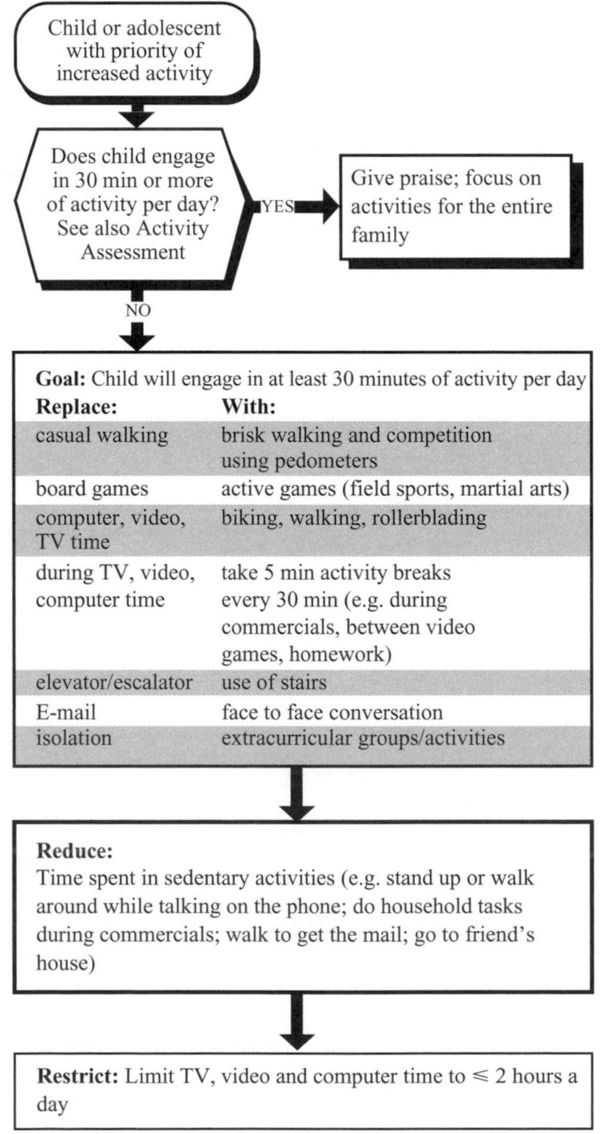

Figure 5.8 Weight Management: Activity

actions in such a manner as to make certain that the major factors are addressed. The assessment begins with understanding the eating habits of the patient. Since snack foods contribute a substantial number of empty calories and are often at the center of poor nutrition, the clinical decision-making identifies the current snacking habits and seeks to replace each snack with a reasonable and healthy substitute (Figure 5.6). After snacks are addressed, the next area to consider is what the child or adolescent is drinking (Figure 5.7). Once snacks and drinks are addressed physical activity is reviewed (Figure 5.8). With the first three areas completed, it is possible to 'routinize' some of the behaviors. Setting times for meals and snacks helps to establish a pattern for future behaviors (Figure 5.9). Establishing a target list of preferred foods, making certain that the child or adolescent is eating healthy food choices such as fruits and vegetables needed for proper growth and development is the next step (Figure 5.10). Finally, addressing issues such as dining out and 'fast food' habits completes the comprehensive approach (Figure 5.11).

Exercise assessment

The importance of exercise in restoring a balance between energy intake and expenditure is paramount in weight management. Increased activity level improves insulin sensitivity, which has a direct impact on the disorders associated with obesity and the metabolic syndrome. Developing a physical activity prescription for children and adolescents must take into account 'normal' daily

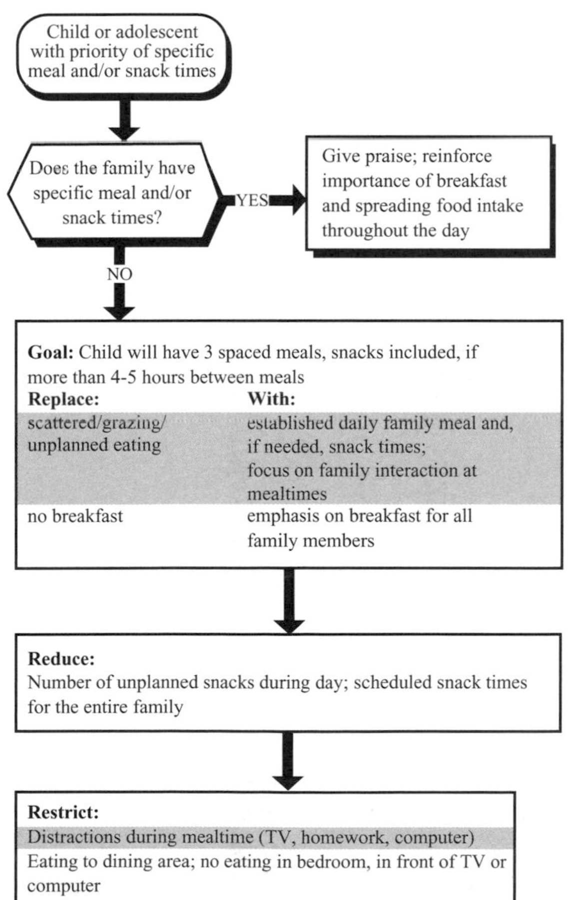

Figure 5.9 Weight Management: Timing of Meals/ Snacks

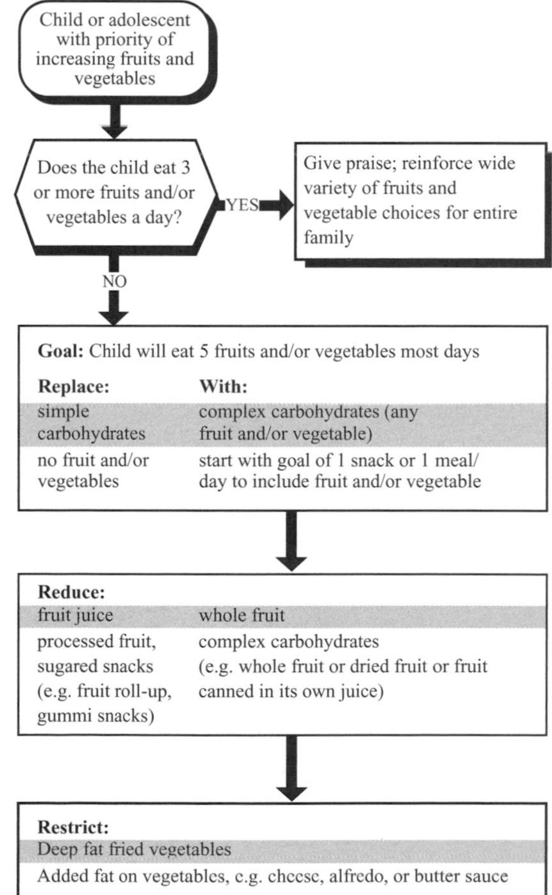

Figure 5.10 Weight Management: Fruits and Vegetables

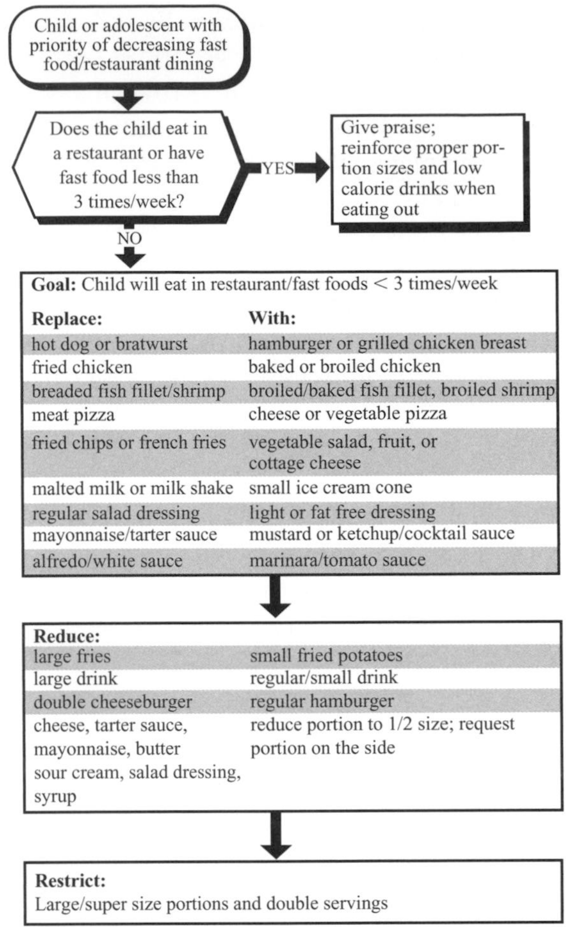

Figure 5.11 Weight Management: Fast Food

BMI %	Recommended Activities	Intensity	Frequency
<85th	No activity or intensity restrictions		
85th–95th	Brisk walking, stair climber, field sports, hiking, aerobic dance, rollerblading, bicycling, basketball, martial arts, swimming, strength/aerobic circuit training	Moderate to vigorous (60–85% of maximum heart rate)	1–2×/week (weeks 1–4), 3–4×/week (weeks 5–10), 4–6×/week (weeks 10+)
95th–97th	Swimming, bicycling, strength/aerobic circuit training, recumbent bike, interval walking (walking with frequent rests as necessary, increase work/rest ratio each week)	Low to moderate (< 50–70% of maximum heart rate)	1–2×/week (weeks 1–4), 3–4×/week (weeks 5–10), 4–6×/week (weeks 10+)
>97th	Weekly supervised training by an exercise professional **Recommended non-weight bearing aerobic activities:** swimming, recumbent bike, strength/aerobic circuit training, seated aerobics, arm ergometry (use interval strategy when appropriate, increase work/rest ratio each week as tolerated)	As tolerated	1×/week or as tolerated (weeks 1–4), 3–4×/week (weeks 5–10), 4–6×/week (weeks 10+)

Figure 5.12 Activity recommendations for children and adolescents

activities and then use these activities as the basis for improvement. In general, there is no need for an extensive assessment of the child's cardiovascular fitness. However, severely obese children may have underlying cardiovascular disease, thus it is recommended that for any obese child or adolescent for whom a major increase in activity is being recommended a baseline cardiovascular profile be completed. Activities should be comfortable, frequent, consistent, and reasonable. They should be based on the child's usual schedule, ability and motivation. Fitting exercise into the lifestyle of most children requires some innovative thinking. Benefiting from school based and after school activities should be strongly considered.

In general, no restrictions are placed on children and adolescents with a BMI less than the 85th percentile. However, as the BMI percentile increases the amount and types of activity must be considered (Figure 5.12). For example, children with a BMI between the 85th and 95th percentiles should be able to achieve the goal of activities that reach between 60 and 85 per cent of maximum heart rate four to six times each week within 10 weeks of the onset of the activity regimen. This contrasts significantly with children who have severe obesity (> 97th percentile BMI). For these children, activity level should only be under professional guidance. They should be encouraged to exercise up to their own limitations as often as is possible. The exercises should be low impact, such as swimming or walking, with adequate rest upon completion.

If the exercise prescription is ineffective, consider re-setting the goals. Determine the patient's readiness to do exercise, re-educate as to the relationship between exercise and weight control, and consider referral to an exercise specialist.

Type 2 diabetes in children and adolescents

(The following guidelines are for non-pregnancy. Type 2 diabetes complicated by pregnancy and gestational diabetes are discussed in Chapter 7.)

This section provides the basis for screening, diagnosis and the treatment of type 2 diabetes in children and adolescents. It begins with the Type 2 Diabetes Practice Guidelines, followed by the Master DecisionPath. The latter lays out an orderly sequence of therapeutic stages shown to improve glycemic control. Specific DecisionPaths for each stage (treatment options) as well as Diabetes Management Assessment DecisionPaths (medical visit, education, nutrition, adherence assessment) along with a complete description of each item and the rationale for decisions are also presented.

As this section is reviewed, note the following.

- Diagnosis of diabetes should be documented in the chart and meet criteria set by the American Diabetes Association or other similar national organization and the World Health Organization.[8]

- All individuals with diabetes should be treated with medical nutrition therapy, either as a primary therapy or in combination with pharmacologic agents.

- At diagnosis, metformin needs careful consideration since some factors such as underlying renal impairment or pregnancy may preclude its use.

- If oral agent therapy fails to improve and eventually restore glycemia to within target goals a regimen including combination oral agent and insulin may be required.

- Severe hyperglycemia (BG $>$ 300 mg/dL or 16.9 mmol/L; and/or HbA_{1c} $>$ 11 per cent) requires immediate initiation of insulin therapy.

- Reversing direction in the Master DecisionPath is possible. Patients started on insulin can, with appropriate lifestyle modifications, stop insulin and start metformin therapy or medical nutrition therapy alone to control blood glucose levels. This is especially true in children and adolescents once glucose toxicity is reduced, allowing for improved β-cell function.

- Diabetes should be treated from a multidisciplinary approach. The Diabetes Management Assessment DecisionPaths review the practices of dietitians, nurse educators, and psychologists.

- Type 2 diabetes is part of a metabolic syndrome; such patients are at higher risk for developing hypertension, dyslipidemia, and renal disease and should therefore be carefully evaluated and closely monitored thereafter.

Type 2 Diabetes Practice Guidelines

The practice guidelines for type 2 diabetes are divided into seven sections: screening, diagnosis, treatment options, targets, monitoring, follow-up, and complications surveillance (Figure 5.13).

Screening

Identifying the child or adolesent with type 2 diabetes begins with surveillance for risk factors, which are listed in Figure 5.13. There are two different screening approaches. The most economical screening method is to use capillary blood measured by a reflectance meter. This is not a replacement for a laboratory measurement, but is sufficiently accurate to justify diagnostic testing. If capillary BG is used, it should be first adjusted for differences between plasma and whole blood (if the meter has not already been calibrated to plasma). A casual capillary value of

Screening Screen all at-risk patients who have 2 or more risk factors every 2 years or more frequently if symptomatic

Risk Factors
- Family history of type 2 diabetes in a 1st or 2nd degree relative
- Overweight: BMI $>$ 85th percentile for age and gender, central obesity, or weight $>$ 120% of ideal for height
- Sedentary lifestyle (persons with no or irregular leisure time activity)
- Hypertension: BP $>$ 95th percentile for gender, age, height percentile (see BMI Tables)
- Dyslipidemia: HDL $\leqslant$ 40 mg/dL (1.0 mmol/L) and or triglyceride $\geqslant$ 250 mg/dL (2.8 mmol/L)
- Previous IFG (BG 100–125 mg/dL [5.6–6.9 mmol/L])
- Previous IGT (2 hour BG 140–199 mg/dL [7.8–11.0 mmol/L)
- Birthweight $>$ 4000 g or $<$ 2000 g at term
- Child of mother with GDM in any pregnancy
- Acanthosis nigricans
- American Indian; Alaska Native; African-American; Asian-American; Native HawaiianPacific Islander; Mexican-American
- Premature pubarche, oligomenorrhea, hirsutism
- PCOS

Diagnosis

Plasma Glucose Casual $\geqslant$ 200 mg/dL (11.1 mmol/L) plus symptoms, fasting $\geqslant$ 126 mg/dL (7.0 mmol/L), or 100 gram oral glucose tolerance test (OGTT) 2 hour glucose value $\geqslant$ 200 mg/dL (11.1 mmol/L); if positive, confirm diagnosis within 7 days

Symptoms Often none
Common: blurred vision; UTI; fatigue; increased urination and thirst, depression
Occasional: increased appetite; nocturia; weight loss; yeast infection; dry, itchy skin,secondary enuresis

Urine Ketones Can be positive

Treatment Options Medical nutrition and activity therapy; metformin; Insulin: Stages 2, 3, 4

Targets

Self-Monitored Blood Glucose (SMBG)
- $>$ 50% of SMBG values within target range
- Pre-meal: 70–140 mg/dL (4.4–6.6 mmol/L)
- Post-meal: (2 hrs after starting meal): $<$ 160 mg/dL ($<$ 8.9 mmol/L)
- Bedtime: 100–160 mg/dL (5.5–8.9 mmol/L)
- No severe (assisted) or nocturnal hypoglycemia. Adjust pre-meal target upwards if hypoglycemia unawareness, decreased cognitive ability, or renal disease.

Glycosylated Hemoglobin HbA_{1c}
- Within 1 percentage point of uppper limit of normal (e.g., normal 6.0%; target $<$ 7.0%)
- Frequency: every 3–4 months
- Use HbA_{1c} to verify SMBG data

Blood Pressure
- Adjusted for age and height

Lipids
- LDL $<$ 100 mg/dL (2.6 mmol/L), HDL $\geqslant$ 35 mg/dL (0.090 mmol/L), triglycerides $<$ 150 mg/dL (1.7 mmol/L)

Weight
- BMI $<$ 85th percentile for gender, age, and height

Targets Meter with memory and log book

SMBG 2–4 times per day (e.g. before meals, 2 hours after start of meal, bedtime); may be modified due to cost, technical ability, activity, availability of meters; if on insulin, check 3 AM SMBG as needed

Growth and Development Normal, as determined using anthropometric scales/growth charts and indices of pubertal development

Follow-up

Monthly Office visit during adjust phase (weekly phone contact may be necessary)

Every 3 Months Review hypoglycemic episodes; medications; height, weight, and BMI; review medical nutrition/activity therapy; BP; SMBG data (download and check meter); HbA_{1c}; diabetes/nutrition education

Yearly In addition to the 3 month follow-up complete the following: history and physical; fasting lipid profile; microalbuminuria screen; dilated eye examination at diagnosis and annually; dental examination; neurologic assessment; complete foot examination (pulses, nerves, ABI and inspection); patient satisfaction evaluation; smoking cessation and family planning as needed

Complications Surveillance Cardiovascular, renal, retinal, neurological, foot, oral, and dermatological (necrobiosis lipoidicia diabeticorum, diabetic shin spots, onychomycosis, acanthosis nigricans), limited joint mobility

Figure 5.13 Type 2 Diabetes Practice Guidelines for Children and Adolescents

> 140 mg/dL (7.8 mmol/L) or a fasting > 100 mg/dL (5.6 mmol/L) would be sufficient evidence to require follow-up with a diagnostic test. The alternative is to use the more costly, but more accurate, laboratory fasting or casual plasma glucose value as the screening test (if positive, it also serves as one of two diagnostic tests).

Symptoms. Children and adolescents often present with no symptoms of type 2 diabetes. This is most probably because the hyperglycemia is not severe nor has it been prolonged. Frequently, fatigue, urinary tract infections, yeast infections, skin irritations, and other vague complaints often accompany type 2 diabetes. Only when hyperglycemia is severe (glucose values > 250 mg/dL [13.9 mmol/L]) do patients develop the classical symptoms of diabetes: weight loss, dehydration, polyuria, polyphagia, and polydipsia.

Urine ketones. Type 2 diabetes in adults is generally distinguished from type 1 diabetes by the absence of ketonuria at diagnosis. However, in children and adolescent, ketones may be found in either type of diabetes. Severe insulin resistance may result in the inability to utilize sufficient amounts of glucose for energy, thus forcing the body to utilize fats for energy. A byproduct of this increased fat metabolism is ketones. On rare occasions, when patients are under stress (exercise, low-calorie diet, high-protein ketogenic diets) and experiencing high blood glucose levels, ketones may be detected.

> Note: The majority of children with type 2 diabetes are obese with an age/gender BMI > 95 per cent. There is a strong genetic predisposition – individuals with siblings with type 2 diabetes are at especially high risk; identical twins have an 80–95 per cent concordance rate. For high-risk ethnic groups such as American Indians and Hispanics, the age of onset lowers to as early as 5 years of age. Many develop type 2 diabetes as part of the ametabolic syndrome. Early teenage pregnancy in obese girls adds greater risk of developing type 2 diabetes. American Indian, Alaska Native, African-American, Hispanic, Asian, and Native Hawaiian and other Pacific Islander children have between three and ten times greater risk of developing type 2 diabetes than age matched Caucasian children and adolescents.

Medical emergencies. Rarely, type 2 diabetes presents as a medical emergency requiring appropriate treatment. See 'Hyperglycemic Hyperosmolar Syndrome (HHS)' in Chapter 10 for further discussion and treatment DecisionPaths.

Diagnosis

In recent years the number of individuals under the age of 18 with type 2 diabetes has increased dramatically. The first principle is that blood glucose alone, as the basis for screening and diagnosis in children, does not differentiate between type 1 and type 2 diabetes. Since the overall incidence of type 2 diabetes is thought to be equal to or higher than the incidence of type 1 diabetes in children and adolescents, it is critical to ascertain whether the patient belongs to a high-risk group. In general, Caucasian children (especially of Scandinavian descent) are at a higher risk of developing type 1 diabetes, while children of certain ethnic groups (American Indian, Alaska Native, African-American, Asian-American, Latino, Mexican-American) are at higher risk of type 2 diabetes. Lean children are more likely to have type 1 and obese children are at greater risk of type 2 diabetes. Despite these trends, exceptions are common. Thus, an underlying principle is to immediately treat the hyperglycemia. When in doubt of a clear distinction between types of diabetes, insulin therapy should be initiated. Surveillance for urine ketones should be considered paramount in this process as moderate to high ketones (associated with diagnosis of either type 1 or type 2 diabetes) indicate the need to immediately initiate insulin therapy (see Figure 5.14).

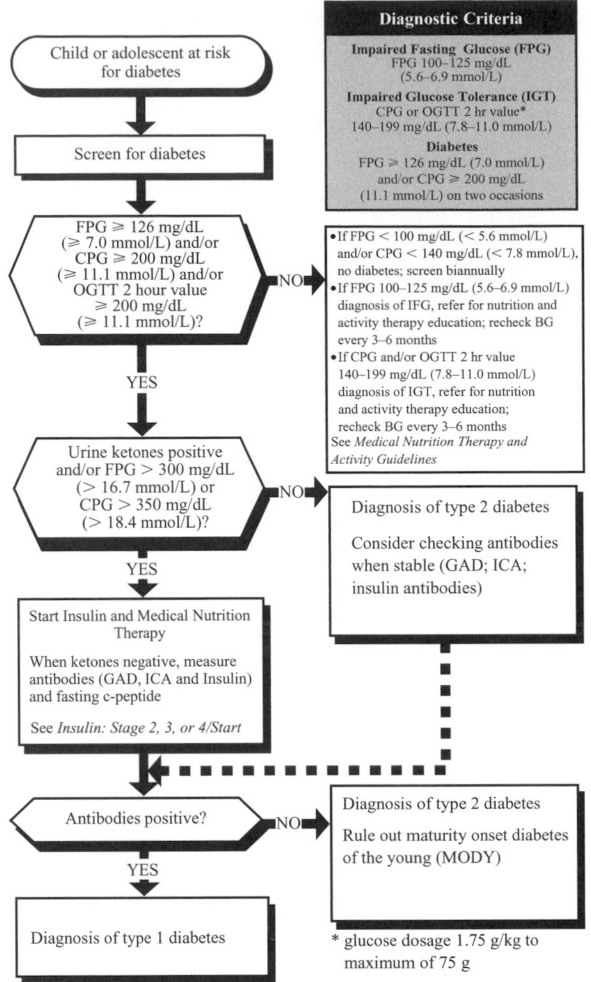

Figure 5.14 Screening and Differential Diagnosis of Diabetes in Children and Adolescents

Once ketones are negative the differential diagnosis requires measuring antibodies to islet cells and C-peptide levels. Insulin C-peptide measures the amount of endogenous insulin in the blood. This assay measures the connecting "C" part of the peptide chain that is removed from proinsulin to form biologically active "mature" insulin because it is produced as part of the insulin peptide. It is equivalent to the amount of insulin secreted. Since the C-peptide is not found in exogenous (vial) insulin, it can be used as a basis for differentiation between endogenous (secreted) and exogenous (injected) insulin. Measuring insulin levels determines the amount of both endogenous and exogenous insulin in the blood (thus is not useful in patients already using exogenous insulin). Elevated or normal levels of C-peptide are indicative of type 2 diabetes, whereas low insulin levels generally mean type 1 diabetes in children. Laboratory tests for anti-insulin, anti-GAD and islet cell antibodies will help determine whether an autoimmune destruction of the pancreatic β-cells is underway, which would confirm type 1 diabetes. These measures are increasingly in use for the differentiation between type 1 and type 2 diabetes in children.

Maturity onset diabetes in youth (MODY)

A very rare autosomal dominant form of diabetes that occurs in young people usually before age 25 is called maturity-onset diabetes of the young (MODY). This form of diabetes results from mutations in genes critical for normal β-cell function and insulin secretion. Many health professionals are quick to diagnoses any young person with non-ketosis-prone diabetes with MODY, when in reality they very likely have type 2 diabetes that has developed at a young age. Genetic testing is available for MODY.

Malnourishment-related diabetes

Yet another clinical syndrome of diabetes has been described in young, malnourished individuals in developing countries, establishing the concept of malnutrition-related diabetes mellitus. Because the lack of evidence supporting the direct role of protein deficiency (malnourishment) in the development of diabetes, this classification of diabetes is rarely found.

Some children will not meet the diagnostic criteria for diabetes. They will, however, meet the criteria for impaired glucose homeostasis (IGH) or prediabetes. Since these children may be developing type 1 diabetes, they must undergo careful surveillance until antibodies to islet cells or to insulin are measured. This is especially the case in children who are lean or not members of ethnic or racial groups at high risk for type 2.

If IGH is present, the appropriate treatment is

to follow medical nutrition therapy. A plan that balances food intake with energy output is vital to prevent IGH from progressing to type 2 diabetes. A complete history and physical should be done and a baseline HbA_{1c} measured. The HbA_{1c} should be within the normal range for the laboratory. To establish a medical nutrition therapy, as with weight management, begin with determining the target BMI. On the basis of this information, a food and exercise/activity plan can be recommended by following the weight management DecisionPaths.

Glycosylated hemoglobin (HbA_{1c}) and the detection of type 2 diabetes. Glycosylated hemoglobin HbA_{1c} or simply HbA_{1c} is not used in the diagnosis of diabetes. HbA_{1c} can be measured by several different methods and as such has not been sufficiently standardized. Some laboratories report total glycosylated hemoglobin (HbA_{1a}, HbA_{1b}, and HbA_{1c}), while others report only the "1c" fraction. One method is equated to the other and by measuring the difference between the upper limit of normal and the reported value. The delta for total glycosylated hemoglobin and HbA_{1c} is approximately equivalent. In general, any delta above the upper limit of normal or any value reported above the upper limit of normal suggests the presence of hyperglycemia. The opposite is not necessarily the case. When HbA_{1c} is normal, although indicative of normoglycemia, when there is a rapid onset of type 1 diabetes, the HbA_{1c} may initially appear normal. In rare instances the abnormally high or low HbA_{1c} may be due to a hemoglobinopathy (such as Sickle-cell trait).

Treatment options

Treatment of type 2 diabetes often requires both behavioral and pharmacological interventions. Independent of the final therapy, medical nutrition therapy and exercise are considered integral to successful outcomes. Generally, treatment for type 2 diabetes has been divided into three periods: (1) medical nutrition alone; (2) oral pharmacological agent – metformin; and (3) insulin. Each period is often seen by both the provider and patient as a major milestone in the progression of diabetes. This is an error. The means of treatment does not necessarily reflect the degree of severity. Two measures, hyperglycemia and complications, are truer reflections of severity of disease.

The overall purpose of medical nutrition therapy is to improve metabolic control by reducing the glycemic effect of excessive carbohydrate intake and decreased energy expenditure. Thus, for medical nutrition therapy to be effective, alterations in food and increase in activity are required. Both steps improve insulin sensitivity and thus lower blood glucose levels. Current food and exercise plans seek to alter the composition and quantity of calories to (1) gradually lower glycemia, (2) maintain or reduce weight, (3) increase physical activity, and (4) promote healthful eating for optimal nutrition.

Only one of the five classifications of oral agents is currently approved by the U.S. Food and Drug Administration for use in children and adolescents – the biguanide metformin. Considered an insulin sensitizer, metformin reduces hepatic glucose output, resulting in lower fasting glucose levels. Metformin may be given alone or in combination with insulin. Such regimens use the metformin to reduce overnight hyperglycemia without risking hypoglycemia and pre-meal insulin to supplement β-cell function.

Insulin therapies include rapid-acting (RA), short-acting (R), intermediate-acting (N), prolonged intermediate (U) and long-acting (G). They are currently delivered by injection or infusion pump and research is being conducted to determine the safety and efficacy of implantable pumps and inhaled versions. Designed to replace or supplement endogenous insulin, oxogenous insulin therapies overcome both insulin resistance and insulin deficiency.

Targets

Numerous studies have demonstrated that, while any improvement in glycemic control is beneficial, near-normal levels of blood glucose

(HbA_{1c} < 7 per cent) afford the best protection against the development and progression of microvascular disease in type 2 diabetes. To achieve this goal, more than 50 per cent of self-monitored blood glucose values should be between 70 and 140 mg/dL (3.9 and 7.8 mmol/L) pre-meal, < 160 mg/dL (8.9 mmol/L) 2 hours after the start of the meal, and between 100 and 160 mg/dL (5.6 and 8.9 mmol/L) at bedtime. Achieving these SMBG targets normally correlates with an HbA_{1c} target of within one percentage point of the upper limit of normal (see Table 5.1).

Monitoring

As with adults, appropriate management of type 2 diabetes in children and adolescents includes SMBG. Three different patterns of SMBG correspond to starting, adjusting, and maintaining the treatment goal. During the start phase, independent of the type of therapy, data gathering is an essential early step in ensuring that the blood glucose levels are responding to the prescribed regimen. SMBG should be performed at defined times throughout the day to collect data on fasting, pre-meal, 2 hours post-meal, and overnight blood glucose levels. During the adjust phase, SMBG should be synchronized to the action of the principal therapy – medical nutrition therapy, metformin, or insulin action curves – to determine where hyperglycemia or hypoglycemia (in the case of insulin) occur. SMBG should be performed at least three times each day to ensure continued improvement in blood glucose levels until targets are achieved. Patients should perform SMBG at different times throughout the day, including fasting, before meals, 2 hours after the start of meals, bedtime, and 3 AM as needed. The goal is to adjust therapy based on blood glucose patterns. During the maintain phase, SMBG can be reduced. For example, if the child is treated by medical nutrition therapy only, testing might be limited to three times per day, two days per week. If circumstances change, such a increased activity, alteration in food plan, or sudden alterations in therapy during illness events, increased testing is recommended to enhance clinical decision-making.

Because many studies have shown that adults (no study in children) may falsify or fail to record their SMBG results, meters with a memory should be used.[10,11] These meters directly record the blood glucose value with the corresponding time and date of test. Some devices can provide a running average of the blood glucose data. More importantly, they can be connected to a computer, which will display the data in several formats that can facilitate clinical decision-making. Whether used routinely or more frequently for special situations, SMBG data provide patients and their care givers with direct feedback on how well the therapy is working and assist clinicians with information needed to make appropriate decisions about therapy. The absence of SMBG data makes clinical decision-making almost impossible for both the patient and the clinician. Determining appropriate diet, exercise, metformin, or insulin dose requires a source of constant, accurate feedback. Currently only SMBG can provide such feedback.

Table 5.1 HbA_{1c} and average SMBG correlation[9]

If HbA_{1c} is	Average SMBG is
1 percentage point above normal	150 mg/dL (8.3 mmol/L)
2 percentage points above normal	180 mg/dL (10.0 mmol/L)
3 percentage points above normal	210 mg/dL (11.7 mmol/L)
4 percentage points above normal	245 mg/dL (13.6 mmol/L)
5 percentage points above normal	280 mg/dL (15.5 mmol/L)
6 percentage points above normal	310 mg/dL (17.2 mmol/L)

Follow-up

For children and adolescents starting treatment for type 2 diabetes, initial follow-up is based on the type of therapy. Treatment with insulin requires 24-hour health provider availability (by phone) and an office visit within one week of initiation. With both metformin and medical nutrition therapy (MNT) the scheduled follow-up may be biweekly or monthly. An important element of SDM is that treatment options that are ineffective should be detected early and changes made rapidly. More frequent phone contact may be required, especially when adjusting insulin doses. *The overall expectation is a monthly decrease in average blood glucose of 15–30 mg/dL (0.8–1.7 mmol/L), which would convert to a monthly reduction in* HbA_{1c} *of 0.5–1.0 percentage point.* This should continue until targets are reached. However, not until the end of the second month will the impact of the initial therapy be fully reflected in the HbA_{1c} levels. This is a safe rate of decline and generally does not place the child at risk of either absolute or relative hypoglycemia (especially if MNT or metformin are used). During the maintain phase, quarterly visits should be scheduled, where weight, glycemic control (HbA_{1c}), and adherence to MNT can be assessed.

Annually, a fasting lipid profile, albuminuria screen, complete foot examination (pulses, nerves, and inspection), dental examination, and dilated eye examination are recommended. Additionally, nutrition and diabetes skills review and evaluation of other risk factors (smoking, alcohol intake, and weight management) are beneficial. Completing this evaluation (with appropriate referral) is necessary to meet national standards for diabetes management.

Type 2 Diabetes complications surveillance

Additionally, surveillance for disorders associated with insulin resistance (such as hypertension and dyslipidemia) as well as microvascular and macrovascular complications of diabetes should occur (see end of this section). For example, a foot check with a 10 g, 5.07 monofilament for sensation and an examination for pressure points, injuries, vibratory sensation and ulcers is a necessity. As many as 80 per cent of adults with type 2 diabetes have a serious co-morbidity. These complications are initially less likely in children and adolescents because it is believed that type 2 diabetes has been discovered early in its natural history. However, as the complications are often associated with persistent hyperglycemia, a child whose diabetes actually began at age 8 and was discovered at age 15 may have the same risk of complications as an adult with 7 years duration of diabetes. In many cases the complication can be managed and its progression slowed if found early. Staged Diabetes Management provides explicit protocols for the detection and treatment of the major microvascular and macrovascular complications in children and adolescents. Periodic screening, rapid intervention, and close follow-up can significantly reduce the consequences of these complications.

Type 2 Diabetes Master DecisionPath

Note: This DecisionPath is for non-pregnancy. Type 2 diabetes complicated by pregnancy is reviewed in Chapter 6.

Once the diagnosis has been confirmed, the next step is to choose the appropriate treatment modality. Staged Diabetes Management provides a Master DecisionPath for type 2 diabetes to facilitate rapid selection of the starting therapy and to lay out the options if the therapy fails to improve glycemic control. Staged Diabetes Management stresses the need to reach an agreed-upon therapeutic goal, which may entail moving the child or adolescent from simple to more complex regimens. It also allows for movement from more complex to less complex regimens as long as glycemic targets are maintained. A principle of SDM is to share the Master DecisionPath and the therapeutic goals with the patient and key family members. Through this process, the family knows the options and the therapeutic goal.

The Type 2 Diabetes Master DecisionPath is shown in Figure 5.15. Three general treatment alternatives (medical nutrition and activity, oral

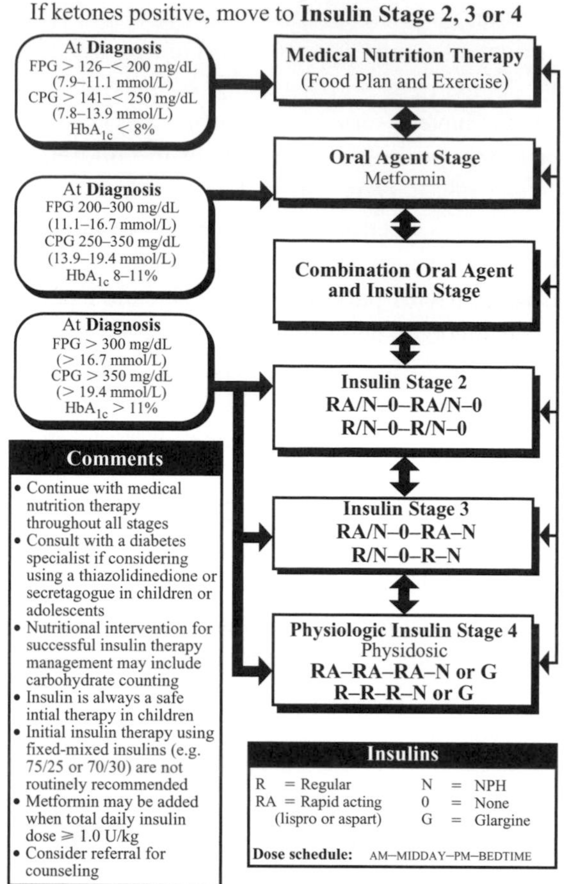

Figure 5.15 Type 2 Master DecisionPath for Children and Adolescents

agent [metformin], and insulin) are available *at diagnosis*. Selection should be based on both a realistic assessment of the patient and parents' or guardian's willingness to follow the regimen and scientific rationale. Acceptance is most related to understanding the regimen, cost, comfort, and specific fears related to certain types of treatment. This contrasts with the medical view, which seeks the most effective treatment from a scientific and clinical perspective. Balancing the two views is important.

While SDM is designed to be customized by the community, *it is important to note that there is a scientific basis for selecting a starting therapy.* It is recognized that limited resources, patient willingness, or ability to follow a specific regimen may not enable the clinician to initiate the most efficacious therapy. Staged Diabetes Management has a built-in mechanism in the Specific DecisionPath that evaluates a therapy against set goals. If the therapy does not meet the goals, it is adjusted until maximum clinical effectiveness is obtained. If targets are not achieved, a new therapy is initiated. The sequential movement to new therapies has timelines to assure that no patient remains on a therapy that is failing.

There are few studies in children and adolescents related to therapeutics in type 2 diabetes. Most of the information is derived from studies of type 1 diabetes in children and type 2 diabetes in motivated adults. From a scientific perspective, if at diagnosis the fasting plasma glucose is < 200 mg/dL (11.1 mmol/L) or the casual plasma glucose is < 250 mg/dL (13.9 mmol/L), medical nutrition and activity therapy should be initiated. Anecdotal reports suggest that most nutritional interventions have a maximum limited effective range of 100 mg/dL (5.6 mmol/L) reduction in SMBG. On average, the benefits of nutritional intervention are a reduction in blood glucose of 30–50 mg/dL (1.7–2.8 mmol/L) or approximately 1.0–2.0 per cent HbA_{1c}. Should the diagnostic value be fasting plasma glucose between 200 and 300 mg/dL (11.1–16.7 mmol/L) or casual plasma glucose between 250 and 350 mg/dL (13.9–19.4 mmol/L), which corresponds to an HbA_{1c} between 8 and 11 per cent, then metformin should be used initially. While there is no evidence that oral agents are dangerous in children and adolescents, neither is there ample evidence of their safety and efficacy. The exception is metformin, which has limited data from small prospective studies that have shown that it is safe and efficacious in the pediatric population.[12,13] The U.S. Food and Drug Administration has recently approved the use of metformin in patients 10 years of age or older for the treatment of type 2 diabetes. It is clear that, as with adults, the initiation of metformin requires careful evaluation of renal function (serum creatinine), and assessment for underlying liver disease, and alcohol intake. Additionally, as metformin passes the placental barrier, it should not be used in adolescents who are sexually active and not practicing birth control. When plasma blood glucose levels exceed

300 mg/dL (16.7 mmol/L) fasting or 350 mg/dL (19.4 mmol/L) casual, or in the presence of ketones, insulin should be initiated. SDM uses one of three regimens to start the insulin therapy. The choice depends a great deal on the patient, parent, and health care provider preference. However, most data suggest that the greater the number of injections the closer one comes to mimicking normal physiology and therefore achieving glycemic targets.

Medical nutrition and activity therapy (MNT)

Medical nutritional interventions are behavioral in their approach. MNT should be intiatied by the diabetes team as quickly as possible after diagnosis (Figure 5.16). Begin by establishing a set of targets and the period of time it should take to reach this goal. MNT as a solo therapy is reserved for children and adolescents with $HbA_{1c} < 8$ per cent. The vast majority of children and adolescents with type 2 diabetes will be overweight or obese. If this is the case, follow the weight management protocols presented in the preceding section of this chapter. If the child or adolescent has a BMI within the normal range, then the principal purpose of the MNT will be to stress healthy food choices and regular activity/exercise. For children and adolescents (and their families), the readiness to change eating and activity behaviors is a function of knowledge. Parents, guardians, and the patient must first understand the disease, treatment options, and long-term prognosis before they are ready to accept a therapeutic choice and make significant changes to their lifestyle. The SDM section on patient education addresses this point and provides details regarding the approach to education.

SDM uses three basic principles to create a food plan as part of effective MNT: replace, reduce, and restrict (see Figures 5.6–5.11). The first step in designing an effective food plan is to replace high carbohydrate foods and drinks with substitutes that are similar in volume, taste, and texture. *Replacing* regular soft drinks with diet soft drinks is one example: the same size portion and the same consistency. Replacing full-fat ice

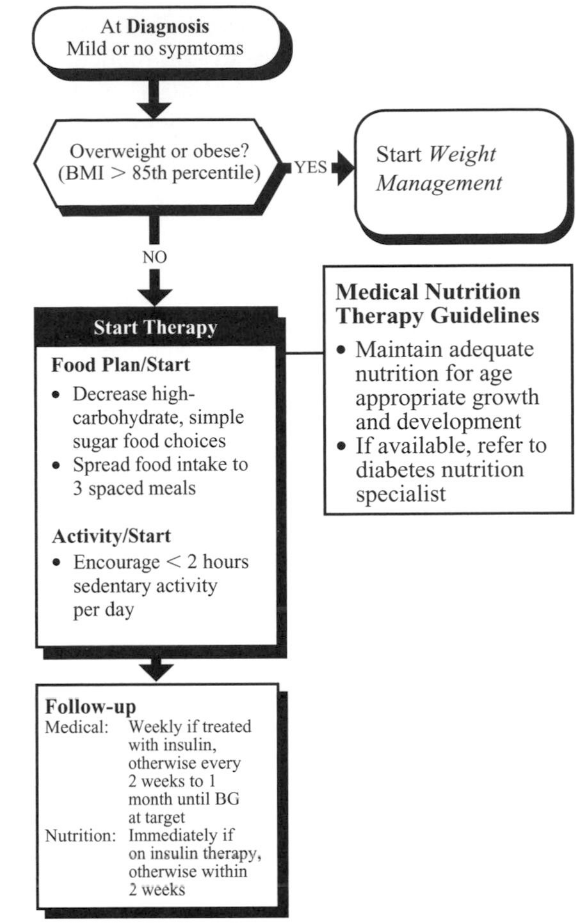

Figure 5.16 Type 2 medical nutrition and activity therapy/start for children and adolescents

cream with a low-fat, low-sugar substitute is another example. In general, children and adolescents are willing to do this as it causes the least inconvenience and is easy to fit into their current lifestyle. If this fails to adequately lower blood glucose (expect a drop of 20–30 mg/dL (1.2–1.7 mmol/L) within the first two to three weeks then move to the second principle: *Reduction* of intake of foods and drinks high in carbohydrate content. This is accomplished by reducing the portion size of these foods and drinks. Begin with a total reduction of approximately 10 per cent. If weight reduction is not a goal, then replace these foods with protein rich (low-fat) substitutes. If the child or adolescent is overweight, then some weight loss at the same time will have a beneficial effect on reducing insulin resistance. For these children reduce all portions during meals and snacks. Keep slowly reducing portion size by 5 per cent/week until intake reaches 75 per cent of the original intake. A weekly weight reduction of approximately 1 pound/week is desired. Blood glucose should continue to improve. If this fails, significant *restrictions* need to be placed on intake of certain food or drinks, for example, total omission of regular soda pop, high-fat milk, cheese, butter, ice cream, salad dressing, and sweetened syrups may be required.

The replace, reduce, restrict approach is a simple strategy. A far more comprehensive approach is usually needed if MNT is to work for a long period of time. Referral to a dietitian is critical and, if available, one specializing with educating a pediatric population is desirable. The regimen can be modified for both daily activity level and age. Children with a sedentary lifestyle generally need fewer calories to maintain their metabolic rate. Typically, an obese and sedentary child requires one-third less calories to maintain the same body weight as an active leaner child. As detailed in the preceding section devoted to weight management, a careful analysis of snacking, drinks, activity, meal timing, healthy food, and fast food habits needs to be undertaken to assure that the MNT approach is optimized. Again the same principles of replace, reduce, restrict apply. Children and adolescents depend on snacks as a major source of energy. This is generally the first area that has to be addressed. Replacing high-fat, high-carbohydrate snacks with fruits and vegetables or simply foods with fewer carbohydrates is often the initial step in changing behavior. If this fails, or is insufficient, then drinks, meal timing, activity, and fast foods are each addressed. As much as possible short-term measurable goals should be agreed upon.

Staged Diabetes Management recommends the food plan be individualized according to a person's lifestyle, eating habits, and concurrent medical conditions. Educating individuals about food planning involves teaching basic concepts of nutrition and diabetes nutrition guidelines, and discussing ideas for altering current food plans to meet these guidelines.

Points of focus include the following:

- *When and how much to eat.* Space food throughout the day to avoid long times between meals and snacks. Choose smaller portions. Eat smaller meals and snacks. Avoid skipping meals and snacks (if part of food plan).

- *What to eat.* Choose a variety of foods each day. Choose foods lower in fat. Avoid foods high in added sugar based sweeteners such as soda pop, syrup, candy, and desserts.

- *How to make food choices.* Include a simple definition of carbohydrate, protein, and fat, with examples of food sources of each; discuss nutrition guidelines, such as eating less fat and carbohydrates, using less added sweetener, eating more fiber, and reducing total caloric (fat) intake for weight loss if appropriate; and suggest grocery shopping tips for making these changes in their current eating pattern.

- *Changes in food plan when taking medications.* Since patients may eventually be placed on metformin or insulin therapy, it is appropriate to indicate that some changes in the food plan may take place when these therapies are initiated. Additional attention to food and eating awareness is recommended for obese individuals. This can be achieved by discussing the connection between portion size and carbohydrates; the calorie and fat content of foods; and the importance of self-monitoring behaviors, such as food records designed to increase awareness of total food consumption and stimuli that promote overeating.

Carbohydrate counting. Carbohydrates are quickly broken down to glucose in the digestive tract and thus have the greatest immediate impact on blood glucose levels. Therefore, accounting for the amount of carbohydrate intake is of particular concern when generating a food plan for the individual with diabetes. One approach, called *carbohydrate counting*, has patients consume a specific number of carbohydrate choices (15 g carbohydrate/choice) at each meal or snack.

Carbohydrate counting also allows for synchronization of pharmacologic therapy to the glucose patterns that emerge from following an established food plan (see the Appendix, Figure A.14). Patients using pre-meal rapid-acting insulin can be taught to adjust the pre-meal dose based on the number of carbohydrates they plan to ingest at the next meal. After experimentation, many patients can become adept at these adjustments (often with excellent results). This approach is best when packaged foods are used with the nutritional labels that contain the amount of calories coming from carbohydrates. The approach is least effective when portion sizes are hard to estimate and the composition of the food or drink is unknown.

Reinforcement, doctor/patient relationship. In order to support and sustain medical nutrition interventions there are many areas that need to be addressed by the patient, family members, and the health care provider. Some of these are listed here.

- *Agreement on short-term goals.* Short-term goals should be specific, "reasonable and realistic," and achievable in 1–2 weeks. Goals should be limited to a maximum of 3 and address eating, exercise, and blood glucose monitoring behaviors. The focus should be to change one or two specific behaviors at a time in each area, e.g. eat breakfast and use less margarine, walk for 15 minutes twice a week, test blood glucose before and after the main meal three times a week.

- *Collection of important clinical data.* Provide instructions on how to record food intake (actual food eaten and quantities, times of meals), exercise habits (type, frequency, and duration), and blood testing results.

- *Documentation.* Include in the patient's permanent record the assessment and intervention. The report should include a summary of assessment information, long-term goals, education intervention, short-term goals, specific actions recommended, and plans for further follow-up, including additional education topics to be reviewed.

Coordinated exercise/activity plan. Medical nutrition therapy incorporates a food plan with exercise or activity designed to optimize glucose uptake and insulin utilization. The approach to exercise and activity is detailed later in this chapter.

Glucose monitoring. Although children and adolescents may be started on a regimen based solely on MNT to improve glycemic control, it is especially important not to omit SMBG. In general, SMBG is used too infrequently in children. This places the healthcare professional at an enormous disadvantage. Lacking SMBG data, it is almost impossible for the diabetes team to have adequate data to determine how well the nutrition therapy is working. Patient and parent or guardian knowledge of target blood glucose ranges and blood glucose testing technique need to be assessed. During the start treatment phase, when data are being collected to determine whether medical nutrition therapy and increased activity/exercise are reasonable choices, SMBG must occur at least two to four times each day. The testing schedule of fasting, before meals, 2 hours after the start of the meal, and before bedtime should be used in order to develop patterns of blood glucose levels throughout the day. This should be combined with testing before and after exercise (at least twice during the initial treatment phase). Testing using a SMBG meter with memory is the only certain way to ensure accurate data. Do not employ SMBG as a punitive measure. Patients are likely to fabricate results to please the diabetes team if SMBG is used punitively.

HbA_{1c} should be used in association with SMBG, but not as a replacement. HbA_{1c} data should be used to corroborate SMBG and vice versa (Table 5.1). Since several assays for glycosylated hemoglobin exist, each with a slightly different normal range, one way to standardize the HbA_{1c} is to report the difference between the reported value and the upper limit of normal.

Thus, when the upper limit of normal is 6 per cent, an HbA_{1c} of 10.0 per cent is 4.0 per cent above normal. As shown in Table 5.1, this would equate to average blood glucose of approximately 245 mg/dL (13.6 mmol/L). The average SMBG value for a period of at least 1 month with two to four tests per day should correlate with the HbA_{1c} level. Minimally, the SMBG values and HbA_{1c} should move in the same direction. If this is not the case, suspect error in SMBG logbook reporting or a meter requiring calibration.

During the start phase (1–2 weeks), all SMBG data should be reviewed weekly. Focus on fasting BG control first because it is the key to initial success. Examine blood glucose records for the incidence of hyperglycemia and number of blood glucose values in target range. If several fasting values exceed 250 mg/dL (13.9 mmol/L), consider initiating metformin. A follow-up contact within 2 weeks of the initial visit should be made. At that time, review baseline SMBG data. A 5–10 per cent reduction in mean blood glucose should have been possible by this time. If this level is reached, a second appointment 2 weeks later should show continued reduction. If, after the second follow-up visit, blood glucose levels (based on verified data) do not show at least 15 mg/dL (0.8 mmol/L) improvement, adjust the food plan, reassess the exercise prescription, and consider starting metformin. If greater than 10 per cent of fasting BG values exceed 300 mg/dL (16.7 mmol/L), consider starting insulin therapy.

Medical nutrition therapy/adjust. Evaluate progress. Optimally, patients should be seen two weeks after the start of MNT to review their progress (Figure 5.17). At this visit, weigh the patient and determine whether there have been changes in diet, alterations in medication, and changes in exercise habits. Review SMBG records for frequency of testing, time of testing, and results. Assess blood pressure and obtain any pertinent laboratory data. As it is too early to uncover a change in HbA_{1c}, measure blood glucose by reflectance meter during the visit. Obtain the patient's food records completed since initial visit or take a 24 hour food recall.

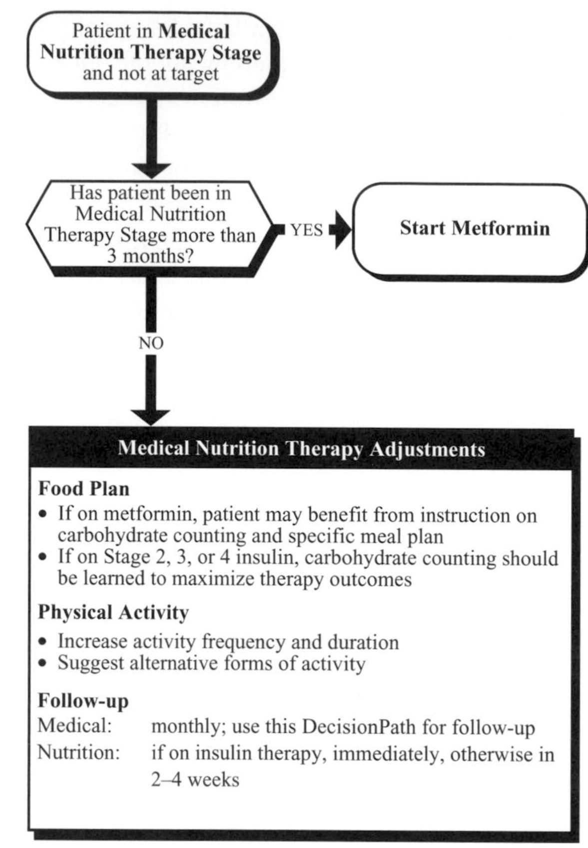

Figure 5.17 Type 2 Medical Nutrition and Activity Therapy/Adjust for Children and Adolescents

To determine whether the therapy is effective, examine the SMBG records for patterns of reduced blood glucose levels. Patterns are generated with at least three values at the same time. To corroborate the blood glucose values check the reflectance meter's memory. This can be accomplished by either downloading the stored glucose data or scrolling though the device. If there is a pattern of high blood glucose, then alterations in the food plan are necessary. If SMBG demonstrates targets have been achieved 50 per cent or more of the time, this is evidence the regimen is working. However, these values must be corroborated by HbA_{1c}. Since only two weeks have passed, the HbA_{1c} will not change to any appreciable degree. Thus, wait at least another two weeks before a second HbA_{1c} assay is performed or consider a fructosamine assay.

If there have been episodes of hypoglycemia,

they are related to exercise or skipped meals. If there is a pattern of hyperglycemia, generally it will appear as post-prandial blood glucose values > 160 mg/dL (8.9 mmol/L). Alterations in food plan should continue for up to three months. Staged Diabetes Management provides the general guideline of between 0.5 and 1 percentage point improvement in HbA_{1c} and a parallel lowering of average blood glucose of 15–30 mg/dL (0.8–1.7 mmol/L) monthly. If this target has not been achieved by at least three months, then the addition of metformin or insulin to MNT should be considered.

Corrective measures are as follows:

- *Changes in exercise and/or activity levels.* Patient should have gradually increased physical activity with a minimum goal of 20 to 30 minutes of physical activity six times a week. Is the patient willing or able to do more?
- *Change in food habits.* Patient eats meals and snacks on a regular basis and makes appropriate food choices in reasonable portions. If caloric intake has been excessive, can patient reduce intake of empty calories by moderate amounts (approximately 250–500 calories per day)? Can patient make further improvements in the overall quality of the diet?
- *Change in weight.* Weight maintenance or modest weight loss would be an appropriate outcome. If patient's weight increases, have positive changes in food selection and/or exercise been made? Or is weight gain related to re-hydration as a result of improved glycemic control?
- *Achievement of short-term goals.* Determine whether patient has achieved short-term goals established in previous visits and whether he or she is willing to set new goals.
- *Intervention.* Identify and recommend the changes in food and exercise that can improve the outcome, such as meal spacing; appropriate portions and choices; meal and snack schedule; and exercise frequency/duration/type/timing, including exercise after meals to reduce post-prandial hyperglycemia. Adjust food plan if necessary based on patient feedback. Reset short-term goals based on recommendations.

Self-management skill review. Do any survival self-management skills need to be reviewed (e.g., hypoglycemia prevention, illness management)? Are continuing self-management skills needed (e.g. use of alcohol, restaurant food choices, label reading, handling special occasions, and other information to promote self-care and flexibility)?

Set follow-up plans. A second follow-up visit within one month is recommended if:

- the patient is newly diagnosed
- there is difficulty making lifestyle changes
- additional support and encouragement is required
- the major goal is weight loss

If no immediate follow-up is needed, schedule the next appointment within 3–4 months.

Communication/summary to referral source. A written documentation of the nutrition assessment and intervention should be completed and placed in the patient's medical record. This documentation should include summary of assessment information, education intervention, short-term goals, specific actions recommended, and plans for further follow-up including additional education topics to be reviewed.

Follow-up visits. All follow-up visits should include weight (in light clothing without shoes); changes in medication; and changes in exercise habits. Review SMBG records including frequency of testing, time of testing and results; current blood pressure level; HbA_{1c}; 24-hour food recall; and problems with current food plan.

Again, evaluate whether therapy is working or whether change is needed, based on the following:

- HbA_{1c} improved or at target.

- Changes in blood glucose values – is there a downward trend in blood glucose values? Have there been episodes of hypoglycemia? Is this related to exercise or skipped meals? Is there a pattern of hyperglycemia? Are post-prandial blood glucose values less than 160 mg/dL (8.9 mmol/L)? What per cent of blood glucose values are within the target range? An overall decrease in blood glucose values of 15–30 mg/dL (0.8–1.7 mmol/L) per month should be obtained until targets are met.

- Changes in exercise and/or activity levels – patient has gradually increased physical activity with a minimum goal of 15–20 minutes of physical activity three to four times a week. Is the patient willing or able to do more?

- Change in food habits – patient eats meals and snacks on a regular basis and makes appropriate food choices in reasonable portions. If calorie intake has been excessive, can patient reduce calorie intake by moderate amounts (approximately 250–500 calories per day)? Can the patient make further improvements in the overall quality of the diet?

- Weight maintenance or modest weight loss would be an appropriate outcome. If patient's weight has increased, have positive changes in food selection and/or exercise been made? Don't make specific weight loss amount a goal (e.g. lose 10 pounds).

- Determine whether patient has achieved short- and long-term goals. Do these goals remain appropriate for the patient, or should new ones be established?

- During the adjust phase, therapy is modified to accelerate reaching the target blood glucose level. Increase in exercise levels, decrease in caloric intake, and other strategies may be enlisted to ensure further glucose reduction at an accelerated rate. The period of experimentation with steps to reduce blood glucose requires SMBG four times per day and monthly visits. HbA_{1c} levels should begin to respond to the overall lower blood glucose during the first month. However, not until the end of the second month will the impact of the initial therapy be fully reflected in the HbA_{1c} levels. From there on, reduction by at least 0.5 percentage points in HbA_{1c} per month should continue until targets (HbA_{1c} within 1.0 percentage point of the upper limit of normal) are achieved.

> Note: If laboratory data show no improvement and/or the patient is not willing to make food plan and exercise/activity behavior changes, a change in therapy will be required. Review the Master DecisionPath to select the next therapy. Otherwise, consider referral to a specialty team. If medical nutrition therapy fails, be certain that long-term goals, ongoing care, weight maintenance or loss, and overall glucose and lipid control are discussed. Reset short-term goals and review self-management skills. Determine whether any survival or continuing level self-management skills need to be addressed or reviewed. Additional follow-up visits are recommended if the patient needs and/or desires assistance with additional lifestyle changes, weight loss, and/or further self-management skill training. Written documentation of the intervention should include a summary of outcomes of nutrition intervention (medical outcomes, food and exercise behavior changes), self-management skill instruction/review provided, recommendations based upon outcomes, and plans for follow-up.

Follow-up intervention. Too often members of the diabetes health care team other than the physician are reluctant to recommend changes in therapy. This leads to both reduced efficiency and needless error in treatment. If any of the following are uncovered by any team member (especially dietitian or nurse), consider contacting provider for immediate alteration in therapy:

- SMBG and/or HbA_{1c} have not shown a downward trend
- SMBG and/or HbA_{1c} targets not achieved within 3–6 months
- hypertension (blood pressure > 130/80 mmHg) and/or dyslipidemia that have not responded to dietary changes, weight loss, and/or exercise changes

Medical nutrition therapy/maintain. This may prove to be the most difficult phase to sustain. During this phase, SMBG and HbA_{1c} target levels have been achieved. Patients often reduce SMBG testing and abandon their food and exercise plans. If at any time the patient exceeds the SMBG or HbA_{1c} levels, return the patient to the adjust treatment phase. Consider referral for diabetes and nutrition education every 6–12 months. Ongoing education that reinforces the importance of a food and exercise/activity plan is a critical factor in helping patients maintain glycemic control.

Metformin

Metformin should be considered under three circumstances. First, consider it for the newly diagnosed patient with type 2 diabetes and a fasting plasma glucose between 200 and 300 mg/dL (11.1 and 16.7 mmol/L) or a casual plasma glucose between 250 and 350 mg/dL (13.9 and 19.4 mmol/L). This would equate to an HbA_{1c} in the range of 8–11 per cent. When plasma glucose reaches these levels, insulin resistance and excess hepatic glucose output are likely causes of persistent hyperglycemia. Since MNT usually will lower glucose by no more than 50–75 mg/dL (2.8–4.2 mmol/L), a pharmacologic agent is needed. Second, consider metformin when medical nutrition therapy fails to improve HbA_{1c} by at least 0.5 percentage points monthly. Third, consider metformin as a therapy to replace low-dose insulin (< 0.1 U/kg) if the patient has achieved glycemic targets.

Oral agent selection and contraindications

Before considering initiation of an oral agent, certain factors must be addressed:

Step 1. The first step should be a review of the contraindications, regulations and other factors that might remove an agent for consideration. In the United States, the Food and Drug Administration (FDA) regulates the use of pharmacological agents. In general, the regulations are applicable to other countries. However, each country may have its own regulations, which need to be considered:

- Currently, metformin is the only oral agent that has been approved by the FDA for use in non-pregnant individuals under the age of 18 with type 2 diabetes or insulin resistance (polycystic ovary syndrome). SDM recommends consulting a Diabetes specialist if considering using a thiazolidinedione or secretagogue in children or adolescents:
- Since metformin is metabolized in the liver it is contraindicated for children or adolescents with severe liver disease or at risk for hepatitis (e.g. use of illicit drugs or alcohol).
- Only when serum creatinine is below 1.4 mg/dL (120 μmol/L) can metformin be initiated.
- The gastro-intestinal side effects of metformin can be significant and should be explained in detail before initiation.

Step 2. The second step is to determine whether the underlying defect is primarily related to fasting plasma glucose levels (caused by excessive and unregulated hepatic glucose output), generalized insulin resistance, or insulin deficiency. At diagnosis most children and adolescents with insulin resistance are overweight or obese – BMI > 85th percentile – and therefore would be started on metformin. Because metformin suppresses hepatic glucose output, it is often targeted at fasting plasma glucose. Since metformin is non-hypoglycemic, there is little concern for low blood glucose levels. Metformin may have some cardiovascular benefit by improving the lipid profile and studies in adults have shown that it does not cause weight gain and may result in modest weight loss. Recently metformin has been successfully used for women with PCOS who are seeking to ovulate.

Metformin/Start
0–0–M–0

Initiation of metformin should begin with the minimum dose (250 mg) independent of the patient's weight and given at the time of the largest meal. Since metformin does not stimulate pancreatic insulin secretion, it is not considered a hypoglycemic drug. However, since it may be used in the future with insulin, precautions should be taken to monitor blood glucose frequently when starting metformin.

For patients with no pre-existing contraindications (especially no liver or kidney disease), the choice of metformin should be based on the degree of obesity and the presence of fasting hyperglycemia. If, however, the child or adolescent has a history of gastrointestinal problems, metformin may exacerbate this condition and should either be avoided or used cautiously. The food plan and exercise program for an individual starting at diagnosis on metformin follows the same principles as for the patient on MNT alone. Special attention should be paid, however, to gastric distress from metformin.

Follow-up. During the first week the patient should do SMBG four times each day, preferably at varying times in order to produce a complete picture of metabolic response to the metformin. At the end of 1 week's testing, review SMBG data to determine whether the blood glucose has been altered. If average blood glucose decreases by more than 10 per cent continue with the minimum dose. Schedule the next visit for 2 weeks following initiation of the oral agent.

Metformin/Adjust
M–0–M–0

If the SMBG has not been lowered significantly (approximately 20 per cent) after 2–4 weeks, increase the dose of metformin by 250 mg and give it at breakfast time. Be sure to confirm that the original medical nutrition therapy is being followed. Continue this therapy for 1–2 weeks using SMBG data to determine impact. Metformin can be adjusted weekly. At most no more than two weeks should elapse without adjustment in metformin if blood glucose does not respond. Staged Diabetes Management is designed to permit up to eight dosage increases before the maximum dose is reached. Note that the clinically effective dose is not necessarily the maximum dose. For example, the clinically effective dose of metformin is 2000 mg/day, not the maximum dose of 2550 mg/day. Because individual differences to dose response exist, close monitoring with verified SMBG data is essential during this phase.

Glycosylated hemoglobin values should begin to decrease due to lowered blood glucose levels within 4–8 weeks following initiation of treatment. If HbA_{1c} level shows no improvement, consider the following:

- A hemoglobinopathy, such as sickle cell trait
- Increase daily testing
- Patient not adhering to diabetes regimen (taking medication meal planning)

The long-term HbA_{1c} target should be set to within 1 percentage point of the upper limit of normal with at least a 0.5 percentage point reduction each month. If the current average SMBG is > 250 mg/dL (13.9 mmol/L), expect a 30 mg/dL (1.7 mmol/L) decrease in blood glucose over the next month and a 1 percentage point decline in HbA_{1c}. If this is not accomplished, increase the dose of the oral agent as described above. If the maximum clinically effective dose is reached, consider combination therapy or insulin therapy.

Oral Agent/Maintain
M–0–M–0

If the patient has reached the therapeutic goal on the oral agent, treatment now turns to maintenance. During this phase, attempt to maintain glycemic control within target range without making significant demands on the patient. SMBG testing schedules and frequency of contact with the healthcare professional are individualized. Insufficient contact may cause the patient to lose interest in the intensified treatment and become less likely to follow the therapeutic regimen, thereby worsening glycemic control. For some patients close contact, frequent visits, and careful assessment of behaviors related to the treatment regimen are the cornerstones of good care. Minimally, all patients should be seen every 3–4 months. Assessment for complications (Chapters 8 and 9) and evaluation of the overall impact of the therapy on glycemic control should be continued.

The addition of insulin to metformin

In patients previously treated by metformin, insulin may be introduced as an adjunctive therapy. This is preferable for those patients who were started on metformin, reached the maximum effective dose, but still were not able to achieve glycemic targets. For most other patients, especially those in whom mean fasting SMBG exceeds 300 mg/dL (16.7 mmol/L), starting insulin as the monotherapy is appropriate. For the latter circumstance, skip this step and follow the DecisionPaths for insulin therapy. In the section following insulin therapies, rationale and methods for the addition of metformin to the current insulin therapy are reviewed.

Combination Metformin–Insulin Therapy/Start
M–0–M–N or G

For some time researchers and clinicians have been examining the efficacy of bedtime insulin and metformin. While virtually every oral agent has undergone some evaluation with insulin, the most frequently tested are metformin and the sulfonylureas.[16] Since insulin is an effective means of lowering blood glucose levels, metformin, which targets insulin resistance by decreasing hepatic glucose output, can be used in combination with insulin. When metformin fails to restore near euglycemia, combination therapies that include bedtime intermediate (N) or long-acting (G) insulin are often considered. It is well recognized that insulin, when used properly, will significantly improve glycemic control at virtually any level of hyperglycemia. However, this is at the risk of hypoglycemia and increased weight gain, especially when high doses of insulin are required or when the patient chooses to skip a meal. It is for this reason that bedtime low-dose insulin is combined with an oral agent to lower blood glucose overnight while reducing the risk of hypoglycemia. It is also well known that multiple defects are at work in type 2 diabetes. While insulin resistance may be addressed by metformin, often it is insufficient to overcome an absolute reduction in endogenous insulin secretion or a failure of β-cell response. In such cases, addition of bedtime low-dose insulin will supplement endogenous insulin. Note that this regimen does not provide for meal related (bolus) insulin requirements, and bolus insulin may be required if post-meal SMBG targets are not achieved.

The current bedtime insulins have substantial differences that should be considered before they are used. N is an intermediate-acting insulin with a peak action at between 4 and 8 hours after administration. Taken overnight, it may lead to early morning hypoglycemia. Glargine (G) is a long-acting insulin analog, which lasts up to 24 hours and has no peak action. Data from use in adults demonstrate that glargine results in improved fasting blood glucose control with a lower incidence of nocturnal hypoglycemia (see Chapter 3 or 4). The latter, therefore, acts more like basal insulin and may be used as such. Use of either insulin places more responsibility with the patient. It is, for example, necessary to monitor blood glucose before each insulin injection. With NPH it may be necessary to measure blood glucose at 2 or 3 AM (or whenever hypoglycemic symptoms appear).

Both the N and G insulins are begun by giving 0.1 unit/kg at bedtime (Figure 5.18). Both the child and family member (parent or guardian) should be taught how to draw up and inject insulin. Education about insulin administration, hypoglycemia and food planning is advisable. As this is generally not a medical emergency it can be scheduled after the child and parent agree to initiation of insulin therapy. Most patients and their families are unaware of how thin the currently available insulin needles are and do not realize that injection of insulin is relatively painless. Prior to drawing up the insulin, the patient and family should be re-evaluated for SMBG. Even low-dose long-acting insulin can contribute to hypoglycemia.

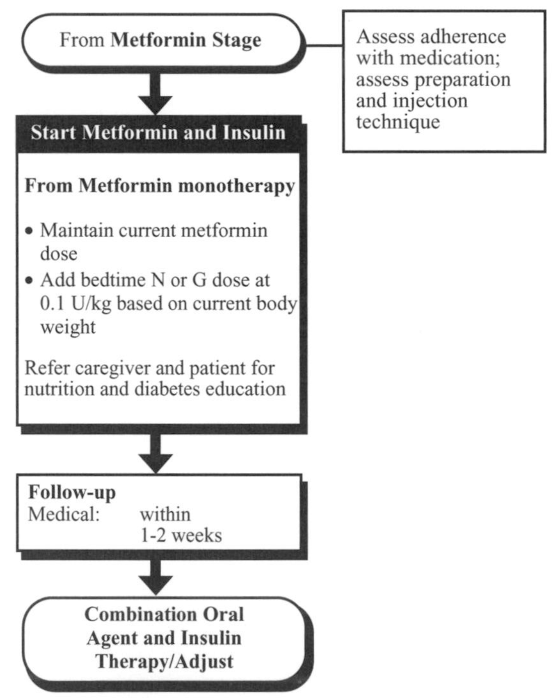

Figure 5.18 Type 2 Combination Oral Agent and Insulin Therapy/Start for Children and Adolescents

Combination Metformin–Insulin Therapy/Adjust
M–0–M–N or G

If fasting blood glucose > 140 mg/dL (7.8 mmol/L) for three consecutive days increase the N or G by 1–2 units or up to 10 per cent of dose (Table 5.2). This process can be continued until the total bedtime dose reaches 0.4 U/kg. Note that often a significant amount of bedtime insulin is required due to the combination of insulin resistance and excess hepatic glucose output. Throughout the metformin–insulin therapy period, be prepared to reduce or increase the insulin as dictated by blood glucose levels and to maintain the current dose of the oral agent. If the intent is to transition the patient to insulin only therapy, slowly reduce the oral agent and replace with regular short-acting (R) or rapid-acting insulin (RA) insulin before meals. It is becoming more common to use G insulin for basal insulin combined with RA insulin before meals because this regimen is more physiologic. Within 1 month both daily blood glucose and HbA_{1c} should show improvement. If no improvement in fasting blood glucose has been noted, insulin-only therapies should be considered (see guidelines for initiating insulin therapy found in the next section).

Table 5.2 Type 2 Combination Oral Agent and Insulin Therapy/Adjust for Children and Adolescents

Recommended Insulin Adjustments		
TIME	BG mg/dL	ACTION
AM	< 80 (< 4.4 mmol/L)	↓ BT N or G by 1–2 U or 10% of dose
	> 140 (> 7.8 mmol/L)	↑ BT N or G by 1–2 U or 10% of dose
PM	> 140 (> 7.8 mmol/L)	Move to **Insulin Stage 2, 3 or 4**
BT	> 160 (> 8.9 mmol/L)	Move to **Insulin Stage 2, 3 or 4**

Combination Oral Agent–Insulin Therapy/Maintain
M–0–M–N or G

Because metformin–insulin therapy is generally not used as a "final" treatment, the long-term impact on the patient is unknown. Theoretically, it should help the patient in two ways: exogenous insulin should rest the pancreas while ensuring improved glycemic control; metformin should reduce insulin resistance. If patients make lifestyle changes that result in weight loss and increased activity, they will often not require movement on to multiple daily injections of insulin and may be able to maintain glucose control with MNT alone or in combination with metformin. Lacking controlled studies, it remains to be determined whether combined therapy is better than insulin alone. An important point to keep in mind is to not eliminate SMBG during the maintain phase and to monitor for weight gain.

Failure of combination therapy. When combination therapies fail, the next stage is insulin. Reasons for lack of success should be explored (e.g. depression, difficulty following MNT, taking medications as directed). The Type 2 Diabetes Master DecisionPath should have already been shown to the patient and family members, and insulin therapy should have been discussed as an option if combination therapy failed to bring the patient into glycemic control. If this is not the case, it is important to reiterate the need to consider alternative therapies, since it is unlikely that continuing with combination therapy will improve control.

Insulin therapy

Because initiation of insulin is a major step in diabetes therapy, it may be helpful to review with the patient and the family some key principles of care and the Type 2 Diabetes Master DecisionPath for Children and Adolescents (see Figure 5.15). It is important to note that patients starting insulin may need a revised food plan and exercise program synchronized to insulin action, and referral to a dietitian is strongly encouraged.

Hyperinsulinemia, hypoglycemia, and weight gain. Introducing exogenous insulin to improve glycemic control raises concerns about hypoglycemia and weight gain. While hyperglycemia may indeed be rectified, if insulin is introduced too rapidly at high doses patients may experience symptoms of relative or "true" hypoglycemia. It is not uncommon to lower blood glucose by $>$ 100 mg/dL (5.6 mmol/L) when high-dose insulin is used. In SDM, insulin is started at the lowest safe dose and is adjusted slowly so that HbA_{1c} decreases at a rate of 0.5–1 per cent HbA_{1c} per month (or average SMBG of 15–30 mg/dL [0.8–1.7 mmol/L]). At this rate of improvement there is time to address weight gain issues. For newly diagnosed patients with severe hyperglycemia prior to the initiation of insulin, there may have been modest weight loss (both by volume of fluid loss and glucose excretion). Using insulin to restore near-normal glycemia is often accompanied by a 3–10 lb (1.5–5 kg) weight gain. This is normal and can be minimized by modifying diet or increasing exercise/activity at the start of insulin therapy. As part of an intensive regimen, the exogenous insulin may cause some "hunger". There is a tendency to chase the insulin with food, which results in added caloric intake. This can be prevented by maintaining the same carbohydrate intake and moving the carbohydrate to synchronize with insulin action and/or adjusting the insulin regimen. (For example, if due to the peak action of intermediate-acting insulin the patient experiences mid-afternoon hypoglycemia, reduce the caloric intake at the midday meal and use some of these calories [carbohydrate] for a mid-afternoon snack. The net effect is to maintain the same caloric intake, but to distribute it more effectively to reduce hypoglycemia.)

Treatment options. Insulin therapy in type 2 diabetes is similar to that for type 1 diabetes because the same insulins and regimens are used (although pump therapy is relatively rare in type 2 diabetes). Where the two differ is how the insulin is used to overcome the underlying defect. In type 1 diabetes the destruction of the pancreatic β-cell results in an absolute insulin deficiency, requiring total reliance on exogenous insulin. This is rarely the case in type 2 diabetes. Depending upon the duration of disease and the severity of insulin resistance and relative insulin deficiency, exogenous insulin has varying functions. Individuals with type 2 diabetes retain the ability to produce and secrete insulin although it may not be enough to meet the metabolic demands of insulin resistance. The defect may be in the timing of insulin secretion (defects in first-phase insulin secretion), amount of insulin that can be produced by the β-cell resulting in a relative insulin deficiency, or insulin resistance. Thus the choice of therapy first takes into consideration the underlying defects. In most children and adolescents requiring insulin at diagnosis, the underlying defect is related to both a relative insulin deficiency and insulin resistance. Thus, the exogenous insulin will have to address both of these defects and generally calls for higher-dose insulin compared with a child or adolescent with type 1 diabetes.

There are several approaches to insulin therapy. SDM divides each insulin regimen into two components: basal or background and bolus or meal related. Combinations of basal and bolus insulin can be used for conventional and intensive management. In conventional insulin therapy, insulin action is matched to carbohydrate intake (see Chapter 3 for insulin action curves). This regimen relies on a consistent schedule of food intake and exercise/activity. Since insulin is given to anticipate when food is ingested, it is important to maintain a consistent eating schedule and carbohydrate intake that is synchronized to insulin action. Typically the conventional regimens require fewer injections and mixing of different types of insulin (see Table 5.3). Once the most popular regimen, it is now being replaced by a more physiologic insulin delivery regimen: intensive insulin therapy. In this regimen, insulin is altered to match energy intake and expenditure. The regimens consist of three or more injections of insulin per day and are co-ordinated with food intake and activity level. Because it comes closer to mimicking the normal physiologic state, intensive insulin therapy provides a better chance of optimizing blood glucose control. Typical of this approach are frequent changes in insulin dose and more frequent SMBG. The goal of both approaches is to optimize glycemic control with fewer episodes of hypoglycemia.

In general, regimens requiring administration of insulin before meals and large snacks are far more physiologic, generally require less total insulin, and usually result in a more flexible schedule for the patient. Many physicians and patients are concerned with the discomfort of multiple-injection insulin regimens. Studies have repeatedly shown that the newer fine-gauge needles (30 and 31 gauge) are nearly painless if proper injection technique is followed. Additionally, needleless insulin delivery devices are available to help patients with needle phobia. Currently studies are underway testing the feasibility, safety, and efficacy of inhaled insulin preparations, which may make multiple insulin administration more acceptable to patients (and health care providers).

For consistency, the insulin therapies supported by SDM use pre-meal (bolus) and bedtime (basal) as the times to administer insulin. Whether basal or bolus, conventional or intensive, generally insulin may be given at four specific times during a day related to meals, activity, and sleep. The times are before breakfast (fasting), midday meal, evening meal, and at bedtime (3–5 hours after the evening meal). The insulins are denoted as short-acting regular (R), rapid-acting (RA), intermediate-acting (N), and long-acting glargine (G). SDM recommends writing out insulin regimens using these specific times and types of insulin. For example, R/N–0–R–N denotes breakfast regular and intermediate insulin, no insulin before lunch,

Table 5.3 Selecting insulin: Stage 2, 3, or 4

	Primarily fasting hyperglycemia	Primarily post-prandial hyperglycemia	Fasting and post-prandial hyperglycemia	Cannot detect problem
Stage 2	X			
Stage 3	X			
Stage 4 (Physiologic)	X	X	X	X

regular insulin before the evening meal, and intermediate insulin before bedtime. See Chapter 3 for a complete review of insulin action curves.

Medical nutrition therapy is continued throughout all stages of therapy. In newly diagnosed patients, MNT is instituted along with insulin initiation and generally follows the carbohydrate counting method. MNT with insulin follows the same general principles as stated in the weight management section of this chapter.

Short-acting insulin: choosing between regular or rapid-acting. No clear criteria currently exist for choosing between regular short-acting and rapid-acting insulin for type 2 diabetes. However, in clinical practice, some principles have emerged that may be helpful in choosing between these two forms of insulin. For patients whose lifestyle makes food and activity planning very difficult, RA, which is injected just prior to eating and has a more predictable action curve (peak within 1 to $1\frac{1}{2}$ hours, overall action 3 hours), is the preferred choice. For patients already under treatment for whom regular insulin before each meal has not resulted in improved post-prandial glucose levels, replacement of R with RA is recommended. This maintains the patient on the same number of injections. For all other patients, at diagnosis or in treatment, either R or RA could be used at the same dose. RA is preferred in SDM because it is generally more predictable and can be more easily adjusted. For children and adolescents with type 2 diabetes the major criteria are twofold: convenience and predictability. Fewer injections of regular insulin are more convenient, but require that meals and snacks be taken at the same time each day. R has a variable peak action and a long-lasting "tail" that make it difficult to predict its action curve. RA insulin is more predictable because of its shorter action curve, but would require insulin administration prior to each meal (and sometimes before snacks). Some would argue that children cannot be expected to do this. In actuality children with type 1 diabetes have been administering their own insulin throughout the day, even in school. When starting insulin in a child with type 2 diabetes it may be helpful for health professionals to consider the manner in which a child with type 1 diabetes would be treated.

Intermediate or long-acting insulin: choosing between N and glargine. In general glargine is superior to N in terms of both predictability and convenience. One injection per day of G at bedtime should provide sufficient basal insulin for a 24 hour period without any peak action. However, some patients may require splitting the dose of G for optimal basal insulin coverage. In contrast, N requires two injections and each may peak at between 6 and 9 hours after administration. When taking N it must be certain that food is available during its peak action to prevent hypoglycemia. Patients tend to overreact, eating snacks throughout the day to anticipate a hypoglycemic reaction.

Starting insulin with a new diagnosis of type 2 diabetes. At diagnosis of type 2 diabetes, initiation of insulin therapy should occur immediately, without regard to symptoms, if fasting plasma glucose is > 300 mg/dL (16.7 mmol/L), casual plasma glucose is > 350 mg/dL (19.4 mmol/L), or ketones are present. At these high plasma glucose levels, medical nutrition therapy alone or in combination with an oral agent (metformin) will not normally sufficiently lower the blood glucose level into the target range. Furthermore, patients with persistent hyperglycemia at these levels experience glucose toxicity. Therefore they are at increased risk for hyperglycemic hyperosmolar syndrome (HHS). Finally, some children may be developing type 1 diabetes, for whom insulin therapy will prevent diabetes ketoacidosis.

Determine whether insulin will be initiated on an inpatient or outpatient basis.

Many institutions have developed systems that allow for the safe initiation of insulin on an outpatient basis. If resources for education and medical follow-up are not available, the patient should be hospitalized. If the patient is at risk for HHS (see Chapter 10), if there is uncertainty as to type of diabetes, or if the individual cannot care for him or herself, consider hospitalization immediately.

Preparing the patient to use insulin: multiple injections and insulin adjustment. *Blood glucose monitoring.* All patients or their family caregiver should be performing SMBG, independent of the number of injections. These data are necessary for meaningful communications between the patient and the health care professional. The type of meter to be used for SMBG varies. However, SMBG should have these important attributes. First, the SMBG meter should have a memory, making it possible to record and store data for retrieval. This also increases the accuracy and reliability of the patient's information. Second, the skills needed by the patient should be simple, with regard to use of the device. Third, testing should be scheduled to coincide with meals, activity, and insulin adjustments to optimize collecting data for clinical decision-making. Fourth, testing should take into account the need to adjust insulin doses based on changes in blood glucose.

Unlike the case with oral agent regimens, patients or their caregivers are expected to play a very important role in the daily adjustments in insulin dose. There are two approaches to adjusting treatment using SMBG data – pattern or immediate response. The two are meant to address most situations. When they do not, it is generally necessary to collect more SMBG data and to confirm that the patient's behavior is consistent with the instructions. Pattern response suggests that each individual has a consistent set of blood glucose/insulin relationships. This consistency is characterized by predictable patterns in which specific insulin doses are related to known glycemic levels. For example, increasing the morning intermediate-acting N insulin will consistently result in a decrease in late-afternoon (pre-evening meal) blood glucose levels. Therefore, the purpose of initial SMBG is to determine whether such a pattern can be easily identified. When, after trial and error (even within 3 days) such a pattern has been identified, treatment of type 2 diabetes may follow a predictable path. Generally, however, identifying a specific pattern takes substantially longer. Because of changes in food plan, exercise/activity, seasons, and so on, patterns may change. Therefore, the concept of patterned response should be continually reassessed.

Immediate response recognizes that an acute situation has developed requiring an immediate action such as hypoglycemia (insulin reaction), hyperglycemia, or an anticipated change in food plan or exercise. This occurs whenever blood glucose is below 60 mg/dL (3.3 mmol/L) or greater than 250 mg/dL (13.9 mmol/L). Refer to "Hospitalization for Problems Related to Glycemic Control" in Chapter 10 for additional information.

Insulin stage 2, 3 or Physiologic Insulin Stage 4? For newly diagnosed children or adolescents starting insulin therapy, the Type 2 Diabetes Master DecisionPath (see Figure 5.15) indicates three insulin regimens using rapid or short-acting and intermediate or long-acting insulins. The conventional approach is to begin with Stage 2 and proceeds to the next stages if this two-injection regimen fails to bring the patient into glycemic control. An alternative approach which SDM has been found to be very effective is to begin with bedtime long-acting (G) insulin with subsequent addition of injections of RA before each meal as needed for daytime management of post-prandial hyperglycemia (i.e. 0–0–0–G built up to RA–RA–RA–G). Basically this is the most physiologic of the insulin regimens supported by SDM. This section discusses each regimen beginning with Stage 2. However, it should be noted that children and adolescents generally have a variable schedule characterized by unpredictability. Unless the scheduled can be fixed, it is recommended that the patient be given an opportunity to try the most flexible regimen – modified Stage 4 beginning with bedtime G. This will require a substantial number of SMBG tests over the first several weeks to assure adequate insulin coverage for each meal. In the long term it should fit into the variable schedule of most children.

Insulin stage 2: conventional approach. *This is the most conservative approach using the smallest number of injections. Its only major limitation is that the child or adolescent cannot skip meals and activity levels must also be regimented.* Following a thorough history, physical, and laboratory evaluation and after review of the target blood glucose levels, the decision as to whether to hospitalize to start the patient on an insulin regimen should be made. In most cases hospitalization is unnecessary. Assuming that insulin will be started on an ambulatory basis, the time of insulin initiation becomes the next question.

> Note: For all insulin therapies the starting dose formula has been carefully selected to meet the immediate metabolic requirements of the individual while reducing the risk of hypoglycemia and severe hyperglycemia.

At **Diagnosis** or from **Oral Agent Stage**, or **Oral Agent and Insulin Stage**
If acutely ill, hospitalize and start insulin immediately; otherwise, start insulin within 1 week and consider hopitalization if outpatient (and caregiver) education not available

Start Insulin Stage 2

RA/N–0–RA/N–0
R/N–0–R/N–0

Calculate total dose at 0.3 U/kg based on current weight

	AM	MIDDAY	PM	BT
Distribution of daily dose	2/3	0	1/3	0
RA/N or R/N ratio	1:2	–	1:1	–

Pre-mixed insulin may be used for patients unable to draw insulin correctly or who have less than optimal caregiver involvement/support.

Refer patient and caregiver for nutrition and diabetes education

Start Medical Nutrition Therapy

Follow-up
Medical: daily phone contact for 3 days, then office visit within 1 week; 24-hour emergency phone support needed
Education: within 24 hours, then office visit in 2 weeks
Nutrition: within 1 week

Insulin Stage 2/Adjust

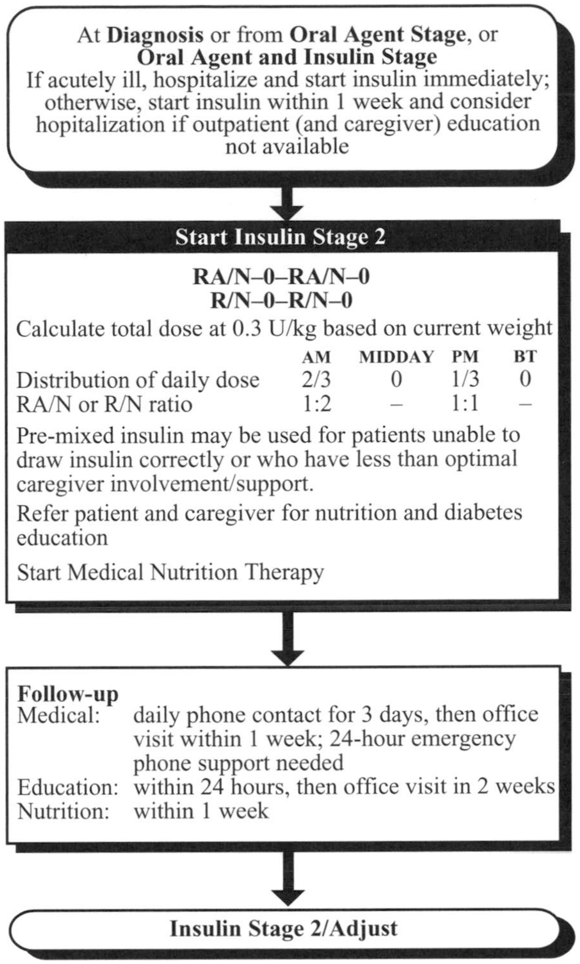

Figure 5.19 Type 2 Insulin Stage 2/Start for Children and Adolescents

Insulin Stage 2/Start
R/N–0–R/N–0 or RA/N–0–RA/N–0

Morning insulin start. If the first time the patient starts this therapy is in the morning, the total daily dose is calculated as 0.3 U/kg (see Figure 5.19). The total daily dose is divided into two periods roughly associated with breakfast and the evening meal (approximately 10 hours apart). The pre-breakfast dose is two-thirds of the total daily requirement. This is further divided into one-third R or RA and two-thirds N. The small amount of R or RA is to cover breakfast. The intermediate-acting insulin is to cover lunch and the afternoon period. Review the insulin action curves described in Chapter 3. Note the likely times of peak action. Glucose excursions after lunch will have to be measured by SMBG between 2 and 4 hours post-meal to determine whether adequate insulin is available. Daytime activity will also affect blood glucose levels. *With adolescents and children it is very important that SMBG be done before and following activity to gauge the impact of the physical activity on glucose level. Because week-days (in school) and weekends differ substantially, it may be necessary to readjust the insulin regimen.* The pre-evening meal insulin is calculated as one-third of the total daily dose equally split between R or RA and intermediate-acting insulin and given as one injection before the evening meal. For example, a patient with a current weight of 100 lb (45 kg) would receive 14 total units of insulin. Of the 14 units, nine would be given in the AM and five in the PM. Of the nine units in the AM, six units would be N and three units would be R or RA. The PM dose would be three units N and two units R or RA (due to rounding the R or RA was kept at less than 1:1 ratio with the N). Note that if premixed insulins is used it cannot easily be adjusted.

Afternoon or evening insulin start. If the therapy is being started in the afternoon or evening, the starting dose is one-third the normal total daily dose (0.1 U/kg), which is equally divided between N and R or RA insulin and administered just prior to the evening meal. The next day the patient would be on the total daily dose (0.3 U/kg) as described above. The patient should be taught both insulin administration technique and how to monitor blood glucose. SMBG should be performed every 4 hours until the next day. If blood glucose levels are > 250 mg/dL (13.9 mmol/L), consider additional small doses (1–2 units) of R or RA with SMBG 2 hours after the insulin injection. This therapy is temporary. Have the patient return the next morning to initiate daily insulin administration (see previous section).

Immediate follow-up. Self-monitored blood glucose is the best way to assess the impact of insulin therapy. The minimum SMBG for this treatment regimen is five times per day (before meals, at bedtime, and at 3AM). An evening snack may be necessary to prevent overnight hypoglycemia. One or two carbohydrate choices taken from earlier in the day and moved to bedtime can be provided as a snack.

During the first several days it is imperative to maintain glucose levels at a point that will avoid both hypoglycemia and hyperglycemia. Additionally, co-management with the various health professionals (nurse educator and dietitian, if available) who will be involved in diabetes care must be established. This is especially important in ambulatory management. The guidelines for insulin adjustments begin immediately, along with making arrangements for follow-up diabetes and nutrition education and establishing target blood glucose levels.

Although near euglycemia is the overall goal of treatment to prevent microvascular and macrovascular complications (see the end of this chapter and Chapters 8 and 9 for further information), any improvement from baseline benefits individuals with type 2 diabetes. Setting the initial goal at fasting < 200 mg/dL (11.1 mmol/L) and post-meal < 250 mg/dL (13.9 mmol/L) is the first step in ensuring eventual near-normal levels of blood glucose. This interim target was established to promote the overall goal of gradual (safe) reduction in blood glucose. While any improvement in blood glucose is acceptable, the overall long-term goal is to achieve near-normal glycemic control. Thus, it is appropriate to react to consistent patterns of high blood glucose with increased insulin after assessing adherence issues.

Medical nutrition therapy. As with all pharmacologic therapies, medical nutrition therapy is part of the overall treatment approach. Start as if the person were treated solely by nutrition therapy (see Medical Nutrition and Activity Therapy/Start and Weight Management Start for children and adolescents). Modifying the nutrition therapy to avoid hypoglycemia may be necessary. To do this, consider altering the timing of both food intake and exercise to synchronize with the insulin action curve. Some *initial* weight gain may occur with the introduction of insulin. This is due to the uptake and metabolism of glucose as glycemic targets are being reached or as a result of rehydration. Subsequent weight gain, however, may be due to chasing insulin with food or poor adherence to MNT recommendation. Since children and adolescents are in an active growing period, "normal" weight gain needs to be differentiated from weight gain due to the insulin regimen. The key is to utilize the growth-related curves and to differentiate between symmetrical and asymmetrical growth. Individuals whose height and weight are in the 90th percentile are experiencing symmetrical growth patterns, whereas individuals whose weight is in the 90th percentile and height in the 50th percentile are asymmetrical and likely to have a BMI > 85th percentile.

In SDM, alterations in the timing of meals, snacks, and exercise are the principal tools by which hyperglycemia and hypoglycemia are prevented. If persistent hyperglycemia or hypoglycemia do occur, immediately consider changing the insulin regimen.

Insulin Stage 2/Adjust
R/N–0–R/N–0 or RA/N–0–RA/N–O

Adjustments to Insulin Stage 2 are based on patterns of SMBG values (see Table 5.4).

Follow these general principles:

- Look for a pattern – at least 3 days of similar blood glucose values.

- Make initial adjustments to target the consistently low blood glucose first. Follow this by targeting patterns of high blood glucose.
- Normally, target only one insulin at a time – either N, R, or RA) – at one time point (AM or PM).
- Change dose by 1–4 units depending on the level of hyperglycemia.
- Become familiar with insulin action curve principles (see Chapter 3).
- Avoid adding calories to total food intake to prevent hypoglycemia. Instead, move carbohydrate choices (e.g. save dessert for bedtime snack).

Target blood glucose and insulin adjustments. During the first several months of insulin therapy, the patient should demonstrate improved glycemic control. HbA_{1c} should drop by approximately 0.5–1 percentage point per month and mean SMBG 15–30 mg/dL (0.8–1.7 mmol/L). If these rates are met, the same insulin doses are kept. If the rates are not met, increase the insulin doses following the adjustment guidelines.

Table 5.4 Insulin stage 2 pattern adjustment guidelines (see Figure 5.20 for letter designations)

Insulin Stage 2 Pattern Adjustments
RA/N–0–RA/N–0 or R/A–0–R/N–0

	< 70 mg/dL (< 3.9 mmol/L)	140–250 mg/dL (7.8–13.4 mmol/L)	> 250 mg/dL (> 13.4 mmol/L)
AM or 3 AM	↓PM N 1–2 U (a,b)	↑PM N 1–2 U (a,k)	↑PM N 2–4 U (a,k)
MIDDAY (MID)	↓AM RA or R 1–2 U (c,e)	↑AM RA or R 1–2 U (f,g,k)	↑AM RA or R 2–4 U (f,g,k)
PM	↓AM N 1–2 U (d,e)	↑AM N 1–2 U (f,h,k)	↑AM N 2–4 U (f,h,k)
	< 100 mg/dL (< 5.5 mmol/L)	160–250 mg/dL (8.9–13.9 mmol/L)	> 250 mg/dL (> 13.9 mmol/L)
BEDTIME (BT)	↓PM RA or R 1–2 U (e)	↑PM RA or R 1–2 U (f,k)	↑PM RA or R 2–4 U (f,k)

Adjust insulin based on BG patterns

May increase or decrease dose by 1–2 U or 10% of dose

Follow-up
Medical: weekly while adjusting insulin, then office visit within 1–2 months

How to Use These Tables
1. Find current insulin stage
2. Find the pattern of blood glucose problem (column)
3. Identify time of day (row) pattern occurs
4. Recommended adjustment is given where the column and row intersect
5. See notes for additional considerations

Insulin Pattern Adjustments
- Adjust insulin from 3 day pattern of typical schedule
- Determine which insulin is responsible for pattern
- Adjust by 1–2 units or 10% of dose
- Adjust only one dose at a time
- Correct hypoglycemia first
- If total dose > 1.0 U/kg, consider adding metformin
- If hyperglycemia throughout day, correct highest average tartget SMBG first; if all within 50 mg/dL (2.7 mmol/L) of target, correct AM first

Notes
a. Evaluate nocturnal hypoglycemia; check 3 AM BG
b. Consider adjusting bedtime snack
c. Consider adding or adjusting mid-morning snack
d. Consider adding or adjusting afternoon snack
e. Evaluate if prior activity is causing hypoglycemia
f. Consider adding activity
g. Consider decreasing mid-morning snack
h. consider decreasing afternoon snack
i. No mid-morning snack usually needed with RA
j. No afternoon snack usually needed with RA
k. Use of regular insulin in place of rapid-acting (RA) necessitates snacking. If possible, use RA insulin in children and adolescents.

Figure 5.20 Type 2 diabetes insulin adjustment considerations for children and adolescents

Insulin Stage 2/Maintain
R/N–0–R/N–0 or RA/N–0–RA/N–0

When SMBG and HbA_{1c} targets are met, alterations to the insulin, food plan, and exercise regimens are still likely to be required to maintain near-normal blood glucose levels. To prevent both hyperglycemia and weight gain, encourage a schedule of blood glucose and weight monitoring. While neither need be as regimented as during start and adjust phases, both are required to detect either increasing blood glucose or weight. At a minimum, SMBG should occur prior to each insulin injection, with at least one daily 2-hour post-prandial (at varying meals each day). Weight should be monitored weekly. Some changes in insulin dose and timing should be expected. The patient might be provided with some general rules for making insulin adjustments based on consistent patterns of blood glucose.

Moving to Insulin Stage 3

Insulin Stage 3/Start: from Insulin Stage 2 R/N–0–R–N or RA/N–0–RA–N

Three conditions can be addressed by Insulin Stage 3 that may have been encountered in Insulin Stage 2:

- morning fasting blood glucose consistently above target range
- nocturnal hypoglycemia
- varying time of evening meal

Morning fasting blood glucose may be high for several reasons. The principal causes relate to a high bedtime glucose, early AM excessive glucose output (dawn phenomenon), Somogyi effect, insufficient exogenous basal insulin and lack of adherence to MNT (large bedtime snacks). One consequence of relative insulin deficiency may be excess hepatic glucose production (gluconeogenesis). The second factor, high evening blood glucose, is usually the result of a larger evening meal or proportionately higher carbohydrates at the evening meal and at bedtime. The third cause for high fasting plasma glucose, dyschronized insulin peak action, may result in low blood glucose from 2 to 4 AM and a rebound to hyperglycemia (Somogyi effect) by morning. The latter is often the cause of nocturnal hypoglycemia. Alternatively, nocturnal hypoglycemia may result from too much intermediate-acting insulin at dinner coupled with insufficient bedtime snack. If adjustments to the Insulin Stage 2 regimen have failed to overcome these problems, moving the intermediate-acting insulin to at least 3 hours after the evening meal (this bedtime injection is shown as BT in figures and tables) should provide some resolution. Before doing this, however, be certain that overinsulinization has not occurred (> 1.0 U/kg). If this is suspected, consider reducing the total daily insulin dose to 1 U/kg and redistributing it according to Insulin Stage 3 (see Figure 5.21).

To start Insulin Stage 3, move the current dose of evening meal N insulin to bedtime. Make

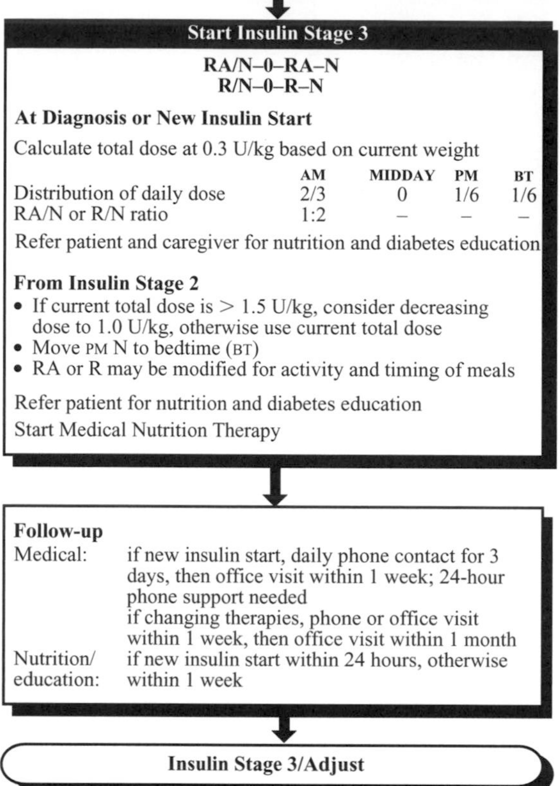

Figure 5.21 Type 2 Insulin Stage 3/Start for Children and Adolescents

certain SMBG occurs at this time. One or two carbohydrate choices from earlier in the day can be moved as a bedtime snack. Readjust both the evening R or RA and the morning R or RA after 3 days on this regimen. Most probably the morning R or RA will be reduced and the evening R or RA will be increased. The total daily dose should still follow the pattern of a maximum of 1.5 U/kg.

Before beginning pattern adjustment, determine which insulin is responsible for the glucose pattern. Intermediate-acting insulin (N) is meant to reach its peak near the morning to lower the fasting blood glucose value. The overlap of R and N between midnight and 2 AM may require adjusting the evening snack. This should not be the case in individuals using RA because of its shorter action curve. In addition, residual bedtime

N may be present when the morning R or RA is administered. Measurement of blood glucose post-breakfast thus becomes important when starting Stage 3.

Insulin Stage 3

Most newly diagnosed patients do not start with three injections because historically this is used in patients who were started on Insulin Stage 2 and ultimately required bedtime intermediate-acting insulin. There is no reason that the three-injection regimen could not be used at diagnosis (this is often the case in gestational diabetes). If Insulin Stage 3 is used at diagnosis, make certain that a thorough history, physical, and laboratory evaluation are completed and that the target blood glucose levels are reviewed.

> Note: For all insulin therapies the starting dose formula has been carefully selected to meet the immediate needs of the individual while reducing the risk of hypoglycemia as well as hyperglycemia.

Insulin Stage 3/Start: at diagnosis
R/N–0–R–N or RA/N–0–RA–N

Morning insulin start. If the patient starts this therapy in the morning, the total daily dose is calculated as 0.3 U/kg (see Figure 5.21). The total daily dose is divided into three periods associated with breakfast, the evening meal (approximately 10 hours apart), and bedtime (at least 3 hours after dinner). The pre-breakfast dose is two-thirds of the total daily requirement. This is further divided into one-third R or RA and two-thirds N. The R or RA insulin is to cover breakfast and the intermediate-acting insulin N is to cover lunch and the afternoon period. The evening dose is calculated as one-third of the total daily requirement and evenly split between R or RA at dinner and intermediate-acting insulin N at bedtime. By placing N insulin at bedtime, its principal action is moved closer to the morning.

Afternoon or evening insulin start. If the therapy is being started in the afternoon or evening, the starting dose is one-third the normal starting dose (0.1 U/kg) equally split between N and R or RA. The short-acting insulin is given before dinner and the intermediate-acting insulin before bedtime. The next day the patient would be on the total daily dose as described above for starting Insulin Stage 3 in the morning. The patient or family caregiver should be taught both insulin administration technique and how to monitor blood glucose. Blood glucose should be monitored (SMBG) every 4 hours. If blood glucose levels are $>$ 250 mg/dL (13.9 mmol/L), consider additional small doses (1–2 units) of R or RA with SMBG an hour after the insulin. This therapy is temporary. Have the patient return the next morning to initiate daily insulin administration (see previous section).

During the first several days it is imperative to maintain glucose levels at a point that will avoid both hypoglycemia and hyperglycemia. Have the patient SMBG at least five times per day (before meals, at bedtime, and at 3AM). Additionally, co-management with the various health professionals who will be involved in diabetes care must be established. If feasible a nurse educator and dietitian should be incorporated into care as soon as possible. The guidelines for insulin adjustments begin immediately. Along with making arrangements for both nurse and dietitian follow-up, establish target blood glucose levels.

Insulin Stage 3/Adjust
R/N–0–R–N or RA/N–0–RA–N

The patient should realize that it will be necessary to frequently adjust the morning short-acting insulin. The first sign of too much morning R or RA will be post-breakfast or midday hypoglycemia. Reduction in morning R or RA (see Table 5.5) will resolve this problem. An additional adjustment in breakfast carbohydrate intake or mid-morning snack may be needed. If the pre-evening meal glucose goes up, use the same formula as

Table 5.5 Type 2 insulin stage 3/adjust for children and adolescents (See Figure 5.20 type 2 diabetes insulin adjustment considerations for children and adolescents)

Insulin Stage 3 Pattern Adjustments RA/N–0–RA–N or R/A–0–R–N			
	< 70 mg/dL (< 3.9 mmol/L)	**140–250 mg/dL** (7.8–13.4 mmol/L)	**> 250 mg/dL** (> 13.4 mmol/L)
AM or 3 AM	↓PM N 1–2 U (a,b)	↑PM N 1–2 U (a,k)	↑PM N 2–4 U (a,k)
MIDDAY (MID)	↓AM RA or R 1–2 U (c,e)	↑AM RA or R 1–2 U (f,g,k)	↑AM RA or R 2–4 U (f,g,i,k)
PM	↓AM N 1–2 U (d,e)	↑AM N 1–2 U (f,h,k)	↑AM N 2–4 U (f,h,k)
	< 100 mg/dL (< 5.5 mmol/L)	**160–250 mg/dL** (8.9–13.9 mmol/L)	**> 250 mg/dL** (> 13.9 mmol/L)
BEDTIME (BT)	↓PM RA or R 1–2 U (e)	↑PM RA or R 1–2 U (f,k)	↑PM RA or R 2–4 U (f,k)
Adjust insulin based on BG patterns			
May increase or decrease dose by 1–2 U or 10% of dose			
Follow-up			
Medical:	weekly while adjusting insulin, then office visit within 1–2 months		

before, i.e., raise the morning N. This will increase the amount of insulin available to cover carbohydrate intake at lunch. Alternatively, if the bedtime N lowers the fasting blood glucose, the intermediate-acting insulin requirements during the daytime may need to be reduced. If the predinner blood glucose is < 70 mg/dL (3.9 mmol/L) for three consecutive days, consider lowering the morning N. Keep in mind the impact of exercise on both when there is too much or too little insulin. Exercise in the mid-afternoon should be closely followed by SMBG before and after the exercise period. If possible, avoid adding additional calories in order to prevent weight gain. The third adjustments are related to the bedtime blood glucose levels. These are affected most by food intake at dinner and by the amount of short-acting insulin used. In addition, many people snack from supper to bedtime without having a discrete evening meal. This may influence the type of short-acting insulin selected and/or the dose administered. Blood glucose at bedtime should not exceed 160 mg/dL (8.9 mmol/L). Consider increasing R or RA before dinner or changing the meal content. Hyperglycemia at bedtime will often result in a high fasting blood glucose (see Insulin Stage 2 for general principles).

Insulin Stage 3/Maintain

R/N–0–R–N or RA/N–0–RA–N

When patients reach their metabolic targets using Insulin Stage 3, they enter the maintain treatment phase. In this phase changes in insulin, food plan, and exercise regimens are likely to be less frequent. Despite this reduction in changes to therapy, surveillance with SMBG is necessary. Because of the addition of a third injection and perhaps fear of hypoglycemia overnight, some patients may add too many calories as part of the evening snack. A schedule of consistent weight monitoring should be encouraged. While neither SMBG nor weight monitoring need be as regimented as during start and adjust phases, both are required to detect trends of either increasing blood glucose or weight. At minimum, SMBG should occur prior to each insulin injection with at least one post-prandial (at varying meals each day). Because this would mean no fewer than four tests a day, for patients who have maintained their metabolic goal for at least 1 month, consider alternate day testing or reducing the number of tests to two a day at different times each day. Some changes in insulin dose and timing should be expected. Food plan should consider further alterations in timing and size; carbohydrate and/or caloric intake should not increase by an appreciable amount. The patient should be reminded of the general rules, such as relying on 3 day patterns before changing insulin dose.

Moving from Insulin Stage 3 to Physiologic Insulin Stage 4

R–R–R–N or G or RA–RA–RA–N or G

The Stage 4 regimen makes insulin adjustments very easy. Each blood glucose determination has a direct relationship to the previous insulin dose. For example, if the bedtime blood glucose level is high, increase the PM R or RA insulin. Similarly, if the fasting blood glucose is high, increase the bedtime N or G.

Before initiating this regimen from Stage 3, make certain the total daily insulin dose has not reached > 1.5 U/kg, which is indicative of overinsulinization. If overinsulization has occurred the total daily dose can be reduced to 1 U/kg (leaving room for subsequent adjustments). Begin by re-calculating the total daily dose at 1 U/kg. Bedtime N should be recalculated so that it is 30 per cent of the total daily dose. The remaining 70 per cent of the insulin should be given in the form of R or RA before each meal. Thus, for the 100 lb (45 kg) child whose current Stage 3 Insulin was comprised of 55 U reduce this to 45 U and give 15 U as bedtime N and 10 U as R or RA before each meal. If the plan is to change to G insulin then reduce the total daily dose by 20 per cent (45 − 9), resulting in 36 U for this 100 lb child. Next divide the total dose into 50 per cent (18 U) of G at bedtime and 6 U of R or RA before each meal. This per cent is a reverse of the earlier regimens. In this case R or RA is used to cover all meal related increases in blood glucose, while bedtime N or G is used to provide a basal insulin.

Physiologic Insulin Stage 4: mimicking normal secretion insulin

Multiple injection regimens are far more adjustable and will most likely result in a more flexible schedule for the patient. Dividing the insulin into smaller doses reduces the chance of local discomfort and provides a more consistent time action profile. Additionally, regimens with more injections generally require less insulin overall.

If Insulin Stage 3 failed to move the patient into the maintain phase of therapy after 6 months of experimentation, or if the patient *at diagnosis* is willing to try a more intensive regimen then a four-injection regimen should be considered. The patient and family should already have been introduced to the Type 2 Diabetes Master DecisionPath for Children and Adolescents, and alternate therapies, requiring an increased number of injections, should have been discussed. Stage 4 is the most physiologic regimen and offers the patient more flexibility regarding timing of meals. Staged Diabetes Management encourages providers to discuss the advantages of Stage 4 with their patients and family caregivers, especially those starting insulin at diagnosis or after metformin has failed.

Physiologic Insulin Stage 4/Start: at diagnosis R–R–R–N or G or RA–RA–RA–N or G

If starting Stage 4 at diagnosis, ask the patient to do SMBG four times/day (before each meal and at bedtime (plus overnight one to two times during the first week). Two approaches can be used to initiate this therapy: formula or experiential (see Figure 5.22). For the formula method calculate the total daily dose at 0.3 U/kg. If using N insulin, calculate the amount as 30 per cent of the total daily dose (of all insulins). Divide the remaining 70 per cent equally and administer as either R or RA before each meal. Thus, for a 100 lb (45 kg) child, 14 total units of insulin would be given. Five units (rounded from 4.5) of N would be given at bedtime and 3 units of R or RA would be given before each meal. If using G insulin, 50 per cent

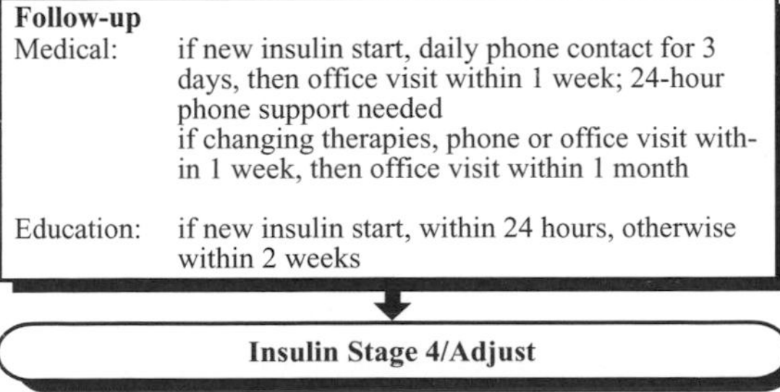

Figure 5.22 Type 2 Physiologic Insulin Stage 4/Start for Children and Adolescents

of the total dose (7 units) would be given at bedtime as G and 2 units (rounded) of R or RA would be given before each meal, resulting in a total of 13 units. Adjustments to this regimen may be made after 3 days of a consistent pattern.

If the plan is to follow an experiential approach, start with N or G at bedtime calculated at 0.1 U/kg (0–0–0–G or N). During the next 7–10 days make 1–2 unit adjustments in the dose until 0.3 U/kg has been reached or fasting plasma glucose (without any hypoglycemia is reduced by at least 60 mg/dL (3.2 mmol/L)). Next, review all blood glucose values to identify the pattern of blood glucose that consistently is highest over more than 3 days (e.g. midday, PM, or bedtime). Add an injection of RA or R insulin (0.1 U/kg) to the preceding meal. Thus if the pre-evening-meal BG is consistently the highest add RA or R insulin prior to the mid-day meal. The new regimen would be 0–RA–0–G. Adjust this insulin every 3 days by 1–2 units until 0.2 U/kg or the pre-evening-meal BG has reduced by least 60 mg/dL (3.2 mmol/L). Repeat this for the next highest blood glucose pattern. Eventually, the patient will be on a regimen of RA–RA–RA–G at the minimum amount of insulin necessary to physiologically mimic insulin requirements.

This gradual introduction of pre-meal insulin based on SMBG data reinforces the experiential aspects of diabetes self-management. The child or adolescent quickly learns how small increments of insulin given at the appropriate time affect BG level. By relying on low-dose basal insulin initially to improve fasting plasma glucose, an added benefit is that the patient begins the day with improved glucose levels. Meal related BG excursions become less dramatic. By identifying the most serious pattern of hyperglycemia first, the insulin can be targeted and thereby used more sparingly. The result is generally a total insulin dose of < 1 U/kg.

Physiologic Insulin Stage 4/Adjust
R–R–R–N or G or RA–RA–RA–N or G

Because this regimen allows for targeting the insulin action to particular postprandial blood glucose excursions, make certain that SMBG occurs before each insulin administration. The blood glucose value determined at that point will help decide how well the insulin given before the last meal worked and will help calculate the insulin to be given at the current meal. Start by identifying the highest blood glucose. Increase by 1–4 units the insulin prior to the high blood glucose (see Table 5.6). Continue until this blood glucose is lowered to within target. Now find the next highest blood glucose. Repeat until all blood glucoses are within target. For example, if the highest blood glucose is fasting, then increase N or G by 1–4 units. Once the fasting has been resolved, turn to the next blood glucose that is persistently highest. Assume it is the pre-evening-meal blood glucose. Increase the midday R or RA by 1–4 units.

Table 5.6 Type 2 Physiologic Insulin Stage 4/Adjust for Children and Adolescents (See Figure 5.20 type 2 diabetes insulin adjustment considerations for children and adolescents)

Insulin Stage 4 Pattern Adjustments
RA–RA–RA–N or G or R–R–R–N or G

	< 80 mg/dL (< 4.4 mmol/L)	140–250 mg/dL (7.8–13.4 mmol/L)	> 250 mg/dL (> 13.4 mmol/L)
AM or 3 AM	↓ PM N 1–2 U (a,b)	↑ PM N 1–2 U (a,k)	↑ PM N 2–4 U (a,k)
MIDDAY (MID)	↓ AM RA or R 1–2 U (c,e)	↑ AM RA or R 1–2 U (f,g,k)	↑ AM RA or R 2–4 U (f,g,k)
PM	↓ AM N 1–2 U (d,e)	↑ AM N 1–2 U (f,h,k)	↑ AM N 2–4 U (f,h,k)
	< 100 mg/dL (< 5.5 mmol/L)	**160–250 mg/dL** (8.9–13.9 mmol/L)	**> 250 mg/dL** (> 13.9 mmol/L)
BEDTIME (BT)	↓ PM RA or R 1–2 U (e)	↑ PM RA or R 1–2 U (f,k)	↑ PM RA or R 2–4 U (f,k)

Adjust insulin based on BG patterns

May increase or decrease dose by 1–2 U or 10% of dose

Follow-up
Medical: weekly while adjusting insulin, then office visit within 1–2 months

Physiologic Insulin Stage 4/Maintain
R–R–R–N or G or RA–RA–RA–N or G

Upon reaching their glycemic targets, patients enter the maintain treatment goal phase. Normally, fewer alterations to insulin, food plan, and exercise regimens will be required. However, surveillance with SMBG is necessary. To prevent both hyperglycemia and weight gain, encourage a schedule of blood glucose and weight monitoring. At a minimum, SMBG should be done prior to each insulin injection with at least one post-prandial (at varying meals each day). Because this would mean no fewer than four tests a day, for patients who have maintained their metabolic goal for at least 1 month, consider alternate-day testing or reducing the number of tests to two a day at different times each day. Some changes in insulin dose and timing should be expected. Monitor weight at least weekly. Food plan should consider further alterations in timing and portion size, keeping in mind that the total caloric intake should not increase appreciably. The patient should be reminded of the general rules for changing insulin doses – a minimum of 3 days of the same pattern. Patients and caregivers should be reminded to contact their healthcare provider if blood glucose levels begin to rise. HbA_{1c} should continue to be determined every 3–4 months.

Metabolic syndrome in children and adolescents

In this section the macrovascular and microvascular diseases that comprise the metabolic syndrome (insulin resistance syndrome) in children and adolescents are highlighted. A more complete review of all associated complications of diabetes is provided in Chapters 8 and 9.

The exact number of children and adolescents with the metabolic syndrome is unknown. Currently, there are seven separate disorders that may be included in the syndrome:

1. overweight–obesity
2. acanthosis nigricans
3. polycystic ovary syndrome
4. hyperglycemia–pre-diabetes or type 2 diabetes
5. dyslipidemia
6. hypertension
7. nephropathy

It is unclear as to how many children and adolescents have one or more of these disorders. Since a child with any one of these disorders is then at increased risk for the others, it is incumbent upon health care providers to maintain close surveillance of any child or adolescent who has evidence of metabolic syndrome. SDM provides an assessment guide and a Master DecisionPath for insulin resistance, which reviews the steps and tests that should be part of the comprehensive, ongoing surveillance. Surveillance begins with evaluation of BMI. All children whose BMI $>$ 85th percentile for age and gender should be evaluated annually for the other elements of the metabolic syndrome. Similarly, all individuals with acanthosis nigricans should be evaluated for co-morbidities associated with insulin resistance. In both instances, they should be immediately screened for hyperglycemia, hypertension, renal disease, and dyslipidemia. For females, discovery of PCOS should be followed by these tests; alternatively, if other insulin resistance disorders are discovered first, female adolescents should be evaluated for PCOS.

Assessment for metabolic syndrome

Figure 5.23 contains a comprehensive assessment for the metabolic syndrome in children and adolescents. Briefly, assessment for the following conditions is required.

Overweight/obesity

Determination of the weight status of children and adolescents requires use of specially designed growth and BMI charts (Figure 5.3 and 5.4). See

Complication	Patient Complaints	Clinical Evidence	Action
Overweight	Irritability, fatigue, sleep apnea, depression	BMI > 85th percentile for age and gender > 120% ideal body weight Pulmonary hypertension Central adiposity	*Refer to BMI Tables*, A–7, A–11 See *Medical Nutrition Therapy and Activity Therapy Guidelines*
Acanthosis nigricans	Often none or cosmetic	Dark, thickened skin due to hyperkeratosis of the skin folds; most common in young individuals of color, clinical sign of insulin resistance	Consider obtaining fasting insulin level to ascertain if hyperinsulinemic
Polycystic ovary syndrome (PCOS)	Oligomenorrhea, hirsutism, acne, infertility, rapid weight gain, acanthosis nigricans	Increased total testosterone, hirsutism, acanthosis nigricans, obesity, hyperinsulinemia, dyslipidemia, oligomenorrhea, amenorrhea, acne	See *PCOS Practice Guideline and Master Decision Path*
Hyperglycemia	Often none Secondary enuresis	**Pre-diabetes: FPG** 100–125 mg/dL (5.6–6.4 mmol/L) **CPG or OGTT 2 hour value** 140–199 mg/dL (7.7–11.0 mmol/L) **Diabetes: FPG** ⩾ 126 mg/dL (7.0 mmol/L) and/or **CPG** ⩾ 200 mg/dL (11.1 mmol/L) on two occasions	See *Screening and Differential Diagnosis*

Figure 5.23 Assessment for insulin resistance syndrome in children and adolescents

the beginning of this chapter for a full discussion of weight management.

Acanthosis Nigricans

Insulin resistance in peripheral tissue induces a chronic state of hyperinsulinemia. The high levels of insulin cause cells found in the skin called keratinocytes to proliferate and produce excessive amounts of keratin. This hyperkeratosis results in a symmetrical, velvet-like, dark hyperpigmentation of the skin folds on the neck and under the arms, in the arm folds and behind knees. The condition is more often diagnosed in people of color.

Polycystic ovary syndrome (PCOS)

PCOS is a chronic condition that is usually marked by anovulation, infertility, and hyperandrogenism. Patients present with irregular menstrual cycles, oligomenorrhea, or amenorrhea and will report excessive vaginal bleeding. They are often obese and have hirsutism. Another early indicator of PCOS is facial acne that does not respond readily to treatment. In adolescents of color there is a high correlation between PCOS and acanthosis nigricans due to hyperandrogenism.

Hyperglycemia

Children and adolescents with insulin resistance may not have elevated blood glucose. Although they produce as much as twice the normal amounts of insulin, initially this is sufficient to overcome hyperglycemia related insulin resistance. However, eventually such individuals will become hyperglycemic if they remain obese and insulin resistant. There is no way, however, to predict when this occurs, therefore surveillance is necessary.

Dyslipidemia

Insulin resistance is often marked by decreased HDL cholesterol and elevated triglycerides. This dyslipidemia has been associated with fatty streaks and fibrous plaques found in the coronary arteries, contributing to increased risk for cardiovascular disease.

Hypertension

The exact cause of hypertension in children with insulin resistance is unknown. It may be related to underlying kidney disease, obesity, hyperinsulinemia, hyperglycemia, or other, as yet undiscovered factors. What is known is that detection is important. Determination of hypertension in children and adolescents is a function of age, gender, and height. Generally there are no symptoms at presentation.

Renal disease

Concern about hypertension in obese children is in part a reflection of the results of some studies that indicate a close association between renal disease and insulin resistance. Since it is uncertain as to whether kidney disease and hypertension occur independently it is important to screen for both entities.

Children and adolescents Master DecisionPath for insulin resistance

Any child discovered to have any of the conditions that are correlated with insulin resistance or any of the risk factors should undergo an annual assessment for the other correlates. This can be carried out efficiently and systematically by following the SDM Master DecisionPath for Metabolic Syndrome (Figure 5.24). In most cases obesity will be the first of the correlates to be noticed. As mentioned in an earlier section clinical obesity is defined as exceeding the 95th percentile BMI based on age and gender. It is recommended, however, that any child above the 85th percentile BMI be evaluated on an annual basis for the other correlates of insulin resistance. The next step is to screen for type 2 diabetes. This is done by either capillary blood glucose or plasma glucose in a laboratory. The screening test can only serve to determine who needs further evaluation. To be diagnosed with diabetes, two tests on different days are required. Afterwards the child will fall into one of three categories: overt diabetes, impaired glucose homeostasis (prediabetes) or normal glycemia. The definitions are not age dependent and are the same for adults. Next is measurement for hypertension. This requires three blood pressure measurements on separate days and meeting the age, gender, and height criteria. Although in most cases hypertension (HTN) would signal the need to evaluate for renal disease, in children suspected of insulin

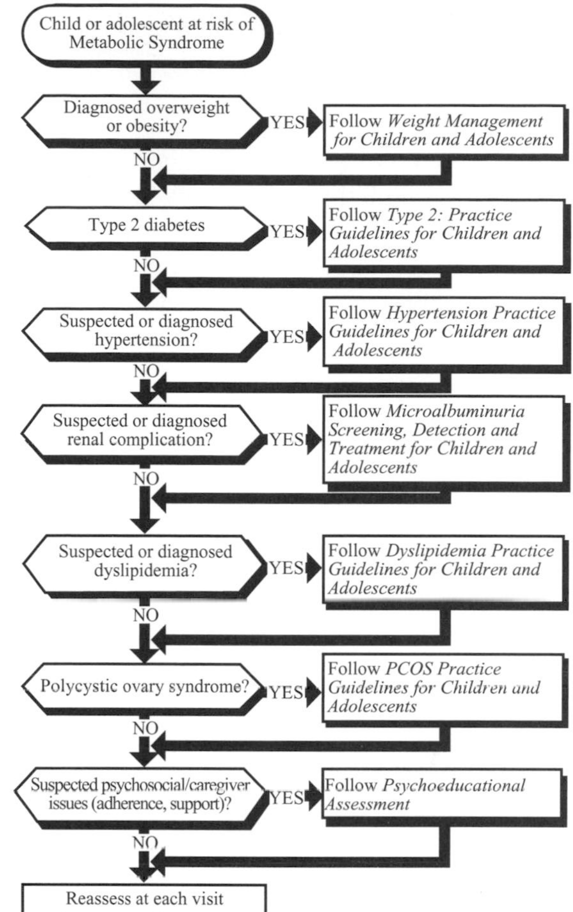

Figure 5.24 Children and Adolescents Master DecisionPath for Insulin Resistance Syndrome

resistance screening for microalbuminuria should be carried out without regard to blood pressure. Renal disease can be assessed initially with a semiquantitative test strip or by quantitative measure in the laboratory. If positive, more detailed examination is in order. Finally, in adolescent females with any suspicion of insulin resistance determine whether they have a history of oligomenorrhea, amenorrhea, or signs of hyperandrogynism.

SDM provides specific Practice Guidelines and DecisionPaths for each of the disorders on the Master DecisionPath. In the following section the key elements of each path as they refer specifically to children and adolescents are discussed. Greater detail is provided in the chapters devoted to metabolic syndrome.

Hypertension

Hypertension Practice Guidelines

As with most co-morbidities associated with insulin resistance, both the detection and the treatment of HTN are modified for children and adolescents. Hypertension Practice Guidelines for children and adolescents are shown in Figure 5.25.

Screening and risk factors. All children ⩾ 2 years of age should be evaluated for hypertension (HTN) at least annually. If the blood pressure (BP) meets the criteria for HTN (adjusted for age, gender, and height), then a full diagnostic series of BPs should be undertaken. Children with risk factors such as obesity, type 2 diabetes, renal disease, or dyslipidemia should be screened at each visit. Generally, HTN in children is without

Screening

Annual blood pressure measurement children ⩾ 2 years of age

Diagnosis

Average systolic and diastolic ⩾ 95th percentile for age and gender (see *BP Tables*) on 3 or more occasions; **use height percentiles rather than chronologic age**.

Rule out renal parenchymal disease, coarctation of the aorta or renal artery stenosis, use of street drugs or ETOH, anabolic steroids, diet drugs, tobacco use/cigarette smoking, oral contraceptive pills (OCP), use of chronic cold remedies and excess caffeine or sport drink intake.

Consider secondary causes such as: with decreased potassium, consider hyperaldosteronism; check TSH to rule out hyper- or hypothyroidism; if positive clinical features consider screening for Cushing's with 24 hour UFC; consider pheochromocytoma

Symptoms

Often none; blurred vision, fatigue, palpatations, sleeping difficulties, dysuria, polyuria, chest pain, abdominal pain, headache, malaise, weight loss, epistaxis, facial palsy

Risk Factors

- Overweight BMI > 85th percentile for age and gender (see *BMI Tables*).
- Waist-to-hip ratio > 1.0
- Positive family history of hypertension, PVD, CVD, stroke, MI, endocrine disease or renal insufficiency or failure
- Microalbuminuria
- Smoking
- History of urinary tract infection
- Hyperinsulinemia
- Child abuse
- Diabetes, IGT, or IFG

Treatment Options

Medical nutrition and activity therapy alone or in combination with pharmacologic agents (ACE inhibitor, angiotensin II receptor blocker, calcium channel blocker, low-dose diuretic, β-blocker); caregiver participation; cardiovascular conditioning, weight loss when appropriate; stress reduction

Targets

Hypertension BP < 90th percentile for gender, age and height percentile (*BP Tables*)

Microalbuminaria ⩾ 2 yrs of age, adult standards apply (< 30 mg albumin/g)

Monitoring

Self-monitor blood pressure 4 times per day (twice prior to prescribed medication) while in adjust phase with oscillometric home blood pressure monitor; one time per day during maintain phase; blood presssure at every office visit

Follow-up

Weekly–Monthly With diastolic blood pressure 5 to 9 mmHg above the 95th percentile Q 4–6 weeks; with diastolic blood pressure ⩾ 10 mmHg above the 95th percentile, in one week

Every 3 Months With marginal elevation, every 3–6 months

Yearly (in addition to 3–4 month visit) History and physical; self-monitored blood pressure profile, screen for albuminuria; fundoscopic eye exam; dental examination; medical nutrition and cardiovascular conditioning continuing education; fasting lipid profile, glucose screen, smoking cessation as needed; consider 24 hour ambulatory blood pressure monitoring

Figure 5.25 Hypertension Practice Guidelines for Children and Adolescents

symptoms, thus risk factor assessment is important.

Diagnosis. The correct BP measurement technique is essential. The patient should be allowed to rest at least five minutes in the office and should be seated at the time of the measurement. The cuff size should be appropriate and carefully placed. Measurement should be made at least twice with 2–5 minutes between determinations. If there is any suspicion that the in-office BP may be compromised by patient anxiety provide the patient with a means of monitoring BP at home (SMBP). The accurate assessment of BP is clearly a necessity if appropriate interventions are to be instituted.

Children and adolescents can be placed in one of four BP categories: normal, high risk, HTN, and severe HTN. With the exception of severe HTN, the criteria for HTN under the age of 18 are based on age and gender adjusted for height (Figures 5.26 and 5.27). Normal BP is both systolic and diastolic BP below the 90th percentile. High risk are either systolic or diastolic by between the 90th and 95th percentiles; HTN is the

Girls

		Systolic BP (mmHg) by percentile of height							Diastolic BP (mmHg) by percentile of height						
Age (yr)	%	5%	10%	25%	50%	75%	90%	95%	5%	10%	25%	50%	75%	90%	95%
1	90th	98	98	99	101	102	103	104	52	52	53	53	54	55	55
	95th	101	102	103	104	106	107	108	56	56	57	58	58	59	60
2	90th	99	99	101	102	103	104	105	57	57	58	58	59	60	60
	95th	103	103	104	106	107	108	109	61	61	62	62	63	64	64
3	90th	100	101	102	103	104	105	106	61	61	61	62	63	64	64
	95th	104	104	106	107	108	109	110	65	65	66	66	67	68	68
4	90th	101	102	103	104	106	107	108	64	64	65	65	66	67	67
	95th	105	106	107	108	109	111	111	68	68	69	69	70	71	71
5	90th	103	103	105	106	107	108	109	66	67	67	68	69	69	70
	95th	107	107	108	110	111	112	113	71	71	71	72	73	74	74
6	90th	104	105	106	107	109	110	111	69	69	69	70	71	72	72
	95th	108	109	110	111	113	114	114	73	73	74	74	75	76	76
7	90th	106	107	108	109	110	112	112	71	71	71	72	73	74	74
	95th	110	111	112	113	114	115	116	75	75	75	76	77	78	78
8	90th	108	109	110	111	112	114	114	72	72	73	74	74	75	76
	95th	112	113	114	115	116	117	118	76	77	77	78	79	79	80
9	90th	110	111	112	113	114	116	116	74	74	74	75	76	77	77
	95th	114	115	116	117	118	119	120	78	78	79	79	80	81	81
10	90th	112	113	114	115	116	118	118	75	75	76	77	77	78	78
	95th	116	117	118	119	120	122	122	79	79	80	81	81	82	83
11	90th	114	115	116	117	119	120	120	76	77	77	78	79	79	80
	95th	118	119	120	121	122	124	124	81	81	81	82	83	83	84
12	90th	116	117	118	119	121	122	123	78	78	78	79	80	81	81
	95th	120	121	122	123	125	126	126	82	82	82	83	84	85	85
13	90th	118	119	120	121	123	124	124	79	79	79	80	81	82	82
	95th	122	123	124	125	126	128	128	83	83	84	84	85	86	86
14	90th	120	121	122	123	124	125	126	80	80	80	81	82	83	83
	95th	124	125	126	127	128	129	130	84	84	85	85	86	87	87
15	90th	121	122	123	124	126	127	128	80	81	81	82	83	83	84
	95th	125	126	127	128	130	131	131	85	85	85	86	87	88	88
16	90th	122	123	124	125	127	128	129	81	81	82	82	83	84	84
	95th	126	127	128	129	120	132	132	85	85	86	87	87	88	88
17	90th	123	123	124	126	127	128	129	81	81	82	83	83	84	85
	95th	127	127	128	130	121	132	133	85	86	86	87	88	88	89

Rosner et. al., *Pediatrics* 1996; **98**: 653–654

Figure 5.26 Female blood pressure level percentile by age and percentile of height

Boys

Age (yr)	%	Systolic BP (mmHg) by percentile of height							Diastolic BP (mmHg) by percentile of height						
		5%	10%	25%	50%	75%	90%	95%	5%	10%	25%	50%	75%	90%	95%
1	90th	94	95	97	99	101	102	103	49	49	50	51	52	53	54
	95th	98	99	101	103	105	106	107	54	54	55	56	57	58	58
2	90th	98	99	101	103	104	106	107	54	54	55	56	57	58	58
	95th	102	103	105	107	108	110	110	58	59	60	61	62	63	63
3	90th	101	102	103	105	107	109	109	59	59	60	61	62	63	63
	95th	105	106	107	109	111	112	113	63	63	64	65	66	67	68
4	90th	103	104	105	107	109	110	111	63	63	64	65	66	67	67
	95th	107	108	109	111	113	114	115	67	68	68	69	70	71	72
5	90th	104	105	107	109	111	112	113	66	67	68	69	69	70	71
	95th	108	109	111	113	114	116	117	71	71	72	73	74	75	76
6	90th	105	106	108	110	112	113	114	70	70	71	72	73	74	74
	95th	109	110	112	114	116	117	118	74	75	75	76	77	78	79
7	90th	106	107	109	111	113	114	115	72	73	73	74	75	76	77
	95th	110	111	113	115	117	118	119	77	77	78	79	80	81	81
8	90th	108	109	110	112	114	116	116	74	75	75	76	77	78	79
	95th	112	113	114	116	118	119	120	79	79	80	81	82	83	83
9	90th	109	110	112	114	116	117	118	76	76	77	78	79	80	80
	95th	113	114	116	118	119	121	122	80	81	81	82	83	84	85
10	90th	111	112	113	115	117	119	119	77	77	78	79	80	81	81
	95th	115	116	117	119	121	123	123	81	82	83	83	84	85	86
11	90th	113	114	115	117	119	121	121	77	78	79	80	81	81	82
	95th	117	118	119	121	123	125	125	82	82	83	84	85	86	87
12	90th	115	116	118	120	121	123	124	78	78	79	80	81	82	83
	95th	119	120	122	124	125	127	128	83	83	84	85	86	87	87
13	90th	118	119	120	122	124	125	126	78	79	80	81	81	82	83
	95th	121	122	124	126	128	129	130	83	83	84	85	86	87	88
14	90th	120	121	123	125	127	128	129	79	79	80	81	82	83	83
	95th	124	125	127	129	131	132	133	83	84	85	86	87	87	88
15	90th	123	124	126	128	130	131	132	80	80	81	82	83	84	84
	95th	127	128	130	132	133	135	136	84	85	86	86	87	88	89
16	90th	126	127	129	131	132	134	134	81	82	82	83	84	85	86
	95th	130	131	133	134	136	138	138	86	86	87	88	89	90	90
17	90th	128	129	131	133	135	136	137	83	84	85	86	87	87	88
	95th	132	133	135	137	139	140	141	88	88	89	90	91	92	93

Rosner et. al., *Pediatrics* 1996; **98**: 653–654

Figure 5.27 Male blood pressure level percentile by age and percentile of height

average systolic and diastolic BPs taken on three separate occasions ⩾ 95th percentile. Severe HTN (requiring referral to a cardiologist) is dependent solely on age range. For example, an 8 year old boy whose height places him in the 50th percentile would have normal BP if the BP < 111/74 mmHg; he would be at high risk if the systolic BP were ⩾ 111 to 115 mmHg or the diastolic BP were ⩾ 74 to 78 mmHg; if he exceeded an average BP of 116/81 mmHg but not > 129/85 mmHg, he would be HTN. If he exceeds 129/85 mmHg on any occasion he would be considered to have severe HTN. Since there may be underlying (or contemporaneous) causes other than insulin resistance a thorough evaluation is needed (generally by a cardiologist).

Treatment options. Treatment for HTN in children is similar to that in adults. The use of medical nutrition therapy (MNT) to manage HTN is the cornerstone of treatment. Weight management, reduction in sodium intake, and increased physical activity are crucial elements. Replacing, reducing and restricting foods and drinks high in sodium, carbohydrate, and/or fats is a fundamental strategy. MNT is the same as would be used in diabetes and dyslipidemia. Generally MNT as a solo therapy is reserved for children in the at risk category. For children meeting the criteria for HTN, pharmacological therapy *plus MNT* is recommended (Figure 5.28). ACE inhibitors are the preferred therapy as they provide a renal protective benefit. However, angiotensin II receptor blockers, calcium channel blockers, low-dose diuretics, and β-blockers are acceptable. Physical activity should be part of therapy after completing a fitness evaluation.

Targets. Intensive management to pre-set and agreed upon targets (treat-to-target) is a hallmark of the SDM approach. For children with insulin resistance it is vital that BP be returned to below the 90th percentile (or less than 130/80 mmHg in children over 11 years of age). This has been shown to reduce the risk of renal disease or slow its progression in cases where it already exists.[14] Because of the close association between these disorders screening for microalbuminuria and, if negative, yearly surveillance is recommended.

Monitoring. Although in-office measurement of BP has been considered the basis for most decisions related to diagnosis and treatment, recent evidence suggests that a far more accurate and reliable method is home or self-monitoring BP (SMBP). Because this method provides vital information related to hourly and daily excursions in BP and more closely resembles BP under normal conditions, it is recommended as part of SDM monitoring for children in the high-risk, HTN, and severe HTN categories. The use of oscillometric monitors should begin with an in-office demonstration and evaluation of technique against in-office BP determinations by sphygmomanometer or office-based oscillometric device. Once it is clear that the patient or caregiver can operate the device, a testing schedule of 4/day at varying times should be initiated. As many of the devices have an onboard memory, the patient need not keep records. The data can be offloaded in the office. If this is not available then patients can use a logbook to record their values. Generally, the accumulated data are averaged and the same BP criteria as mentioned above are used. For a complete discussion of how to interpret BP data from self-monitoring devices see Chapter 9 on HTN.

Follow-up. During the initial treatment phase, patients should have 24-hour telephone access and should be seen at least monthly. In the more severe cases, weekly contact and review of self-monitored BPs will assure timely interventions should the current therapy be inadequate. Quarterly visits and annual reassessment for co-morbidities of insulin resistance are recommended. Special attention to weight, blood glucose, HDL cholesterol, triglycerides, and proteinuria is essential.

Hypertension Drug Therapy/Start Treatment

Most antihypertensive drugs have had limited testing in children and adolescents, thus careful surveillance for contraindications is necessary. Following the history and physical examination make the selection of pharmacological agent based on whether the child has diabetes and/or underlying renal disease. If the child was not evaluated for all disorders associated with insulin resistance, first complete the steps in the Master DecisionPath for Insulin Resistance. Before selecting the therapy also make certain that the patient and family understand the significance of the clinical findings, the goal of treatment and the importance of the antihypertensive drug and SMBP. It is imperative that all of those involved in the child's care agree on the target BP, how it is to be measured and how long it will take to reach. As best as possible, determine the role of each family member and the patient related to administering the antihypertensive agent and measuring BP. Finally, it should be made very clear that some antihypertensive drugs may fail to achieve the agreed upon goal; under such circumstances, the family should be informed that there are many alternative drugs.

For children > 2 years of age and non-pregnant adolescents with diabetes and/or renal disease, the first drug of choice is an ACE inhibitor; for those > 13 years of age either an ACE (non-pregnant only) or ARB may be initiated (Figure 5.28). Both antihypertensive agents have renal protective functions as well as BP lowering ability. For individuals without diabetes or renal disease dihyroperiodones are recommended. For all drugs generally begin at the lowest dose based on body weight.

Independent of the medication, all patients and their caregivers should be taught about HTN, the importance of the medication, the role of medical nutrition therapy, and the contraindications or side effects. Within one week of initiation of and ACE-I repeat both potassium and creatinine measures. Check for any indication of persistent cough, hypotension, rash, or leukopenia. If these occur consider switching to an ARB.

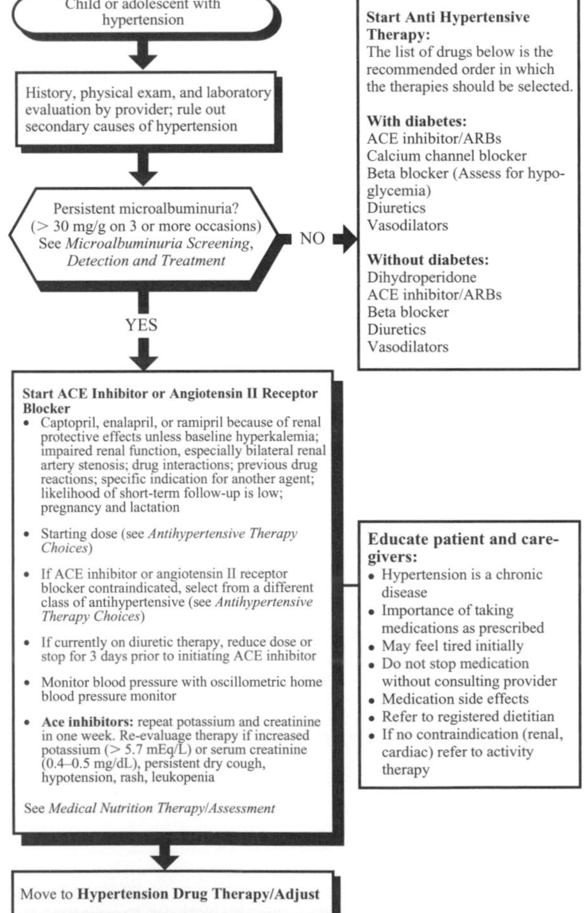

Figure 5.28 Hypertension drug therapy start/treatment for children and adolescents

As soon as feasible, MNT should be initiated following the weight management protocols provided by SDM. The focus of MNT is to optimize the effectiveness of the pharmacological intervention by reducing foods high in salt, lowering the carbohydrate load, and preventing unnecessary weight gain or, in obese children, promoting weight control.

Finally, SMBP should be encouraged. The variability in BP throughout the day and from day to day is a major factor associated with underlying cardiovascular disease. Little is known about the patterns of BP in children and adolescents. However, it has been well established that SMBP is a reliable and accurate indicator of BP control. Some studies have demonstrated that it is more reliable and accurate than in-office measurements, correlating very well with ambulatory 24-hour monitoring. The optimal schedule for SMBP is four tests daily at varying times over a period of one month. This provides adequate data to determine whether the therapy is successful and whether there are any BP patterns that require attention. As with in-office measurements, the goal is to maintain the patient below the 95th percentile for both systolic and diastolic BP.

Hypertension Drug Therapy/Adjust

The principal strategy by which SDM operates is to set a mutual goal with the patient and family within a set timeframe. Initially, the goal is to achieve consistent BPs ≤ 90th percentile (as measured by SMBP) within 4 weeks and sustain this over a period of 6 months (Figure 5.29). If this is accomplished and corroborated by four in-office BP measurements over the 6 months, the patient enters the Maintain Phase of treatment. The antihypertensive drug therapy can now be re-examined and slowly withdrawn. SMBP should be used to confirm that as the medication is reduced BP values remain within target. The justification for regular visits during this period is

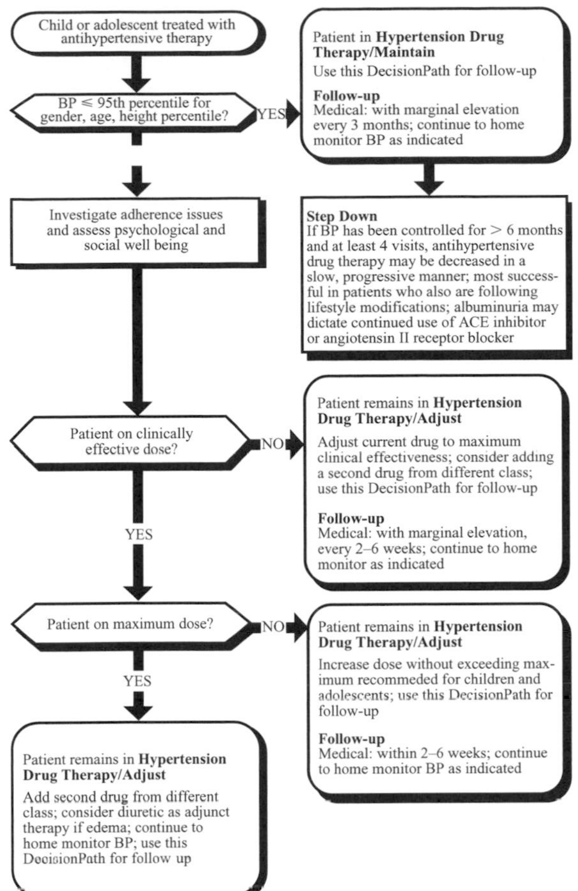

Figure 5.29 Hypertension drug therapy adjust/treatment for children and adolescents

to make certain that microalbumin levels remain within the normal range. If they do not, then ACE-I therapy should continue (see Microalbuminuria Screening, Detection and Treatment for Children and Adolescents).

If BP levels do not achieve the initial target, then consider whether the key factor is adherence to the regimen. In many cases the initial emotional stress from the diagnosis may result in both patient and family dysfunction. This, in turn, may lead to a lack of adherence to taking medications and to monitoring BP. Often the root cause is a lack of understanding about the disease process, the goals of treatment, and the effect of non-adherence (see Adherence DecisionPath). The first step is to assess whether the patient and family still agree with the goals that were mutually established at the first visit. Often, after a period of time to reflect on the changes in lifestyle required by treatment and to understand each family member's responsibilities, the stresses related to the diagnosis reflect themselves in a lack of adherence to the drug and testing regimens. If this occurs consider re-setting the goals. This requires reducing the number of goals. Thus, the initial goal may be limited to taking the ACE-I according to the prescribed schedule without SMBP and MNT. Once this is achieved, then MNT may be initiated. Finally, the SMBP goals may be re-instituted.

If adherence is not the principal issue and if the maximum dose has not been reached, the choice is to continue to increase the current medication until the maximum dose is reached or to maintain the current dose and add a different classification of antihypertensive agent. In most instances, a calcium channel blocker would be the next drug to add. Although β-blockers and diuretics are effective, they present some problems for individuals with or at risk for diabetes that make them less optimal. β-blockers interfere with feedback during hypoglycemic events (only likely in children or adolescents treated with insulin) and diuretics have been associated with increased blood glucose levels. Thus, in this population, β-blockers and diuretics should be considered after other drugs have failed. Each adjustment should be given at least 2 weeks, but no more than 6 weeks, before it is re-evaluated. Most drugs allow for four to six dose adjustments, thus it may take as long as half a year to reach the maximum dose. If a second drug is initiated, this may add another half year. Since the children are growing at the same time be certain to recalculate the dose based on weight changes.

If a number of the drugs have been tried, if MNT has not successfully managed weight, or if the family remains dysfunctional related to treatment, consider referral to a multi-disciplinary care team. The management of HTN as part of the overall metabolic syndrome is very complex and may require the expertise of specialists, nurse educators, dietitians, and psychologists to address each of the underlying issues.

Nephropathy

Nephropathy practice guidelines

Practice guidelines for nephropathy are shown in Figure 5.30.

Screening, risk factors, and diagnosis. Too often the development of renal disease in children and adolescents is related to other conditions that give rise to their discovery. The presence of either diabetes or hypertension is often a signal to screen for microalbuminuria. Nonetheless, often these disorders proceed renal disease. Thus, all children with insulin resistance should be screened annually. There are however, in addition to diabetes and hypertension, less apparent risk factors that increase the chance that renal disease is present. They are principally related to the genetic predis-

Screening	See *Microalbuminuria Screening, Detection and Treatment Guidelines*
Diagnosis	
Incipient Nephropathy	Persistent microalbuminuria (on 2 out of 3 occasions) Random urine collection 30–300 mg albumin/g creatinine
Overt Nephropathy	Macroalbuminuria (proteinuria indicated by a positive dipstick test) Random urine collection >300 mg albumin/g creatinine Note: albumin/creatinine ratio not sensitive when urine protein > 2–3 g/24 hours
Hypertension	Average systolic and diastolic > 95th percentile for age, gender, and height percentile
Glomerular Disease	Evidence includes mesengial cell matrix expansion, increased basement membrane thickness, and loss of glomerular capillary surface area
Risk Factors	• HbA_{1c} > 2 percentage points above upper limit of normal • Sibling with nephropathy • Smoking • Duration of diabetes > 5 years • Family history of hypertension and/or dyslipidemia • American Indian or Alaska Native; African-American; Asian; Native Hawaiian or other Pacific Islander; Hispanic
Treatment Options	If hyperglycemia, intensify metabolic control
Hypertension	Medical nutrition and activity therapy; ACE inhibitors; angiotensin II receptor blockers; calcium channel blockers; low-dose diuretics; β-blockers
Dyslipidemia	Medical nutrition and activity therapy; bile acid sequestrants (for other medication therapies refer to a pediatric specialist)
Targets	Near euglycemia; BP < 95th percentile for age, gender, and height percentile; glomerular filtration rate (GFR) decrease < 0.2 mL/minute/month acceptable
Monitoring	Self-monitoring of blood pressure (SMBP) and SMBG daily while adjusting treatment
Follow-up	
Monthly	Office visit during adjust phase (weekly phone contact may be necessary)
Every 3 Months	Urinalysis with dipstick test for proteinuria; determine HbA_{1c}
Yearly	Serum creatinine and blood urea nitrogen (BUN) annually in patients with albuminuria; if macroalbuminuria present, consider consult with pediatric endocrinologist, diabetologist, of nephrologist

Figure 5.30 Nephropathy Practice Guidelines for Children and Adolescents

position in some minority groups to insulin resistance, notably American Indian, African-American, and Hispanic. Diagnosis is confirmed by repeated albumin/creatinine (A/C) ratio after ruling out possible transient and benign causes. Incipient nephropathy is defined by an A/C ratio of 30–300 mg/g, while overt nephropathy (macroalbuminuria) is >300 mg/g.

Treatments and targets. The treatment of nephropathy in the presence of diabetes and hypertension coordinates medical nutrition therapy and anti-hyperglycemia and anti-hypertensive regimens to assure optimization of each approach and to reduce redundancies. Thus, generally therapy begins with an ACE-I and intensive control of blood glucose most likely using insulin. In the absence of HTN and diabetes, an ACE-I is still used along with some alteration in diet either for obesity or protein.

Monitoring and follow-up. For children with diabetes, close surveillance using SMBG is fundamental to long-term management. When the disease is complicated by HTN close monitoring by SMBP is also necessary. In all situations, annual dipstick urinalysis and serum creatinine should be measured. As with all children and adolescents with insulin resistance an annual evaluation for all co-morbidities should be undertaken.

Microalbuminuria screening, detection and treatment

In children and adolescents with insulin resistance, renal disease may occur prior to the earliest sign of hyperglycemia (see Figure 5.31). Furthermore, BP measurements may not be sufficiently accurate to signal possible underlying kidney involvement. Thus, it is imperative that screening for microalbuminuria (by either semiquantitative or quantitative methods) be undertaken annually in asymptomatic persons. If the screening is positive, an A/C ratio should be performed on a first morning urine specimen. Children are subject to

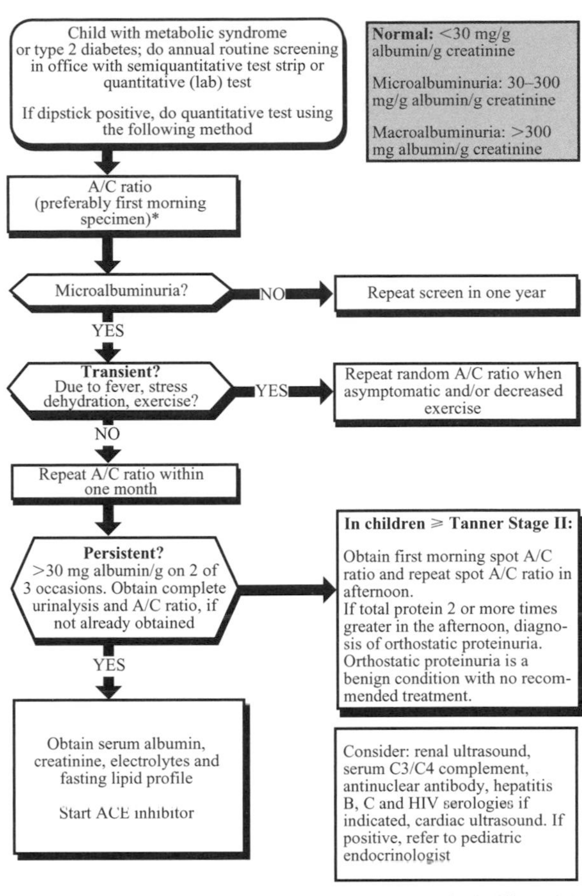

Figure 5.31 Microalbuminuria Screening, Detection and Treatment in Children and Adolescents

the same criteria as adults for albumin/creatinine: normal (<30 mg/g), microalbuminuria (30–300 mg/g), and macroalbuminuria (>300 mg/g). The finding of microalbuminuria requires ruling out such causes as physical activity, stress, dehydration, or fever. Thus, repeat the A/C ratio within one month of resolving these possible causes. Otherwise, repeat the A/C ratio within a month of the original measurement.

In children ≥ Tanner Stage 2 the explanation for a positive A/C ratio may be a benign condition called orthostatic proteinuria, which is determined by comparing the first morning urine sample with an afternoon sample. If the afternoon total protein is more than twice the morning value then the diagnosis is confirmed and no treatment is required. Referral to a pediatric nephrologist should be considered to verify the diagnosis.

If orthostatic proteinuria has been ruled out, obtain serum creatinine, electrolytes, and a fasting lipid profile. An ACE-I should be initiated immediately along with SMBP. Because this condition is serious in children with insulin resistance, it is further recommended that renal ultrasound, serum C3/C4 complement, and cardiac ultrasound be considered. Referral to a pediatric endocrinologist, nephrologist, or cardiologist is also advised.

Ongoing treatment for microalbuminuria depends a great deal as to whether HTN and/or diabetes (or any hyperglycemia) is present. With regards to diabetes, the fundamental treatment is to aim for euglycemia without any significant BG excursions. Mean BG as well as significant variations from the mean are closely associated with progression of renal disease. If type 2 diabetes is present then follow the children and adolescent DecisionPaths. Since intensive treatment of type 2 diabetes ($HbA_{1c} < 7$ per cent) is required, and because metformin is contraindicated when there is renal disease, initiating insulin therapy should be considered. Modifications in MNT for diabetes may also be necessary as diets low in protein have been shown to have renoprotective effects and to slow the progression of overt diabetic nephropathy (macroalbuminuria). Although no conclusive evidence has shown that low-protein diets slow the progression from incipient diabetic nephropathy to overt diabetic nephropathy, it is hypothesized that excess protein in the diet causes glomerular hyperfiltration, renal vasodilatation, and changes in intraglomerular pressure, all of which are associated with proteinuria. Reduction in the proportion of total daily calories comprised of protein to 15 per cent initially, and to 10 per cent if overt diabetic nephropathy is present, is recommended. Where possible, vegetable based protein should be used in place of animal protein.

With respect to BP management, once again intensive management is necessary. The target should be set for between the 30th and 60th percentile BPs based on age, gender and height. SMBP should be used. If significant excursions of more than 10 mmHg appear in systolic or diastolic BP on three consecutive days at the same hour, or at different hours on the same day, consider altering the timing of the agent by splitting the dose or adding a second anti-hypertensive agent from another classification. Consider consultation with a pediatric nephrologist or cardiologist as needed for more complex cases.

Dyslipidemia

Dyslipidemia practice guidelines

Dyslipidemia is a common co-morbidity of insulin resistance and is most often found in those children and adolescents with obesity, diabetes, and HTN. There are, in general, no overt signs of dyslipidemia that would be readily recognized by the patient or caregiver. Additionally, total cholesterol is often normal. Because of this, it is important to maintain a program of careful evaluation by lipid profiles of those individuals at high risk. SDM has established practice guidelines for the detection and treatment of dyslipidemia in children and adolescents (Figure 5.32).

Screening, risk factors, and diagnosis of dyslipidemia. Screening is generally limited to children greater than 2 years of age with at least two risk factors associated with coronary artery disease. Along with the co-morbidities of insulin resistance the principal risk factor is genetic. If the family history is positive for CAD and the child is insulin resistant then he/she should be evaluated. Because the type of dyslipidemia often found in these children is characterized by normal cholesterol, low HDL, and high triglycerides, SDM recommends using the screening as the basis for diagnosis by using a fasting fractionated lipid profile. The diagnostic criteria are based on the American Diabetes Association recommendations for management of dyslipidemia in children and adolescents with diabetes:[15]

- LDL-cholesterol $\geqslant$ 100 mg/dL (2.6 mmol/L)
- HDL-cholesterol $\leqslant$ 35 mg/dL (0.9 mmol/L)
- triglyceride level $\geqslant$ 150 mg/dL (1.7 mmol/L)

Screening Screen for dyslipidemia with a fasting lipid profile for all children starting at age 2 annually who have 2 or more risk factors for CAD

Risk Factors

- Overweight BMI > 85th percentile for age and gender (see *BMI Tables*)
- Waist-to-hip ratio > 1.0
- Hypertension
- Elevated mean LDL concentration
- Increased saturated fats/cholesterol in diet
- Nephrotic syndrome
- Elevated glucose
- Use of anticonvulsant medication
- Smoking
- Positive family history of CAD with symptom onset ⩽ 55 years of age; MI, angina pectoris, PVD, cerebrovascular disease, sudden cardiac death, type 2 diabetes or metabolic syndrome
- Unobtainable family history or parents with unknown cholesterol levels

Diagnosis LDL ⩾ 100 mg/dL (2.6 mmol/L), Triglycerides ⩾ 150 mg/dL (1.7 mmol/L), HDL ⩽ 35 mg/dL (0.9 mmol/L)

Symptoms Often none, corneal arcus, skin xanthomata

Treatment Options

- **Achieve blood glucose control first in patients with diabetes**
- Ages 2–10 years: with BMI > 85th percentile for gender and age
- Age > 10 years; with BMI > 85th percentile for gender and age: weight management and medical nutrition therapy and pharmacologic agents after 6 months–1 year trial of diet alone
- With LDL > 160 mg/dL (4.1 mmol/L) start bile acid sequestrants (if considering statins, refer to pediatric diabetes specialist)

Targets LDL < 100 mg/dL (2.6 mmol/L), Triglycerides < 150 mg/dL (1.7 mmol/L), HDL > 35 mg/dL (0.9 mmol/L)

Monitoring Medical nutrition and activity therapy alone: appropriate growth for age, fasting lipid profile every 3 months
Pharmacologic agents: baseline liver function tests, CPK, family planning/contraception for sexually active females due to unknown use in pregnancy; if pregnancy is planned ⩽ 18 years of age discontinue therapy

Follow-up

Monthly	Phone or office contact until lipid targets met
Every 3 Months	Fasting lipid profile until targets reached, then at provider discretion
Yearly (in addition to 3–4 month visit)	History and physical; screen for albuminuria; dental examination; medical nutrition and activity therapy continuing education, fasting lipid profile; glucose screening; preconception planning for females of childbearing age as indicated

Figure 5.32 Dyslipidemia Practice Guidelines for Children and Adolescents

Since any abnormal value is diagnostic and since LDL or triglyceride levels may be abnormal even when the total cholesterol level is normal a fasting fractionated lipid profile for diagnosis is recommended. The National Cholesterol Education Program has recognized that very low levels of HDL increase the risk of vascular disease. Therefore, low HDL is also a lipid abnormality.

Treatment options and targets. The current therapies are based on severity of the dyslipidemia, presence of diabetes, and/or HTN and are age dependent. In the presence of diabetes or HTN control of BG and BP is essential. Generally treatment for dyslipidemia begins with medical nutrition therapy aimed at weight reduction by alteration of the proportion of fats in the diet. If this fails or if LDL > 160 mg/dL (4.1 mmol/L) then bile acid sequestrants (cholestyramine, colestipol, colesevelam) are recommended. For initiation of other lipid lowering agents such as statins or ezetimibe, it is recommended that the patient be referred to a pediatric specialist. The goal is to reach the 'normal range for children' within one year of initiation of therapy.

Monitoring and follow-up. Fundamentally, close surveillance of adherence to the medical nutrition and pharmacological therapies requires evaluation of BG, BP, and weight in children and adolescents with co-morbidities. At 3 month intervals a lipid profile is recommended. For children without HTN and/or diabetes, annual reassessment is necessary. Since most drugs for dyslipidemia are contraindicated in pregnancy, make certain that sexually active adolescent females are using birth control.

Dyslipidemia/Diagnosis and Start Treatment

The discovery of lipid abnormalities in children and adolescents with insulin resistance, frank type 2 diabetes, or HTN is generally characterized by elevated triglyceride level, low HDL, and normal to moderately elevated LDL-cholesterol. The targets for treatment of children and adolescents with diabetes and/or the metabolic syndrome are

- LDL-cholesterol < 100 mg/dL (2.6 mmol/L)
- HDL-cholesterol > 35 mg/dL (0.9 mmol/L)
- triglyceride level < 150 mg/dL (1.7 mmol/L)

These targets are consistent with the American Diabetes Association. If the diagnosis is not met then repeat in one year and annually thereafter. Children with insulin resistance are always at greater risk of dyslipidemia.

Upon diagnosis of dyslipidemia, medical nutrition therapy should be initiated for normal weight and obese children (Figure 5.33). For normal weight children the purpose is to modify intake of saturated fats to < 10 per cent of the daily fat intake (which should be less than 30 per cent of total calories), increase soluble fiber intake to > 10 g/day and increase intake of Omega-3 fatty acids. This is accomplished by following the

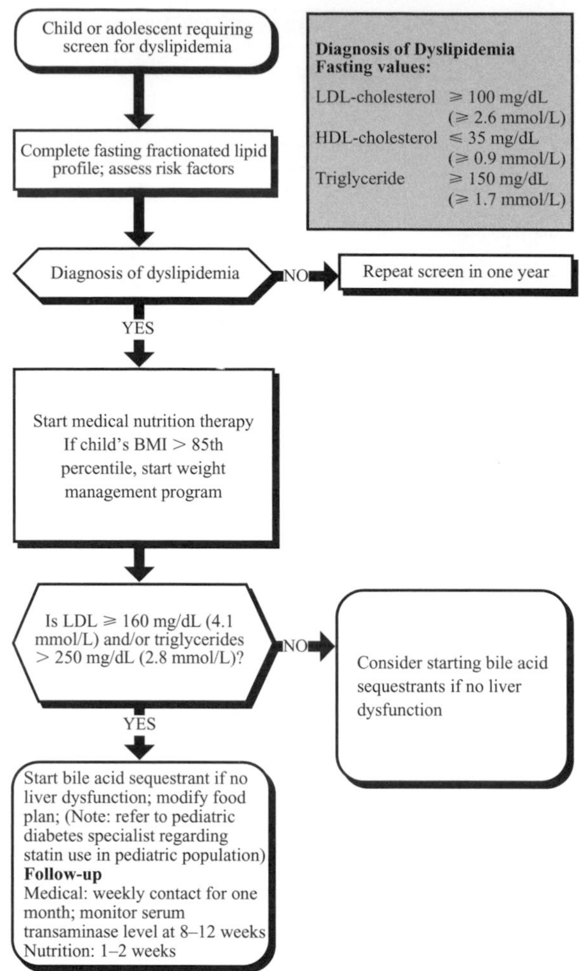

Figure 5.33 Dyslipidemia/diagnosis and start treatment for children and adolescents

principles of replace, reduce, and restrict. For example, replace fried foods with baked, broiled, or microwaved foods; reduce reliance on vegetable shortenings for cooking and baking; restrict high-fat fast foods and snacks. Simultaneously a plan for increased physical activity should be instituted. Should the child be overweight (85th–95th percentile BMI) or obese (95th percentile BMI) institute a program of weight management. This requires a comprehensive review of lifestyle. Following the weight management protocols for obese children and adolescents (modified for dyslipidemia).

For patients with type 2 diabetes, treatment of lipid abnormalities usually will not require a change in therapy if the HbA_{1c} is within 1.0 percentage point of the upper limit of normal range. In those patients on medical nutrition therapy only, some minor alterations in food plan (as already mentioned) are required. Finally, weight management and weight loss may have to be further emphasized if it is desirable to avoid the addition of pharmacologic agents for BG management.

The next step is to determine the severity of the cholesterol level. If the LDL $\geqslant$ 190 mg/dL (4.9 mmol/L) in the absence of a genetic predisposition to coronary artery disease (CAD) or LDL-cholesterol $\geqslant$ 160 mg/dL (4.1 mmol/L) with a positive family history for CAD or triglyceride $\geqslant$ 250 mg/dL (2.8 mmol/L) then a bile acid sequestrant should be started (after obtaining liver function tests). If diabetes or HTN is present, bile acid sequestrant should be initiated when there is any dyslipidemia. Next, alter the treatment for diabetes if the $HbA_{1c} > 1.5$ percentage points above upper limit of normal. Start metformin unless there is underlying renal disease otherwise initiate insulin therapy. Treat HTN intensively (see Hypertension Management).

Adjust/Maintain Medical Nutrition Therapy

Improvement in the abnormal lipid levels should occur within 3 months of initiation of treatment and continue until normal levels of total cholesterol and LDL cholesterol are reached. Continued modification in diet and increase in activity level should be encouraged to maintain improved lipid levels. If improvement is not occurring, consider evaluation for adherence and introduction of drug therapy no later than one year after initiation of MNT and provided the dyslipidemia does not worsen. Otherwise, initiate bile acid sequestrant therapy. Another option is the intiation of ezetimibe therapy in patients greater than 10 years of age. Consider referral to diabetes specialist or cardiologist if starting statin therapy.

The best results occur when alterations in food and exercise occur over time and are planned. Slow changes in behavior provide both immediate and long-term feedback. Moderating food intake and increasing activity provide rapid positive feedback. Weight management in children and adolescents, especially during periods of accelerated growth is complex. Adequate nutrients must be present with appropriate calories. However, in the obese child or adolescent moderation of caloric intake, especially fats, is necessary. Careful surveillance of weight and BMI will assure that appropriate calories are consumed for growth. If caloric reduction is necessary to manage weight keep in mind that a reduction of no more than 250 calories per day will result in a 2 lb (1 kg) loss per month. If increased exercise of 30 minutes per day, three times per week is added, the patient may lose up to 4 lb per month. Reduction in calories should be accompanied by modification in both fat and sodium intake. Since fat provides more than twice as many calories as an equivalent quantity of carbohydrate or protein, further reduction in weight can be realized by replacing fat with carbohydrate and protein.

General recommendations include:

- fat at less than 30 per cent of total calories
- saturated fat, less than 10 per cent of total calories
- fat limited to monounsaturated and polyunsaturated (avoid animal fats)
- meat limit to 6 ounces per day (avoid high-fat products)
- dairy limit to low-fat variety
- eggs limit to 2–3 per week
- breads, whole grain variety
- alcohol, avoid if high triglyceride level

Adjust/Maintain Drug Treatment

At the 3 month visit cholesterol, LDL, HDL, and triglyceride levels are measured to identify any current lipid abnormality. If the therapy has resulted in reaching the target, the patient moves into the maintain phase. Continue to monitor the patient every 3 months. After 1 year in the maintain phase, reduction in drug therapy may be considered.

If the patient has not reached target, first determine whether the lipid abnormality is the same as before. If it is the same, assess overall adherence to the prescribed regimen. This should address changes in lifestyle as well as whether the medication dose and timing are followed. Lifestyle changes should be reflected in alteration in diet, activity level, weight, and blood glucose levels. Increase the dose of the bile acid sequestrant until 1.1 g/kg/day is reached. If the maximum dose is reached do not add another drug classification before consultation with a pediatric specialist.

Polycystic ovary syndrome

Polycystic ovary syndrome (PCOS) develops in females with the onset of menarche. It is found at a disproportionately high incidence among adolescents with insulin resistance (with the highest incidence among obese females). It is a syndrome characterized by hyperandrogenism, chronic anovulation, and infertility. Related to insulin resistance, PCOS is characterized by derangements in gonadotropin releasing hormone and increased luteinizing hormone and decreased follicle stimulating hormone. SDM has developed guidelines for screening, diagnosis, and treatment of PCOS (Figure 5.34).

Practice guidelines

Screening, risk factors and symptoms. Screening for PCOS is based on the presence of risk factors and clinical signs or symptoms. With the onset of puberty all females with irregular menstrual cycles, oligomenorrhea or amenorrhea should be screened. Additionally, excessive hair (hirsutism) should be assumed to be related to PCOS. Finally, as PCOS is part of the insulin resistant syndrome, any other component of insulin resistance should be considered a risk factor necessitating diagnostic testing.

Diagnosis and treatment. The first diagnostic test is measurement of total testosterone and free testosterone by radioimmunoassay. If total testosterone is between 50 ng/dL and 200 ng/dL above normal (<2.5 ng/dL) PCOS is present. If >200 ng/dL then serum DHEA-S should be measured. If total testosterone or DHEA-S > 700 μg/dL then rule out an ovarian or adrenal tumor. These tests should be followed by tests for hypothyroidism, hyperprolactinemia, and adrenal hyperplasia.

The treatment of PCOS is directed primarily at its clinical manifestations: menstrual irregularity, infertility, and hirsutism. The choice of treatments is related to the co-morbidities associated with insulin resistance. Generally the choices are low-androgen-activity oral contraceptive pills or anti-androgen therapy (non-obese and hirsutism) or metformin (obese).

Targets, monitoring, and follow-up. Normal menstrual cycles and fertility are the principal targets of treatment. Close monitoring of menstrual cycles with follow-up every 3 months with testosterone and liver function tests is recommenced. Annually, the patient should be evaluated for all co-morbidities of insulin resistance.

Polycystic ovary syndrome DecisionPath

Female adolescents with insulin resistance, especially those who have type 2 diabetes, obesity, dyslipidemia, or HTN, should be evaluated for PCOS (see Figure 5.35). Irregular menses, hirsutism, and unresolved acne are often symptomatic of PCOS. Any of these signs require that total and free testosterone be measured. If the values is between 50 and 200 ng/dL above normal then the diagnosis of PCOS is confirmed. If the value exceeds 200 ng/dL then further tests are necessary to rule out other potential causes. Referral to endocrinologist is recommended.

Once the diagnosis of PCOS has been made the selection of treatment is in part dependent upon the degree of insulin resistance as measured by a fasting insulin/glucose ratio. If the ratio exceeds

Screening

Screen all adolescent females, with history of oligomenorrhea or amenorrhea (primary or secondary) without delayed puberty

Risk Factors

- Overweight (> 85th percentile for age & gender)
- Central adiposity
- Elevated triglycerides
- Positive family history of type 2 diabetes, PCOS, or infertility
- Acanthosis nigricans
- Premature adrenarche
- Smoking
- Female relative with hirsutism or infertility
- Hyperinsulinemia
- Being a member of a high-risk group; American Indian or Alaska Native; African-American; Asian; Native Hawaiian or other Pacific Islander; Hispanic
- Birthweight > 4000 g (or > 90th birth percentile) or < 2000 g (or < 10th birth percentile) at term
- Child of a mother diagnosed with GDM during any pregnancy

Symptoms

- Oligomenorrhea (≤ 8 menses/yr)
- Dysmenorrhea/amenorrhea
- Rapid weight gain
- Hirsutism
- Family history of infertility/oligomenorrhea
- Type 2 diabetes IGT, or IFG (pre-diabetes)
- Alopecia (frontal hair loss)
- Hypercholesterolemia
- Hypertension
- Elevated triglycerides
- Premature pubarche
- Acne

Diagnosis

Total testosterone > 50 ng/dL (normal female < 2.5 ng/dL)
Rule out:

- Ovarian or adrenal tumor. Total testosterone > 200 ng/dL or DHE-S > 700 μg/dL
- Hypothyroidism (TSH); Hyperprolactinemin (prolactin)
- Incomplete on non-classic adrenal hyperplasia ("Late onset").
  If 17-hydroxyprogesterone > 2 ps/mL needs confirmation with ACTH stimulation test

Screen for PCOS-associated disorders; fasting or 2 hour glucose/insulin ratio, fasting lipid profile, hypertension; Consider referral to specialist

Treatment Options

Lean without hyperinsulinemia, use low-androgen-activity oral contraceptive pills (Yasmin); obese and/or hyperinsulinemic or dyslipidemic treat with metformin, the OCP with low androgen activity and antiandrogen. Refer to multidisciplinary team.
Medical nutrition therapy, family planning, and psychological support are essential componenets

Targets

Decreased fasting insulin; normolipidemia, normotension
Clarify goal with patient; if goal is pregnancy, discuss preconception planning and related health issues; if goal is restoration of fertility without pregnancy, discuss preconception planning

Monitoring

Track menstrul cycles

Follow-up

Monthly Track menstrual cycles
Every 3 Months Testosterone and LFTs, weight, hirsutism, and menstrual cycles
Yearly (in addition to 3-4 month visit) History and physical; screen for albuminuria; eye examination with dilation; dental examination;
Medical nutrition and activity therapy continuing education; fasting lipid profile, glucose screening; preconceptual planning for females of childbearing age as indicated, psychological support, depression screening

Figure 5.34 Polycystic Ovary Syndrome Practice Guidelines for Children and Adolescents

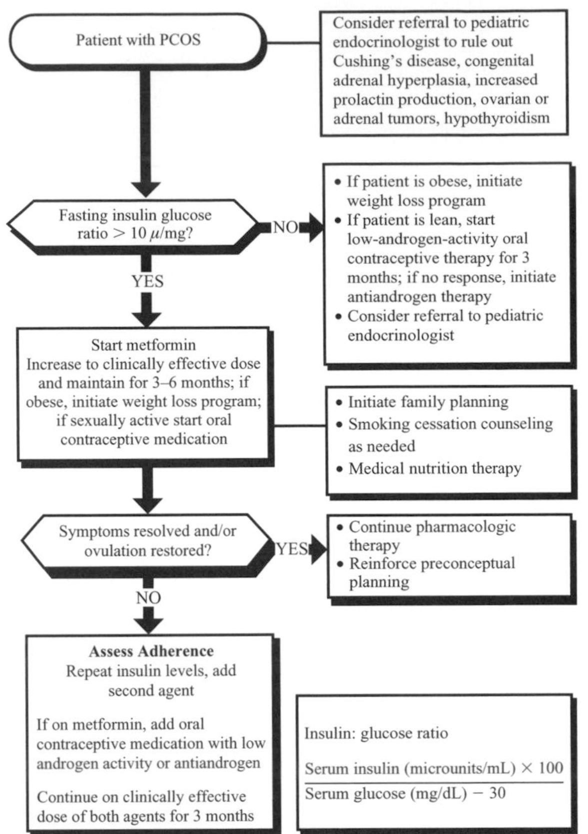

Figure 5.35 Polycystic ovary syndrome diagnosis and treatment options for children and adolescents

10 μ/mg then it is recommended that the biguanide metformin be considered. Before metformin can be initiated the patient must be evaluated for renal disease and liver disease. Metformin should be started using no more than 250 mg/day given with the largest meal. If the patient is already treated for type 2 diabetes with insulin then the addition of metformin therapy should be considered. Weekly increases of 250 mg can continue, alternating between morning and evening meals, until normal menstrual cycles or 2000 mg/day of metformin is reached. If after 3 months normal menstrual cycle has not begun then oral contraceptive pill with low androgen activity may be added.

If the insulin/glucose ratio is ≤10 μ/mg then the treatment depends upon BMI. For obese adolescents medical nutrition therapy to manage weight precedes use of oral contraceptive therapy. If normal or lean body mass then the patient is given low-androgen-activity oral contraceptive therapy for 3 months. If this does not resolve symptoms, then antiandrogen therapy is initiated. If MNT, metformin, and oral contraceptive therapies have failed to ameliorate the PCOS symptoms refer the patient to a pediatric endocrinologist.

Psychosocial and Educational Assessment for Children and Adolescents

The diagnosis of any of the components of insulin resistance carries with it the risk of psychological and social dysfunction. The realization that a child or adolescent has a chronic disease or a set of inter-related chronic diseases combined with the added burden of life-long responsibilities for the patient and the family present a unique dilemma. On the one hand the individual and the family are expected to return to normal life as quickly as possible; on the other hand the child and family are expected to immediately take on the major responsibilities of care. The list of responsibilities range through changes in lifestyle, drug therapy, monitoring, and surveillance. The initiation of a new approach to treatment (such as introducing insulin therapy) may also cause both psychological and social dysfunction. This is often reflected in how the individual and family adjust to changes in lifestyle brought about by treatment.

The patient's and family's ability to acquire new knowledge and skills needed to manage the disease(s) is related to their psychological and social adjustment. Such psychological factors as depression and anxiety and social factors such as conduct disorders significantly interfere with acquiring self-care skills or caregiver skills as well as with the ability to accept the seriousness of insulin resistance and associated disorders. If the psychological and social adjustment of the individual or family proves to be dysfunctional, it will most likely be reflected in poor disease management. This, in turn, raises the risk of acute and chronic complications, which contribute still further to the psychological and social dysfunction. To break this cycle, it is necessary to identify the earliest signs of dysfunction and to intervene as soon as possible.

Identification of psychological and social problems generally begin with the primary care physician only after symptoms of anxiety or depression occur. SDM has a Psychosocial and Educational Assessment for Children and Adolescents (Figure 5.36). In anticipation of such symptoms, it might be appropriate for primary care physicians to refer newly diagnosed patients and their families to a psychologist or social worker trained to detect the earliest symptoms of psychological or social dysfunction and to intervene before they result in destructive behaviors. Often one or two counseling sessions are required to detect underlying psychological or social problems and to intervene effectively.

Assessment

Family System
- Religious or cultural influences
- Who is present in the home
- Relationships of those individuals
- Who is involved in care of the child
- Who buys groceries and does the cooking
- Who is involved in setting guidelines and discipline
- Closeness of family relationships
- Who makes healthcare decisions?
- Are there any other health care conditions?

Progress in School
- Grades
- Extra-curricular activities
- Peer relationships
- Behavior in class
- Latch-key children: what does the child do after school?

Stress in Family
- Parents' relationship
- Financial
- Recent crises
- Work related stress for parents
- Level of independence of child

Emotional Reaction to Diagnosis
- Child
- Parents
- Siblings
- Grandparents
- Peers
- Extended family

History of Coping Strategies
- Has the family dealt with crises before?
- What is the family's preferred style of coping (seek information vs. limit information; seek support vs. avoid other people?)

History of Depression or Other Psychiatric Concerns
- History of counseling or medications
- Current treatment
- Do medications interfere with self-care regimen?

For Children and Adolescents with Diabetes
- Other family members with diabetes?
- How does the family divide diabetes responsiblities?
- Any deaths from diabetes in the family?
- Can they test blood glucose as needed? Can they test in classroom?
- Told peers or teacher about diabetes?
- Can the child eat when they want to or have to?
- Any major complications?

Figure 5.36 Psychosocial and Educational Assessment for Children and Adolescents

Recognizing these early warning signs requires a complete psychological and social profile of the individual, which should include any family caregiver. One approach to obtaining this information is to begin the patient encounter with the idea that insulin resistance will be co-managed by the patient, the family caregiver (where appropriate), and the physician (and team), and that the patient, if capable, will be empowered to participate in all decisions. Most children and adolescents begin interactions with physicians assuming the power to make all clinical decisions rests with the physician. Setting reasonable goals and establishing a clear plan for the child or adolescent is critical (Figure 5.37).

Goals and Plan

Goals
- A balanced support system with family involvement
- Recognition of the burden of metabolic syndrome and/or diabetes in relationship to the stresses within the family
- Recognition of the limits of the family's coping behavior and needed support
- Be aware of and diminish barriers to the child making behavioral change
- Identify and treat depression, if existent
- Positive emotional adjustment for child and family
- Avoidance of guilt, improve self-esteem

Plan
- Educate the family and child re metabolic syndrome/diabetes as a family disease
- Give an appropriate amount of information
- Problem solve with the child and family the barriers to treatment
- Listen and validate feelings
- Make a referral to mental health professional and consider anti-depressant medication

Figure 5.37 Psychosocial and Educational Goals and Plan for Children and Adolescents

For successful chronic disease management where children or adolescents are involved, giving them self-care responsibilities as early as they are capable is considered crucial. Co-empowerment of the child or adolescent with the healthcare team effectively brings the patient onto the team and ensures that the patient understands and takes on clinical care responsibilities. Co-empowerment recognizes that the child or adolescent and physician may have a different view of the seriousness of the disease, the responsibilities of each healthcare professional, and the expectations of the patient's performance. The individual with insulin resistance may feel the physician will make all decisions related to care and the patient should be passive. Alternatively, the physician may feel the patient and family should make daily decisions about diet, insulin, and exercise.

Co-empowerment is an agreement between the patient, the family, and the health care team that delineates the responsibilities and expectations of each participant in care and also establishes the DecisionPath that all team members have agreed to follow. From a psychosocial perspective, it may be seen as a contract in which the patient and family detail their expectations and in which health care professionals have an opportunity to determine how well those responsibilities and expectations fit with the management plan. It presents an opportunity to review behaviors that may be detrimental to the overall treatment goal. The person who refuses to test, who is hyperactive at school, or who binge eats must be encouraged to share this information with the health team. Similarly, the physician who believes in strict adherence to regimens or the dietitian who expects 100 percent compliance to a restrictive food plan must be able to state these expectations and have them challenged by the patient. Through this process of negotiation, a consensus as to goals, responsibilities, and expectations can be reached that will benefit the person with diabetes as well as the healthcare team members.

References

1. Kaufman FR. Type 2 diabetes mellitus in children and youth: a new epidemic. *J Pediatr Endocrinol Metab* 2002; Suppl 2: 737–744.
2. Fagot-Campagna A. Emergence of type 2 diabetes mellitus in children: epidemiological evidence. *J Pediatr Endocrinol Metab* 2000; Suppl 6: 1395–1402.
3. American Diabetes Association (ADA). Type 2 Diabetes in Children and Adolescents. *Pediatrics* 2000; **105**: 671–680.
4. LeRoith D. Beta-cell dysfunction and insulin resistance in type 2 diabetes: role of metabolic and genetic abnormalities. *Am J Med* 2002; **113**: 3S–11S.
5. Neel, JV. Diabetes mellitus: a 'thrifty' geno-type rendered detrimental by 'progress?' *Am J Hum Genet* 1962; **14**: 353–362.
6. Klein R, Klein BEK, Moss SE and Cruickshanks KJ. Relationship of hyperglycemia to the long-term incidence and progression of diabetic retinopathy *Arch Intern Med* 1994; **154**: 2169–2178.
7. Sothern MS. *Trim Kids Harper Resource*. 2001.
8. American Diabetes Association (ADA). Report of the Expert Committee on the Diagnosis and Classification of Diabetes Mellitus. *Diabetes Care* 2003; **26**: S5–S20.
9. Nathan DM, Singer DE, Hurxthal K and Goodson JD. The clinical information value of the glycosylated hemoglobin assay. *N Engl J Med* 1984; **310**: 341–346.
10. Mazze RS, Shamoon H, Parmentier R, *et al*. Reliability of blood glucose monitoring by patients with diabetes. *Am J Med* 1984; **77**: 211–217.
11. Mazze RS. Computers and diabetes therapy; key variables and quality of data for clinical decision making. *Horm Metab Res Suppl* 1990; **24**: 97–102.
12. Kaufman FR. Effect of metformin in children with type 2 diabetes. *Curr Diab Rep* 2001; **1**: 9–10.
13. Jones KL, Arslanian S, Peterokova VA, Park JS and Tomlinson MJ. Effect of metformin in pediatric patients with type 2 diabetes: a randomized controlled trial. *Diabetes Care* 2002; **25**: 89–94.
14. Soergel M and Schaefer F. Effect of hypertension on the progression of chronic renal failure in children. *Am J Hypertens* 2002; **15**: 53S–56S.
15. American Diabetes Association Consensus Statement. Management of dyslipidemia in children and adolescents with diabetes. *Diabetes Care* 2003; **26**: 2194–2197.
16. Yki-Järvinen H. Combination therapies with insulin in type 2 diabetes. *Diabetes Care* 2001; **24**: 758–767.

6 Type 1 Diabetes

Type 1 diabetes (formerly known as insulin-dependent diabetes mellitus (IDDM) or juvenile onset diabetes) is found in approximately 750,000 Americans.[1] Each year about 35,000 new cases are discovered and approximately 30,000 individuals die with type 1 diabetes as an underlying cause. Worldwide the number of people with type 1 diabetes varies markedly. In the countries that comprise Scandinavia and northern continental Europe the prevalence is high, while in countries near the equator (with the exception of Israel) the prevalence is less than 0.01 per cent.[2] Originally it was thought that the onset of the disease was limited to children (juvenile onset). It is now known that diagnosis of type 1 diabetes can occur at virtually any age, with onset reaching a peak frequency during pre- and early adolescence. The immediate cause of type 1 diabetes is believed to be progressive pancreatic β-cell destruction. The cause of β-cell destruction appears to be an autoimmune response to antigens expressed by the β-cell. The exact mechanism by which the autoimmune response is triggered is a subject of intense scientific research. Currently, it is thought that β-cell destruction results from genetic factors coupled with (an) environmental trigger(s).

Etiology

Human leukocyte antigen (HLA) typing has identified two alleles, HLA-DR3 and HLA-DR4, in the major histocompatibility complex (MHC), that are considered diabetogenic. The presence of at least one of these alleles is found in the vast majority of individuals diagnosed with type 1 diabetes.[3] However, HLA-DR3 and HLA-DR4 alleles have been found in as many as 40 per cent of people without diabetes, indicating that other factors besides a genetic predisposition are involved in the development of type 1 diabetes. Studies in identical twins have confirmed a 36 per cent concordance of type 1 diabetes after 24 years of follow-up investigations.[4] It is, however, the discordance of 64 per cent among identical twins that supports the theory that some type of environmental trigger acts on one of the genetically predisposed twins to initiate autoimmune β-cell destruction. Interestingly, the HLA-DR2 allele appears to be negatively associated with the development of the disease, because this allele is found in very few individuals with type 1 diabetes.[5]

The destruction of islet β-cells occurs via direct autoimmune response against β-cell antigens, resulting in infiltration of lymphocytes into the islets of Langerhans (insulitis). Antibodies directed against islet cell autoantigens are called

Staged Diabetes Management: A Systematic Approach (2nd Edition) R. S. Mazze, E. S. Strock, G. D. Simonson and R. M. Bergenstal
 ISBN: 0 470 86576 8

cytoplasmic islet cell antibodies (ICAs). Screening for cytoplasmic ICAs has demonstrated that they are clearly present in the circulatory system prior to diagnosis of the disease.[6] While many autoantigens exist, one has received much attention. Autoantibodies against glutamic acid decarboxylase (anti-GAD), the enzyme responsible for the production of gamma-aminobutyric acid, have been implicated as a key autoantigen in the development of type 1 diabetes.[7] In addition, autoantibodies against human insulin are often present at the onset of type 1 diabetes.

What triggers the autoimmune response against the islet cells is the subject of much research and debate. Viral infections have been implicated as a possible triggering mechanism setting off the autoimmune response. Congenital rubella virus infection has been linked to the onset of type 1 diabetes.[8] Other viruses (Coxsackie, mumps, and herpes) have also been suggested as factors in the development of type 1 diabetes, but the association of the latter group is much less clear. For this reason, recent research focused on the possibility of preventing diabetes in those at high risk. In 1994 the National Institutes of Health established the Diabetes Prevention Trial-1 (DPT-1), that set out to test the hypothesis that type 1 diabetes may be prevented by early and sustained use of low-dose insulin (injected twice daily) in individuals at high risk for its development. Family members of those with type 1 diabetes were studied for several years due to the relatively low incidence of type 1 diabetes and the rate of conversion from ICA positive to type 1 diabetes. To date, the results have not been promising.[9] The use of low-dose insulin does not appear to prevent the onset of type 1 diabetes. However, the DPT-1 did demonstrate that large prevention trials for type 1 diabetes are feasible and future studies may be considered as this area of clinical science expands.

The physiologic state of type 1 diabetes

Type 1 diabetes develops over different time periods based upon age. In children and adolescents type 1 diabetes usually appears quite suddenly (over several days to weeks). In adults it may take several years before the appearance of acute symptoms, such as polyuria, polydipsia and polyphagia with consequential weight loss. This set of symptoms marks the final phase of the complete destruction of pancreatic β-cells, and if left unchecked will lead to diabetic ketoacidosis.

Note: Before continuing, it might be helpful to review the structure of Staged Diabetes Management for type 1 diabetes. The Master DecisionPath presents the stages and phases of diabetes diagnosis and treatment. The phases refer to three specific periods in diabetes management – start treatment (diagnosis and initial insulin dose), adjust treatment (experimentation with the type of insulin, dose, and timing of injection), and maintain treatment (reaching the therapeutic goal). Stages are the treatment options. This information should be shared with the patient and family members.

Type 1 diabetes detection and treatment

The following sections provide the means of diagnosis and the treatment choices for type 1 diabetes. They begin with the practice guidelines, followed by the Master DecisionPath, which lays out an orderly sequence of stages shown to foster improved glycemic control. Specific DecisionPaths for each stage (treatment option) as well as Diabetes Management Assessment DecisionPaths (medical visit, education, nutrition, adherence assessment) along with a complete description of each item and the rationale for decisions are also presented.

Type 1 diabetes practice guidelines

While no group is immune to the development of type 1 diabetes, certain age groups and ethnic populations are at higher risk for its development. The highest-incidence group is pre- and early adolescents of Scandinavian descent with siblings who have developed type 1 diabetes. The incidence is lowest in adults of African-American or Native American heritage (see Figure 6.1).

Diagnosis

Although type 1 diabetes can occur at any age, the vast majority of cases occur in children and adolescents with no family history of the disease. Among these two groups taken collectively, approximately 2 per cent of children with diabetes are diagnosed as infants, 37 per cent between 2 and 5 years of age, 41 per cent between 6 and 12 years of age, and 20 per cent as adolescents between 13 and 19 years of age.[10,11] While the overall risk in the general population is between 1/400 (in children) and 1/1000 (in young adults under age 40), the offspring of adults with type 1 diabetes and the siblings of individuals with type 1 diabetes are at increased risk, with an approximate 5 per cent prevalence.[12] The benefits of early detection of type 1 diabetes in a general pediatric or family practice setting are based on evidence that many acute complications are directly related to the severity of persistent hyperglycemia prior to diagnosis. In particular, timely diagnosis avoids further metabolic decompensation and the risk of diabetic ketoacidosis (DKA).

While in the past many patients with type 1 diabetes presented in DKA, this can and should be avoided through better surveillance. Insulin is necessary for the normal metabolism of glucose. In its absence the body has an excess of glucose in the blood, resulting in dehydration due to "spilling" of glucose in the urine and a reliance on fat metabolism as the major source of energy. Ketones are a byproduct of fat catabolism. If left undetected, patients will present with DKA, which constitutes a medical emergency. Most patients should be diagnosed earlier. Astute observers may note one or more of the classic symptoms of type 1 diabetes:

- polyuria (excess urination)
- polyphagia (excess eating)
- polydipsia (excess thirst)
- unequivocal hyperglycemia (fasting plasma glucose $\geqslant$ 126 mg/dL or 7.0 mmol/L and/or casual plasma glucose $\geqslant$ 200 mg/dL or 11.1 mmol/L)
- unexplained weight loss
- blurred vision

Children present a special challenge to the primary care clinician. Diabetes mellitus is one of *many conditions* that cause these symptoms in children. The clinician should always consider diabetes when there is no obvious explanation for polyuria or failure to thrive. While polyuria is more commonly associated with urinary tract infection, diuretic abuse, psychogenic polydipsia, or renal disease, diabetes should be ruled out. Questions pertaining to bed-wetting and frequent nocturia may help reveal urinary frequency. Type 1 diabetes must be seriously considered in the child with clinical dehydration who continues to urinate regularly. Failure to thrive may be the result of neglect of other non-organic factors, however, it may also be due to severe and prolonged hyperglycemia due to insulin insufficiency and its consequent loss of calories. Additionally, approximately 10 per cent of children with type 1 diabetes are asymptomatic at time of diagnosis. Finally, type 2 diabetes may be confused with type 1 diabetes in overweight children who are Hispanic, African-American, or Asian-American. Although more likely to have type 2 diabetes, any child present with the florid symptoms associated with type 1 diabetes should be treated as having-type 1 diabetes until definitive evidence (C-peptide assay) proves otherwise.

Diagnosis	Majority < 30 years old and not obese
Plasma Glucose	Casual $\geqslant 200$ mg/dL (11.1 mmol/L) plus symptoms, fasting $\geqslant 126$ mg/dL (7.0 mmol/L), or oral glucose tolerance test (OGTT) $\geqslant 200$ mg/dL (11.1 mmol/L) at 2 hours; if acute metabolic decompensation (positive ketones), make diagnosis immediately; in the absence of acute metabolic decompensation, confirm with fasting plasma glucose within 24 hours
Symptoms	Increased urination, thirst, and appetite; nocturia; weight loss Occasional: blurred vision; urinary tract infection; yeast infection; fatigue; acute abdominal pain; flulike symptoms
Urine Ketones	Usually positive, with or without diabetic ketoacidosis
Treatment Options	Insulin: Stages 2, 3A, 4A, 3B or pump synchronized with medical nutrition therapy **These patients require insulin therapy and should not be treated with an oral agent**
Targets	
Self-Monitored Blood Glucose (SMBG)	• More than 50% of SMBG values should be within target range • Age < 6 years: 100–200 mg/dL (5.6–11.1 mmol/L) pre-meal and bedtime • Age 6–12 years: 80–180 mg/dL (4.4–10.0 mmol/L) pre-meal and bedtime • Age > 12 years: 70–140 mg/dL (3.9–7.8 mmol/L) pre-meal; , 160 mg/dL (8.9 mmol/L) 2 hours after start of meal; 100–160 mg/dL (5.6–8.9 mmol/L) at bedtime • No severe (assisted) or nocturnal hypoglycemia; Adjust pre-meal target upward if hypoglycemia unawareness or repeated severe hypoglycemia occurs
Hemoglobin HbA_{1c}	• Age < 6 years: within 2.5 percentage points of upper limit of normal (e.g. normal 6%; target $< 8.5\%$) • Age 6–12 years: within 2 percentage points of upper limit of normal • Age > 12 years: within 1.0 percentage point of upper limit of normal • Frequency: 3–4 times per year • Use HbA_{1c} verify SMBG data or to adjust therapy when data unavailable
Monitoring	
SMBG	Minimum 4 times per day (before meals, 2 hours after start of meal, and at bedtime) Check 3 AM as needed (AM hyperglycemia, nocturnal hypoglycemia)
Method	Meter with memory and log book
Urine Ketones	Check if unexplained BG > 250 mg/dL (13.9 mmol/L) on 2 consecutive occasions, or if any illness or infection present
Growth and Development	Normal, as determined using anthropometric scales/growth charts
Follow-up	
Monthly	Office visit during adjust phase (weekly phone contact may be necessary)
Every 3 Months	Hypoglycemia; medications; weight; height; growth rate; medical nutrition therapy; BP; SMBG data (download meter); glycosylated hemoglobin; eye screen; foot screen; diabetes/nutrition continuing education; smoking cessation counseling, aspirin therapy for age > 30
Yearly	In addition to the 3 month follow-up, complete the following: history and physical; dental examination; fasting lipid profile within 6 months of diagnosis In patients $>$ age 12 with diabetes for 5 years complete the following: albuminuria screen; dilated eye examination; neurologic assessment; complete foot examination (pulses, nerves, and inspection); patient satisfaction evaluation
Complications Surveillance	Cardiovascular, renal, retinal, neurological, oral, dermatological and foot disease

Figure 6.1 Type 1 Diabetes Practice Guidelines

Adults present a different set of challenges. Because type 1 diabetes develops over a prolonged period of time, they are unaware of the common symptoms, which have occurred with such subtlety as to have gone unnoticed. When their hyperglycemia is discovered it is often initially classified as type 2 diabetes. This is especially true in adults between 40 and 50 years of age. For instance, Zimmet and coworkers found that as many as 10 per cent of the adults participating in the United Kingdom Prospective Diabetes Study who were classified as having type 2 diabetes may actually have latent autoimmune diabetes of adults (LADA).[13] This subset of patients in the study had classic markers of autoimmune diabetes (type 1) such as anti-GAD antibodies and islet cell antibodies (ICA) and tended to be younger and leaner compared with the other patients in the study. Interestingly, these individuals with LADA may be treated effectively with medical nutrition therapy alone or in combination with oral agents for several years before progressing to the point of requiring insulin to maintain normoglycemia. This presumably occurs due to a slow rate of β-cell destruction. In either case, diagnosis of diabetes is based on either casual or fasting blood glucose as shown in the Screening and Diagnosis Decision-Path (see Figure 6.2).

Diagnostic criteria

A fasting plasma glucose $\geqslant 126$ mg/dL (7.0 mmol/L) or a casual plasma glucose $\geqslant 200$ mg/dL (11.1 mmol/L) with symptoms is sufficient for diagnosis of diabetes in the presence of acute metabolic decompensation (positive ketones). A 2 hour post 75 g oral glucose tolerance test value of 200 mg/dL (11.1 mmol/L) is used when neither the fasting nor casual plasma glucose levels are conclusive. Subnormal insulin release (C-peptide analysis) may be used as early markers of type 1 diabetes, but for now the current criteria remain intact. In the unique case of an adult 40 years or older developing what appears to be type 1 diabetes, differential diagnosis in the absence of diabetes ketoacidosis is based on C-peptide analysis as well as assays for immune markers of type 1 diabetes. At the time of diagnosis of type 1 diabetes, both non-stimulated and glucose stimulated insulin secretion are very low. In contrast, individuals with type 2 diabetes normally have a significant post-prandial rise in insulin. Assays for islet cell antibodies (ICAs), insulin autoantibodies, or anti-GAD (glutamic acid decarboxylase) may also be utilized to differentiate between type 1 and type 2 diabetes. Whenever there is doubt about the type of diabetes and persistent hyperglycemia, the use of insulin is recommended until a differential diagnosis can be made.

Treatment options

Treating type 1 diabetes requires administering exogenous insulin in a way that mimics physiologic requirements. There are currently five types of insulin defined according to their length of action: rapid acting, short acting, intermediate acting, prolonged intermediate acting, and long acting. Since the early 1990s, insulin produced by recombinant DNA has been available. In 1996 the first insulin analog, lispro, was introduced in an effort to more precisely control the starting time, peak action, and duration of short-acting insulin. Two amino acids in regular human insulin were transposed to generate an insulin (lispro) with a faster subcutaneous absorption rate compared with regular insulin. A second rapid-acting insulin, aspart, was introduced in 2000. Both are comparable (with slight variations) in their action curves. In 2001, the first long-acting insulin analog, glargine, was introduced. All of these insulins may be injected using standard syringes or insulin pen devices. An externally worn insulin infusion pump can also administer the short- and rapid-acting insulins. Current research studies are underway to test the safety and efficacy of insulin administered by inhalation device.

Conventional insulin therapy versus physiologic insulin therapy

The two general methods of insulin administration are (1) conventional therapy and (2)

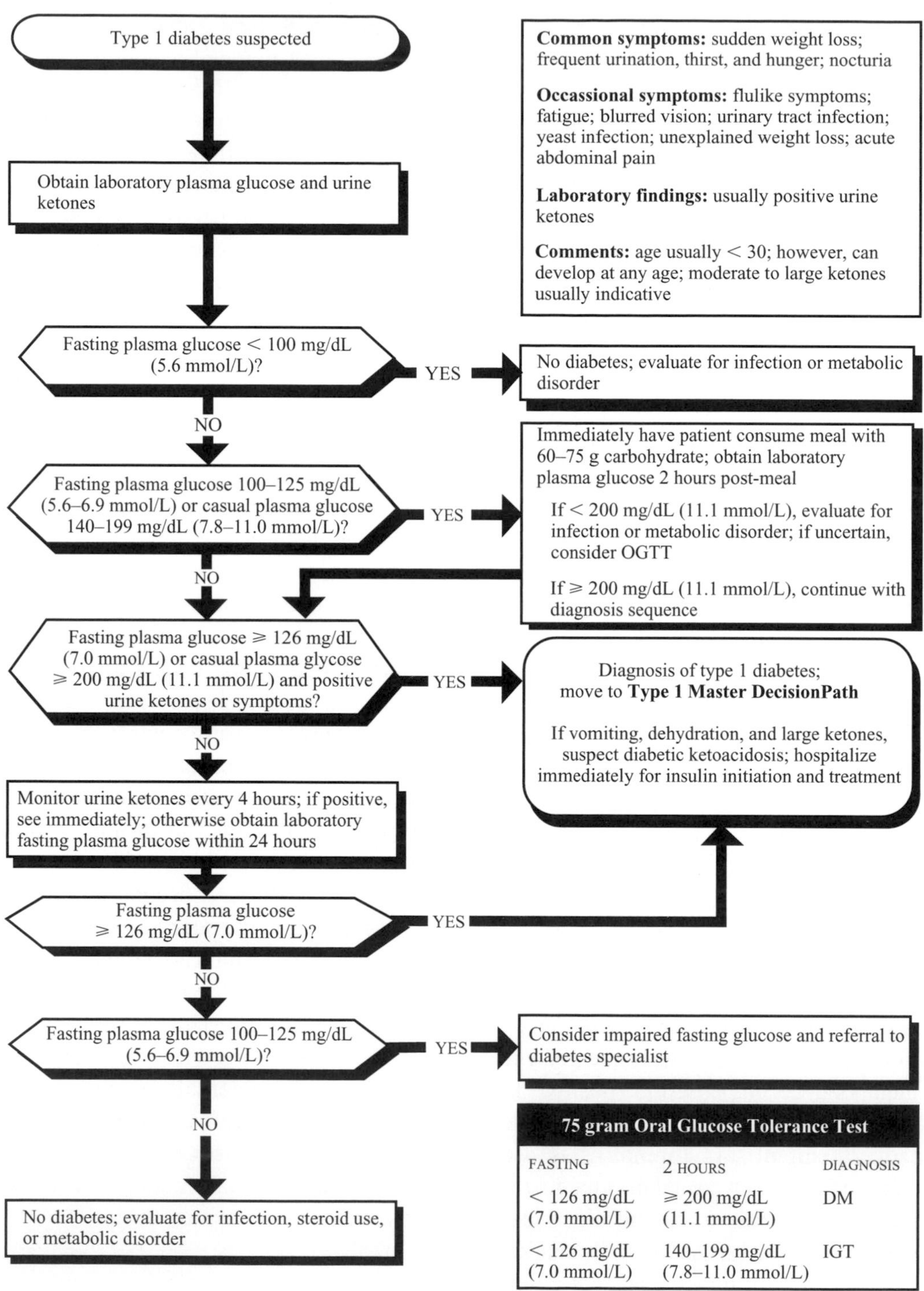

Figure 6.2 Type 1 Diabetes Screening and Diagnosis DecisionPath

intensive therapy. In conventional insulin therapy, food intake is timed to match insulin action. These regimens consist of at least two injections of mixed insulins (rapid or short acting and intermediate or long acting) per day, three meals at specific times throughout the day, and snacks as required. In intensive insulin therapy, insulin is altered to match the food plan and the lifestyle of the individual. These regimens generally consist of bolus (short- or rapid-acting) insulin with meals (not necessarily at specific times) and snacks, and basal (prolonged intermediate- or long-acting) insulin at bedtime. Because intensive insulin therapy comes closer to mimicking the normal physiologic state, it provides a better chance of optimizing blood glucose control and provides the most flexibility for those motivated to make adjustments in insulin dose throughout the day.

Targets

In 1993, the multicenter United States, National Institutes of Health study, the Diabetes Control and Complication Trial (DCCT), reported that any improvement in glycemic control was beneficial. It went on to show that near-normal levels of blood glucose afforded the best protection against the development and progression of microvascular disease.[14] During the following decade these findings were sustained by numerous other studies. Currently the target is to come as close to normal blood glucose as is feasible without experiencing debilitating hypoglycemia. To achieve this level of blood glucose the patient must sustain an HbA_{1c} of < 7 per cent with greater than half of the SMBG values falling between 70 and 140 mg/dL (3.9 and 7.8 mmol/L) pre-meal and < 160 mg/dL (8.9 mmol/L) 2 hours after a meal. While individual differences due to age and ability should be considered, these targets are both realistic and achievable (see Figure 6.1). Blood pressure and lipids levels must also be sustained at normal levels for people with diabetes.

Monitoring

Appropriate therapy for type 1 diabetes always includes SMBG and testing for urine ketones. Three different patterns of SMBG correspond to initiating treatment, adjusting treatment, and maintaining the treatment goal. During the start phase, data gathering is an important early step to ensure that blood glucose levels are responding to the insulin regimen and dietary adjustments. Self-monitoring of blood glucose should be timed to collect important data on fasting, 2 hours post-prandial, and overnight blood glucose level, along with pre-injection blood glucose determinations. Throughout the adjust phase, SMBG should be synchronized with the insulin action curves to determine where insulin action peaks. This is in addition to SMBG pre-insulin injections. During the maintain phase, SMBG can be modified to two to four times per day to ensure continued stability in blood glucose level. Patients should perform this daily before meals and at bedtime. Additional special circumstances for changes in SMBG patterns are to determine the impact of exercise, changes in MNT, and sudden alterations in therapy during intercurrent events. Under such circumstances, increased testing is recommended to enhance clinical decision-making. Because many studies have shown that patients may falsify their SMBG results, or fail to log results in a record book, meters with a memory should be used.[15] These meters discourage fabrication of results by directly recording the blood glucose value with the time and date of test. Some devices average the data and can be downloaded to a computer that displays the data in graphic format.

Whether used routinely or more frequently for special situations, SMBG data provide patients with direct feedback on how well their individual therapy is working and assists the team with information needed to make appropriate decisions about the therapy. Absence of SMBG data makes clinical decision-making almost impossible for both the patient and the clinician. Determining insulin dose, evaluating the impact of the insulin on glycemic control, and assessing diet and exercise all require a source of constant, accurate feedback. Currently only SMBG provides such feedback.

Urine ketones should also be part of the self-monitoring program. Whenever BG > 240 mg/dL (13.3 mmol/L) on two consecutive tests, urine ketones should be measured. If urine ketones are positive, patients should supplement with rapid-acting insulin and retest. Persistent positive ketones need to be treated to prevent possible DKA. In addition, urine ketones should be monitored if any illness or infection is present.

Growth and development

Perhaps no concern is greater for the parents of a child with type 1 diabetes than the impact of diabetes on growth and development. Insulin insufficiency, with accompanying diabetes out of control, can contribute to retarded growth, which may contribute to developmental problems. Generally, children with diabetes treated to maintain near-normal glycemia have normal growth and development. Frequent DKA with consequential hospitalization can contribute to long-term developmental problems.

Follow-up

During the diagnosis and start treatment period, daily communications are necessary to assure that the patient (or caregiver) is adjusting to diabetes and is fully capable of self-care. Next, weekly telephone contact with biweekly to monthly visits will be necessary in order to analyze SMBG data to develop a personal algorithm for daily management. Data from SMBG and frequent (quarterly) HbA_{1c} determinations are vital to determine the impact of the therapy. Additional data needed at follow-up include weight and height (for BMI); changes in schedule, food, and/or insulin; changes in exercise/activity habits; frequency of SMBG testing, time of testing, and results; frequency of hypoglycemic episodes; current blood pressure level if hypertension is present; new or updated laboratory data; food records completed since initial visit or 24 hour food recall; food plan problems; and other psychological issues that may influence diabetes management. Since all newly diagnosed patients, as well as many currently treated patients, require substantial diabetes education and nutrition counseling, this should be an integral part of the follow-up plan.

Complications surveillance

Generally, chronic complications of diabetes occur several years after its onset. However, unclear histories, slow onset (as in patients with LADA), and other factors support the practice of an annual complete complications surveillance. Retinal, kidney, neurological, cardiovascular, oral, and dermatological surveillance should be part of the annual examination (see Chapters 8 and 9).

Screening and Diagnosis DecisionPath

There is no standard protocol for screening for type 1 diabetes. Generally a fasting plasma glucose (FPG) is favored over a casual plasma glucose (CPG) especially when there are no symptoms. If the fasting plasma glucose < 100 mg/dL (5.6 mmol/L) there is no need to continue to screen. If the FPG is between 100 and 125 mg/dL (5.6–6.9 mmol/L) or the CPG is between 140 and 199 mg/dL (7.8–11.0 mmol/L) then immediately provide a meal consisting of 60–75 g carbohydrate (or a glucose challenge of 75 g glucola). If 2 hours after the test the BG ⩾ 200 mg/dL (11.1 mmol/L), continue with the diagnostic test.

With hyperglycemia in the presence of ketones or other signs of metabolic decompensation, the diagnosis of type 1 diabetes does not require an additional diagnostic test. Insulin therapy must be initiated immediately. A second diagnostic test is necessary to confirm type 1 diabetes in the absence of metabolic decompensation (ketones) and should be performed within 24 hours. To assure the patient is not at risk for DKA, monitor both urine ketones and BG every 4 hours. If the FPG meets the criteria then type 1 diabetes is confirmed; if not, then the patient either has impaired glucose homeostasis or is currently "normoglycemic."

Note: There is also the slight possibility that the patient is slowly developing type 1 diabetes (LADA). This would generally be a lean adult and may have been misdiagnosed and treated for type 2 diabetes. Close surveillance, C-peptide, or SMBG should be considered.

Type 1 diabetes Master DecisionPath

In this section, use of rapid-acting (RA), short-acting (R), intermediate-acting (N), and prolonged intermediate acting (UL) and long-acting (G) insulins is discussed. For a complete discussion of their action curves, see Chapter 3. In most cases, patients are started on two- or three-injection regimens (see Figure 6.3). In rare instances, such as the "honeymoon" period, Insulin Stage 1 is used. This assures that when the honeymoon period is over there is available exogenous insulin. Once the diagnosis of type 1 diabetes is made, insulin initiation must occur immediately (maximum time lapse of 24 hours). Determine whether insulin will be initiated on an inpatient or outpatient basis. Many institutions have developed systems that allow for safely initiating insulin on an outpatient basis. If resources for education and medical follow-up are not present, the patient should be hospitalized. If the patient is in DKA or at high risk for coma, hospitalize immediately (see Diabetic Ketoacidosis in Chapter 10).

The selection of the initial insulin therapy favors minimizing the complexity of the treatment while meeting lifestyle needs of the patient. Thus, beginning with Insulin Stage 2 (mixed rapid- or short- and intermediate-acting insulin in the morning and before the evening meal) makes sense. However, all patients should be offered three or more injections if rapid achievement of tight glycemic control is desired, or lifestyle issues would make a two-injection regimen difficult to follow. The fundamental principle is that the patient does not fail; only therapies fail. Furthermore, the patient should be made aware of each of the options, including pump therapy, so that an informed decision can be made. Because it is unclear which stage may allow a patient to achieve glycemic targets, SDM provides general guidelines for how long a patient should remain on a given regimen before starting another (see Table 6.1). In all cases, when the patient exceeds 1.5 U/kg total daily insulin the next stage should be considered. MNT should always accompany insulin initiation with an emphasis on synchronizing the meal and activity plans with the insulin injection schedule.

Insulin Stage 2

At diagnosis, it is recommended that individuals be started on Insulin Stage 2 or 3A. Much depends on the patient's willingness and ability to administer insulin and SMBG several times each day. In general, the more injections, the more closely the injected insulin mimics normal physiologic release of insulin. A complete discussion of Insulin Stage 3A follows this section.

Insulin Stage 2/Start
R/N–0–R/N–0 or RA/N–0–RA/N–0

In the absence of DKA, patients with newly diagnosed type 1 diabetes should be started on insulin in the office. Initial insulin injection should be administered by the patient or family member (for younger children). All patients should be started on human insulin.

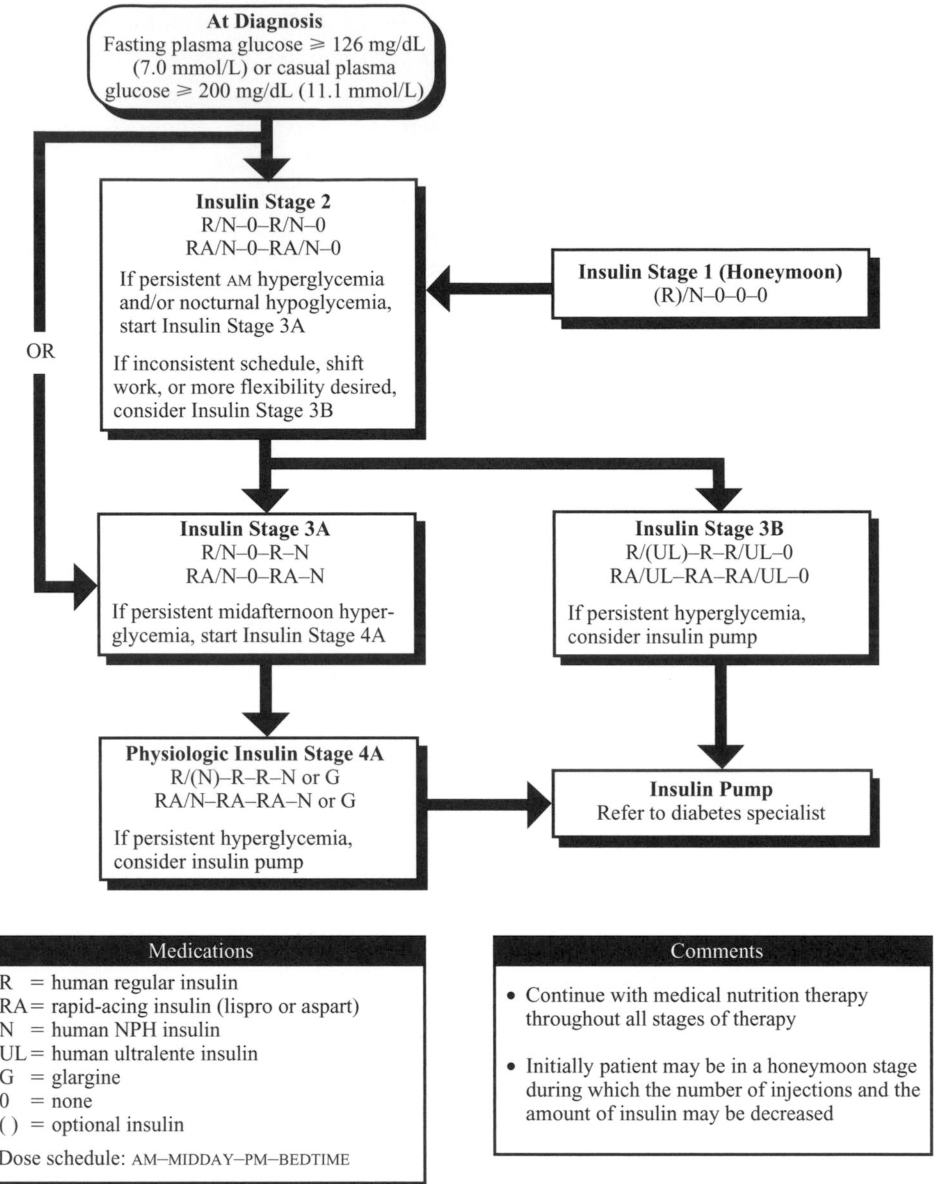

Medications
R = human regular insulin
RA = rapid-acing insulin (lispro or aspart)
N = human NPH insulin
UL = human ultralente insulin
G = glargine
0 = none
( ) = optional insulin
Dose schedule: AM–MIDDAY–PM–BEDTIME

Comments
• Continue with medical nutrition therapy throughout all stages of therapy
• Initially patient may be in a honeymoon stage during which the number of injections and the amount of insulin may be decreased

Figure 6.3 Type 1 Diabetes Master DecisionPath

Table 6.1 Timelines to reach management goals

Insulin Stage	Time
Stage 2	12 months
Stage 3A/3B	6 months
Stage 4A	6 months
Pump	12 months

Determining the initial insulin dose. The total daily insulin requirement at diagnosis is a function of the current weight and urine ketones – an early sign of significant insulin deficiency and possible impending DKA – see Figure 6.4. Insulin is calculated in Units/kg based on current weight. If ketones are large, 0.7 U/kg total dose is recommended; for negative to moderate ketones

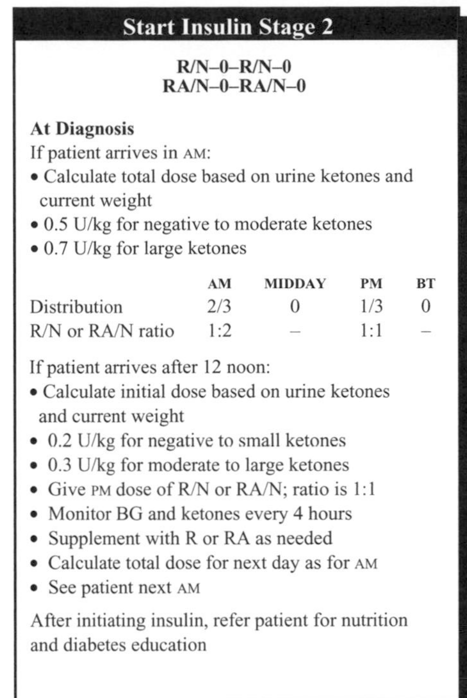

Start Insulin Stage 2

R/N–0–R/N–0
RA/N–0–RA/N–0

At Diagnosis
If patient arrives in AM:
- Calculate total dose based on urine ketones and current weight
- 0.5 U/kg for negative to moderate ketones
- 0.7 U/kg for large ketones

	AM	MIDDAY	PM	BT
Distribution	2/3	0	1/3	0
R/N or RA/N ratio	1:2	–	1:1	–

If patient arrives after 12 noon:
- Calculate initial dose based on urine ketones and current weight
- 0.2 U/kg for negative to small ketones
- 0.3 U/kg for moderate to large ketones
- Give PM dose of R/N or RA/N; ratio is 1:1
- Monitor BG and ketones every 4 hours
- Supplement with R or RA as needed
- Calculate total dose for next day as for AM
- See patient next AM

After initiating insulin, refer patient for nutrition and diabetes education

Figure 6.4 Dosing recommendation for starting Insulin Stage 2

0.5 U/kg is suggested. The total daily dose is divided into two periods roughly associated with breakfast and the evening meal (approximately 10 hours apart). The pre-breakfast dose is two-thirds of the total daily requirement. This is further divided into one-third R or RA and two-thirds N. The small amount of rapid- or short-acting insulin covers breakfast. The intermediate-acting insulin covers lunch and afternoon snack. Review the insulin action curves for the AM mixed insulin (see Chapter 3). Note that by the time of the evening meal most insulin has been cleared. The PM dose (one-third total) is divided equally between R or RA and N. Again, the bolus insulin is meal related and the intermediate-acting insulin is designed to provide for basal insulin requirements for overnight hepatic glucose output.

Patients with newly diagnosed type 1 diabetes present at various times of the day, e.g., midmorning or late afternoon. After calculating the total requirement, if the patient is diagnosed in the morning, begin with the morning dose (two-thirds total). If the patient is diagnosed any time after noon, it will be necessary to start with a small amount of short-acting insulin to bring the patient to the time of the evening meal. At the time of the evening meal begin with the PM dose (one-third of total). If RA is used, make certain that the patient has a small snack available. Since SMBG is a necessity in any insulin regimen, until the patient is able to learn SMBG, it is suggested that he/she return to the office the next morning to continue blood glucose management.

Medical nutrition therapy. See the section "Medical Nutrition Therapy and Education," at the end of this chapter, for a complete discussion of the medical nutrition therapy for type 1 diabetes. It covers starting and adjusting food and exercise plans. Figure 6.5 provides some essential information to be considered when a food plan is being developed.

Glucose monitoring: HbA_{1c} and SMBG. HbA_{1c} should be measured at the onset of treatment to serve as a baseline. It should then be repeated monthly to assess progress toward target. Self-monitoring of blood glucose should start at the onset of treatment to assess the effect of treatment (changes in blood glucose due to insulin dose and lifestyle changes), and should be timed to the action of insulin. In addition to testing prior to insulin administration to determine the appropriate dose, it is also necessary to assess the impact of meals and physical activity to determine whether adequate insulin has been administered. The minimum SMBG is four times per day (before each meal plus at bedtime, just before the patient has a snack). A bedtime snack is designed to prevent overnight hypoglycemia. To ensure insulin is working accurately, the patient should also measure BG at 3 AM at least once or twice per week and any time there are severe enough symptoms (night-time sweating or shaking) to wake up.

Education and behavioral issues. Diabetes education should begin immediately. A

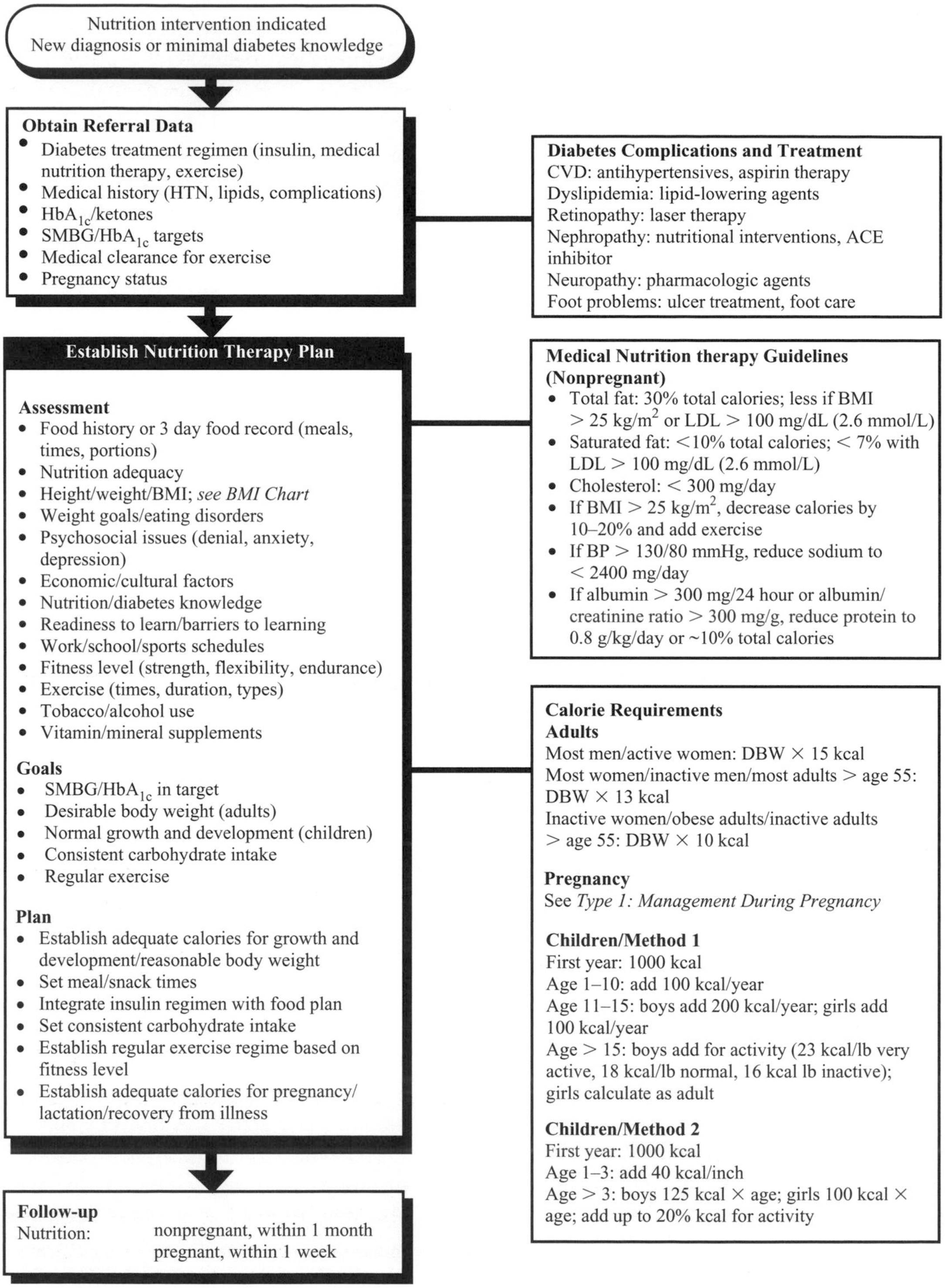

Nutrition intervention indicated
New diagnosis or minimal diabetes knowledge

Obtain Referral Data

- Diabetes treatment regimen (insulin, medical nutrition therapy, exercise)
- Medical history (HTN, lipids, complications)
- HbA_{1c}/ketones
- SMBG/HbA_{1c} targets
- Medical clearance for exercise
- Pregnancy status

Diabetes Complications and Treatment
CVD: antihypertensives, aspirin therapy
Dyslipidemia: lipid-lowering agents
Retinopathy: laser therapy
Nephropathy: nutritional interventions, ACE inhibitor
Neuropathy: pharmacologic agents
Foot problems: ulcer treatment, foot care

Establish Nutrition Therapy Plan

Assessment

- Food history or 3 day food record (meals, times, portions)
- Nutrition adequacy
- Height/weight/BMI; *see BMI Chart*
- Weight goals/eating disorders
- Psychosocial issues (denial, anxiety, depression)
- Economic/cultural factors
- Nutrition/diabetes knowledge
- Readiness to learn/barriers to learning
- Work/school/sports schedules
- Fitness level (strength, flexibility, endurance)
- Exercise (times, duration, types)
- Tobacco/alcohol use
- Vitamin/mineral supplements

Goals

- SMBG/HbA_{1c} in target
- Desirable body weight (adults)
- Normal growth and development (children)
- Consistent carbohydrate intake
- Regular exercise

Plan

- Establish adequate calories for growth and development/reasonable body weight
- Set meal/snack times
- Integrate insulin regimen with food plan
- Set consistent carbohydrate intake
- Establish regular exercise regime based on fitness level
- Establish adequate calories for pregnancy/lactation/recovery from illness

Medical Nutrition therapy Guidelines (Nonpregnant)

- Total fat: 30% total calories; less if BMI > 25 kg/m^2 or LDL > 100 mg/dL (2.6 mmol/L)
- Saturated fat: $<10\%$ total calories; $< 7\%$ with LDL > 100 mg/dL (2.6 mmol/L)
- Cholesterol: < 300 mg/day
- If BMI > 25 kg/m^2, decrease calories by 10–20% and add exercise
- If BP $> 130/80$ mmHg, reduce sodium to < 2400 mg/day
- If albumin > 300 mg/24 hour or albumin/creatinine ratio > 300 mg/g, reduce protein to 0.8 g/kg/day or ~10% total calories

Calorie Requirements
Adults
Most men/active women: DBW × 15 kcal
Most women/inactive men/most adults > age 55: DBW × 13 kcal
Inactive women/obese adults/inactive adults > age 55: DBW × 10 kcal

Pregnancy
See *Type 1: Management During Pregnancy*

Children/Method 1
First year: 1000 kcal
Age 1–10: add 100 kcal/year
Age 11–15: boys add 200 kcal/year; girls add 100 kcal/year
Age > 15: boys add for activity (23 kcal/lb very active, 18 kcal/lb normal, 16 kcal lb inactive); girls calculate as adult

Children/Method 2
First year: 1000 kcal
Age 1–3: add 40 kcal/inch
Age > 3: boys 125 kcal × age; girls 100 kcal × age; add up to 20% kcal for activity

Follow-up
Nutrition: nonpregnant, within 1 month
pregnant, within 1 week

Figure 6.5 Type 1 Diabetes Medical Nutrition Therapy DecisionPath

discussion of education issues is found in the section Patient Education Secion. Consider referring the patient to a diabetes educator.
The standards for patient education are very rigorous, encompassing survival skills, daily management, diet and exercise, adjustment to diabetes, and surveillance for acute, such as diabetic ketoacidosis, and long-term complications.

Insulin Stage 2/Adjust
R/N–0–R/N–0 or RA/N–0–RA/N–0

Fundamental to this phase is the slow adjustment to insulin to achieve glucose levels that avoid both hypoglycemia and hyperglycemia. Additionally, linkages to the different health professionals involved in diabetes care must be established. The nurse educator and dietitian are vital components of the health care team and, where feasible, should be involved in care. This is especially important in ambulatory management of diabetes. The guidelines for the adjustments begin on the second day (see Table 6.2). Along with arranging for both nurse and nutritionist follow-up, target blood glucose levels should be established.

Table 6.2 Insulin Stage 2 pattern adjustment guidelines (see Figure 6.6 for letter designations)

Time	< 70 mg/dL (< 3.9 mmol/L)	> 140 mg/dL (> 7.8 mmol/L)
AM or 3 AM	↓PM N 1–2 U (a,b)	↑PM N 1–2 U (a)
MIDDAY (MID)	↓AM R or RA 1–2 U (c,e)	↑AM R or RA 1–2 U (f,g)
PM	↓AM N 1–2 U (d,e)	↑AM N 1–2 U (f,h)
	< 100 mg/dL (< 5.6 mmol/L)	> 160 mg/dL (> 8.9 mmol/L)
BEDTIME (BT)	↓PM R or RA 1–2 U (e)	↑PM R or RA 1–2 U (f)

The target blood glucose level for patients aged > 12 years of age should initially be set as more than 50 per cent of the SMBG values between 120 mg/dL and 180 mg/dL (6.7 and 10 mmol/L),

Notes
a. Evaluate nocturnal hypoglycemia; check 3 AM BG
b. Consider increasing bedtime snack
c. Consider adding or adjusting mid-morning snack
d. Consider adding or adjusting afternoon snack
e. Evaluate whether previous exercise is causing hypoglycemia
f. Consider adding exercise
g. Consider decreasing mid-morning snack
h. Consider decreasing afternoon snack
i. No mid-morning snack usually needed with RA
j. No afternoon snack usually needed with RA
k. Consider adding AM N if long interval between midday and evening meal or afternoon hyperglycemia.

Calculate AM N as 50 per cent
MIDDAY R or RA dose.
Lower MIDDAY R or RA by 50 per cent
do not change AM R or RA.

Figure 6.6 Type 1 diabetes insulin adjustment considerations

with negative ketones. This will assure a slow and steady improvement, while minimizing the risk of relative hypoglycemia. This target should be sustained for the next several days. This interim target promotes the overall goal of gradually reducing blood glucose to near-normal levels. While any blood glucose within this range is acceptable, the goal is to reduce more than half of the blood glucose values. It is appropriate to react to episodic high blood glucose (> 250 mg/dL or 13.9 mmol/L) with small supplements of bolus insulin (immediate response). During the adjust phase, modification of insulin doses will be based on a 3 day pattern (termed pattern control) using SMBG data. Pattern control is based on the principle that each individual has a consistent set of glucose/insulin relationships. This consistency is characterized by predictable patterns in which specific insulin doses are related to known glycemic responses. For example, increasing the morning intermediate-acting insulin results consistently in a decrease in late afternoon (pre-evening meal) blood glucose levels. This initial data collection determines whether such a pattern can be easily identified. When, after trial and error (even within 3 days), such a pattern has been identified, treatment of type 1 diabetes may follow a predictable path. Generally, however, identifying a specific pattern takes substantially longer. Because of changes in food plan, exercise, seasons, and so on, patterns may change. Thus, glucose patterns should be continually reassessed.

Have the patient try to maintain a consistent food and exercise plan and make changes only to the insulin dose and amount. With the Insulin Stage 2 regimen, pattern response should anticipate the insulin action curves of both short-acting and intermediate-acting insulin. Recall that R peaks between 2 and 3 hours, but may last as long as 8 hours. In contrast, RA peaks at 1–1.5 hours and has a duration of approximately 3 hours. Finally, N peaks at 5–9 hours and lasts up to 22 hours. The problems likely to be encountered and suggested pattern responses are listed in Table 6.3. Pattern response is not limited to insulin adjustments alone. Be certain to consider adjustments in the food and exercise plan. Recall that exercise directly affects metabolic control depending on two factors: prandial state and available insulin.

At times, it may be necessary to use an immediate response when an acute situation such as hypoglycemia (insulin reaction) or hyperglycemia occurs. This happens whenever blood glucose is below 70 mg/dL (3.9 mmol/L) or greater than 240 mg/dL (13.3 mmol/L). Blood glucose levels are like measures of velocity; they are constantly changing. A blood glucose of 60 mg/dL (3.3 mmol/L) may be coming from 50 mg/dL (2.8 mmol/L) and heading toward 90 mg/dL (5.0 mmol/L) or the reverse. In such situations, a second blood glucose measurement 15–30 minutes after the first test should be performed to determine the direction of blood glucose. For patients experiencing hypoglycemia, providing juice or glucose tablets is advisable. Make certain the direction is known before subjecting the patient to a needless sudden rise in blood glucose. If the patient has a pattern of these events, either low or high blood glucose, be sure to consider pattern response for long-term corrections. Compensatory adjustments should be used to target very specific situations.

As the patient proceeds beyond the first several days, new targets should be set. Ultimately near-normal glycemia should be the goal. Using SDM should result in a monthly reduction in mean SMBG of between 15 and 30 mg/dL (0.8 and 1.7 mmol/L) and a parallel reduction in HbA_{1c} of 0.5–1 per cent. If these changes are not occurring, review the regimen with the patient. Refer to the Adherence Assessment Section, to systematically review possible explanations when there is a lack of improvement.

Follow-up data should include height; weight in light clothing without shoes; changes in schedule, food, and/or insulin; changes in exercise habits; review of SMBG records including frequency of testing, time of testing, and results; frequency of hypoglycemic episodes; current blood pressure level if hypertension is present; new or updated laboratory data; food records completed since initial visit or 24 hour food recall; food plan problems and/or concerns. During the adjust phase, therapy is modified to accelerate reaching a premeal target blood glucose between 70 and 140 mg/dL (3.9 and 7.8 mmol/L). Changes in insulin, synchronization of insulin with medical nutrition therapy, and other strategies may be enlisted to ensure further accelerated glucose reduction. SMBG four times per day and monthly

Table 6.3 Suggested pattern response for Insulin Stage 2

Problem	Insulin	Action
Midday hyperglycemia	R or RA	Increase AM dose
Late afternoon hyperglycemia	N	Increase AM dose
Fasting hyperglycemia	N	Increase PM dose
Bedtime hyperglycemia	R or RA	Increase PM dose
Mid-afternoon hypoglycemia	N	Decrease AM dose

office visits (contacts) are necessary in order to reduce blood glucose during this period. HbA_{1c} levels should begin to respond to the overall lower blood glucose during the first month. However, not until the end of the second month will the impact of the initial therapy be fully reflected in HbA_{1c} levels. From then on, at least 0.5–1 percentage point reduction should continue monthly until HbA_{1c} is within 1.0 percentage points of the upper limit of normal for patients >12 years of age. A change in regimen may be required if glycemic control is not achieved within a reasonable period of time.

Insulin Stage 2/Maintain
R/N–0–R/N–0 or RA/N–0–RA/N–0

The patient should have reached a level of metabolic control consistent with preventing microvascular complications (HbA_{1c} within 1.0 percentage points of the upper limit of normal). Implicit in SDM is the realization that not all patients can achieve near-normal blood glucose levels, thus supporting individualized metabolic goals. Assuming the patient has reached an agreed-upon goal, what changes in routine should be undertaken? Self-monitoring of blood glucose must still be carried out. During the maintenance phase, the SMBG pattern may be reduced as long as sufficient data are collected to ensure continued stability.

Some alternate patterns of SMBG are (1) every other day, (2) random measurements each day, and (3) slight reduction in the number of times per day. This should be done with the patient, to support and reward improved control. Under no circumstances should SMBG be stopped. In fact, there is good reason to argue for more vigorous testing to detect any deterioration in control. Early discovery makes it far easier to reinstitute tighter metabolic control.

Insulin therapy: Path A and Path B

If Insulin Stage 2 therapy fails to provide improved glycemic control after up to 12 months of adjusting treatment (or before if the maximum safe dose – 1.5 U/kg – has been reached), or if at any time the patient is experiencing persistent AM hyperglycemia and/or nocturnal hypoglycemia, move the patient to Insulin Stage 3. In addition, if at diagnosis the patient is willing to inject three times per day, consider starting with Insulin Stage 3. Remind the patient that almost everyone with type 1 diabetes has a better chance of achieving and maintaining near-normal fasting blood glucose levels, without overnight hypoglycemia, with N taken at bedtime compared with N taken before supper. The patient should have already seen the Master DecisionPath and, therefore, may agree to alternate therapies requiring increased injections and SMBG.

Now, two paths are available: Path 3A or Path 3B. Both should provide improved glycemic control (over two-injection regimens). The choice of one path over the other relates to the problems the patient is currently encountering and the desired level of flexibility in insulin administration. Path 3A slightly modifies the dose timing of Insulin Stage 2 by moving the evening meal intermediate-acting insulin (N) to bedtime. This should improve the fasting blood glucose level and reduce the likelihood of overnight hypoglycemia. Path 3B is an alternative that is used infrequently. It introduces a new insulin – prolonged intermediate acting (UL) – that requires some adjustments in testing and dosing. UL insulin provides basal insulin requirements (with a slight peak action for periods of 12 to 24 hours. It is combined with rapid- or short-acting insulin, which acts as the bolus or meal related insulin. The choice should be discussed fully with the patient. Once the decision to go to either 3A or 3B is made, changes in the insulin regimen should remain within the selected path. If the choice is 3A and it has failed to improve control, then moving to 4A may be needed. If the choice is 3B and this fails to improve control, changing to a four-injection regimen or an insulin infusion pump may be necessary.

Insulin Stage 3A

Three conditions that may have been encountered in Insulin Stage 2 can be addressed by Insulin Stage 3A:

- fasting blood glucose greater than target
- varying times and caloric intake in the evening meal
- nocturnal hypoglycemia

Fasting blood glucose may be above target for several reasons. The principal causes relate to overnight hepatic glucose output, high evening blood glucose, and early peak action of the PM intermediate-acting insulin. Excessive hepatic glucose output is a consequence of insulin deficiency and many investigators have argued that, along with β-cell destruction, liver involvement may result in desynchronized glucose secretion. This mis-timing of glucose release contributes to higher than normal levels of glycemia. The second factor, high evening blood glucose, is usually the result of proportionately higher carbohydrate intake at the evening meal and bedtime snack. The increased glucose load may not be overcome by the PM short-acting insulin, which results in high blood glucose at bedtime that is further exacerbated by the bedtime snack. Together these factors raise overnight blood glucose levels that are reflected in the fasting blood glucose measurement. Finally, nocturnal hypoglycemia may result from too much intermediate-acting insulin prior to the evening meal with insufficient carbohydrate overnight. Usually, the caloric and carbohydrate content of the evening meal along with either mistiming or improper insulin dosing result in high fasting blood glucose as well as nocturnal hypoglycemia. Moving the intermediate-acting insulin to 2 or 3 hours later should provide some resolution of these problems. Before doing this, however, be certain overinsulinization has not occurred. Overinsulinization is defined as > 1 U/kg for those under age 12 and over age 18. For adolescents and older teenagers, a level > 1.5 U/kg is considered overinsulinization. This age group normally requires more insulin. If this is suspected, consider reducing the total daily insulin dose before changing the therapy. Then recalculate the new daily dose as three injections with one-sixth of the total as N at bedtime.

Insulin Stage 3A/Start
R/N–0–R–N or RA/N–0–RA–N

To move from Insulin Stage 2 to Insulin Stage 3A, maintain the same total daily dose (assuming < 1.5 U/kg) and move the evening meal intermediate insulin (N) to bedtime (approximately 9–10 PM). When starting Insulin Stage 3A at diagnosis, the initial dose of insulin is calculated at 0.5 U/kg body weight with negative to moderate ketones and 0.7 U/kg with large ketones. The pre-breakfast dose is two-thirds the total dose, which is further divided into one-third R or RA and two-thirds N. One-sixth of the total insulin dose is R or RA administered before the evening meal and the remaining one-sixth total insulin dose is N taken at bedtime. Note that an SMBG test at bedtime is also necessary. Once initiated, adjusting both the evening R or RA and the morning R or RA will likely be required. Typically, the morning R or RA insulin will be reduced and the evening insulin will be increased.

For medical nutrition therapy see the discussion in "Medical Nutrition Therapy and Education," at the end of this chapter.

Insulin Stage 3A/Adjust
R/N–0–R–N or RA/N–0–RA–N

The key to the adjust phase is to identify blood glucose patterns that are consistently either too high or too low and adjust the appropriate insulin in order to achieve glycemic targets (see Table 6.4). With this regimen, generally it will be necessary to adjust the morning short-acting insulin. The first sign of too much morning R or RA is Midday hypoglycemia. Because these insulins have different peaks and durations, expect to find the hypoglycemia earlier with the RA than with the R. In fact, the R effect is often additive to the morning N, causing hypoglycemia in the mid-afternoon. Reduction in morning R or RA resolves this problem. It may also be necessary to readjust the breakfast meal and to move some calories to a mid-morning snack. A second problem is that pre-evening meal blood glucose may rise. If this is the

Table 6.4 Insulin Stage 3A pattern adjustment guidelines (see Figure 6.6 for letter designations)

Time	< 70 mg/dL (< 3.9 mmol/L)	> 140 mg/dL (> 7.8 mmol/L)
AM or 3 AM	↓BT N 1–2 U (a,b)	↑BT N 1–2 U (a)
MIDDAY (MID)	↓AM R or RA 1–2 U (c,e)	↑AM R or RA 1–2 U (f,g,i)
PM	↓AM N 1–2 U (d,e)	↑AM N 1–2 U (f,h)
	< 100 mg/dL (< 5.6 mmol/L)	> 160 mg/dL (> 8.9 mmol/L)
BEDTIME (BT)	↓PM R or RA 1–2 U (e)	↑PM R or RA 1–2 U (f)

situation, consider raising the morning N. This tends to increase the duration of the peak action. Alternatively, if the morning N leads to mid-afternoon hypoglycemia, then lower the morning dose. However, if the bedtime N results in lower fasting blood glucose levels, the insulin requirements during the daytime may need to be reduced. If the PM blood glucose is less than 70 mg/dL (3.9 mmol/L), consider lowering the morning N. Other factors, such as exercise, may also lower blood glucose. Exercise in the mid-afternoon should be closely monitored with SMBG before and after activity.

Be careful not to "chase" insulin with changes in the food plan. Attempt to keep food consistent initially. Only after changes in insulin are exhausted should changes in the food plan be tried.

Further adjustments are related to the bedtime (9–10 PM) blood glucose levels. These are affected most by the evening meal and the amount of short-acting insulin. Blood glucose at bedtime should be between 100 mg/dL (5.6 mmol/L) and 160 mg/dL (8.9 mmol/L). Consider adding more R or RA before the evening meal or changing the meal content. Hyperglycemia at bedtime often carries over, resulting in a high fasting blood glucose.

Insulin Stage 3A/Maintain
R/N–0–R–N or RA/N–0–RA–N

Large proportions of patients benefit from this regimen and may achieve a level of glycemic control not possible with a two-injection regimen. Improvement may be gradual at first. Once the patient has stabilized at near-normal levels of glycemic control, alterations in SMBG may be appropriate. Using exercise and food plan to enhance stability is an option at this point. With two different insulins and three time periods, minor adjustments are likely to be needed. Make certain sufficient information is available from SMBG to ensure maintaining treatment goals.

If the target blood glucose cannot be stabilized or if the maintain phase cannot be held, consider dropping or reducing N in the morning and adding regular or rapid-acting insulin at Midday. Note that for patients using RA in the morning the AM intermediate-acting insulin cannot be dropped because it provides a basal insulin throughout the late morning and afternoon. In this case, consider switching to glargine (G) insulin which is given as one injection either in the evening or in the morning.

Physiologic Insulin Stage 4A

Balancing basal and bolus insulin requirements in a physiological manner is the goal of Stage 4A. To accomplish this the intermediate-acting insulin N or the long-acting insulin G is used as the basal or background insulin. R or RA is used as the bolus insulin. In general, such regimens tend to require less total insulin and are thus least likely to result in overinsulinization.

Physiologic Insulin Stage 4A/Start
R/(N)–R–R–N or RA/N–RA–RA–N
R–R–R–G or RA–RA–RA–G

The first decision is whether to continue with the Stage 3A insulins and make some minor adjustments or to move directly to RA–RA–RA–G. In the former, consider the overall daily dose and check for overinsulinization. If the overall daily dose is < 1.5 U/kg, the new regimen will simply add a mid-day insulin injection and reduce the amount of AM intermediate- and short-acting insulin. If the decision is to move to a regimen with G as background insulin, then a recalculation of the dosing will be necessary. This provides a more manageable approach for adjustments to meal related hyperglycemia and mid-afternoon hypoglycemia.

With respect to therapies that continue with N and R or RA, the insulin action curves for Stage 4A produce a pattern that initially optimizes the short-acting insulins for both Midday and mid-afternoon glycemic control. Retention of the evening N should provide for overnight basal insulin requirements. Because there is no endogenous insulin production in type 1 diabetes, the option of continuing N at breakfast is present to overcome any lack of insulin late in the morning. Note that AM N is required with the use of rapid-acting insulin. Recalculating the insulin dose is required. For regimens using R insulin, drop the morning N. Next, calculate the Midday R at 20 per cent of the morning N. The Midday dose may initially prove to be too low unless the individual consistently eats a small lunch. Next, increase the morning R or RA by 1 unit to compensate for lack of N at breakfast. If currently using morning N then reduce (do not completely drop) the dose by 50 per cent. Next, adjust doses following the insulin adjustment guidelines for Stage 4A. Table 6.5 shows the recalculation based on 44 total units of insulin. Note that the DecisionPath shows an exact percent for each dose. This is a guide to enable the patient to experiment with the dosage without experiencing hypoglycemia in mid-afternoon. This, of course, assumes the pre-lunch blood glucose is within target range. Two different examples are shown. The first continues with R and drops N in the morning. The R has a long enough action curve to cover some of the late morning. In contrast, the second example replaces the R with RA and continues morning N at half the original dose. This allows for coverage late in the morning and mid-afternoon.

If switching to glargine as the basal insulin, then start bedtime G as 80 per cent of the total N (both morning and bedtime doses) from Stage 3A. Stop AM and PM N and add a Midday R or RA. The starting dose of Midday insulin is generally based on 50 per cent of the morning N. If no morning N, then use the same amount as is used for the morning R or RA. Adjust following the 4A Pattern Adjustments.

Physiologic Insulin Stage 4A/Adjust
R/(N)–R–R–N or RA/N–RA–RA–N
R–R–R–G or RA–RA–RA–G

The first target should be the fasting blood glucose (see Table 6.6). Note that the evening N or G is usually the key insulin. If the fasting blood glucose level is below target, reduce the N or G. If it is above target, increase the N or G. Use 1–2 units of insulin at a time. Wait 3 days after each change to determine the effect. These adjustments are straightforward for the patient.

If overnight hypoglycemia is suspected, have the patient test blood glucose at 3 AM. If confirmed and the patient is using N insulin, switch to G if possible; otherwise, reduce N and/or provide a bedtime snack. If the patient is already

Table 6.5 Example of conversion from Insulin Stage 3A to Insulin Stage 4A

	AM	Midday	PM	Bedtime	Dose
Stage 3A	10R/20N	0	7R	7N	44 units
Stage 4A	11R	10R	7R	7N	35 units
or	11R/10N	4R	8R	7N	40 units
or	10RA/10N	4RA	7RA	7N	38 units

Table 6.6 Physiologic Insulin Stage 4A pattern adjustment guidelines (see Figure 6.6 for letter designations)

Time	< 70 mg/dL (< 3.9 mmol/L)	> 140 mg/dL (> 7.8 mmol/L)
AM or 3 AM	↓BT N 1–2 U (a,b)	↑BT N 1–2 U (a)
MIDDAY (MID)	↓AM R or RA 1–2 U (c,e)	↑AM R or RA 1–2 U (f,g,i)
PM	↓MID R or RA 1–2 U (d,e)	↑MID R or RA 1–2 U (f,h,j,k)
	< 100 mg/dL (< 5.6 mmol/L)	> 160 mg/dL (> 8.9 mmol/L)
BEDTIME (BT)	↓PM R or RA 1–2 U (e)	↑PM R or RA 1–2 U (f)

treated with G, consider reducing the dose, adding a bedtime snack, or moving G to AM.

Since R or RA insulin is used in this regimen to cover each meal, blood glucose levels measured prior to the next meal should guide changes in the R or RA insulin dose. For patients using RA, blood glucose should be determined 2 hours post-meal to guide changes in the insulin dose. In this as in other insulin regimens, medical nutrition therapy can aid tremendously in making adjustments. Since identifying the problem also pinpoints the cause, begin by identifying the consistently highest blood glucose. Change insulin dosage first, then food plan. Once the adjustment has improved control for the targeted blood glucose, go to the next highest blood glucose. SMBG is important here as it is the best data source. Be sure to increase testing if necessary. Expect adjustments to take several weeks before they begin to affect overall glycemic control.

Physiologic Insulin Stage 4A/Maintain
R/(N)–R–R–N or RA/N–RA–RA–N
R–R–R–G or RA–RA–RA–G

Because Stage 4A relies heavily on short- or rapid-acting insulin to cover each meal, fine changes (1–2 units) from time to time can be made and should be encouraged. If the amount of food or timing changes, R or RA can be easily adjusted. This is also true for evening N or G. In all cases, use SMBG to determine when to change insulin dose and to measure overall effectiveness.

Insulin Stage 3B

Insulin Stage 3B introduces long-acting ultralente (UL), which requires some adjustments in testing and dosing. This prolonged intermediate-acting insulin provides basal or background insulin requirements, with R or RA insulin used to cover each meal. It is an alternative to using G insulin as basal with three instead of four injections per day. The choice should be discussed fully with the patient.

Human UL has only a slight peak action. Review the action curves for UL and short-acting insulin in Chapter 3. Note the necessity to monitor blood glucose before each meal. Since this is a new therapy, it is advisable to initially increase SMBG to six times per day to obtain blood glucose levels at mid-afternoon and at 2–3 AM.

Insulin Stage 3B/Start
R/(UL)–R–R/UL–0 or RA/UL–RA–RA/UL–0

UL insulin is generally given as two injections totaling 50 per cent of the daily insulin requirement, based on the current insulin requirements (See Table 6.7). One-third is given in the morning with R or RA insulin and two-thirds is given PM with pre-meal R or RA. The rapid- or short-acting insulin comprises 50 per cent of the total requirements, distributed as 35 per cent AM, 25 per cent Midday, and 40 per cent PM.

If the patient is using only UL insulin in the evening, then 40 per cent of the total insulin requirement is given as PM UL, with the remaining 60 per cent distributed as RA or R with 35 per cent AM, 25 per cent Midday, and 40 per cent PM. Thus, 60 per cent of the insulin is in the form of short-acting insulin to compensate for postprandial rise in blood glucose, and 40 per cent is in the form of UL to meet basal insulin requirements. When considering Insulin Stage 3B,

Table 6.7 Example of conversion from Insulin Stage 2 to Insulin Stage 3B

	AM	Midday	PM	Bedtime	Dose
Insulin Stage 2	10R/20N	0	7R/7N	0	44 units
Insulin Stage 3B	9R/6UL	7R	10R/12UL	0	44 units

RA may be substituted at the same dose for R.

re-examine the total daily insulin requirements to make certain overinsulinization (> 1.0 U/kg in under 12 and over 18 year olds, > 1.5 U/kg in 12–18 year olds) has not occurred. Adjustments should be easy to calculate. If the regimen still results in afternoon hypoglycemia and pre-evening meal hyperglycemia, consider replacing UL with G given at bedtime.

Insulin Stage 3B/Adjust
R/(UL)–R–R/UL–0 or RA/UL–RA–RA/UL–0

Daily adjustments of R or RA insulin in Insulin Stage 3B are more frequent than in Insulin Stage 2 (see Table 6.8). Since ultralente has only a slight peak action, adjustments to this prolonged intermediate-acting insulin should be few and should be at a low dose. Think of ultralente as providing a base for R or RA insulin when making an adjustment. The usual problem confronted after initiation of this regimen is elevated post-prandial blood glucose (measured before the next meal).

Adjustment of R or RA is straightforward since its action is within a narrow time period. For all post-prandial blood glucose measurements, consider the interaction between the meal and R or RA insulin. When post-prandial hyperglycemia is present, increase the R or RA immediately preceding that meal and instruct the patient to test blood glucose 2–4 hours after starting the meal. Do not adjust the morning UL unless the patient is known to consistently skip breakfast. In that case reduce morning R or RA and increase by 1–2 units UL in the morning. Fine adjustments in this regimen should significantly improve blood glucose levels. For more persistent problems such as overnight hyperglycemia or hypoglycemia, adjust the UL or consider switching to 4A. For morning hyperglycemia, for example, add 1–2 units PM ultralente. Overall control should improve within 1–2 weeks.

In the absence of improvement, many explanations are possible. The first is to determine whether the patient is taking the short-acting insulin as prescribed and is testing frequently. If the patient is not following the regimen, consider re-education. Often patients require a period of retraining when a totally new regimen is introduced. This is especially true when more work is required. Emphasize the benefits of Insulin Stage 3B in terms of flexibility, more varied food plan, and reduction in overnight hypoglycemia. Use the pattern adjustments in the Insulin Stage 3B DecisionPath, summarized in Table 6.8, as a guide for pinpointing problems.

Insulin Stage 3B/Maintain
R/(UL)–R–R/UL–0 or RA/UL–RA–RA/UL–0

As with the other stages, maintaining the goal allows for a period of fine-tuning. Reducing SMBG should be accompanied by assurance of sufficient information to confirm that the patient has remained stabilized. Limit reduction in SMBG to maintain at least one test before each insulin injection. Providing patients with this information permits them to continue a flexible schedule while at the same time controlling blood glucose levels. Since the basal dose remains relatively stable, changes in this phase should be limited to the short-acting insulin. If the patient cannot maintain stability and is moving back into the adjustment phase, consider an insulin infusion pump. See the next page for details.

Table 6.8 Insulin Stage 3B pattern adjustment guidelines (see letter designations below)

Time	< 70 mg/dL (< 3.9 mmol/L)	> 140 mg/dL (> 7.8 mmol/L)
AM or 3 AM	↓BT UL 1–2 U (a,b)	↑BT UL 1–2 U (a)
MIDDAY (MID)	↓AM R or RA 1–2 U (c,e)	↑AM R or RA 1–2 U (f,g)
PM	↓MID R or RA 1–2 U (d,e)	↑MID R or RA 1–2 U (f,h)
	< 100 mg/dL (< 5.6 mmol/L)	> 160 mg/dL (> 8.9 mmol/L)
BEDTIME (BT)	↓PM R or RA 1–2 U (e)	↑PM R or RA 1–2 U (f)

Notes

a. Evaluate nocturnal hypoglycemia; check 3 AM BG
b. Consider increasing bedtime snack
c. Consider adding or adjusting mid-morning snack
d. Consider adding or adjusting afternoon snack
e. Evaluate whether previous exercise is causing hypoglycemia
f. Consider adding exercise
g. Consider decrease in mid-morning snack
h. Consider decrease in afternoon snack
i. AM UL is a basal insulin and usually does not require adjusing. If PM BG > target due to a long interval between midday and evening meal, consider increasing UL by 1–2 units

Co-management option. SDM emphasizes co-managing the individual with diabetes by seeking advice and assistance from diabetes specialists when therapies are not working. This does not mean abandoning the patient. The specialist should be familiar with SDM and understand the progression through the stages that the patient has already completed. The referral should be very specific. Details on the history of the disease and the progression through the therapies are important, if the advice is to be useful. In some cases, the therapies may have been exhausted and the specialist may confirm that the limit of therapy has been reached. If the decision is to place the patient on an insulin infusion pump or an experimental therapy, make certain that you are aware of the basis for the decision, understand how it works, and are clear as to your role once the patient is in treatment.

Insulin infusion pump

For some patients, continuous subcutaneous insulin infusion (CSII) may be a necessary consequence of failing to achieve control, lifestyle, or other factors expressed by the patient (see Photo 6.1). CSII or the pump requires a longer baseline period (1 month), more closely supervised therapeutic phase by a diabetes care team, and greater surveillance during stabilization.

Insulin Pump/Start

In preparation for CSII, verify the daily excursions in glycemic control so both basal and

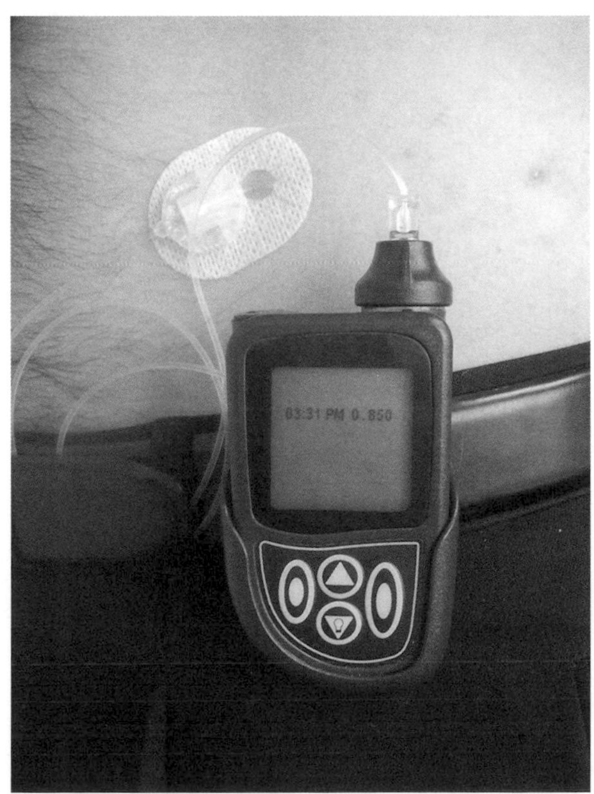

Photo 6.1 Insulin pump

supplemental doses can be calculated. Review the DecisionPaths for the infusion pump before referring the patient to a specialist (see Figure 6.7). Make certain the specialist is following a DecisionPath (either the one provided or another one) that has been shared with you. Make certain the patient has undergone careful education and demonstration on the pump device. Only after the patient demonstrates the ability to work the device should therapy be initiated. Remind the patient

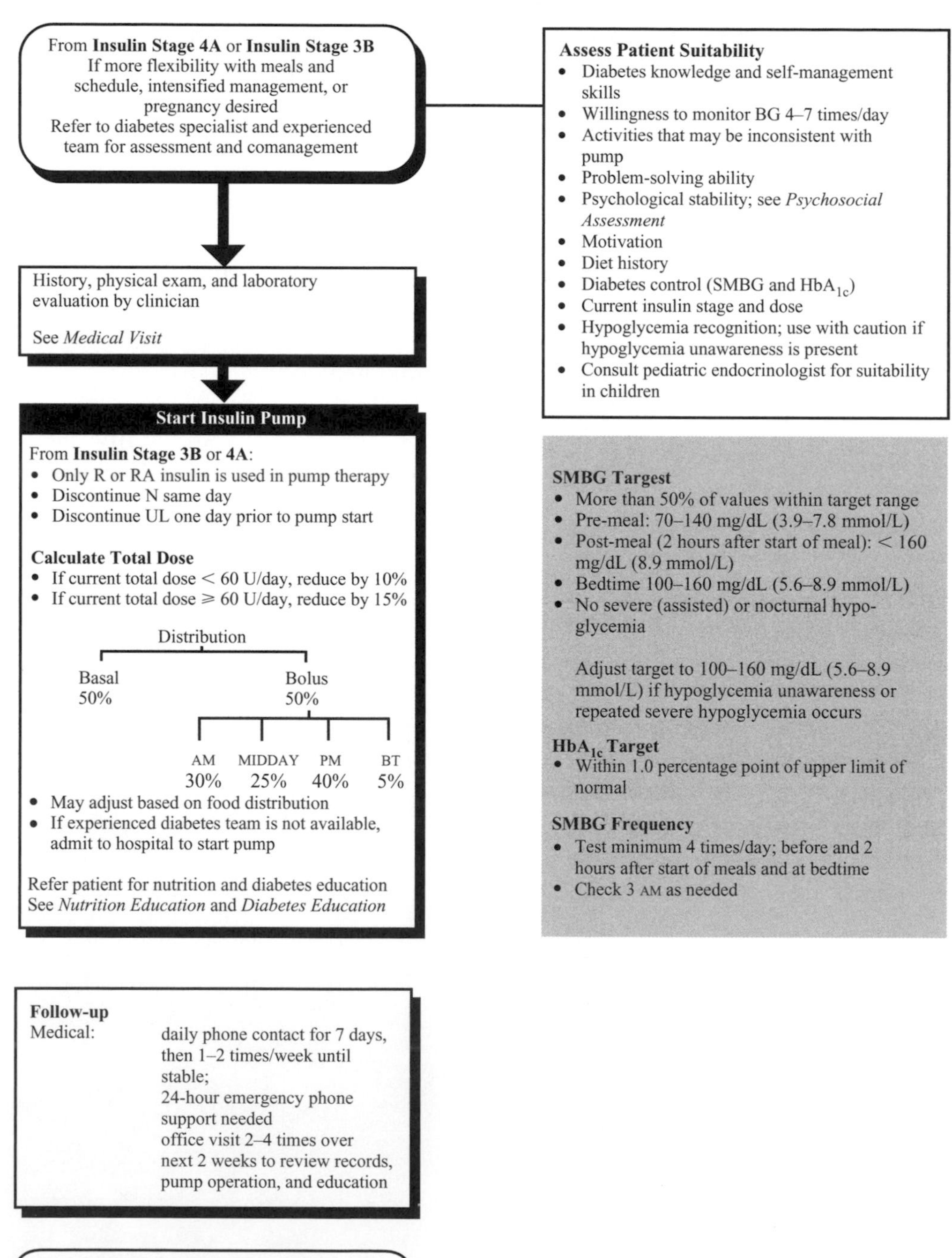

Figure 6.7 Insulin Pump/Start DecisionPath

that SMBG must be performed at least before each bolus dose.

To begin, discontinue the basal insulin on the previous evening. Using the current total daily dose as a basis, if the dose is 60 units or less, reduce this by 10 per cent. If it is greater than 60 units, reduce the total daily dose by 20 per cent. Divide the new dose into 50 per cent basal and 50 per cent bolus. Further divide the bolus into four periods: 30 per cent AM, 25 per cent mid, 40 per cent PM, and 5 per cent BT, or based on carbohydrate intake. Maintain close contact.

Insulin Pump/Adjust and Insulin Pump/Maintain

Start with determining whether to adjust the basal or bolus doses. Adjustments to bolus doses based on a pattern of persistent hyperglycemia occurring after meals should be confirmed by SMBG. If a pattern of hyperglycemia occurs, adjustments in increments of 1–4 units should be made (see Figure 6.8). If they are needed, make certain a discernible pattern is found. While as much as a 50 per cent increase may be necessary, make certain this is done over time. Begin all adjustments to basal insulin 2 hours before the blood

Basal Adjustments
- Fewer adjustments once stabilized, usually only if significant changes in lifestyle

Alternate Basal Adjustments
- Overnight common and necessary if AM and/or 3 AM BG > target
- start 2 hours before BG rise and continue for 4–6 hours
- As much as 50% increase in basal rate may be necessary
- Adjust based on pattern over 2 consecutive days; see table below

TIME	< 80 mg/dL (< 4.4 mmol/L)	> 140 mg/dL (> 7.8 mmol/L)
AM or 3AM	↓by 0.1–0.2 U/hr	↑by 0.1–0.2 U/hr

Compensatory Adjustments
- Pre-meal correction of BG value
- Temporary correction of a low or high BG
- May be added or subtracted based on BG, food, or exercise
- Used **with caution** at bedtime

Blood Glucose Adjustment in mg/dL (mmol/L)	Bolus
< 70 (3.9)	↓1–2 U
140–200 (7.8–11.1)	↑1 U
201–250 (11.2–13.9)	↑2 U
251–300 (13.9–16.7)	↑3 U
> 300 (16.7)	↑≥4 U

How to Use This Table
1. Find the pattern of blood glucose problem (column)
2. Identify time of day (row) pattern occurs
3. Where the column and row intersect, see recommended changes
4. See notes for additional considerations

Notes
a. Evaluate nocturnal hypoglycemia; check 3 AM BG
b. Consider increasing bedtime snack
c. Consider adding or adjusting mid-morning snack
d. Consider adding or adjusting afternoon snack
e. Evaluate whether previous exercise is causing hypoglycemia
f. Consider adding exercise
g. Consider decrease in mid-morning snack
h. Consider decrease in afternoon snack
i. Consider increasing alternate basal overnight; may need to decrease BT R or RA
j. Consider decreasing alternate basal overnight

Bolus Adjustments
- Based on 3-day pattern of consistent compensatory changes; see table below
- Determine which insulin is responsible

	< 70 mg/dL (< 3.9 mmol/L)	> 140 mg/dL (> 7.8 mmol/L)
AM or 3 AM	↓BT 1–2 U (b,e,j)	↑BT 1–2 U (b,i)
MIDDAY (MID)	↓AM 1–2 U (c,e)	↑AM 1–2 U (f,g)
PM	↓MID 1–2 U (d,e)	↑MID 1–2 U (f,h)
	< 100 mg/dL (< 5.6 mmol/L)	> 160 mg/dL (> 8.9 mmol/L)
BEDTIME (BT)	↓PM 1–2 U (b,e)	↑PM 1–2 U (f)

Figure 6.8 Insulin pump adjustment guidelines

glucose rises and continue the dose for 4–6 hours. For example, some patients with type 1 diabetes experience a dramatic rise in blood glucose between 4 AM and 6 AM (called the dawn phenomenon). To adjust for this, increase basal insulin starting at 2 AM through 6 AM. The patient should reach the maintain phase rapidly on pump therapy. If not, consider problems with adherence to the regimen (see the "Adherence Assessment" section in this chapter). Work closely with the specialist for all patients on pump therapy. This complex treatment modality has many technical issues to address.

Insulin Stage 1

Under some circumstances, a patient presents having been prescribed a single injection of intermediate-acting insulin or intermediate insulin combined with R insulin given AM. While it is becoming rarer to find such patients with type 1 diabetes, it does occur and must be addressed. As with all other stages, the first requirement is to make certain sufficient baseline data have been collected to determine whether a single injection has been and continues to be effective. If a patient presents on a single injection of mixed insulin, consider whether to adjust the current dose or to split the dose into two injections (AM and PM).

The principal reason for single-injection therapy is that the patient has normal fasting blood glucose. Thus, any decision to alter the AM dose is related to the PM blood glucose levels. If the PM blood glucose is greater than 150 mg/dL (8.3 mmol/L), consider increasing both the short-acting and intermediate-acting insulin dosages. This can be done only if there is no apparent hypoglycemia mid- to late afternoon (the time of the mixed insulin's peak action). Hypoglycemia is a signal to consider split dosage.

Insulin Stage 1/Adjust

N(R)–0–0–0

Unless the patient presents with verified self-monitored blood glucose values for the preceding month, a recent glycosylated hemoglobin, or other relevant data related to glycemic control, additional data must be collected. The patient should be placed on a memory-based meter and asked to test four times per day for at least 1 week before considering a change in the current regimen. Additionally, an HbA_{1c} should be assessed to gauge the past level of glycemic control. Overnight blood glucose values at 2 AM, 3 AM, and 4 AM on different nights should provide additional data. In elderly patients with type 1 diabetes, the same situation may be necessary, especially among the very old, who often skip meals. In this case, careful attention to post-prandial blood glucose values is necessary. In either extreme, baseline data must be collected before making any changes in therapy.

Therapies based on a single injection of intermediate-acting insulin are, in general, prescribed to newly diagnosed type 1 diabetes and more than likely during the earliest stages. For patients presenting on a single injection of intermediate-acting insulin, if fasting blood glucose is normal and pre-evening meal blood glucose is high, one option is to add short-acting insulin to the AM injection. However, it is very likely that the single-injection therapy will be transient in type 1 management, thus SDM strongly urges moving the patient to a regimen of two injections of mixed insulin (Insulin Stage 2). This regimen is more physiologic and it will be easier to adjust to achieve and maintain glycemic targets.

Considerations for adjusting and maintaining treatment

Throughout the adjust phase, the goal is to identify problems (glycemic control or lifestyle issues) and provide interventions to address them. To accomplish this, general guidelines are necessary. During this phase the target glucose has been narrowed to a range of 70–140 mg/dL (3.9–7.8 mmol/L) pre-meal, with negative ketones. (Individual targets may need to be identified, particularly for children under age 6 and elderly patients.) If this target has been reached and verified by SMBG data from a memory-based meter, continue with pattern response. Follow the DecisionPath and note the following aspects of pattern response.

Up to 60 per cent of patients with type 1 diabetes may experience a significant drop in insulin requirements within the first year following diagnosis. The period may last as long as 6 months and has been referred to as the "Honeymoon Period." For some patients this may require discontinuing the evening insulin injection while maintaining the AM dose at a very low level (1–2 units). In no cases has the honeymoon period resulted in complete remission. Some practitioners omit all insulin during this period. Generally, however, insulin in low doses should be continued for two purposes: (1) to maintain the injection and self-testing schedule and skills, and (2) to anticipate the end of this phase and return to overt diabetes.

Regardless of the therapy, the maintain phase refers to a period during which it is agreed by both provider and patient that no further major changes in therapy are forthcoming. This decision should be based on optimized glucose control for the patient who is satisfied with flexibility related to his or her daily schedule. During the maintain phase, while minor adjustments are likely, significant changes in treatment should not be necessary. To confirm stability SMBG must be continued. Under no circumstances should SMBG be halted.

Management of acute complications

Few events in diabetes management raise as much concern for both the patient and the physician as diabetic ketoacidosis (DKA), hypoglycemia, and illness. This section provides an overview of each of these conditions. *For comprehensive DKA management, see Chapter 10.* Preventing these events, following a step-by-step procedure when they occur, and making certain that they do not occur again are integral to diabetes management. In most instances, DKA and hypoglycemia are preventable. Perhaps more than any other aspect of diabetes management, DKA has benefited most from the introduction of SMBG. There are, however, always exceptions.

Managing diabetic ketoacidosis

When the individual with confirmed type 1 diabetes is first diagnosed, it is important to determine whether ketoacidosis is present as it can result in a medical emergency within less than 24 hours should it remain untreated. DKA is a combination of three events – hyperglycemia, acidosis, and ketosis – all of which result from insulin deficiency. It generally begins with an overproduction of glucose by the liver and kidneys. During insulin deficiency, hepatic and renal glucose production can reach twice normal. This is accompanied by reduction in peripheral tissue uptake of glucose. The most common cause of this reduction in peripheral uptake is insulin deficiency combined with increased counter-regulatory hormone activity. This cycle is further exacerbated by the reduced efficiency of any residual insulin when a state of severe hyperglycemia is present, thus leading to still higher levels of blood glucose. Lack of insulin also leads to increased lipolysis and a rise in ketones exacerbated by the counter-regulatory hormones: glucagon, catecholamines, and cortisol. Finally, due to glycosuria, there is a profound and dangerous loss of fluids, sodium, and potassium, resulting in electrolyte depletion.

Although mild DKA can be managed in an outpatient setting, close monitoring and rapid response are necessary and inpatient management is usually preferred. DKA is based on clinical symptoms, physical examination, and laboratory data. The presence of ketones alone does not necessarily meet the criteria for DKA. Signs of DKA include polyuria, polydipsidia, and polyphagia accompanied by abdominal discomfort, Kussmaul breathing (deep/heavy breathing), vomiting, dehydration, and acetone on the breath. The patients may appear confused or lethargic. Laboratory tests show serum glucose > 250 mg/dL (13.9 mmol/L), pH < 7.3, and bicarbonate < 15 mEq/L. Both urine and serum ketones are positive.

Treatment aims at re-hydration (including stabilized BP and fluid input/output), stabilization of blood glucose (< 200 mg/dL or 11.1 mmol/L), electrolytes (serum bicarbonate $\geqslant 18$ mEq/l), and venous pH > 7.3. Initial treatment is with IV isotonic saline and continuous insulin infusion until metabolic control is regained and serum potassium can be measured. If needed potassium can be added and need for bicarbonate can be assessed. The initial symptoms are usually resolved within 24 hours.

For newly diagnosed patients, once DKA has been successfully treated, initiate Stage 2 or 3A insulin therapy. Use the same formulation as would have been carried out in the absence of DKA. If in an outpatient setting, the patient should not be permitted to leave until survival skills have been taught. Because DKA is a traumatic experience, especially at diagnosis of type 1 diabetes, learning even survival skills at this moment is less than optimal. Make certain that as part of follow-up the survival skills are repeated during the next office visit.

Persistent episodes of DKA

Some patients have repeated episodes of DKA, especially during the first year following diagnosis. This is especially the case in adolescence. Frequently this can be traced to a misunderstanding of how to manage diabetes. Self-monitored blood glucose must be considered an integral part of diabetes management along with ketone testing. Most DKA is preventable. When repeated events occur and education does not seem to be the issue, suspect underlying psychological or social factors to play a role. Referral to a counselor or psychologist, especially after assessment by a diabetes educator, is appropriate. Most adolescents outgrow the dysfunctional behavior resulting in DKA.

Managing hypoglycemia

Low blood glucose (hypoglycemia) is generally the result of overinsulinization and/or not eating often injecting insulin. The first step is to determine whether the patient is having a seizure or is unconscious. If either condition occurs, immediate medical attention is necessary. If SMBG data are available, measure the blood glucose first to make certain the level is low. If SMBG data are not immediately available, administer glucagon and follow by obtaining a blood glucose value as soon as possible. Thereafter monitor blood glucose closely. When the hypoglycemic reaction is controlled, investigate the cause of hypoglycemia. In general, too much insulin, too little food, or no adjustment in food intake or insulin doses when exercising leads to a severe reaction.

If the patient is conscious, the next question is whether the patient requires assistance to overcome the hypoglycemia. Again, measure blood glucose to confirm hypoglycemia. Some patients experience hypoglycemic symptoms when the blood glucose drops rapidly, for example, from 270 mg/dL (15 mmol/L) to 120 mg/dL (6.7 mmol/L). These symptoms should be treated, but they generally do not need medical attention or glucagon.

If the patient is truly hypoglycemic and needs assistance but is conscious and able to swallow, administer fruit juice, a commercial glucose gel, or some form of carbohydrate (regular soda pop, etc.). Once stabilized, investigate the cause of the hypoglycemic episode. Consider re-educating the patient and re-evaluating the food and exercise plan, and insulin dosage and timing.

If patients are having mild to moderate hypoglycemia in which they are symptomatic but able to manage by themselves, again SMBG should be reinforced. Documenting the blood glucose levels during hypoglycemic episodes is necessary. Also, it is important to determine the cognitive state of the individual during such episodes. They should be able to report the symptoms and the action they took to overcome the hypoglycemia.

Treatment of mild to moderate hypoglycemia generally includes ingesting 15 grams of carbohydrate and retesting blood glucose. When the blood glucose reaches 100 mg/dL (5.6 mmol/L), it is safe to cease treatment and monitor every 2 hours until the next meal. The best way to ascertain the response to counter hypoglycemia is SMBG. It is also a good learning tool for future episodes. Remind the patient that glucose is a velocity measure and thus constantly changing as opposed to a static physiologic measure. To rapidly reach a steady state, the individual must counteract the effect of insulin with food. Injectable glucagon may be used to counter hypoglycemia when the person does not respond to repeated treatment with carbohydrate, or is unable to swallow safely. Persistent hypoglycemia should be treated vigorously in consultation with an endocrinologist specializing in diabetes.

Preventing hypoglycemia requires careful reassessment of the possible contributing factors: overinsulinization (generally > 1 U/kg), overaggressive insulin supplements, starvation, increased activity, alcohol intake, and intercurrent illness. To prevent the onset of hypoglycemia, SMBG should be performed at least four times each day. Multiple-injection regimens relying on rapid-acting insulins should replace two-injection regimens.

Management during illness

Blood glucose levels normally increase during illness due to release of stress hormones without regard to prandial state. Patients should be instructed to maintain their usual food plan and insulin regimen. Noncaloric fluid intake (water, broth, diet soda pop) may be increased. If patients have nausea or are vomiting, initiate their sick day food plan (if available). Increase SMBG and urine ketone testing to every 2–4 hours. If SMBG > 240 mg/dL (13.3 mmol/L), patients may have to supplement their current regimen with R or RA insulin (10 per cent of total daily dose) every 2–4 hours as necessary. Patients should be instructed to contact their provider if SMBG > 240 mg/dL (13.3 mmol/L) and/or they develop moderate to large ketones. Since diabetic ketoacidosis can occur at any time, frequent telephone contact may be required to prevent the illness from becoming a medical emergency (see Chapter 9). Very ill patients may need to be managed in a medical facility if the following occur: SMBG persistently above 400 mg/dL (22.2 mmol/L), large ketones for more than 6 hours, persistent vomiting or diarrhea, or inadequate phone contact.

Type 1 diabetes and pregnancy

For a full discussion of preconception planning and treatment of type 1 diabetes in pregnancy see Chapter 7. In general, these principles should always be followed.

- All women actively seeking to become pregnant should be at near-normal blood glucose prior to conception.
- Sexually active women should use some form of contraception until they desire to conceive and have documented adequate blood glucose control.

Management of women with diabetes prior to pregnancy (pregestational) requires very close surveillance (see Figure 6.9). A complete discussion of the significant management issues can be found in the section on diabetes in pregnancy. In Figure 6.10, note the use of various team members, reliance on close surveillance for complications, and attention to diet.

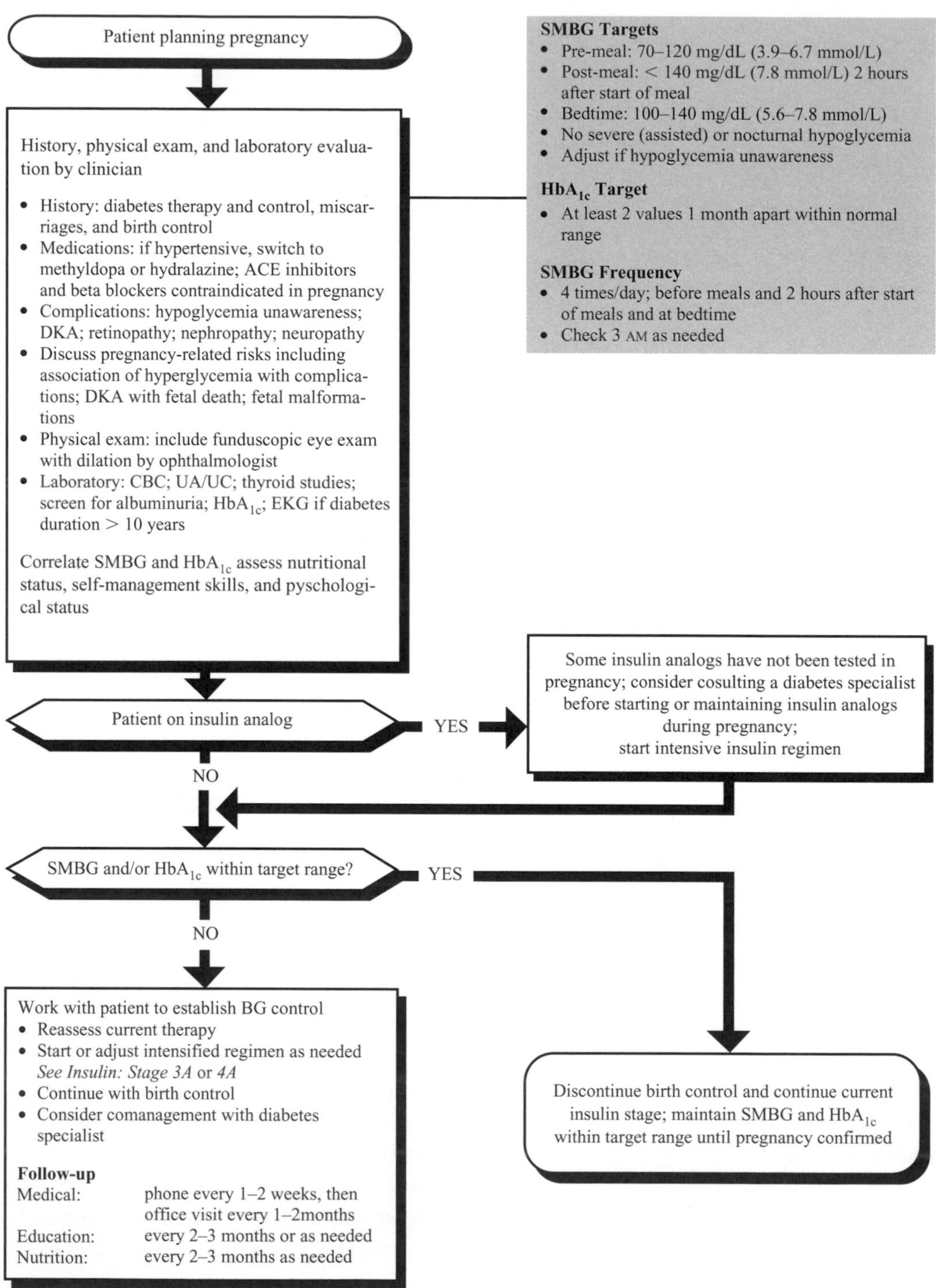

Figure 6.9 Preconception Diabetes Management

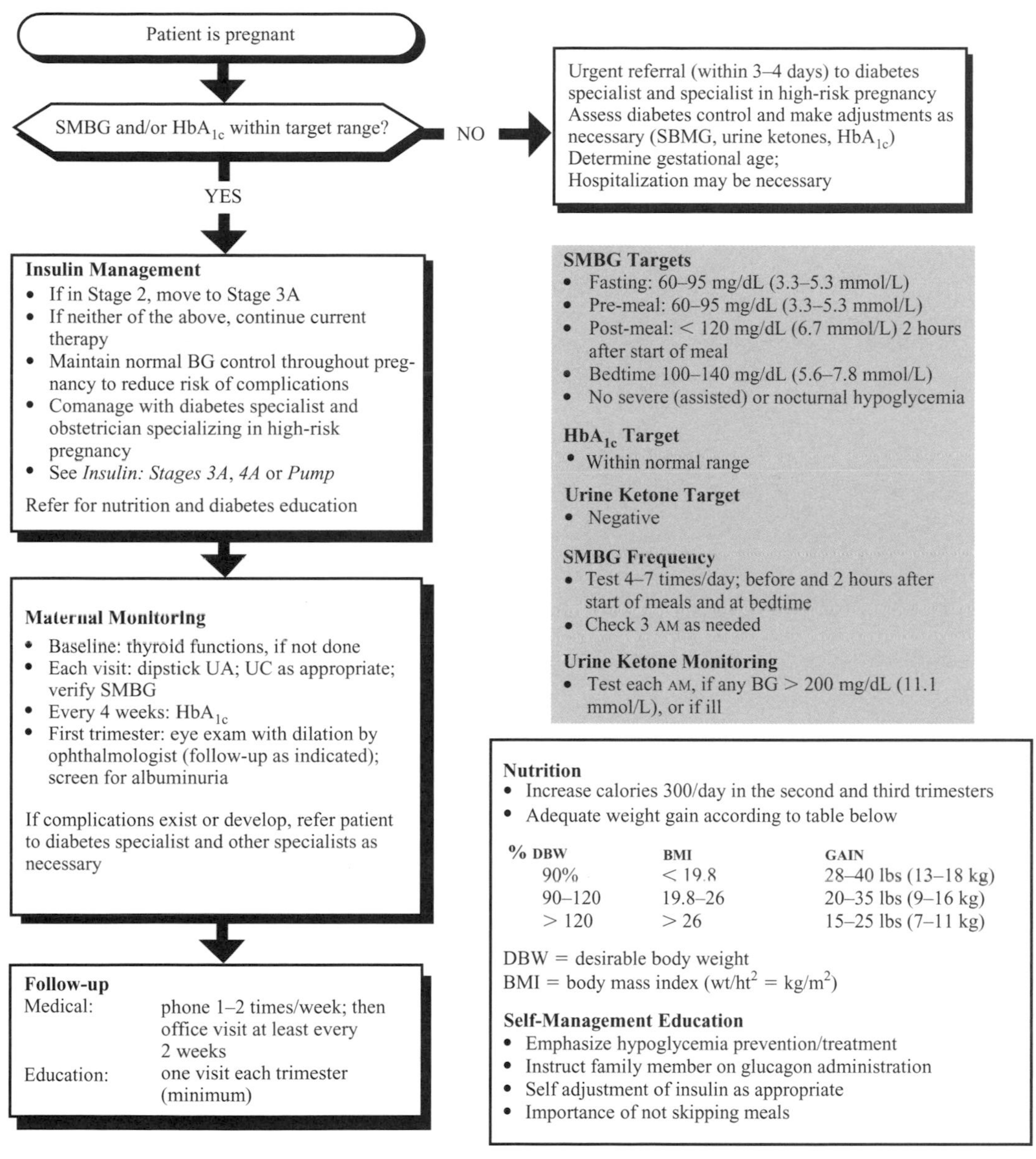

Figure 6.10 Multidisciplinary approach to management of pregnancy

Patient education

Since the patient is in the initial phase of diagnosis and starting treatment, education is needed. Education is also important for the individual with long-standing diabetes.

Diabetes education

The patient and family must be instructed in survival skills for diabetes management, including food plan, exercise, SMBG, techniques for insulin injection (see Photo 6.2), hypoglycemia management, and issues regarding day-to-day care. A thorough nutritional evaluation (preferably by a dietitian) with a diet history and determining an appropriate food plan as well as assistance in food plan and lifestyle issues are necessary. Additionally, information regarding exercise needs to be provided. The education content areas required by the American Diabetes Association (ADA) for program recognition are found in Figure 6.11.

American Diabetes Association Education Content Areas

1. Pathophysiology of diabetes and treatment options
2. Medical nutrition therapy
3. Physical activity
4. Medications
5. Blood glucose monitoring and use of results
6. Prevention, detection, and treatment of acute complications
7. Prevention, detection, and treatment of chronic complications
8. Goal Setting
9. Psychosocial adjustment
10. Preconception care, pregnancy, and gestational diabetes management

Figure 6.11 Required education content areas for American Diabetes Association recognition

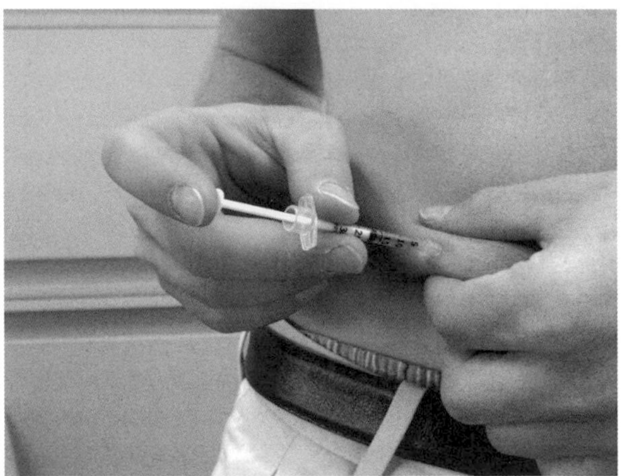

Photo 6.2 Abdomen injection site and technique

Stress and psychosocial adjustment

Patient education both at diagnosis and thereafter is an integral part of diabetes management. Each patient or parent is expected to understand the seriousness of diabetes and its management. Certified Diabetes Educators (CDEs) complete a course of training that includes both didactic and experiential learning to prepare them to educate newly diagnosed diabetic patients. In most instances, hospitals employ such nurses or dietitians. These individuals assess the patient's readiness and ability to learn, review the patient's medical history, examine current lifestyle, and discuss changes necessitated by diabetes regimens.

Many children and adolescents are so well trained that ongoing insulin adjustments may be safely left in their hands. At the initial diagnosis, the patient is trained in insulin administration (drawing up insulin, mixing insulin, selecting an injection site and rotation). Additionally, the patient is taught SMBG technique for the particular meter selected.

The DecisionPaths for diabetes education (see the Appendix, Figures A.8 and A.9) summarize both the initial and ongoing support provided by the diabetes educator. If a CDE is not available, a community or hospital-based nurse educator should be contacted. The DecisionPath defines the areas to be covered. Patients have the principal responsibility in terms of self-management and must leave the office confident in their skills and understanding. A follow-up educational visit should be arranged for no more than 3 days after diagnosis to review understanding and skills. Most likely, the attention will shift from survival skills (insulin administration, hypoglycemia, and SMBG) to meals, exercise, and symptoms – especially hypoglycemia. Increasing the patient's knowledge base incrementally ensures close adherence to the diabetes regimen.

Over the next several days, assess the patient's initial response to diabetes, its treatment, and his or her ability to follow the regimen (see Figure 6.11). SMBG is set at four times per day, preferably before each meal and before the evening snack. Urine ketones continue to be monitored four consecutive times per day until negative. Thereafter, it is done only when two unexplained blood glucose readings exceed 240 mg/dL (13.3 mmol/L) or if the patient is ill.

During the second and third days it is important that the patient report blood glucose values daily either by office visit, telephone, or modem. Patient generated SMBG data should be verified. If possible, each patient should be asked to use a memory based reflectance meter (which provides verified blood glucose data). Where unavailable, the patient's SMBG technique should be observed at an office visit, and, if results are questioned, verified with a laboratory correlation. This ensures that clinical decisions are based on reliable, accurate data. Check technique, strips, blood sample size, and cleanliness of meter window.

Medical nutrition therapy and education

When a registered dietitian is involved in care, patient education tends to be very thorough. Developing a complete food plan is a vital element of diabetes management. The food plan considers the role of food in the overall therapeutic strategy. It is meant to be comprehensive and to accommodate not only the insulin therapy but exercise as well. In general the success of nutrition therapy in type 1 diabetes relies on synchronizing what the patient normally eats (especially carbohydrate choices at each meal) and exercise/physical activity with insulin administration.

Start phase: synchronizing food and insulin

The best treatment of type 1 diabetes requires administering insulin in a way that mimics physiologic requirements. However, insulin therapy alone cannot produce near-normal blood glucose values. The appropriate therapy includes prescriptions for food and exercise synchronized to insulin administration. The patient must match these elements for the best blood glucose control. The prescription, however, may vary from a very detailed and restrictive description of the exact amount and timing of food, exercise, and insulin administration to a series of algorithms or rules on how to match these.

Establishing a food plan. Developing a systematic approach to nutrition management of the individual with type 1 diabetes begins with collecting data on which to base the initial interventions. Whether carried out by a registered dietitian or a physician, the information required is the same (see Figure 6.5).

Assessing height and weight. The initial visit to determine the appropriate nutrition intervention should include a very careful, documented means of assessing height and weight. Height should be measured without shoes and not recorded from patient recall. Weight is recorded without shoes and with the patient in light clothing. For children, plot height and weight on the National Center for Health Statistics growth chart. Use this as a baseline to monitor height and weight at future visits. For adults, height and weight can be expressed as body mass index (BMI), calculated by dividing the body weight measured in kilograms by the square of the height measured in meters ($BMI = kg/m^2$). A person with a BMI of $> 25\ kg/m^2$ to $30\ kg/m^2$ is considered to be overweight and with a BMI $> 30\ kg/m^2$ is considered obese.

Assessing nutritional needs. Once the height/weight ratio has been determined, sufficient data to develop a food plan must be obtained (insulin regimen, laboratory data, medications, medical history, and overall therapeutic goals). A thorough diet history should include past experience with food plans, other diet restrictions, weight history and recent weight change (adjusted for height), weight goals (if appropriate), appetite, eating or digestion problems, eating schedule, who prepares meals, a typical day's food intake (to be evaluated for approximate calories and nutrient composition, other nutritional concerns, and frequency and timing of meals), frequency and choices in restaurant meals, alcohol intake, and use of vitamins or nutritional supplements.

Data from the diet history should be combined with exercise history that includes a review of exercise habits and physical activity level. (What activities does the patient do? Does the patient exercise regularly? When does exercise occur? What limitations does the patient have that would hinder/prevent exercise? Is the patient willing or interested in becoming more physically active?) Psychosocial/economic and family issues must also be assessed (see the "Behavioral Issues and Assessment" at the end of this chapter). Include living situation, cooking facilities, finances, educational background, employment, and ethnic, religious, and belief considerations.

It is especially important to use SMBG to collect data on the effect of food and exercise on overall glycemic control. Lacking SMBG data, it is almost impossible for the patient or professional to have adequate data on which to determine how well the food plan is working. Therefore, it is important to assess patient knowledge of target blood glucose ranges, to review blood glucose testing method and frequency of testing if needed, and to review blood glucose records for incidence of hyperglycemia and hypoglycemia and number of blood glucose values in the target range.

The food plan should be individualized and based on diet history, food patterns, preferences, socioeconomic issues, ethnic/cultural and religious practices, and lifestyle. Calories should be appropriate for growth and development in children and for maintaining ideal body weight in adults (see Figure 6.5).

Macronutrient composition. Food plans should be individualized according to a person's lifestyle and eating habits as well as concurrent medical conditions (e.g. if weight maintenance is a concern, readjust caloric intake; if elevated cholesterol is a concern, reduce saturated fat to less than 10 per cent of total fat; if elevated triglycerides are a concern, moderately reduce carbohydrate content as well as fat content; if kidney disease is of concern, consider reducing protein intake).

Patient education on food planning and survival skills involves teaching basic nutrition, diabetes nutrition guidelines, and beginning ideas for altering current food plans to meet these guidelines. Points of focus are the following:

- *When and how much to eat.* Match insulin administration and food intake throughout the day. Avoid long times between meals and snacks. Choose smaller portions. Avoid skipping meals and snacks.

- *What to eat.* Choose a variety of foods each day. Choose foods lower in fat. Avoid foods high in added sweeteners such as soda pop, syrup, candy, and desserts. The food pyramid is a good general guide. Carbohydrate counting can be very effective to bring consistency to the amount of carbohydrate consumed at meals and snacks (see Carbohydrate Counting in the Appendix, Figure A.14).

- *Definitions and guidelines.* The meaning of carbohydrate, protein, and fat with examples of food sources of each nutrient; a discussion of the nutrition guidelines such as eating less fat, eating more carbohydrate, using less added sweeteners, eating more fiber, reducing total food intake for weight loss if appropriate; and suggestions for making these changes in current eating pattern, such as grocery shopping tips.

- *Record keeping*. To encourage patients to maintain food/exercise/SMBG records, provide record forms for them to complete prior to the next visit. Provide instructions on how to record food intake (actual food eaten and quantities, times of meals), exercise habits (type, frequency, and duration), and blood testing (time and result).

Patient nutrition education. First consider seeking a registered dietitian with experience in diabetes to counsel the patient as soon as feasible. The initial visit should occur within the first 2 weeks of diagnosis at a point in which blood glucose levels have stabilized. During the initial visit a complete diet history is collected. This information is integrated with the laboratory values, current health status, and insulin regimen. A registered dietitian who participates must be provided with the laboratory findings and other relevant medical information prior to seeing the patient.

A complete nutritional assessment, temporary food plan, and general nutrition education should be completed during the first nutrition visit. The food plan should be an extension of the original plan developed at the first medical visit. If no such plan was developed, and the meeting with the dietitian constitutes the first visit for nutrition counseling, see Figure 6.5 and the Appendix, Figures A.11 and A.12.

The next visit should be a reassessment combined with an individualized food plan that reflects the ethnic, socioeconomic, and personal preferences of the patient while addressing the needs of an individual with diabetes. At this point discuss how to integrate blood glucose results and food plan records. Patient education should focus on understanding the importance of appropriate food intake, knowing how to measure caloric intake, and being aware of the effects of different nutrients on blood glucose level.

Physical assessment. Combine data from the food plan with exercise history, including a review of exercise habits and physical activity level.

- What activities does the patient do? Does the patient exercise regularly? When does exercise occur?
- What limitations does the patient have that would hinder/prevent/change the type of exercise prescribed?
- Is the patient willing to become or interested in becoming more physically active?

Together these elements provide a framework for patient education.

Identify and summarize short-term goals. Short-term goals should be specific and achievable within 1 or 2 weeks. Goals should address eating and exercise and should focus on changing only one or two specific behaviors at a time in each area: e.g., eat meals at approximately the same time each day, have a routine evening snack, or eat 10–15 grams of carbohydrate per hour of exercise.

Food/exercise/SMBG records. Provide record forms for the patient to complete before the next visit. Provide instructions on how to record food intake (actual food eaten and quantities, times of meals), exercise habits (type, frequency, and duration) and blood testing (time and result).

Follow-up plans. Arrange the appointment for the next visit. Documentation from each visit should include a written record of the assessment and intervention. The report should include:

1. summary of assessment information
2. short-term goals
3. education intervention
4. long-term goals
5. specific actions recommended
6. plans for further follow-up, including additional education topics to be reviewed

Adjust and maintain phases

Collect follow-up data including weight (and height for individuals under 18 years of age) without shoes in light clothing; changes in schedule, food, and/or insulin; and changes in exercise habits. Review SMBG records, including frequency of testing, time of testing, and results; frequency of hypoglycemic episodes; and current blood pressure level if hypertension is present. Record new or updated laboratory data; food records completed since initial visit or 24 hour food recall; and food plan problems and/or concerns.

Determine whether therapy is working or whether change is needed, based on changes in blood glucose values. Questions to ask include the following:

- Is there a downward trend in blood glucose values?
- Have there been episodes of hypoglycemia? Are the episodes related to exercise or to skipped or delayed meals?
- Is there a pattern of hyperglycemia?
- Are post-prandial blood glucose values less than 160 mg/dL (8.9 mmol/L)?
- What percent of blood glucose values are within the target range? (An overall decrease in blood glucose values of 10 per cent or more may be realistic.)
- Is change needed based on change in exercise and/or activity levels? (Patient has gradually increased physical activity with a minimum goal of 10–15 minutes of physical activity three to four times a week.) Is the patient willing or able to do more?
- Is there a change in food habits? Patient regularly eats meals and snacks consistent with insulin action curves and makes appropriate food choices in reasonable portions; patient is able to adjust delayed meals with appropriate snacks; food adjustments are appropriate to preventing hypoglycemia and hyperglycemia. Can patient make further improvements in the overall quality of the diet?
- Is there a change in weight? If patient is at ideal body weight, is the patient losing or gaining weight? (If obese, 1–2 pounds (1 kg) of weight loss may be an appropriate outcome.) If weight remains stable, have positive changes in food selection and/or exercise been made?
- In children, is growth and development normal? Has the child gained excessive weight with improved glucose control?

Assess achievement of short-term goals and whether patient is willing to make further changes. If therapy is working, continue. If therapy is not working, intervene.

Intervention. Identify and recommend the changes in insulin, food, and exercise that can improve outcome such as:

- consistent meal and snack schedule
- insulin/food synchronization
- meal spacing and timing
- food portions and choices
- exercise frequency/duration/type/timing

Adjust the food plan if necessary based on patient feedback. Reinforce consistency in food plan, especially in timing and snacks. Reinforce methods of adjusting for delayed meals. Reset short-term goals based on recommendations. Do any survival self-management skills need to be reviewed, e.g. exercise, food intake, insulin administration and timing, hypoglycemia, or illness management? Are continuing level self-management skills needed, for example, use of alcohol, restaurant dining choices, label reading, handling special occasions, carbohydrate counting, and other information, to promote self-care and flexibility (see Table 6.9)?

A second follow-up visit is recommended if the patient is having difficulty making lifestyle changes, requires additional support and encouragement, has not met weight goals, or further self-management skills are required. Follow-up should occur within 2–4 weeks. If no immediate follow-up is needed, schedule the next appointment with the dietitian in 3–6 months. See the patient more frequently until near-normal levels of blood glucose are reached. Written documentation of the nutrition assessment and intervention should be completed and placed in the patient's file or medical record. The report should include education intervention, short-term goals, specific actions recommended, and plans for further follow-up, including additional education topics to be reviewed.

Subsequent follow-up. Weigh without shoes in light clothing. Review changes in medication (i.e. dose/frequency of insulin injections) and changes in exercise habits. Review SMBG records including frequency of testing, time of testing, and results; current blood pressure level; and HbA_{1c} and other new or updated laboratory data. Review food records completed since initial visit or 24 hour food recall; food plan problems and/or concerns.

Again, evaluate whether therapy is working or whether change is needed, based on change in:

- HbA_{1c}
- blood glucose values
- exercise and/or activity levels
- food habits
- weight or growth and development
- complications (hypertension, hyperlipidemia, renal disease, etc.)

Assess achievement of short-term goals and whether the patient is willing to make further changes. If therapy is working, continue. If therapy is not working, intervene.

Intervention. Too often members of the health care team are reluctant to recommend changes in therapy. This leads to both reduced efficiency and needless error in treatment. If any of the following are uncovered by any team member (dietitian and nurse especially), consider immediate alteration in therapy:

- Blood glucose levels (average SMBG) have not shown a downward trend of 15–30 mg/dL (0.8–1.7 mmol/L) per month.
- Blood glucose levels (average SMBG) have not reached the target range by 3–6 months.
- HbA_{1c} has not shown a downward trend of 0.5–1.0 per cent per month. HbA_{1c} has not reached target range by 3–6 months.
- Patient has lost or gained weight with no improvement in blood glucose levels.
- Elevated blood pressure has not responded to dietary changes, weight loss, and/or exercise changes.

Table 6.9 Problem-solving

Problem	Solution
Hypoglycemia prevention	Maintain consistent carbohydrate choices
Hyperglycemia and hypoglycemia	Synchronize insulin/food
Improve action of insulin	Meal spacing and timing; food portions and choices
Inefficient use of insulin	Exercise frequency

- Lipids are outside target range after 4–6 months of nutrition intervention.

If there is no improvement in laboratory data and the patient is not willing to make food and exercise changes then further nutrition intervention is unlikely to result in improved medical outcomes.

In addition to the preceding, be certain the physician, the dietitian, or nurse educator reviews long-term goals, discusses ongoing care, assesses growth and development in children, examines additional weight loss if needed, and assesses overall glucose and lipid control. Reset short-term goals and review self-management skills. Determine whether any survival or continuing level self-management skills need to be addressed or reviewed. Additional follow-up visits are recommended if the patient needs or desires assistance with additional lifestyle changes, weight loss, and/or further self-management skill training. If no further follow-up is needed, schedule the next appointment with the dietitian in 6 months. Ongoing nutrition follow-up should be planned. The nutrition plan, once understood and implemented by the patient, should be reviewed at least every 6 months.

Written documentation of the intervention should include a summary of outcomes of nutrition intervention (medical outcomes, food and exercise behavior changes), provision of self-management skill instruction/review, recommendations based on outcomes, and plans for follow-up.

During the adjust phase, therapy is modified to accelerate reaching the target of fasting blood glucose between 70 and 140 mg/dL (3.9 and 7.8 mmol/L). Changes in insulin, synchronization of food plan with insulin and exercise, and other strategies may be enlisted to ensure glycemic control. During the period of experimentation with steps to reduce blood glucose, it will be necessary to SMBG four times per day and have monthly visits. HbA_{1c} levels should begin to respond to the overall lower blood glucose during the first month. However, not until the end of the second month will the impact of the initial therapy be fully reflected in HbA_{1c} levels. From there on reduction by at least 0.5–1 per cent should continue monthly until near-normal levels (within 1.0 percentage point of the upper limit of normal) of HbA_{1c} are achieved.

Exercise program

An exercise prescription to determine appropriateness of exercise as part of diabetes care requires careful evaluation of fitness. Medical clearance should be obtained before starting an exercise program (keeping in mind that many older individuals with type 1 diabetes may not have participated in a regular exercise program for many years). Considerations for medical clearance include hypertension, cardiovascular disease, neuropathy (especially silent ischemic heart disease), severe proliferative retinopathy, stress EKG if over age 40 or over age 30 with diabetes for > 10 years, overall fitness level and blood glucose control. Generally, the patient should be assessed for four parameters: VO_2 max (oxygen intake and conversion), endurance (repetitive movements), strength (lifting weight), and flexibility (reaching). Where this evaluation is not available, contact a community health center or club. The level of exercise is determined individually and must address such questions as when, how often, how long, and at what pace (see Figure 6.13). Evaluation of an exercise plan must consider the impact of exercise when either too much or too little

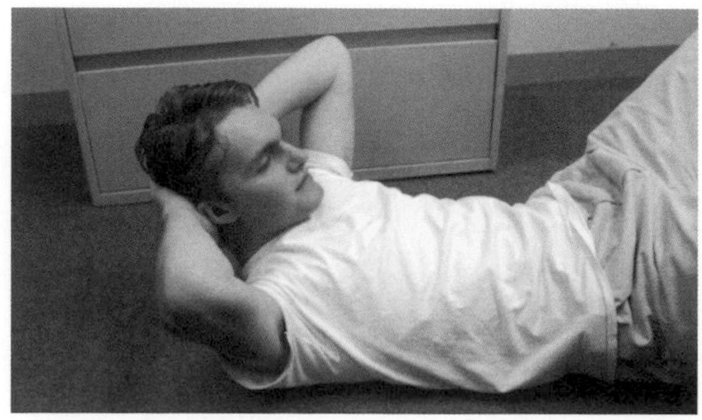

Photo 6.3 Exercise: sit-ups

insulin is available. As mentioned earlier, exercise must be carefully planned.

Patients who participate in regular fitness programs benefit from improved glycemic control as part of their overall treatment regimen as well as improved overall health (see Photo 6.3). To avoid hypoglycemia and hyperglycemia, it is important that individuals self-monitor blood glucose before and after exercise. Note, when exercise occurs in a state of insulin deficiency, blood glucose may actually be elevated.

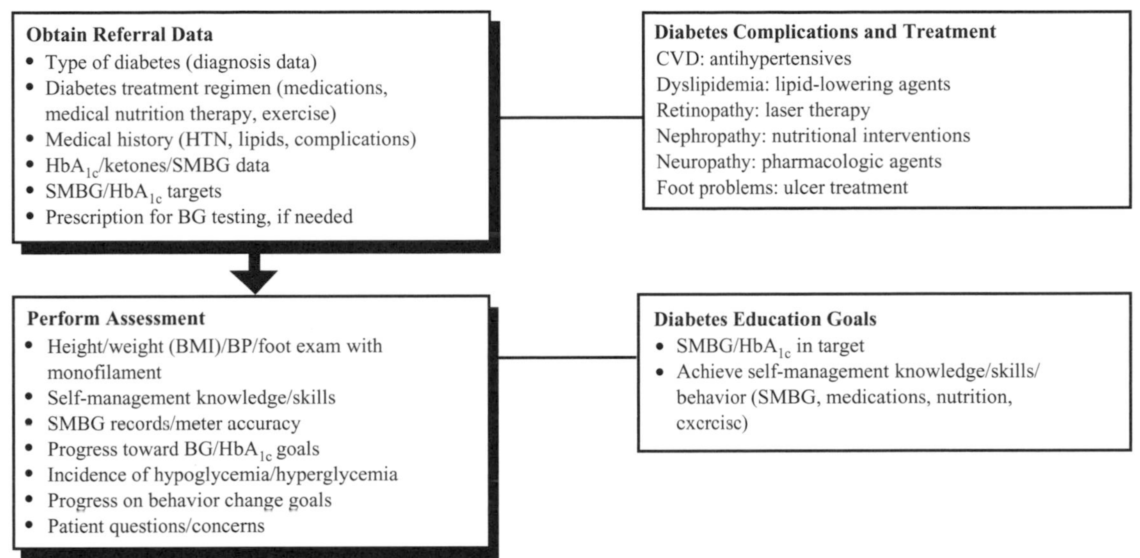

Figure 6.12 Follow-up self-care education

Behavioral issues and assessment

The diagnosis of diabetes requires physical and psychological adjustments. This is especially true of adolescents and young adults. For them, diabetes presents a unique dilemma. On the one hand they are expected to return to normal life; on the other hand they are expected to be responsible for self-care. With the need to restore near euglycemia, this becomes even more problematic. One early sign of a problem is the patient's inability to follow the prescribed regimen. However, before seeking a psychological explanation, the reason for non-adherence may be simply miscommunication between the patient and the provider. Therefore, before seeking a psychological explanation, SDM suggests an evaluation of the non-adherent behavior. DecisionPaths related to behaviors that affect diabetes management are discussed below.

Adherence assessment

Adherence assessment begins with an evaluation of the current level of glycemic control as reported by the patient (SMBG) and the laboratory (fasting plasma glucose or HbA_{1c}). This is neces-

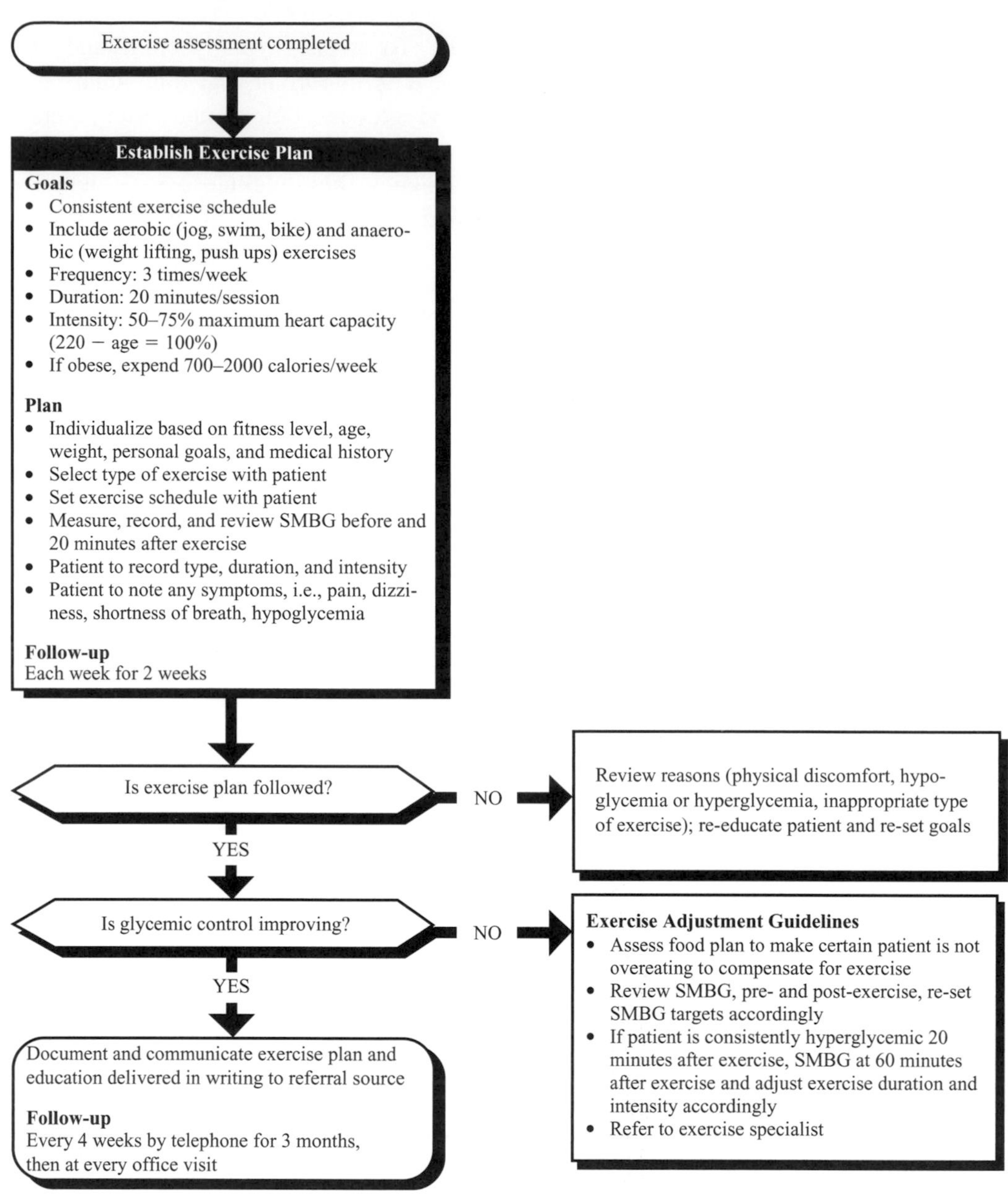

Figure 6.13 Exercise plan

sary because medical intervention is justified when the current therapy is not working. If the correlation (see Figure 6.14) is poor, make certain that technique, device, and reporting by the patient are understood. Have the patient demonstrate technique and at the same time draw a simultaneous blood sample for the laboratory. If the correlation between patient and laboratory data is poor, consider re-education.

Four diabetes related areas of adherence that can be readily assessed in the primary care setting include food plan, medication, SMBG, and exercise. Each area is approached in a similar manner. First, determine whether the patient understands the relationship between the behavior and diabetes. Second, determine whether the patient is prepared to set explicit short-term behavioral goals. Third, determine why the goals are not met; and fourth, be prepared to return to a previous step along this pathway if the current step is not completed.

The Specific DecisionPath for assessing adherence to taking insulin is shown in Figure 6.14. DecisionPaths for assessing adherence to food plan, SMBG, and exercise regimens are located in the Appendix, Figures A.20, A.22, and A.23. Based on the transtheoretical model of behavior change, all of the adherence DecisionPaths begin with whether the patient understands the connection between the behavior and diabetes.[15] It has been found that changing behavior without understanding why it is important is likely to fail. Thus, providing the patient with specifics as to how food, exercise, medication, or SMBG is related to diabetes management and prevention of complications is critical. Next, determine specifically what the patient is willing to do. In most cases, any misunderstanding as to the importance of adhering to the prescribed regimen can be resolved through this systematic approach. The next step involves setting goals with the patient. Set simple, reasonable, and explicit short-term goals such as "add one more SMBG test per day before dinner." Setting impossible goals will assuredly result in failure. Next, determine whether the patient has met or is attempting to meet the goals. Be prepared to reset the goals and move back a step. As the behavior changes, negotiate new explicit goals. Always ask the patient to help set the new goal. There are, however, those patients for whom this approach will not work. Some patients are not ready to change their behaviors. Continued reinforcement for change, combined with education, will sometimes help overcome this reluctance to modify behavior.

As the behavior changes, reset the goals. At each subsequent visit recheck behaviors, determine priorities for adherence assessment, and go through the same steps. If this is ineffective consider referral to a behavioral expert (psychologist or counselor).

Disagreement

The child who refuses to test, the adult who skips taking medications as prescribed, and the teenager who binge eats must be encouraged to share this information with the health care team. Similarly, the physician who believes in strict adherence to regimens, the dietitian who expects 100 per cent compliance to a restrictive diet, and the nurse educator who expects the patient to adjust rapidly to diabetes must state these expectations and have them challenged by the patient. Through this negotiation process a consensus as to goals, responsibilities, and expectations can be reached that will be beneficial to both the patient and the health care team. Table 6.10 compares the initial perspectives of a patient with that of a health care team. Note how consensus is reached on each point. This will reduce both the patient's anxiety and the disappointment many health care professionals experience when a therapy is not followed. The consensus serves as a contract. Used in conjunction with the Master DecisionPath, it documents what is expected by both the patient and the provider.

Psychological and social assessment

Both psychological and social dysfunction may occur with the onset of type 1 diabetes, when initiating a new approach to treatment (such as intensified insulin therapy), or with the discovery of an underlying complication. This is often reflected in how the individual adjusts to changes in lifestyle brought about by type 1 diabetes. At the time of diagnosis or when a new approach to treatment is undertaken, concern focuses on the patient acquiring the knowledge and skills required for immediate survival and long-term self-care. Patients' ability to acquire this new knowledge and skills is related to psychological and social adjustment. Psychological factors, such as depression and anxiety, and social factors, such as conduct disorders, significantly interfere with acquiring self-care skills and accepting the seriousness of diabetes. While depression is more common among individuals with diabetes than in

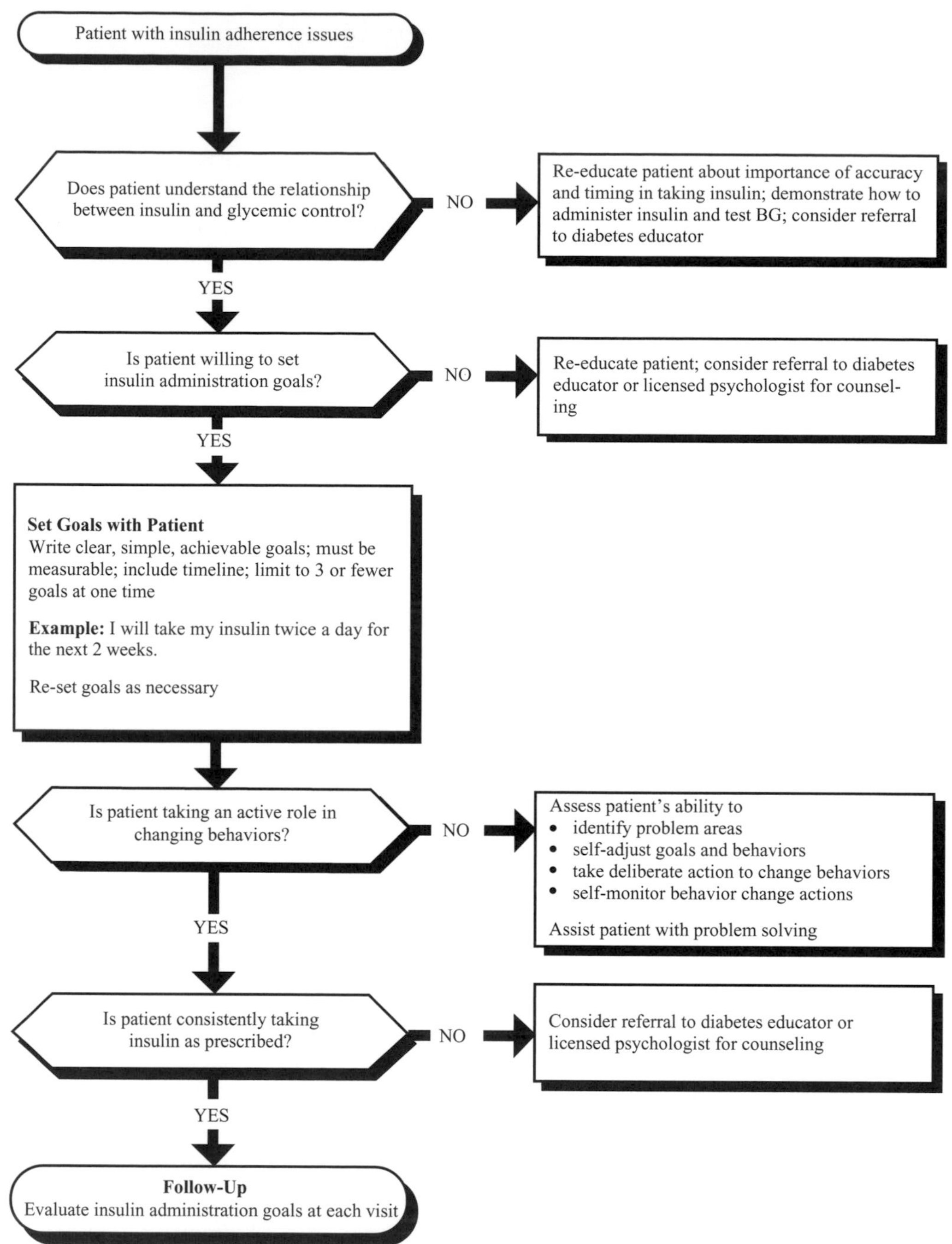

Figure 6.14 Insulin adminstration adherence

the general population, screening is often dependent upon patient self-reported symptoms. As this can be indeterminate, formal screening by a verified depression protocol is recommended. Often the person with diabetes may also suffer from an eating disorder. Diabetes is intertwined with diet and as such poses a unique set of behavioral issues. Since changes in diet may interfere with treatment and may present serious, long-lasting complications, it is important to note any significant weight loss.

If psychological and social adjustment proves

Table 6.10 The negotiation process

	Patient	Provider (team)	Consensus
Insulin injections	2	4	3
SMBG	2/day	5/day	4/day
Blood glucose goal	normal	< 250 mg/dL (13.9 mmol/L)	< 200 mg/dL (11.1 mmol/L)
Food plan	3 meals, no snacks	3 meals, 3 snacks	3 meals, bedtime snack
Exercise	daily 10 minutes	daily 1 hour	daily 30 minutes
Phone contact	whenever	weekly	every 2 weeks until stable
Office visits	every 6 weeks	every 8 weeks	every 6 weeks until stable

dysfunctional, it is ultimately reflected in poor glycemic control. This, in turn, raises the risk of acute and chronic complications, which contribute further to the psychological and social dysfunction. To break this cycle, it is necessary to identify the earliest signs of dysfunction and to intervene appropriately. Psychological and social interventions in diabetes are generally initiated by the primary care physician only after symptoms occur (see Figure 6.15). A newly diagnosed patient (as well as a patient in whom significant changes in therapy are being contemplated) should be considered for referral to a psychologist or social worker trained to detect the earliest symptoms of psychological or social dysfunction and to intervene before destructive behaviors occur. Often one or two counseling sessions are required to detect underlying psychosocial problems and to effectively intervene. Recognizing these early warning signs requires a complete psychological and social profile. One approach to obtaining this information is to begin the patient encounter with the idea that diabetes will be co-managed by the patient and the physician (and team) and that the patient will be empowered to make decisions. Most patients begin interactions with physicians assuming the power to make all clinical decisions rests with the physician.

For successful diabetes management (where > 90 per cent is patient responsibility) co-empowerment of the patient with the health care team effectively brings the patient onto the health care team and ensures that the patient understands and assumes clinical care responsibilities. Co-empowerment recognizes that the patient and physician may have a different view of the seriousness of the disease, the responsibilities of each health care professional, and the expectations of the patient's performance. The patient may feel the physician will make all decisions related to care and the patient should be passive. Alternatively, the physician may feel the patient should be the person to make daily decisions about diet, insulin, and exercise.

Co-empowerment is an agreement between the patient and health care team that delineates the responsibilities and expectations of each participant in care. It also established the DecisionPath all team members have agreed to follow. From a psychosocial perspective, it may be seen as a contract in which the patient spells out in detail his or her expectations and in which the health care professionals have an opportunity to determine how well those responsibilities and expectations fit with the diabetes management plan. It presents an opportunity to review behaviors that may be dysfunctional to the overall treatment goal.

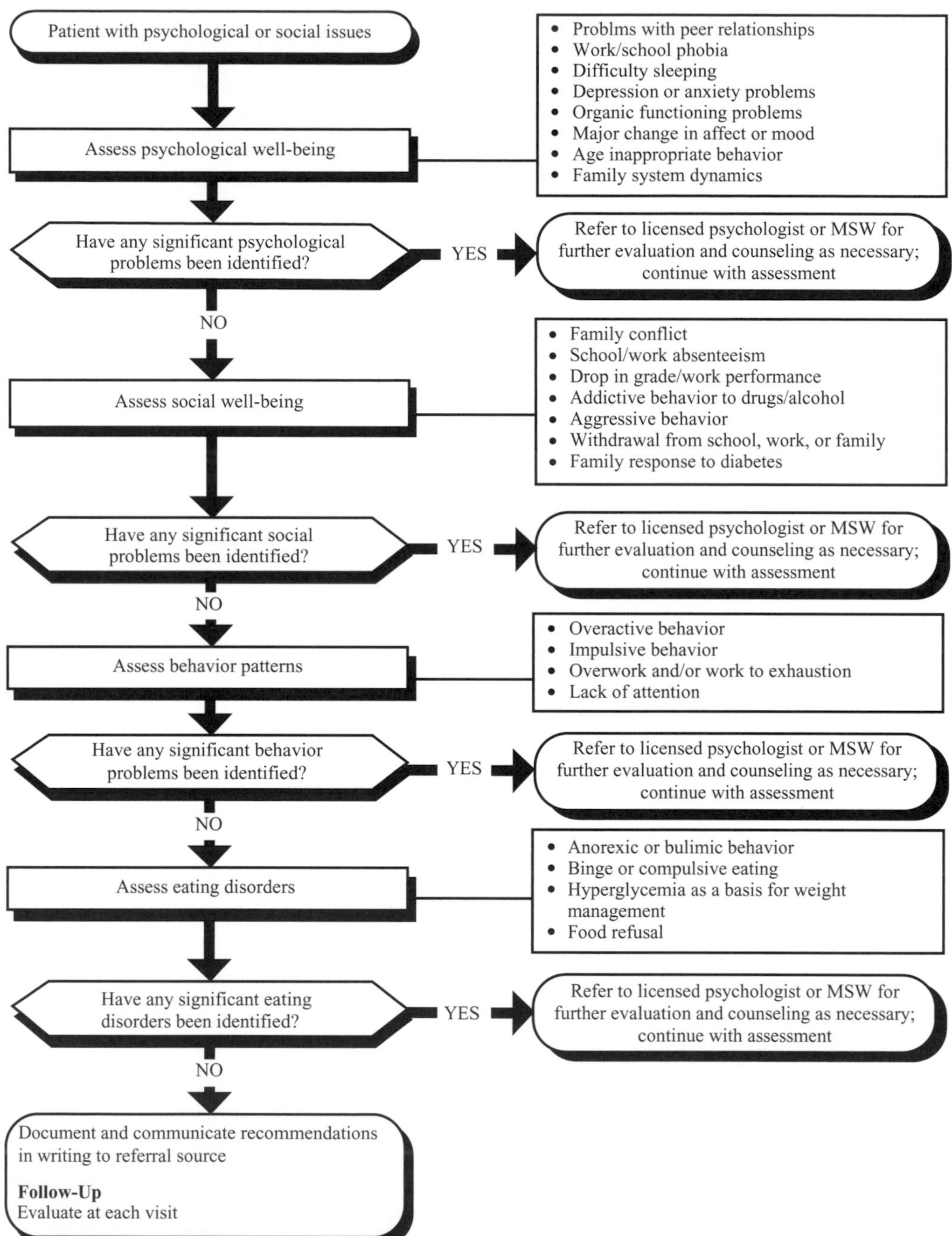

Figure 6.15 Psychological and Social Assessment DecisionPath

References

1. National Institute of Diabetes and Digestive and Kidney Diseases (National Diabetes Information Clearinghouse). *Diabetes Statistics* 1997; 98–3926.
2. International Diabetes Federation. *Diabetes Atlas* 2000.
3. Palmer JR and Lernmark A. Pathophysiology of type 1 (insulin-dependent) diabetes. In: Porte D and Sherwin RS, eds. *Ellenberg and Rifkins Diabetes Mellitus*, 5th ed. Stamford, CT: Appleton and Lange, 1997.
4. Olmos P, A'Hern R and Heaton DA. The significance of concordance rate for type 1 (insulin-dependent) diabetes in identical twins. *Diabetologia* 1988; **31**: 747–750.
5. Sanjeevi CB, Lybrand TP, Landin-Olsson M, *et al.* Analysis of antibody markers, DRB1, DRB5, DQA1 and DQB1 genes and modeling of DR2 molecules in DR2-positive patients with insulin-dependent diabetes mellitus. *Tissue Antigens* 1994; **44**: 110–119.
6. Bottazzo GF, Florin-Christensen A and Doniach D. Islet cell antibodies in diabetes mellitus with autoimmune polyendocrine deficiencies. *Lancet* 1974; **2**: 1279–1283.
7. Myers MA, Rabin DU and Rowley MJ. Pancreatic islet cell cytoplasmic antibody in diabetes is represented by antibodies to islet cell antigen 512 and glutamic acid decarboxylase. *Diabetes* 1995; **44**: 1290–1295.
8. Karounos DG, Wolinsky JS and Thomas JW. Monoclonal antibody to rubella virus capsid protein recognizes a beta-cell antigen. *J Immunol* 1993; **150**: 3080–3085.
9. Pozzilli P. The DPT-1 trail: a negative result with lessons for future type 1 diabetes prevention. *Diabetes Metab Res Rev* 2002 **18**: 257–259.
10. Libman I, Songer T and LaPorte R. How many people in the U.S. have IDDM? *Diabetes Care* 1993; **16**: 841–842.
11. Dokheel TM. An epidemic of childhood diabetes in the United States? Evidence from the Allegheny County, Pennsylvania, Pittsburgh Diabetes Epidemiology Research Group. *Diabetes Care* 1993; **16**: 1606–1611.
12. Dorman JS, McCarthy BJ, O'Leary LA and Koehler AN. Risk factors for insulin dependent diabetes. *Diabetes America* 1995; **96-1468**(2): 166–177.
13. Zimmet P, Turner R, McCarty D, Rowley M and MacKay I. Crucial points at diagnosis. *Diabetes Care* 1999; **22**: B59–B64.
14. Diabetes Control and Complications Trial Research Group. The effect of intensive treatment of diabetes on the development and progression of long-term complications in insulin-dependent diabetes mellitus. *N Engl J Med* 1993; **329**: 977–986.
15. Mazze R, Shamoon H, Parmentier R, *et al.* Reliability of blood glucose monitoring by patients with diabetes. *Am J Med* 1984; **77**: 211–217.
16. Prochaska JO, Norcross JC and Diclemente CC. *Changing for Good*. New York: Avon, 1994.

7 Pregestational and Gestational Diabetes

There are several forms of glucose intolerance found in pregnancy. One category consists of those women who, prior to conception, have type 1 or type 2 diabetes. They are classified as having pregestational diabetes. Because of the existence of diabetes prior to the current pregnancy, they are not subjected to screening or diagnostic tests in pregnancy. The prevalence rate of pregestational diabetes is between one and three per 1000 births, reflecting the relatively low number of women of childbearing age with preexisting diabetes.[1] A second category includes those women whose hyperglycemia is first detected in pregnancy. They are classified as having gestational diabetes mellitus (GDM). These women are subject to screening and diagnostic tests, because the identification of GDM can only be made by measuring blood glucose tolerance during pregnancy. Prevalence rates for GDM vary greatly due both to ethnic and racial differences and variation in diagnostic procedures. GDM has been reported in two to five per cent of all pregnancies. Certain ethnic groups (American Indians, Alaska Natives, African-Americans, Asians, Native Hawaiians and other Pacific Islanders, and Hispanics) are considered at highest risk for GDM with prevalence rates of 8–14 per cent.[2,3] Two other forms of hyperglycemia in pregnancy are impaired glucose homeostasis (IGH) and tocolytic related hyperglycemia. IGH may occur in as many as eight per cent of all pregnancies. These women are often screened positive for GDM, but do not meet the current diagnostic criteria. As many as 10 per cent of the women treated for pre-term labor with a tocolytic agent have subsequent hyperglycemia, often reaching levels that meet the criteria for GDM.

The full significance of elevated blood glucose during pregnancy is recent. Initially, studies of the effects of hyperglycemia in pregnancy focused on the mother with pre-existing diabetes and how elevated blood glucose contributed to her health during and after pregnancy. It was not until the latter half of the last century that investigators studied women whose hyperglycemia was first discovered in pregnancy and how their blood glucose levels affected the developing fetus. Currently, diabetes (especially hyperglycemia) is the second most common complication of pregnancy. It is associated with maternal and fetal complications that may be life-long.

Screening for hyperglycemia in pregnancy was originally proposed when O'Sullivan and Mahan studied the use of the oral glucose tolerance test (OGGT) in pregnancy to predict subsequent development of type 2 diabetes.[4] They found that hyperglycemia in pregnancy was significantly associated with a sixfold increased risk of subsequently developing type 2 diabetes. Since their findings, other investigators have expanded this original research. One path has led to a clearer understanding of the risk factors that predict the development of type 2 diabetes and subsequent GDM. A second path has been to evaluate the

Staged Diabetes Management: A Systematic Approach (2nd Edition) R. S. Mazze, E. S. Strock, G. D. Simonson and R. M. Bergenstal

ISBN: 0 470 86576 8

relationship between hyperglycemia discovered in pregnancy and adverse perinatal outcome. With respect to subsequent development of GDM and type 2 diabetes, along with the significance of GDM itself as a predictor, such factors as multiparity, ethnicity, and pre-existing insulin resistance (HTN, obesity, PCOS) have been identified as important risk factors.[5] With respect to hyperglycemia and adverse perinatal outcome, the findings of O'Sullivan and associates have been substantially elaborated upon.[6] While it has been reported that uncontrolled BG during the first trimester is a leading cause of fetal anomalies, evidence has associated macrosomia, polycythemia, neonatal hypoglycemia, and organomegly with persistent uncontrolled maternal hyperglycemia (BG > 120 mg/dL or 6.7 mmol/L).

Etiology of GDM and hyperglycemia

The exact etiology of gestational diabetes is unknown. It is known that insulin resistance increases throughout the first two trimesters of gestation partially associated with the production of the human placental lactogen (HPL). This is normal, resulting in a 50 per cent reduction in insulin sensitivity by the end of the third trimester.[7] To compensate for this significant insulin resistance, there is up to a threefold increase in pancreatic β-cell insulin secretion over that of the non-pregnant woman in response to the same amount of exogenous glucose. This balance between lower insulin sensitivity and higher insulin production maintains glucose homeostasis in pregnancy. Gestational diabetes occurs when this balance can no longer be maintained. Three possible factors have been identified that may contribute to reducing insulin effectiveness in pregnancy: decreased blood flow, reduced transendothelial transport of insulin between the capillary and target cells, and post-insulin receptor defects. Because these factors are modulated by insulin secretion patterns, their net effect is to reduce maternal glucose uptake to allow, under normal circumstances, for 20 per cent of the maternal nutrients to be shunted to the fetus to allow for appropriate growth and development.[8] During periods of hyperglycemia excess nutrients are shunted to the developing fetus. This accounts for both a higher maternal glucose level and a higher fetal insulin level. The underlying cause of the excess nutrients is most likely a greater level of insulin resistance, which exaggerates the "normal" insulin resistance of pregnancy. Recent evidence may point to pre-existing, pre-pregnancy (but undetected until pregnancy) insulin resistance.

Impaired glucose homeostasis and tocolytic related hyperglycemia

Two other forms of hyperglycemia are found in pregnancy. They are impaired glucose homeostasis (IGH) and hyperglycemia induced by tocolytic therapy. Women diagnosed with IGH do not meet the strict diagnostic criteria for GDM, but they are at a higher risk for adverse perinatal outcome than are women with normoglycemia in pregnancy. It is estimated that as many as 150 000 women have IGH during pregnancy. Hyperglycemia can also be induced by treatment for premature labor with tocolytic therapy. Every year approximately 300 000 pregnancies are complicated by premature labor.[9] Among the most common therapies in use is the β-2-adrenergic agonist, terbutaline sulfate. Although terbutaline's principal role in pregnancy is to prevent premature uterine contractions, it also affects the liver, causing an increase in glycogenolysis.[10] This increase results from the drug binding to β-2-adrenergic receptors in the hepatocyte membrane, which activate intracellular adenyl cyclase, resulting in an increase in intracellular cAMP. The rise in cAMP activates cAMP-dependent protein kinase, setting off a cascade of phosphorylation reactions resulting in glycogenolysis and release of glucose into the bloodstream. Insulin works antagonistically in this process by inducing dephosphorylation of key enzymes involved in this pathway, causing a decrease in glycogenolysis and increasing glycogen formation. Due to insulin resistance, which is not clearly understood, the liver is not able to counteract the effects of terbutaline, which results in tocolytic-induced hyperglycemia.

Adverse fetal and perinatal outcome

Two types of adverse perinatal outcome are related generally to diabetes and more specifically to hyperglycemia. The existence of hyperglycemia during the first trimester of pregnancy raises threefold the risk of fetal anomalies and miscarriage. High maternal glucose ($>$ 150 mg/dL or $>$ 8.3 mmol/L) has been associated with an increase in spontaneous abortions due to fetal and placental anomalies.[11] The association between blood glucose level and abnormalities is specific to the first 9 weeks of fetal development (during organogenesis). Congenital malformations have been found in 25 per cent of the women with pregestational (type 1 or type 2) diabetes when the HbA_{1c} was $>$ 10 per cent (normal 6 per cent). The incidence of these anomalies decreased to 5 per cent when HbA_{1c} was $<$ 8 per cent.[12] Because women with GDM are subjected to hyperglycemia principally limited to the third trimester, their risk of having children with congenital abnormalities is no greater than that of women with normal glycemia in pregnancy.

In women with GDM the complications that may develop include macrosomia, large-for-gestational-age (LGA) infants, neonatal hypoglycemia, hyperbilirubinemia, polycythemia, shoulder dystocia, and traumatic birth injury.[13] The major effect of persistent hyperglycemia is accelerated fetal growth. Although all the factors leading to excessive fetal growth are not yet known, clinical studies have shown the risk of a large infant is as much as nine times greater among women with glucose levels in excess of 105 mg/dL (5.9 mmol/L) fasting and 140 mg/dL (7.8 mmol/L) post-prandial than non-diabetic women and women with gestational diabetes whose glucose level is maintained between 60 and 120 mg/dL (3.3 and 6.7 mmol/L).[14]

Large infants are at greater risk for childhood, adolescent, and adult obesity, and metabolic syndrome.[13] It has been suggested that accelerated fetal growth and maternal hyperglycemia are linked through a process by which maternal circulating glucose passes through the placenta (maternal insulin is blocked) into the developing fetus's circulation, stimulating excessive fetal pancreatic β-cell production of insulin. As a growth hormone, fetal insulin fosters fat deposition, resulting in birth weights above the 90th percentile for a gestational age. Supporting this hypothesis is the high incidence of hypoglycemia following birth in these infants, suggesting that the pancreas has not yet adjusted to the cessation of maternal carbohydrate "shunting." Further supporting the relationship between glucose control and fetal size is evidence that low maternal blood glucose levels increase the risk of intrauterine growth retardation.[15]

Preventing gestational diabetes and subsequent type 2 diabetes

Can gestational diabetes be prevented? Current understanding of the mechanisms that lead to GDM suggest that, like type 2 diabetes, it is a multi-factorial disease with underlying defects that may be amenable to some interventions. Maintaining normal weight and treating impaired glucose homeostasis present two steps that modify the risk of GDM. Because weight gain in pregnancy often leads to obesity following pregnancy, counseling at-risk women to alter caloric intake and increase exercise is yet another step that may prevent GDM. The ability to prevent type 2 diabetes is discussed in detail in Chapter 4. It is important to note that the risk of type 2 diabetes developing after GDM increases substantially. The age of onset also is lower following the GDM index case. The factors that are most predictive are multi-parity, obesity, family history of type 2 diabetes, and level of hyperglycemia in pregnancy. These factors provide added evidence for tight metabolic control and weight management in the treatment of GDM with careful postpartum surveillance.

Pregestational diabetes

Women with type 1 or type 2 diabetes need to restore near-normal levels of blood glucose before conception. Approaches to these forms of diabetes in planning for pregnancy are outlined below.

Type 2 diabetes and pregnancy

Preconception planning

Preconception planning begins with a complete history and physical with special attention on evaluation of complications. Hypoglycemia unawareness, retinopathy, nephropathy, or neuropathy are reasons to confer with a specialist and to counsel continued birth control. After completing the history and physical, evaluate current glycemic control. The range of SMBG should be kept within 70 and 100 mg/dL (3.9 and 5.6 mmol/L) pre-meal and < 120 mg/dL (6.7 mmol/L) 2 hours after the start of the meal. The HbA_{1c} should be within the normal range. Again, unless these criteria are met, counsel continued birth control.

The next step takes into account two factors: current therapy and level of glycemic control. Patients who are treated with medical nutrition therapy only and whose diabetes is well controlled may be maintained on this therapy with adequate SMBG (four to seven times per day). The patient should be taught to notify the healthcare professional if blood glucose is > 100 mg/dL (5.6 mmol/L) fasting or > 160 mg/dL (8.9 mmol/L) post-prandial. If this should occur treatment with either glyburide or insulin should be initiated immediately. If the patient is currently treated with any oral agent, independent of the level of control, if the principal problem is insulin deficiency, glyburide should be initiated. If, however, the problem is insulin resistance or $HbA_{1c} > 9$ per cent Insulin Stage 3 or 4 should be initiated (see Chapter 4). Current studies suggest that all oral agents except glyburide pass through the placenta.[16] Since the exact moment of conception is unknown, the most prudent advice would be to replace the oral agent with glyburide or insulin during the period of preconception planning. If the patient is currently treated with insulin, intensify treatment as needed.

If the blood glucose is confirmed to be within the target range, stop birth control measures and maintain close surveillance of glycemic control (both SMBG and HbA_{1c}) until pregnancy is confirmed. If blood glucose is not at the target range, continue birth control and follow the appropriate DecisionPath. Consider co-management with a diabetes specialist. During the preconception period, weekly phone contact and monthly office visits are important to assess the level of glycemic control (HbA_{1c} and SMBG) and to determine whether conception has occurred. Upon confirmation of pregnancy, change the target range to between 60 and 95 mg/dL pre-meal (3.3 and 5.3 mmol/L) and less than 120 mg/dL (6.7 mmol/L) 2 hours after the start of the meal. Blood glucose targets in pregnancy are approximately 20 per cent lower than in the non-pregnant state. In addition, the discontinuation of medications that are contraindicated during pregnancy should be considered as part of the preconception plan. For example, ACE inhibitor and/or β-blocker therapy must be discontinued and alternative anti-hypertension medications (methyldopa or hydralazine) should be considered.

Clinical presentation

Many women with type 2 diabetes present late in the first trimester of pregnancy. This raises enormous problems since organogenesis has already begun and the impact of persistent hyperglycemia may have already occurred. Under these circumstances, obtain history of glycemic control by patient record and HbA_{1c}. If possible, such patients should be referred to a specialty center with perinatologists and/or endocrinologists to complete the overall assessment. This is especially true if the patient is in poor glycemic control, significantly obese, or already has kidney, eye, or neurological complications of diabetes.

Type 1 diabetes and pregnancy

Preconception planning

Preconception planning begins with a complete history and physical with emphasis on any previous history of miscarriages or anomalies. Miscarriages occur in four to eight per cent of pregnancies complicated by type 1 diabetes. More often than not, the level of glycemic control during the first trimester causes the miscarriage or anomaly. Pay special attention to evaluation of complications. Hypoglycemia unawareness, retinopathy, nephropathy, or neuropathy are reasons to recommend reconsideration of conception. After completing the history and physical, evaluate current glycemic control. SMBG should be kept within 70 and 100 mg/dL (3.9 and 5.6 mmol/L) pre-meal and the HbA_{1c} within the normal range. Again, unless these criteria are met, counsel continued birth control.

Next, consider current therapy and level of glycemic control. Patients treated with an insulin analog may continue this therapy. If not already managed with more intensive regimens, consider moving the patient to Stage 3A or 4A. This will provide adequate time and flexibility to reach the target range. Follow the Insulin Stage 3A/Start or Physiologic Insulin Stage 4A/Start guidelines in Chapter 6. Use of single- and two-injection regimens during preconception planning is not recommended. Since the exact moment of conception is unknown, the most prudent advice is to optimize control with multiple injections in a rapid, safe fashion.

If the blood glucose is confirmed to be within the target range, stop birth control measures and maintain close surveillance of glycemic control (both SMBG and HbA_{1c}) until pregnancy is confirmed. If blood glucose is not in the target range, continue birth control and adjust therapy until glycemic targets are achieved. Consider co-management with a diabetes specialist. During the preconception period, weekly phone contact and monthly office visits are important to assess level of glycemic control and to determine whether conception has occurred. Upon confirmation of pregnancy, change the target range to between 60 and 95 mg/dL (3.3 and 5.3 mmol/L) pre-meal and fasting and < 120 mg/dL (6.7 mmol/L) 2 hours after the start of a meal. Note that blood glucose targets are set $\sim$20 per cent lower during pregnancy than in the non-pregnant state.

Clinical presentation

Women with type 1 diabetes who present in the first trimester of pregnancy in poor glycemic control are at significant risk for adverse fetal and maternal outcome. This raises enormous problems since organogenesis has already begun and the impact of persistent hyperglycemia may result in a fetal anomaly or a miscarriage. Under these circumstances obtain a history of glycemic control by patient record and HbA_{1c}. If the patient has an $HbA_{1c} > 2$ percentage points above the upper limit of normal, evaluation by a perinatologist and neonatologist is necessary. If there is evidence of maternal microvascular or macrovascular disease and/or the patient is not able to achieve good metabolic control, an endocrinologist should be consulted.

Maternal monitoring during pregnancy

Improvement in glycemic control and pregnancy are both associated with weight gain. Individuals who become pregnant at ideal body weight are expected to gain between 20 and 35 pounds (9–16 kg) during the pregnancy to accommodate nutritional needs for adequate fetal growth and development. Obese individuals need not gain as much weight. This is especially important in type 2 diabetes and GDM, where obesity is a factor in insulin resistance. Substantial weight gain will further aggravate the high insulin resistance associated with obesity and pregnancy.

Monitoring follows two specific areas related to diabetes: glycemic control and complications. With respect to glycemic control it is important to detect any instances of hypoglycemia or hyperglycemia and to react immediately. Self-monitoring of blood glucose using a meter with a memory ensures that the reported test results have not been altered. Studies have shown a vast majority of patients will change their blood glucose results in pregnancy to avoid both more intensive therapies and any blame for an adverse outcome. To avoid this, continue to have patients SMBG (download meter to a computer to review data if possible) and measure HbA_{1c} every 4 weeks. The values for HbA_{1c} should be at or near normal since fasting and pre-meal SMBG targets are 60–95 mg/dL (3.3–5.3 mmol/L) and < 120 mg/dL (6.7 mmol/L) 2 hours post-prandial. If this is not the case and the SMBG is reported within the normal range, suspect falsification of data and consider referring the patient to a specialty team.

With respect to complications, both eye- and kidney-related diseases tend to be aggravated during pregnancy. Careful follow-up with an ophthalmologist is very important. Changes in renal function should also be carefully followed by monitoring for albuminuria.

> Note: Before continuing, it might be helpful to review the structure of Staged Diabetes Management (SDM) for gestational diabetes. The Master DecisionPath presents the stages and phases of diabetes diagnosis and treatment. The phases refer to three specific periods in diabetes management – start treatment (diagnosis and initial therapy), adjust treatment (modifying therapy in order to achieve glycemic targets), and maintain treatment (reaching the therapeutic goal). Stages are the treatment options. This information should be shared with the patient and family members.

Gestational diabetes detection and treatment

The following sections discuss the means of identifying those women at risk for GDM, diagnosing GDM, and treatment options. It begins with the overall practice guidelines for gestational diabetes, followed by the screening and diagnosis and Master DecisionPath, which provides the sequence of stages or therapies used to restore euglycemia in GDM. Also presented are DecisionPaths for the initiation and adjustment of each stage.

Gestational diabetes practice guidelines

The practice guidelines (see Figure 7.1) contain the criteria for screening, risk assessment, diagnosis, target, treatment, and follow-up. Women may fit into one of two categories in the development of GDM. The first are those at risk. They include women from high-risk ethnic groups (American Indians and Alaska Natives, African-Americans, Asians, Native Hawaiians and other Pacific Islanders, and Hispanics) and those who present with a family history of type 2 diabetes,

Screening	Screen between 24th and 28th gestational weeks; with any risk factor(s), consider screening at first prenatal visit Screen with 50 gram glucose challenge test: 1 hour plasma glucose ≥ 140 mg/dL (7.8 mmol/L) positive; ≥ 120 mg/dL (6.7 mmol/L) suspected
Risk Factors	• BMI > 25 kg/m² (especially waist-to-hip ratio > 1) • Family history of type 2 diabetes (especially first-degree relatives) • Age > 25 • Multiparity • Previous gestational diabetes (GDM): macrosomic or large-for-gestational-age infant • Previous impaired fasting glucose (IFG) with fasting plasma glucose 100–125 mg/dL (5.6–6.9 mmol/L) • Previous impaired glucose tolerance (IGT) with oral glucose tolerance test (OGTT) 2 hour glucose value 140–199 mg/dL (7.8–11.0 mmol/L) • American Indian or Alaska Native; African-American; Asian; Native Hawaiian or Other Pacific Islander, Hispanic
Diagnosis	100 gram oral glucose tolerance test (OGTT) after 10 hour overnight fast
Plasma Glucose	Fasting ≥ 95 mg/dL (5.3 mmol/L), 1 hour ≥ 180 mg/dL (10.0 mmol/L), 2 hour ≥ 155 mg/dL (8.6 mmol/L), 3 hour ≥ 140 mg/dL (7.8 mmol/L). Two abnormal values required for diagnosis; if one abnormal or high normal consider SMBG for 7 days; if average fasting BG ≥ 95 mg/dL or average 2 hour post-meal ≥ 120 mg/dL (6.7 mmol/L), treat with medical nutrition therapy; see *Medical Nutrition Therapy/Start*
Symptoms	Usually none: rarely, increased urination, thirst, and appetite; nocturia; weight loss
Urine Ketones	Usually negative; positive can indicate starvation ketosis
Treatment Options	Medical nutrition therapy; Insulin: Stages 3, 4; Glyburide
Targets	
Self-Monitored Blood Glucose (SMBG)	• All values within target range • Pre-meal and bedtime: 60–95 mg/dL (3.3–5.3 mmol/L) • Post-meal: < 120 mg/dL (6.7 mmol/L) 2 hours after start of meal; < 140 mg/dL (7.8 mmol/L) I hour after start of meal
Hemoglobin HbA_{1c} or Total Glycosylated Hemoglobin	May be used to evaluate prior hyperglycemia, but is not used in GDM management; should be within normal range
Urine Ketones	Negative
Monitoring	
SMBG	6–7 times/day; before and 1–2 hours after start of meals, and at bedtime Minimum 4 times/day; fasting and 1–2 hours after start of meals
Method	Meter with memory and log book
Urine Ketones (Fasting)	Every AM for 7 days if negatives, then every other AM thereafter
Follow-up	
Pre-natal	Phone 1–2 times a week to review SMBG data; office visit every 2 weeks up to 36 weeks, then weekly; SMBG data (download meter); frequency of hypoglycemia; weight or BMI; medications; blood pressure; medical nutrition therapy; exercise
Fetal Monitoring	Kick counts at 28 weeks; non-stress test at 34 weeks until end of pregnancy
After Delivery	**In hospital:** check fasting BG and 2 hours after breakfast each day **After discharge:** check fasting BG and 2 hours after breakfast 1 day/week until first postpartum visit. If fasting BG > 120 mg/dL (6.7 mmol/L) or post-prandial BG > 160 mg/dL (8.9 mmol/L) evaluate for diabetes immediately **6 weeks:** nutrition education if needed **3–6 months:** evaluate for diabetes

Figure 7.1 Gestational Diabetes Practice Guidelines

previous gestational diabetes, previous large-for-gestational-age (LGA) or macrosomic infant, obesity, multi-parity, metabolic syndrome and/or over the age of 25. Approximately 50 per cent of all cases of GDM will come from amongst those women with one or more risk factors for SDM. The remainder come from women with no apparent risk factors.

Screening

The original criteria for screening for persistent hyperglycemia or gestational diabetes (adopted by both the National Diabetes Data Group and the American Diabetes Association) are based on work performed by O'Sullivan and associates.[17] In their study, a 50 g glucose challenge test (GCT) was administered. Glucose was measured in whole blood 1 hour later by the Somogyi–Nelson method. Support for the O'Sullivan approach was based on the findings that selective screening by risk factors alone identified fewer than 50 per cent of those women with GDM (as determined by the oral glucose tolerance test). The GCT detects approximately 80 per cent of women with GDM when using the glucose cut-off of > 140 mg/dL (7.8 mmol/L). Current screening procedures (see Figure 7.2) recommended by SDM are adapted from the two-step approach supported by the American Diabetes Association.[18] According to SDM recommendations, all women with risk factors should be screened at the first prenatal visit and, if negative, again between 24 and 26 weeks. All other women should be screened initially between the 24th and 26th gestational weeks.

At this point human placental lactogen is nearing its highest level and, thus, this constitutes the time at which insulin resistance is most likely to affect glucose homeostasis. Non-fasting women drink 50 g of glucose suspended in liquid. One hour following ingestion, venous blood is drawn and glucose concentration measured. Values ⩾ 140 mg/dL (7.8 mmol/L) for plasma glucose and ⩾ 120 mg/dL (6.7 mmol/L) for whole blood are considered positive. These women are then followed up (within 1 week) with a 3 hour oral glucose tolerance test to diagnose gestational diabetes. Approximately 25 per cent of the women undergoing the GCT are likely to have a positive screen.

Diagnosis

Diagnostic criteria for GDM were established after the observation was made that women with hyperglycemia in pregnancy were at a significantly higher risk of developing type 2 diabetes than women with normal glycemia in pregnancy. Although the observation that GDM raises the risk of type 2 diabetes is important, the primary purpose of early detection of GDM is to reduce the immediate risk of maternal, perinatal, and neonatal complications. The diagnostic criteria are based on the O'Sullivan–Mahan criteria that have been modified by Carpenter and Coustan and are supported by the American Diabetes Association.[3] The modifications arose from the notion that the O'Sullivan standards relied on whole blood glucose assays while the current GCT and OGTT measure plasma glucose levels using the glucose oxidase method. The conversion from plasma glucose to whole blood is approximately 14 per cent lower, thus requiring a modification from the original O'Sullivan–Mahan criteria. The oral glucose tolerance test requires an overnight, or at least an eight hour, fast. After a fasting venous blood sample is taken, the patient is administered 100 g glucose load (orally) and venous samples are drawn at 1, 2, and 3 hours (see Figure 7.2). Two values for plasma blood glucose must be equal to or greater than 95 mg/dL (5.3 mmol/L) fasting, 180 mg/dL (10.0 mmol/L) at 1 hour, 155 mg/dL (8.6 mmol/L) at 2 hours, and/or 140 mg/dL (7.8 mmol/L) at 3 hours to diagnose GDM.

Some women, despite a normal oral glucose tolerance test, may still be at risk for an LGA infant. Recent evidence suggests that women with a screening value > 140 mg/dL (7.8 mmol/L) can reach as high as a 14-fold greater risk of adverse perinatal outcome in spite of a subsequent "normal" OGTT.[10] It is difficult to determine on the basis of the GCT which women these will be.

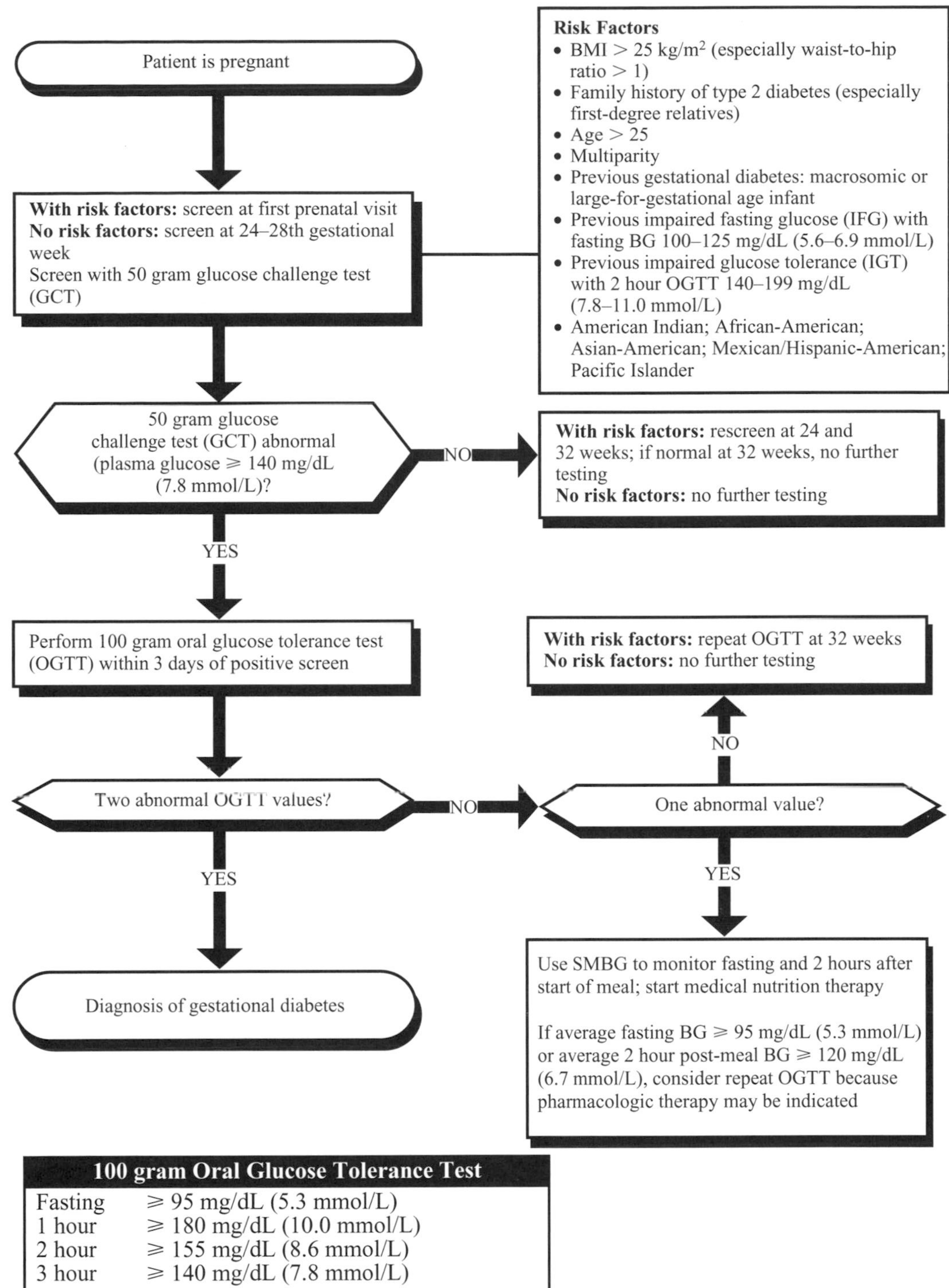

100 gram Oral Glucose Tolerance Test	
Fasting	≥ 95 mg/dL (5.3 mmol/L)
1 hour	≥ 180 mg/dL (10.0 mmol/L)
2 hour	≥ 155 mg/dL (8.6 mmol/L)
3 hour	≥ 140 mg/dL (7.8 mmol/L)

Figure 7.2 Gestational Diabetes Screening and Diagnosis DecisionPath

Other evidence suggests that women with one abnormal value or high normal values during an OGTT are also at increased risk of adverse outcome. For these women re-evaluation by SMBG for 1 week after the OGTT often provides ample evidence of underlying abnormalities in glucose regulation. If the mean fasting SMBG values exceed 95 mg/dL (5.3 mmol/L), the risk of adverse perinatal outcome is sufficiently high to begin medical nutrition therapy and to continue monitoring. Since the OGTT is the only way to "diagnose" GDM, testing by OGTT may be necessary. However, since the OGTT was not originally meant to predict adverse outcomes, it may not be sensitive enough to ensure no risk. Using SMBG in a manner similar to that of women in treatment for GDM is an alternative information source. If the glucose pattern appears to parallel that of untreated GDM, fasting > 95 mg/dL (5.3 mmol/L) and 2 hr post-prandial > 120 mg/dL (6.7 mmol/L), consider treatment even when the OGTT does not corroborate the SMBG findings. Referral to a diabetes specialist for further evaluation should also be considered.

Alternate screening and diagnostic criteria

An alternate method uses the 75 g oral glucose load with two or more values exceeding fasting 95 mg/dL (5.3 mmol/L), 1 hour greater than or equal to 180 mg/dL (10.0 mmol/L) and/or 2 hour greater than or equal to 155 mg/dL (8.6 mmol/L) for a positive diagnosis.

Treatment options

Gestational diabetes has three treatment options: medical nutrition therapy (alone), glyburide, or insulin. The options have the same goal – to rapidly restore euglycemia in pregnancy. Nutrition therapy, which includes regular physical activity, is meant to optimize energy intake and to counter the effect of insulin resistance. Food is divided into smaller and more frequent portions to minimize post-prandial hyperglycemia. Exercise is designed to foster more efficient uptake of glucose by muscle tissue. Neither the food plan nor the exercise plan is meant to reduce maternal weight. Treatment with glyburide (a secretagogue) fosters release of endogenous insulin by improving the response of the maternal pancreatic β-cells to fasting and post-prandial blood glucose excursions. Glyburide does not pass through the placental barrier and has been shown to be a safe and efficacious way to treat women with GDM.[19] Insulin therapies are meant to supplement endogenous insulin to counter insulin resistance. Since exogenous insulin does not pass the placental barrier, it will affect only maternal blood glucose levels and thereby indirectly affect fetal glucose levels. The options range from two to four injections per day, depending on the patient's glycemic pattern. Mixed regular and intermediate-acting insulins are recommended, since they allow for sufficient flexibility to customize the regimen to the patient's lifestyle.

Targets

Because normal pregnancy is a state of insulin resistance (due partly to HPL) in which maternal nutrients are shunted to the developing fetus, the normal range of blood glucose is lower by approximately 20 per cent. Therefore, the target blood glucose should be set between 60 and 95 mg/dL (3.3–5.3 mmol/L) pre-meal and no greater than 120 mg/dL (6.7 mmol/L) 2 hours post-meal. Ample evidence shows that, as blood glucose rises, the risk of adverse perinatal outcome increases. In some studies, this relationship is linear. At fasting blood glucose levels of 95 mg/dL (5.3 mmol/L), the risk of a macrosomic infant is seven times greater than at 75 mg/dL (4.2 mmol/L).[10] At 105 mg/dL (5.8 mmol/L), the risk rises to 14 times greater than normal. It has also been noted that at blood glucose levels less than 75 mg/dL (4.2 mmol/L) intrauterine growth retardation may result. Setting the targets within these narrow parameters appears to be the most effective way to reduce risk of adverse perinatal outcome. The targets refer specifically to self-monitored blood glucose because of the need for continuous data on blood glucose level. These values are for the duration of the pregnancy regardless of the type of therapy. Normal HbA_{1c} should result from reaching these target blood glucose levels. HbA_{1c} may be assessed at the start of therapy as a baseline measure; however, it is generally not used in treatment. HbA_{1c} provides an approximation of the average blood glucose for 8–10 weeks before the test. An elevated HbA_{1c} (> 1.0 percentage points above the upper limit of normal) may suggest that the patient is actually an individual with pregestational diabetes (most likely type 2 diabetes) and had persistent hyperglycemia earlier than the time of screening. Under such circumstances, closer fetal evaluation for abnormalities is advisable. Under most conditions the HbA_{1c} will be at or near normal since increased glycosylation of hemoglobin is not normally detected until blood glucose reaches an average of > 140 mg/dL (7.8 mmol/L) over an extended period of time. Once in treatment, the HbA_{1c} would not be a sensitive indicator of mild hyperglycemia (120–150 mg/dL or 6.7–8.3 mmol/L) and, therefore, is not generally used for clinical decision-making. Because some women with GDM will fast in order to lower their blood glucose (and thereby avoid insulin therapy), ketones should be measured and maintained at negative throughout the pregnancy.

Monitoring

One of the most perplexing problems in the treatment of GDM is the question of SMBG. Should the women with GDM be subjected to frequent monitoring (four to seven tests per day) from the time GDM is diagnosed? Reliance on SMBG for clinical decisions is almost self-evident. Certainly, patients treated with insulin are required to SMBG prior to each injection to adjust the dose. What about women on glyburide or diet only regimens? Regardless of the type of therapy, until hyperglycemia is regulated and restored to euglycemia, rapid deterioration in BG is likely. As many as 50 per cent of those women with low-level hyperglycemia at diagnosis (fasting < 105 mg/dL or 5.3 mmol/L) may, despite dietary only interventions, experience persistent hyperglycemia (post-prandial > 120 mg/dL or 6.7 mmol/L) that would go undetected without frequent SMBG. About 4 per cent of the women initially assigned to glyburide therapy require insulin to restore euglycemia. These women would go undetected without SMBG. Office visits, as often as every 2 weeks, would still be too infrequent to identify persistent, meal-related hyperglycemia and to foster rapid ameliorative interventions. Therefore, SDM recommends that, independent of the type of therapy, SMBG be initiated in all patients. The frequency of testing is noted in Table 7.1.

A meter with a memory is recommended in pregnancy. A number of studies have reported that reliability of patient SMBG reports is less than 20 per cent. To improve reliability of reporting, meters with onboard memories capable of storing the blood glucose test result with the corresponding time and date are necessary. Data can be accessed from these meters in two ways. The meter itself can be scrolled for individual values as well as for a two week average. For more precise data, the meter can be connected to a personal computer and all data off-loaded. Evaluate for urine ketones until seven consecutive days of negative ketones are obtained and every other day thereafter. This will help detect starvation ketosis.

Follow-up

Specific to managing diabetes in pregnancy is the need to rapidly respond to hyperglycemia. Weekly phone contact plus office visits every 2 weeks until 36 weeks is recommended. Evidence suggests that, even as late as the thirty-sixth week, introducing insulin or glyburide therapy can restore euglycemia and slow accelerated fetal growth due to maternal hyperglycemia. Close surveillance by SMBG is very important even as late as the 40th week.

Table 7.1 Frequency of testing

Treatment	Start	Adjust	Maintain
Medical nutrition therapy	4/day	6–7/day	4/day
Insulin Stages	4–6/day	6–7/day	6–7/day*

* May reduce to 4/day after the 32nd gestational week.

The decision in delivery time is based on four factors:

- maternal hypertension (preeclampsia)
- previous stillbirth
- macrosomia
- poor compliance and/or metabolic control

Presence of any of these factors indicates need for early delivery (37–38 weeks). All other cases are encouraged to achieve spontaneous delivery at term.

Postpartum maternal and infant follow-up

Follow-up after delivery takes two courses for the mother. In instances where gestational diabetes resolves itself to normal levels of glycemia immediately after birth, the mother should return for screening by fasting plasma glucose between 3 and 6 months following hospital discharge. Women with GDM are at increased risk for developing type 2 diabetes and should be monitored yearly for the development of the disease. Women with pregestational diabetes, and women with GDM whose blood glucose does not return to normal levels following delivery, should continue to be treated to restore near-normal blood glucose levels. Women with GDM should be treated as type 2 diabetes unless their BG returns to normal. Infants of all patients are assessed at birth for APGAR score and glucose level. Infants are fed within 6 hours, and blood glucose levels are followed closely. Intravenous glucose may be necessary for 24–48 hours. Within 24 hours, additional evaluation includes gestational age, evidence of macrosomic, congenital anomalies, and other diabetes-related morbidity such as polycythemia. Examination over the next several years encompasses evaluation of physiologic, psychomotor, and psychological development.

Gestational diabetes Master DecisionPath

Approximately 50 per cent of the women with GDM will begin treatment by medical nutrition therapy only, based on their diagnostic values during the OGTT. Nutrition therapy encompasses adopting a set of general rules to guide caloric intake and timing of meals (see the next section). If such rules fail to restore normoglycemia, SDM recommends following the principles set out for general dietary management in diabetes and insulin resistance, specifically, to replace high-calorie foods with lower-calorie foods and drinks, to reduce portion sizes if the replacement fails, and to restrict certain foods if the reduction does not achieve lower BG. The remaining women will require either glyburide or insulin based on entry BG and patient preference.

The Master DecisionPath for gestational diabetes, shown in Figure 7.3, contains the criteria for making decisions along with guidelines to assist in the implementation of each decision. The DecisionPath guides the practitioner regarding when to start each therapy and the criteria by which changes in therapy are made. Medical nutrition therapy is part of the overall therapeutic strategy for gestational diabetes. In gestational diabetes, the food and exercise plan is intended to lower blood glucose levels while avoiding excess weight gain or loss. A major problem is balancing caloric intake with caloric expenditure. While the non-obese woman with GDM generally consumes adequate calories, the obese woman with GDM may take in excess calories compared with energy needs. A person who is obese may store three times more energy in the form of fat than the normal-weight individual. Obese individuals tend to have a diet with proportionately more fat and carbohydrate than the normal-weight individual and tend toward less activity, contributing to the overall energy imbalance.

In pregnancy, insulin resistance is already high.

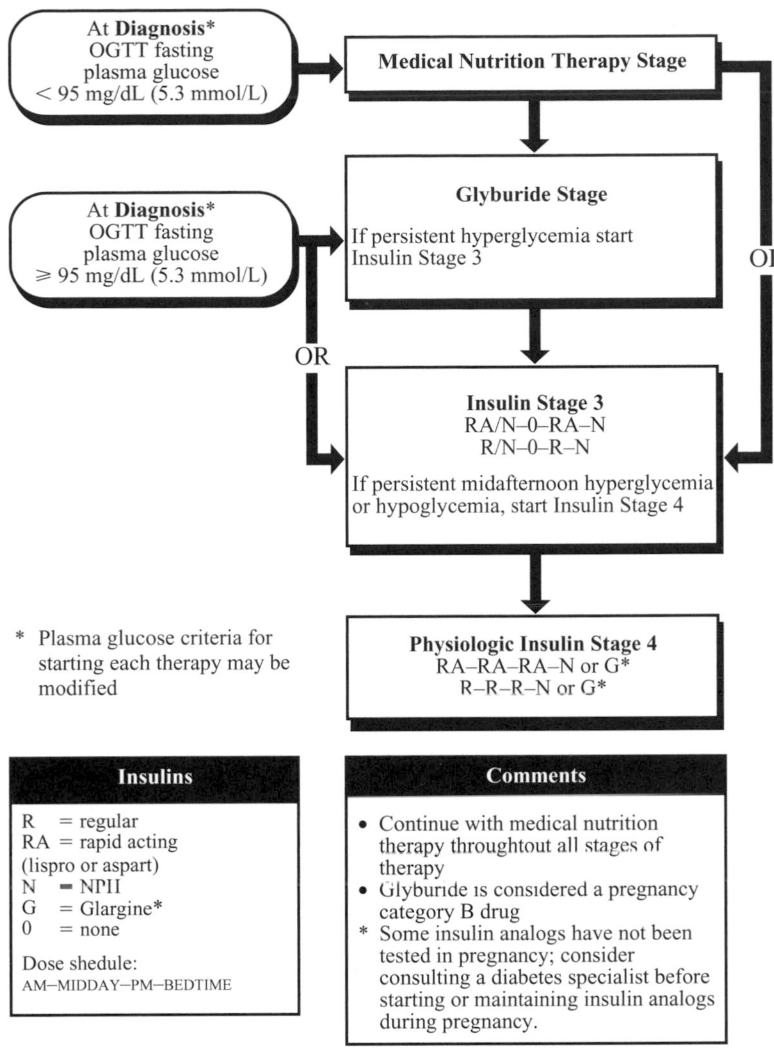

Figure 7.3 Gestational Diabetes Master DecisionPath

In GDM the normally high insulin resistance tends to be exaggerated. Obesity is also part of the metabolic syndrome and therefore further exaggerates the effect of insulin resistance on BG, BP, and lipid abnormalities. Obesity related insulin resistance is probably due to changes that occur in the adipose tissue as cell size increases. It is believed that the number of insulin receptors remains stable while the cell surface area increases, effectively reducing the number of insulin receptors per unit of cell surface area. Simultaneously it has been demonstrated that, although insulin production increases in pregnancy, in GDM insulin production is still lower than that of age and weight matched women without GDM. This gives rise to a state of relative insulin deficiency in pregnancy, which if left untreated results in hyperglycemia.[8]

To reverse the course of hyperglycemia through medical nutrition therapy, the energy balance must shift to an increase in output with a decrease in input. An increase in output not only fosters more efficient use of calories but also begins to use energy stored from the fat depot. The immediate result is improved insulin utilization as adipose tissue reduces in size. With a concomitant reduction in stored energy as fat, the feedback loop favors improved glucose uptake with expended energy on the output side. If the changed caloric intake (from fat to carbohydrates and proteins) is coordinated with an increased level of activity, the imbalance that led to the obesity should be resolved and a balanced or steady state re-instituted. This will help to overcome the insulin resistance and relative insulin deficiency.

When GDM is treated with glyburide or insulin, medical nutrition therapy, which includes regular physical activity, is synchronized with the pharmacologic action of glyburide on the pancreatic β-cells or with action curves of exogenous insulin (see Chapter 3). The major challenge is not to allow the additional endogenous insulin (from the action of glyburide) or the exogenous insulin to justify increased caloric intake in excess of that needed to respond to energy output. This requires adjusting the timing of food, not the amount. The same caloric intake should be maintained to ensure appropriate growth and development of the fetus as would have been recommended in the absence of either pharmacologic agent. Administration of glyburide or exogenous insulin necessitates spreading food intake rather than adding calories. This will require trial and error.

Selecting a treatment regimen

Staged Diabetes Management relies on blood glucose data gathered during diagnosis and initial therapy to characterize the underlying hyperglycemia of pregnancy and to rapidly select a therapy to ensure an orderly progression to euglycemia. In this manner, SDM bases its approach on the scientific rationale for treatment. The underlying principle in managing GDM is to expeditiously initiate therapy to forestall the effect of maternal hyperglycemia on accelerated fetal growth. Gestational diabetes is generally detected during the third trimester at a point when human placental lactogen reaches its highest levels. In GDM, this allows a very short time to identify the correct treatment and intensify the therapy to re-establish normal blood glucose levels (60–120 mg/dL or 3.3–6.7 mmol/L). Aware that any period of hyperglycemia, however brief, may contribute to excessive fetal growth, SDM seeks to reduce the risk of accelerated fetal growth through restitution of normoglycemia.

The goal of SDM is to use the earliest possible criteria to determine the most efficacious therapy. Since the OGTT is the basis of diagnosis in GDM, using the fasting plasma glucose value determined at the start of this test provides a good source for selecting initial therapy. At diagnosis, when the OGTT fasting plasma glucose is less than 95 mg/dL (5.3 mmol/L), medical nutrition therapy has a good chance of restoring euglycemia if followed rigorously. When the OGTT fasting plasma glucose level is $\geqslant$ 95 mg/dL (5.3 mmol/L) at diagnosis, the risk of persistent hyperglycemia increases significantly. At this point, initiating pharmacologic therapy is recommended to prevent further deterioration of blood glucose levels.[18] The choice of therapy is between glyburide and insulin. So long as the fasting BG is less than 150 mg/dL (8.3 mmol/L), there is a chance that glyburide will be effective. Above this point, glyburide cannot effectively lower BG to near-normal levels. If the BG is above the criteria for glyburide or if the newness of this therapy presents any doubts in its efficacy, then insulin therapy should be initiated. While two- and three-injection regimens can be effective, Stage 4 is the most physiologic and therefore likely to achieve tight control using the smallest amount of insulin. Once the therapy is selected SMBG is used to evaluate its continued efficacy.

The Master DecisionPath for GDM contains the sequence of therapies to try if the first therapy fails to achieve glycemic targets. The patient, using SMBG, provides the clinician with the data on which the efficacy of the initial and subsequent therapies is assessed. The criteria for moving from one stage to the next are based principally on identification of patterns of abnormal blood glucose values. For example, movement from MNT stage to glyburide is based on SMBG fasting between 95 mg/dL and 150 mg/dL (5.3 mmol/L and 8.3 mmol/L) or two hour post-prandial between 120 mg/dL and 180 (6.7 mmol/L and 10 mmol/L) occurring twice within a week. Similarly, if the patient is in Stage 3 and experiences persistent mid-afternoon hypoglycemia and/or late afternoon hyperglycemia, movement to Stage 4 is recommended to provide greater flexibility in insulin adjustment. Throughout all therapies, a food plan is maintained. Refer to Table 7.2 for approximate timelines to reach management goals.

Table 7.2 Timelines to reach management goals

Stage	Time
Medical nutrition therapy	7–14 days
Glyburide stage	10–14 days
Insulin Stage 3	14–21 days
Physiologic Insulin Stage 4	14–21 days

Patient education

Initiating treatment for gestational diabetes includes an orientation/education program designed to help the individual recognize the importance of diabetes in pregnancy and to institute the prescribed regimen immediately (see Figures 7.4 and 7.5). This is required because, unlike all other forms of diabetes, during pregnancy the window for effective intervention during which achieving euglycemia is an effective means of tertiary prevention (i.e. prevention of complications) diminishes. During orientation, all patients (regardless of treatment modality) are taught SMBG techniques and given dietary instructions. All women are also taught insulin administration techniques. The objective of therapy is to rapidly achieve euglycemia (fasting blood glucose averaging below 95 mg/dL (5.3 mmol/L)) and postprandial blood glucose averaging below 120 mg/dL (6.7 mmol/L). Concurrently, patients at ideal body weight must gain weight during pregnancy to ensure appropriate growth and development of the fetus. Obese individuals' weight management must consider fetal growth and development and maternal well-being (specifically pregnancy induced hypertension). During follow-up visits education should reinforce treatment goals and emphasize the points found in Figure 7.5.

Medical nutrition therapy

All persons with GDM require a food and activity plan as part of the initial and follow-up treatment for hyperglycemia. If the individual is initially or subsequently placed on pharmacological therapy, she will continue to maintain virtually the same nutritional therapy as if she were following a food plan alone. The term food plan (or medical nutrition therapy) encompasses the total daily required caloric intake (a combination of meals and snacks). The first step in determining the appropriate food plan is to complete the physical examination and, where possible, to consider consultation with a dietitian. The variables that determine appropriate food plan and eventually dietary compliance go well beyond the current physical well-being of the individual. Psychosocial issues and economics must be considered. Thoroughly assess the patient's readiness and ability to follow a food plan to re-establish a balance between caloric input and energy output. Discussing the overall Gestational Diabetes Master DecisionPath, providing the patient with choices, and clearly establishing the metabolic goals are necessary steps in this process.

Medical Nutrition Therapy/Start

Establish an appropriate food plan based on an assessment of the individual's current food intake (see Figure 7.6). A food history or three day food record, with confirmation by another family member (if possible), provides adequate approximations of caloric intake. Choice of food plan depends substantially on the resources of the patient and the physician. The dietary information provided here supports the initial purpose of the food plan – to reduce blood glucose to near-normal levels.

Food planning and nutrient composition. Individualize the food plan. The percentage of carbohydrates, protein, and fat varies depending on the patient's usual food intake. Controlling carbohydrate intake is especially important since

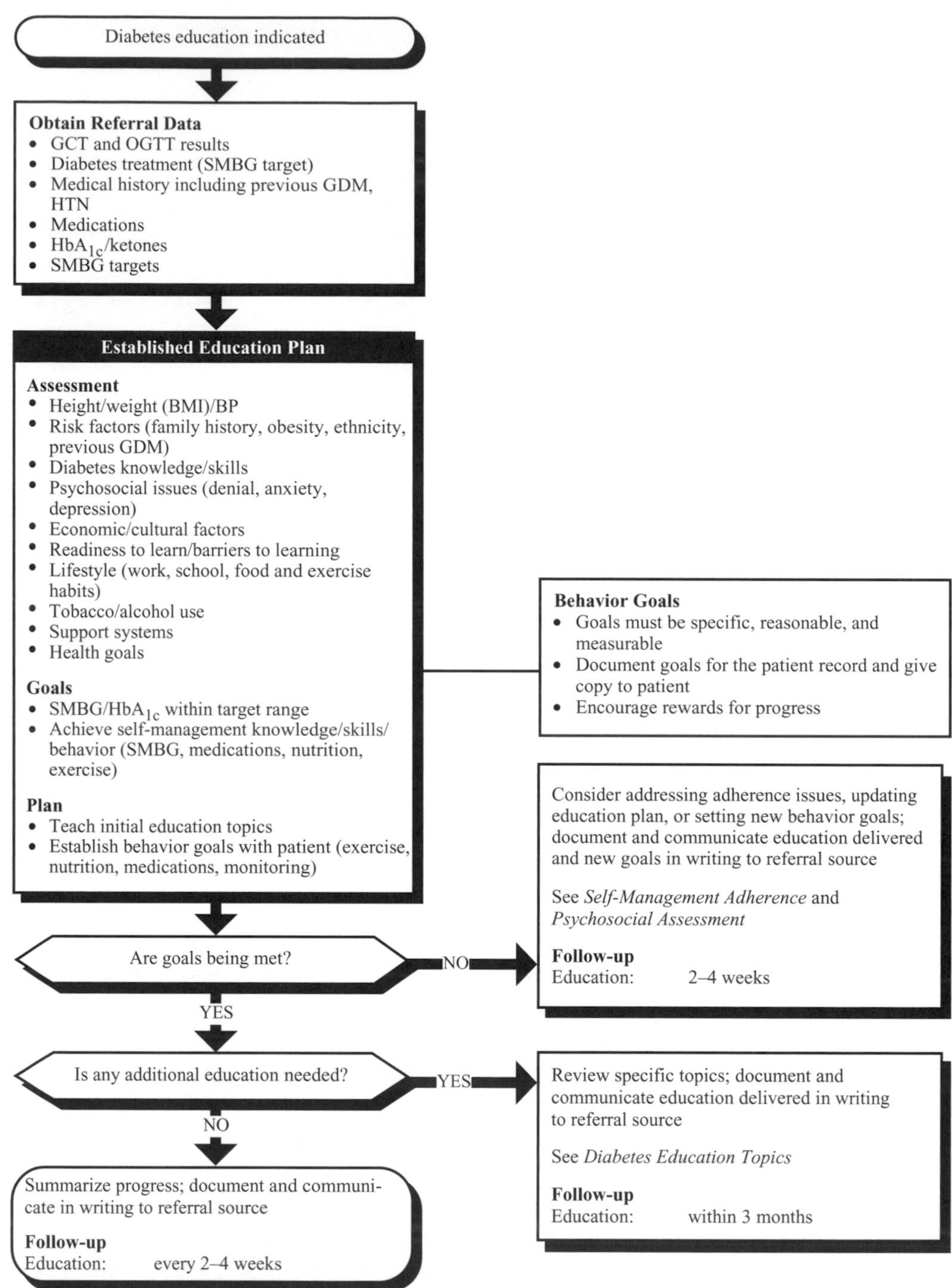

Figure 7.4 Gestational Diabetes Education

the nutrient contributes significantly to blood glucose level. A sample food plan is shown in Figure 7.6. Modifications in nutrient composition will be required for patients with such conditions as hyperlipidemia and/or hypertension (preeclampsia).

Exercise. Recall that the importance of exercise in restoring a balance between food intake and energy expenditure is paramount in managing the non-pregnant woman with diabetes. Developing an exercise plan for pregnancy begins with assessing the patient's fitness. A registered dietitian or

Initial Visit

General Information	Add for Insulin Users
• Explain gestational diabetes, pathophysiology • Discuss risk factors (obesity, family history, age, multiparity, ethnicity) • Discuss risks to mother and baby (macrosomic or large-for-gestational-age infant) • Review treatment plan and Master DecisionPath • Discuss target goals for SMBG and weight • Teach SMBG with memory meter and record-keeping • Hypoglycemia • Daily schedule • Urine ketone monitoring • Alcohol, medications, and drugs • Emergency phone numbers	• Insulin injection technique • Daily schedule • Interaction of food, exercise, and insulin • Insulin action and insulin storage • Medical identification • Syringe disposal • Driving and diabetes

Follow-up Visits

General Information	Add for Insulin Users
• Review first visit topics • Review SMBG/urine ketone results • Check meter accuracy, compare record book and download data • Lifestyle issues (home, work, school) • Hypoglycemia/hyperglycemia • Review use of glucagon for hypoglycemia • Illness management	• Review technical skills in SMBG and injections • Insulin adjustment using SMBG patterns • Insulin site rotation and problems • Travel/schedule changes and the effect on insulin **Add as Needed** • Healthy lifestyles, weight management • Benefits and responsibilities of self-care • Emergencies • Hygiene • Stress management • Travel/schedule changes • Community resources • Psychological adjustments • Food stamps

Postpartum Visit

- Review SMBG since delivery
- Discuss risk factors for developing type 2 diabetes (family history, obesity, previous GDM, multiparity, GDM in future pregnancies)
- Birth control
- Preconception planning for future pregnancies

Figure 7.5 Gestational Diabetes Education Topics

exercise specialist often can be very helpful. In their absence, common sense plays a major role. Exercises should be comfortable, frequent, consistent, and reasonable based on the limitations of pregnancy. Fitting exercise into the lifestyle of most patients requires innovation. Some exercises can be done while sitting, standing, and even lying down. In pregnancy, exercise should be carefully monitored. Preterm labor is a risk in 10–15 per cent of these women. Exercise that stimulates labor should be avoided. Exercise should also take into account seasons. Walking outdoors is fine on days when the weather is good, but walking indoors in shopping centers or a health club is best for inclement weather. One way to reinforce the benefits of exercise and activity is to use SMBG. The next section details how this method of monitoring may support feedback for exercise.

Glucose monitoring. To determine if the nutrition and exercise goals are being met, self-monitoring of blood glucose should be an integral part of treatment. During the start treatment phase when data are being collected to determine whether medical nutrition therapy and increased

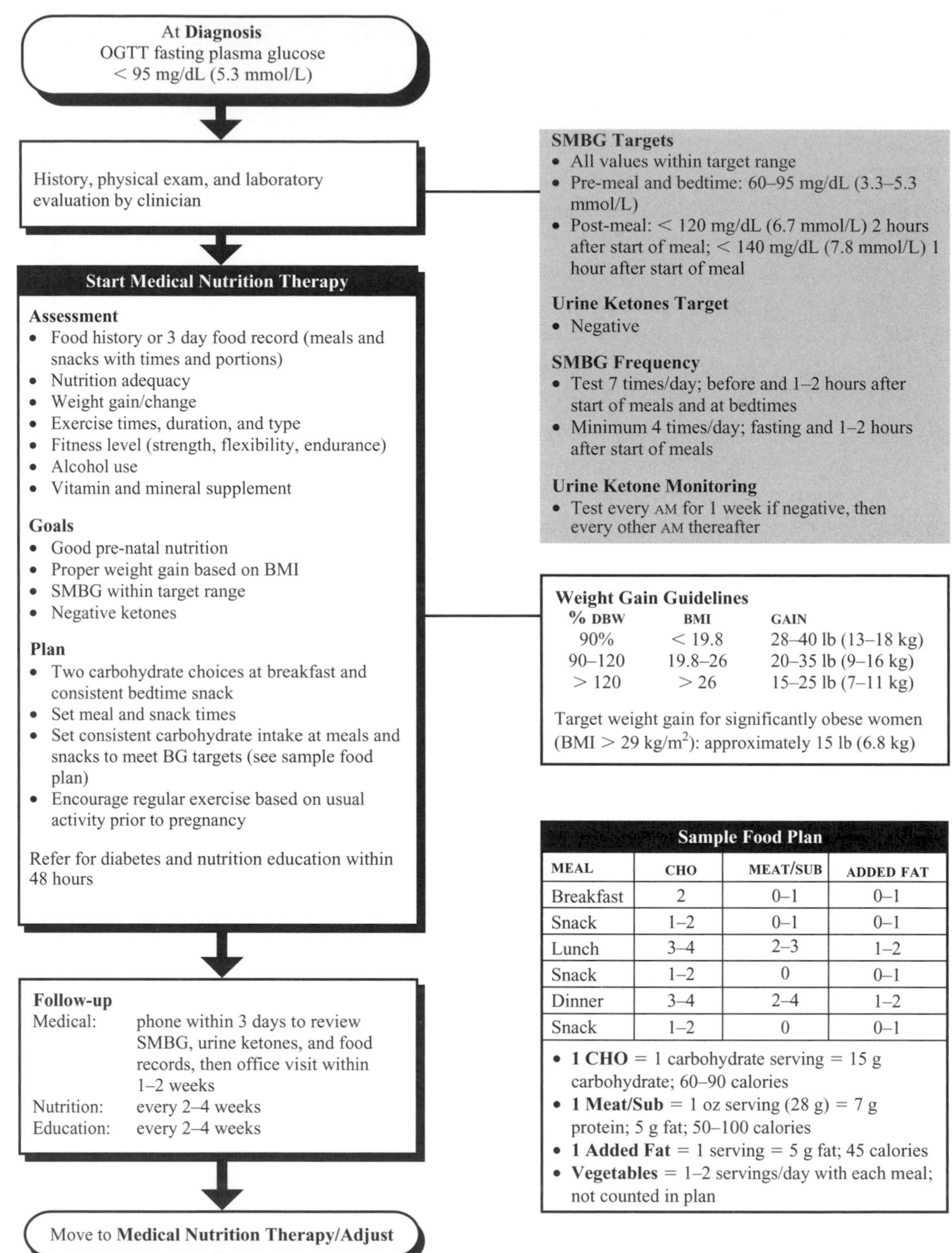

MEAL	CHO	MEAT/SUB	ADDED FAT
Breakfast	2	0–1	0–1
Snack	1–2	0–1	0–1
Lunch	3–4	2–3	1–2
Snack	1–2	0	0–1
Dinner	3–4	2–4	1–2
Snack	1–2	0	0–1

- **1 CHO** = 1 carbohydrate serving = 15 g carbohydrate; 60–90 calories
- **1 Meat/Sub** = 1 oz serving (28 g) = 7 g protein; 5 g fat; 50–100 calories
- **1 Added Fat** = 1 serving = 5 g fat; 45 calories
- **Vegetables** = 1–2 servings/day with each meal; not counted in plan

Figure 7.6 Gestational Diabetes Medical Nutrition Therapy/Start

exercise are reasonable choices, SMBG must occur at least four to six times each day. A schedule of before and 2 hours after the start of each meal provides adequate information on fasting glucose levels as well as post-meal recovery. This should be combined with testing before and after exercise (at least twice during the initial treatment phase). Testing using a memory-based meter is the only certain way to ensure reliable, accurate data. Where memory meters are unavailable, attempt to have a third party witness testing. Whether a memory meter or another method of verification is used, do not employ any technique as punishment. Patients are likely to fabricate results to please the provider.

For some clinicians, using glycosylated hemoglobin (HbA_{1c}) in place of SMBG has become routine practice. In gestational diabetes, HbA_{1c} may be used at the time of diagnosis as a basis to assess overall glycemic control up to this point and to determine whether the patient is at high risk for type 2 diabetes. *It should not be used thereafter since it provides no additional information for clinical decision-making in GDM.* HbA_{1c} measures glycosylation of the hemoglobin in red blood cells over their lifetime (~120 days). As blood glucose concentrations rise, the per cent of hemoglobin that is glycosylated increases. Measuring this fraction makes it possible to estimate the overall blood glucose control for the previous 8–10 weeks (taking into account the half-life of a red blood cell). In GDM, daily monitoring of blood glucose, not HbA_{1c}, is the basis of evaluating the effectiveness of treatment.

During the initial treatment period, all SMBG data should be reviewed weekly. If two unexplained elevations in fasting blood glucose exceed 95 mg/dL (5.3 mmol/L) or two post-prandials exceed 120 mg/dL (6.7 mmol/L), consider starting glyburide or insulin. If the elevations are due to excessive carbohydrate intake, reinforce the importance of following the prescribed food plan.

A follow-up visit within 1–2 weeks of the initial visit should be made. At that time review baseline data (SMBG). If glycemic targets have not been achieved by the follow-up visit, reinforce principles of medical nutrition therapy and consider starting pharmacological therapy.

A systematic approach to nutrition management of GDM begins with collecting data on which the initial interventions will be based. Whether carried out by a registered dietitian or a physician, the information required is the same. It is recognized, however, that where referral is not possible, the physician and nurse may be required to perform this assessment. Evaluate for:

- Diabetes treatment regimen (medical nutrition therapy, or medical nutrition therapy with insulin)
- Medical history – medications that affect diet prescription such as hypertensive medications, lipid lowering medications, gastrointestinal medications, and so on
- Laboratory data: glucose challenge test and oral glucose tolerance test results
- Provider goals for patient care: target blood glucose, method and frequency of blood glucose monitoring or plans for instruction
- Medical clearance for patient to exercise and/or other pertinent information related to exercise, i.e., limitations for exercise, reasons patient cannot exercise

Assessing obesity. The initial visit to determine the appropriate nutrition intervention should include a very careful and documented means to assess body mass index (BMI). Measuring BMI is frequently used because it permits adjustment of nutrient intake for appropriate weight gain during pregnancy. A table for calculating BMI is located in the Appendix, Figure A.5. The recommended weight gain in pregnancy based on BMI is shown in Table 7.3.

Table 7.3 Recommended weight gain during pregnancy

Pre-pregnancy (%DBW)	BMI	Weight Gain
<90%	<19.8	28–40 lb (13–18 kg)
90–120%	19.8–26	20–35 lb (9–16 kg)
>120%	>26	15–25 lb (7–11 kg)

Target weight gain for significantly obese women (BMI > 29 kg/m^2) is approximately 15 lb (6.8 kg).

Once the BMI has been determined, assess whether data are sufficient (diabetes treatment regimen, laboratory data, medications, medical history, and overall therapeutic goals) to develop a food plan. With sufficient data on hand a thorough diet history should include past experience with food plans, other diet restrictions, weight history and recent weight change, weight goals, appetite, eating or digestion problems, eating schedule, who prepares meals, typical day's food intake (to be evaluated for approximate calories and nutrient composition, other nutritional concerns, and frequency and timing of meals), frequency and choices in restaurant meals, alcohol intake, and use of vitamins or nutritional supplements.

Data from the diet history should be combined with exercise habits and physical activity level. (What activities does the patient do? Does the patient exercise regularly? What limitations does the patient have that would hinder/prevent exercise? Is the patient willing to become or interested in becoming more physically active?) Psychosocial/economic issues must also be assessed. During the visit include in the review information about the patient's living situation, cooking facilities, finances, educational background, employment, and ethnic, religious, and belief considerations. While most women experience some mild anxiety when they learn they have gestational diabetes, most women adjust rapidly and will follow the treatment plan. Emphasis on tight control to avoid complications should be balanced with sensitivity to "self-blame." If persistent non-adherence occurs, consider immediate counseling services.

If the patient is to start medical nutrition therapy alone to improve glycemic control, it is especially important not to omit SMBG. Frequently, SMBG is used less often with such patients. This places the patient and health care professional at an enormous disadvantage. Without SMBG data it is almost impossible for the patient or professional to have adequate data to determine how well the nutrition therapy is working. Therefore, it is important to assess patient knowledge of target blood glucose ranges, review blood glucose testing method and frequency of testing if needed, and review blood glucose records for incidence of hyperglycemia and number of blood glucose values in the target range.

Next, to determine goals, develop a plan that includes a combination of patient and health care team goals related to diabetes management, such as target blood glucose levels (lower in pregnancy), weight, and blood pressure (if pre-eclampsia). The nutrition prescription should include a food plan individualized to the patient based on diet history, food patterns and preferences, and other collected data, as well as socioeconomic issues, ethnic/cultural and religious practices, and lifestyle.

Determine caloric requirements. Table 7.4 shows how to estimate caloric requirement.

Table 7.4 Estimation of caloric requirement

To convert to metric system: 2.2 lb = 1 kg
To estimate maintenance calories, use the following formulas:

Weight	Maintenance calories
Underweight	35 kcal/kg
Normal weight	30 kcal/kg
Obese	25 kcal/kg

Next, evaluate the macronutrient composition of the food plan. Food plan should be individualized according to a person's lifestyle and eating habits as well as concurrent medical conditions. (In pregnancy the concerns are to balance fetal nutrition with maternal weight gain. To avoid possible starvation, check ketones daily.)

Once determined, the food plan will remain fairly constant. Specifically, the total caloric plan and energy output are not altered if the patient moves to insulin therapy.

Educating individuals about food planning and survival skills involves teaching basic nutrition, diabetes nutrition guidelines, and beginning ideas for altering current food plans to meet these guidelines. Points of focus are what, when, and how much to eat, based on the following guidelines:

- space food throughout the day to avoid long times between meals and snacks
- choose smaller portions; eat smaller meals and snacks
- avoid skipping meals and snacks
- choose a variety of foods each day
- choose foods lower in fat
- avoid foods high in added sugar such as soda pop, syrup, candy, and desserts

Note. This information may also include simple definitions of carbohydrate, protein, and fat with examples of food sources of each nutrients; a discussion of the nutrition guidelines, such as eating less fat, eating more carbohydrate, using less added sweetener, eating more fiber, and reducing total food intake for weight loss if appropriate; and suggestions for making these changes in their current eating pattern, such as grocery shopping tips.

Since patients may eventually be placed on glyburide or insulin therapy, it is appropriate to indicate that some changes will take place, but that total caloric intake will remain the same. For the obese individual with GDM, additional attention to food and eating awareness is recommended. This can be achieved by discussing the connection between portion size and calories, the calorie and fat content of foods, and the importance of self-monitoring behaviors, such as keeping food records, which are designed to increase awareness of total food consumption and stimuli that promote overeating. Complete the first visit by making certain the following items have been addressed:

- SMBG skills and urine ketones. Verify that the patient has obtained the necessary skills for proper SMBG and measurement of urine ketones.
- Identify and summarize short-term goals. Short-term goals should be specific, "achievable," and completed in 1–2 weeks.
- Goals should address eating, exercise, blood glucose monitoring behaviors, and urine ketones and should focus on changing only one or two specific behaviors at a time in each area, e.g. eat breakfast every day; walk every day for 15 minutes.

Food/exercise/SMBG records. Provide record forms for the individual to complete prior to next visit. Provide instructions on how to record food intake (actual food eaten and quantities, times of meals), exercise habits (type, frequency, and duration), and blood testing (time and result).

Follow-up plans. Arrange the appointment for next visit. Regardless of who undertakes the nutritional intervention, documentation should include a written record of the assessment and intervention completed and should be placed in the patient file or medical record.

The report should include a summary of assessment information, goals, education intervention, goals, specific actions recommended, and plans for further follow-up including additional education topics to be reviewed.

Medical nutrition therapy/adjust

Evaluate progress by collecting data including weight (without shoes in light clothing), changes in diet, alterations in medication, and changes in exercise habits. Review SMBG and urine ketone records including frequency of testing, time of day testing is done, and results. Measure blood pressure at each visit. Assess adherence to food plan by reviewing patient records completed since the previous visit. As a general rule, treatment with medical nutrition therapy should significantly improve blood glucose levels by the time of the first follow-up visit (1 week).

Determine whether food plan adjustments are necessary in order to achieve glycemic targets based on SMBG data. For example, are there patterns of hyperglycemia that may be due to excessive carbohydrate consumption at a particular meal? Are patterns of hypoglycemia related to exercise or skipped meals? Is the patient exercising regularly and is she willing to do more? Does the patient have positive ketones? Figure 7.7 describes some common adjustments to the patient's food plan depending on the answer to these questions. For example, if post morning meal glucose is elevated, consider subtracting one carbohydrate choice from breakfast and adding a meat. If caloric intake has been excessive, patient should reduce calorie intake by 10–20 per cent (checking urine for starvation ketosis) per day. Weight gain of 1–2 pounds (1 kg) would be appropriate between visits.

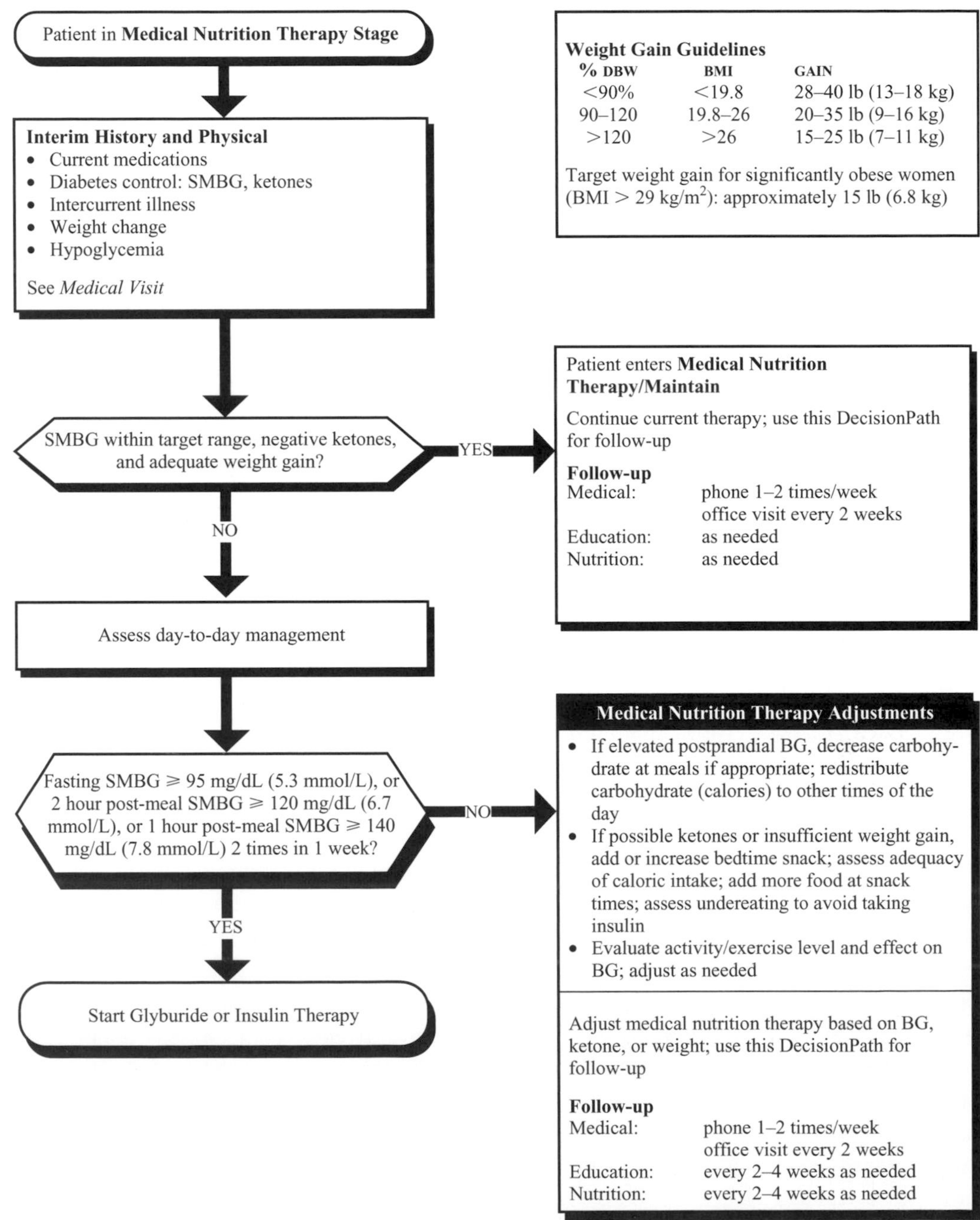

Figure 7.7 Gestational Diabetes Medical Nutrition Therapy/Adjust DecisionPath

If weight remains stable or if there is weight loss, verify that the patient is receiving adequate nutrition and consider the possibility that she may be skipping meals to avoid taking insulin. Whatever the reason, if medical nutrition plan therapy is not working, intervene.

Nutrition interventions. Identify and recommend the changes in nutrition therapy that can improve outcomes such as:

- re-educate patient on appropriate food portions and choices
- establish a consistent meal and snack schedule
- clarify exercise frequency/duration/type/timing (e.g. including exercise/activity after meals to reduce post-prandial hyperglycemia)
- reinforce importance of SMBG and benefit of effective blood glucose control

Glyburide or insulin therapy should be strongly considered if these nutritional interventions *fail* to bring the patient into glycemic control (more than two unexplained fasting blood glucose values 95 mg/dL (5.3 mmol/L) and/or two hour post-prandial blood glucose values 120 mg/dL (6.7 mmol/L) occur within 1 week). SDM recommends initiating glyburide first if the blood glucose excursions do not exceed fasting of 150 mg/dL (8.3 mmol/L). Otherwise, initiate insulin therapy.

Set follow-up plans. A second follow-up visit is recommended if the patient is newly diagnosed or the patient is having difficulty making lifestyle changes and requires additional support and encouragement. If stable, follow up in 2 weeks; if not stable, within 1 week or less.

Communication. A written documentation of the nutrition assessment and intervention should be completed and placed in the patient's medical record. Documentation should include summary of assessment information, education intervention, short-term goals, specific actions recommended, and plans for further follow-up, including additional education topics to be reviewed.

Follow-up intervention. Members of the healthcare team are often reluctant to recommend changes in therapy (i.e. starting insulin). This leads to both reduced efficiency and needless under-treatment. Consider immediate introduction of insulin therapy if blood glucose levels are not within target range. In addition to the preceding, be certain that the physician, dietitian, or nurse review treatment goals and discuss ongoing care, appropriate weight gain, and overall glucose control. Determine whether any survival or continuing level self-management skills need to be addressed or reviewed. Review the nutrition plan and food records at every visit. Written documentation of the intervention should include a summary of outcomes of nutrition intervention (medical outcomes, food and exercise behavior changes), self-management skill instruction/review provided, recommendations based on outcomes, and plans for follow-up.

During this period therapy is modified to accelerate reaching the target of blood glucose between 60 and 95 mg/dL (3.3 and 5.3 mmol/L) pre-meal and $<$ 120 mg/dL (6.7 mmol/L) 2 hours after the start of the meal. Increase in exercise levels in accordance with pregnancy, change in caloric intake, and other strategies may be enlisted to ensure further glucose reduction at an accelerated rate. During the adjust phase self-monitoring of blood glucose four to seven times per day is necessary.

Medical Nutrition Therapy/Maintain

This may prove to be the most difficult phase to sustain. During this phase, the level of blood glucose has reached normal levels, remaining within the normal range of 60–120 mg/dL

(3.3–6.7 mmol/L). Approximately 50 per cent of patients appropriately selected for medical nutrition therapy at diagnosis will achieve these blood glucose targets using a food plan in combination with exercise (activity). However, blood glucose may gradually increase due to increased human placental lactogen. If at any time the patient exceeds these ranges, return to the adjust treatment phase for closer follow-up. Modifications to the food plan and/or initiation of pharmacological therapy will be necessary.

Oral agent therapy – glyburide

Oral agent therapy using the sulfonylurea glyburide should be considered under three circumstances. First, consider it for the newly diagnosed patient with GDM and a fasting plasma glucose between 95 and 150 mg/dL (5.3 and 8.3 mmol/L) or a casual plasma glucose between 120 and 180 mg/dL (6.7 and 10.0 mmol/L). When plasma glucose reaches these levels, insulin resistance, excess hepatic glucose output, and relative insulin deficiency are likely causes of persistent hyperglycemia. Since medical nutrition therapy alone usually will lower glucose by no more than 50–75 mg/dL (2.8–4.2 mmol/L), a pharmacologic agent is needed. Second, consider an oral agent when medical nutrition therapy fails to improve glycemic control to target within one or two weeks of initiation. Third, consider an oral agent as a therapy to replace low-dose insulin (< 0.1 U/kg) if the patient has achieved glycemic targets.

Five classifications of oral agents are currently available, but only glyburide – belonging to the sulfonylurea class of secretagogues – has been shown to be effective and without danger to the developing fetus.

Contraindications for glyburide.

Before considering initiation of an oral agent, certain factors must be addressed. In the United States, the Food and Drug Administration (FDA) regulates the use of pharmacological agents. In general, the regulations are applicable to other countries. However, each country may have its own regulations, which need to be considered.

- *Only one oral agent, glyburide (glibenclamide), has been reported to be effective in controlling hyperglycemia in pregnancy and not to pass the placental barrier*
- Since oral agents are either metabolized in, or cleared by the liver, they are not recommended for patients with severe liver disease
- Only when serum creatinine is below 2.0 mg/dL (170 μmol/L) should glyburide be considered
- Some patients may be allergic to sulfa-based drugs
- Glyburide may induce hypoglycemia

Glyburide/Start
OA–0–(OA)–0

Initiation of glyburide should begin with a low dose (2.5 mg) independent of the patient's weight (see Figure 7.8). Oral agents are generally given before breakfast and/or the evening meal. The code for all oral agent administration is provided above. The first OA (without parenthesis) denotes the most popular time (pre-breakfast) for OA administration. The OA in parenthesis denotes optional or alternate times. Two factors should be considered when using sulfonylureas: (1) risk of hypoglycemia and (2) allergic reaction (rare). Generally, glyburide is safe, in terms of the risk of hypoglycemia, at this low dosage level. Use caution in patients with a history of allergies to sulfa drugs.

Food plan and exercise. Glyburide, food plan, and exercise need to be synchronized. Appropriate glyburide synchronizes carbohydrate intake and exercise. The goal of the food and exercise plan is to match these elements for optimal blood

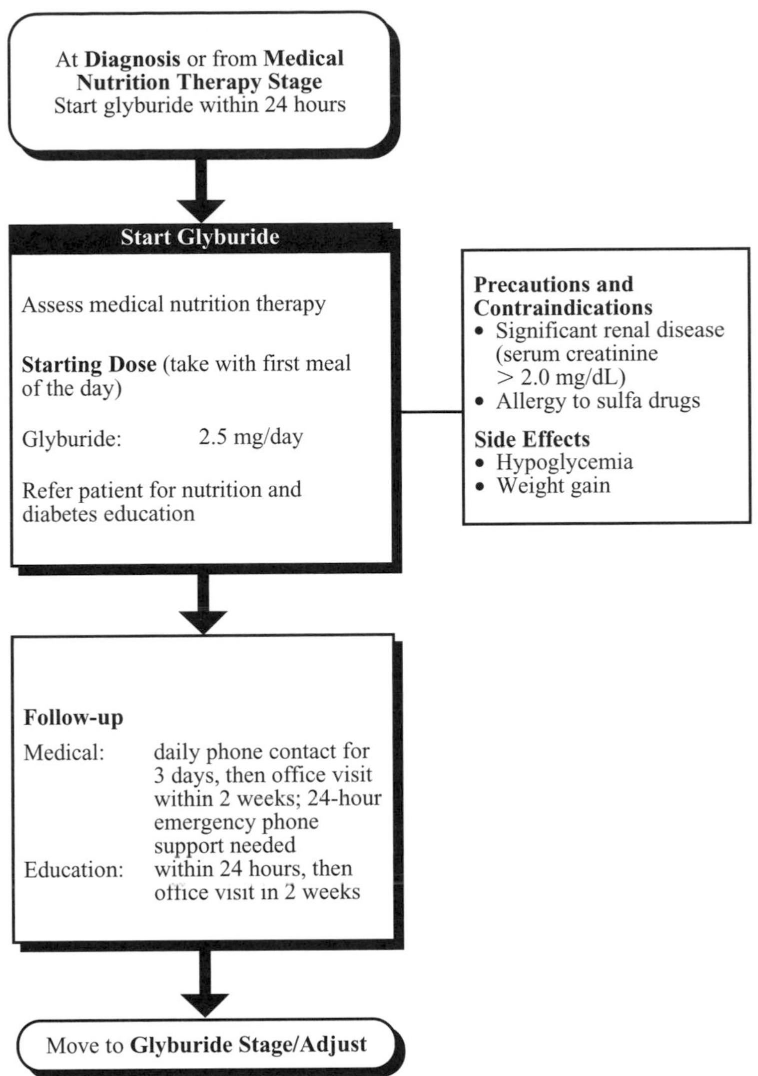

Figure 7.8 Gestational Diabetes Glyburide Stage/Start

glucose control. In order for glyburide to be successful the patient must be taught the relationship between carbohydrate intake, exercise, and blood glucose.

Blood glucose monitoring. All patients should be taught SMBG at the time of diagnosis of GDM. This will enable communication between the patient and the physician or nurse clinician. The meter to be used for SMBG will vary from site to site; however, all meters should have some important attributes. First, the meter should have a memory, making it possible to record and store data for retrieval. This also ensures the accuracy and reliability of the information provided by the patient. Second, the skills the patient needs to use the devices should be simple. Third, testing should be scheduled to coincide with the dose adjustments to optimize data collection for clinical decision-making. Initial testing should consider the need to detect changes in blood glucose due to dose, carbohydrate intake, and lifestyle changes. Patients should perform SMBG testing four to seven times per day including before meals, 2 hours after the start of the meal and at bedtime. The evening snack is designed to prevent overnight hypoglycemia and ketosis. To ensure it is working accurately, at least once or twice per week (or whenever there are symptoms), consider SMBG at 3 AM.

Follow-up. At the end of 1 week's testing, review SMBG data to determine whether the blood glucose has been altered and if any hypoglycemic episodes have occurred. If average blood glucose decreases by more than 20 per cent continue with the current dose. Schedule the next visit for 1 week following initiation of the oral agent.

Glyburide/Adjust
OA–0–(OA)–0

If the SMBG has not been lowered significantly after one week, increase the glyburide to 5 mg in the morning (see Figure 7.9). Glyburide can now be adjusted every 3 days. Staged Diabetes Management is designed to rapidly achieve near normal glycemia in pregnancy by slowly increasing the dose to reach the optimum therapeutic dose without risk of hypoglycemia. The adjustments to glyburide should be in increments of *no more than 2.5 mg*. After reaching between 5 mg in the morning, consider adding 2.5 mg with the evening meal. Then add an additional 2.5 mg in the evening if after 3 days blood glucose has not improved. Keep adding 2.5 mg every 3 days thereafter alternating between morning and evening. Note that clinically effective dose is not necessarily the maximum dose. For example, the clinically effective dose of glyburide is approximately 10–15 mg/day. Because individual differences to dose response exist, close monitoring with verified SMBG data is essential during this phase. The maximum daily dose is 20 mg.

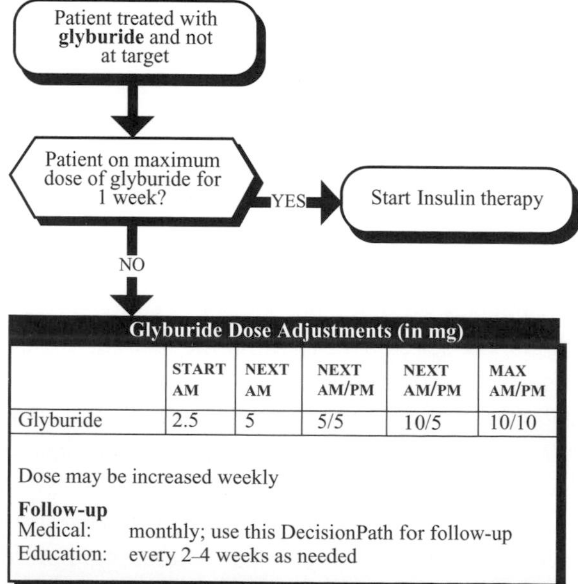

	START AM	NEXT AM	NEXT AM/PM	NEXT AM/PM	MAX AM/PM
Glyburide	2.5	5	5/5	10/5	10/10

Figure 7.9 Gestational Diabetes Glyburide Stage/Adjust

Glyburide/Maintain
OA–0–(OA)–0

If the patient has reached the therapeutic goal on glyburide, treatment now turns to maintenance. During this phase, attempt to maintain glycemic control within target range without making significant demands on the patient. SMBG testing schedules and frequency of contact with the health care professional are individualized. Insufficient contact may cause the patient to lose interest in the intensified treatment and become less likely to follow the therapeutic regimen, thereby worsening glycemic control. For some patients close contact, frequent visits, and careful assessment of behaviors related to the treatment regimen are the cornerstones of good care. All patients should be seen every 2–3 weeks. If the patient reports symptoms of hypoglycemia, consider moving some meal-related carbohydrate to snacks, or add a carbohydrate choice to snacks.

Insulin therapy

One of four criteria was met to initiate insulin therapy: medical nutrition therapy failed to adequately lower the blood glucose; glyburide failed to lower blood glucose to the target; the patient was diagnosed with a fasting plasma glucose > 150 mg/dL (8.3 mmol/L); or the patient was diagnosed with a fasting plasma glucose > 95 mg/dL (5.3 mmol/L) and preferred insulin over glyburide. If newly diagnosed, complete the physical examination and history. Determine whether the patient is obese and what the appropriate caloric intake should be (see previous section on medical nutrition therapy). For newly diagnosed patients starting insulin therapy, refer to the previous section to develop a food plan. All stages of insulin therapy use the same principles of the nutrition therapy in terms of assessment and follow-up.

Use of insulin analogs in women with GDM

With the addition of several new insulin analogs (lispro, aspart, and glargine) the question of safety and efficacy of these pharmacologic agents must be considered before they are used in the treatment of pregestational and gestational diabetes. Ample evidence is currently available to support the use of lispro insulin in both pregestational and gestational diabetes. Studies have shown that lispro has no immunlogic effect (measured by anti-insulin antibody levels) compared with regular insulin for the treatment of GDM.[20] Moreover, lispro therapy did result in improved glycemic control compared with regular insulin that was accompanied with high patient satisfaction with the analog.[21] Currently, there are no well controlled studies demonstrating the safety and efficacy of aspart and glargine insulin during pregnancy. Both aspart and glargine are considered pregnancy category C drugs (based on United States Food and Drug Adminstration classification) and should not be considered for routine management of pregestational or gestational diabetes.

Insulin Stage 3

Insulin Stage 3/Start
R/N–0–R–N or RA/N–0–RA–N

The total daily dose is calculated using 0.4 U of insulin/kg of current body weight (see Figure 7.10). Divide the total daily dose into three periods roughly associated with breakfast, evening meal, and bedtime. The pre-breakfast dose is two-thirds of the total daily requirement and is comprised of a 1:2 ratio of rapid-acting (or short-acting R) with N. The rapid-acting insulin covers breakfast and the intermediate insulin covers lunch and afternoon snack. Review the insulin action curves for the AM mixed insulin (see Chapter 3). The remaining one-third total daily dose is further equally divided into RA or R before the evening meal and N at bedtime. Make certain the patient understands how to mix insulins, proper injection technique, and the importance of timing insulin administration and meals.

Insulin, diet, and exercise – synchronization. The best treatment requires administering insulin in a way that mimics physiologic requirements. Appropriate insulin therapy synchronizes carbohydrate intake and exercise with insulin action. The goal of the food and exercise plan is to match these elements for optimal blood glucose control. In order for insulin therapy to be successful the patient must be taught the relationship between carbohydrate intake, blood glucose, and insulin action.

Blood glucose monitoring. All patients should be taught SMBG at the time of diagnosis of GDM. This will enable communication between the patient and the physician or nurse clinician. The meter to be used for SMBG will vary from site to site; however, all meters should have some important attributes. First, the meter should have a memory, making it possible to record and store data for retrieval. This also ensures the accuracy and reliability of the information provided by the patient. Second, the skills the patient needs to use the devices should be simple. Third, testing should be scheduled to coincide with the insulin adjustments to optimize data collection for clinical decision-making. Initial testing should consider the need to detect changes in blood glucose due to insulin dose, carbohydrate intake, and lifestyle changes.

Patients should perform SMBG testing four to seven times per day including before meals, 2 hours after the start of the meal, and at bedtime.

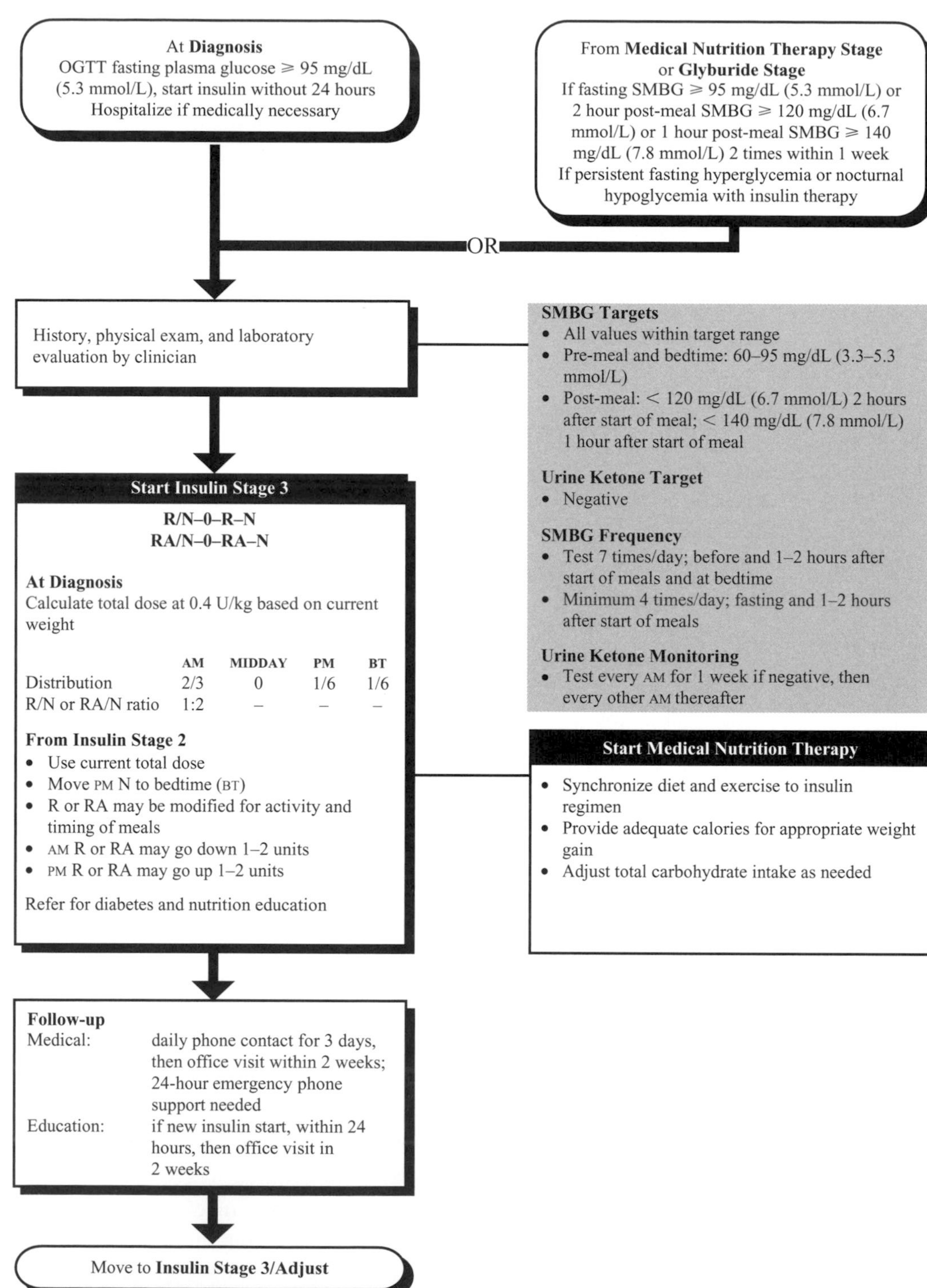

Figure 7.10 Gestational Diabetes Insulin Stage 3/Start

The evening snack is designed to prevent overnight hypoglycemia and ketosis. To ensure it is working accurately, at least once or twice per week (or whenever there are symptoms), consider SMBG at 3 AM.

Insulin Stage 3/Adjust
R/N–0–R–N or RA/N–0–RA–N

Because of this regimen's greater flexibility, increases in insulin dose may be more specific. Instead of increasing total insulin dose, increase each injection independently at intervals of 2 U or 10 per cent, whichever is greater (see Table 7.5). It may be necessary to adjust the morning regular or rapid-acting insulin. The first sign of too much morning R or RA will be midday hypoglycemia. Reducing the morning R or RA will resolve this problem with an additional adjustment in breakfast plus midmorning snack. A second problem may arise: pre-evening-meal blood glucose may rise. Use the same formula as before, i.e. raise the morning N. This will tend to increase the peak action duration. Alternatively, if the bedtime N lowers the fasting level, the insulin requirements during the daytime may need to be reduced. If the pre-evening meal blood glucose is less than 60 mg/dL (3.3 mmol/L), consider lowering the morning N. Be careful not to chase the insulin with changes in the food plan. Encourage the patient to maintain a consistent food plan.

Table 7.5 Insulin Stage 3 pattern adjustment guidelines (see Figure 7.11 for letter designations)

Time	Pattern of BG in mg/dL (mmol/L) Pre-meal < 60 (3.3)	Pre-meal > 90 (5.0)	Post-meal < 90 (5.0)	2 hr > 120 (6.7) 1 hr > 140 (7.8)
AM	↓BT N (a,d)	↑BT N (a,n)	↓AM R or RA (b,k)	↑AM R or RA (f,j)
MIDDAY (MID)	↓AM R or RA (b,k)	↑AM R or RA (j,l)	↓AM N (c,k)	↑AM N (i,j,l)
PM	↓AM N (c,k)	↑AM N (j,m)	↓AM R or RA (k)	↑AM R or RA (j)
BEDTIME (BT)	↓PM R or RA (k)	↑PM R or RA (j)	–	–

Adjust Insulin dose by 10% or 2 units, whichever is greater

Notes
a. Evaluate nocturnal hypoglycemia, check 3 AM BG
b. Consider increasing mid-morning snack
c. Consider increasing afternoon snack
d. Consider increasing bedtime snack
e. Consider giving injection 45 minutes before meal
f. Consider decreasing carbohydrate at breakfast
g. If post AM increase, increase AM snack
h. Consider Insulin Stage 3
i. Consider Physiologic Insulin Stage 4
j. Consider adding exercise
k. Evaluate if previous exercise is causing hypoglycemia
l. consider decreasing mid-morning snack
m. Consider decreasing afternoon snack
n. Consider decreasing bedtime snack

Figure 7.11 Gestational diabetes insulin adjustment considerations

The third adjustments are related to the bedtime or 9–10 PM blood glucose levels. These are affected most by the evening meal and the amount of R or RA insulin given at the evening meal. Blood glucose prior to the evening snack should not exceed 95 mg/dL (5.3 mmol/L). Consider adding more R or RA before the evening meal or reducing the number of carbohydrate choices consumed at this meal. Hyperglycemia at bedtime will often carry over, resulting in high fasting blood glucose. If all blood glucose values continue above the target, increase all insulin doses by 10 per cent every 3 days. Continue adjusting until insulin requirements are reached and glycemic targets met. Move to Stage 4 if targets are not being achieved (especially persistent mid-afternoon hyperglycemia), the patient requires more flexibility in daily schedule, or total daily insulin dose exceeds 1 U/kg.

Insulin Stage 3/Maintain
R/N–0–R–N or RA/N–0–RA–N

Many patients benefit from this regimen and may achieve a level of glycemic control not possible with a two-injection regimen. Improvement should be rapid. Once the patient has stabilized at the near-normal levels of glycemic control, continue SMBG four to seven times per day in order to make certain sufficient data are available to ensure maintenance of treatment goals. Reinforce the importance of following the prescribed food plan. Minor insulin adjustments will continue as insulin requirements increase.

Physiologic Insulin Stage 4

If Insulin Stage 3 insulin therapy has failed to move the patient to near-normal control (blood glucose 60–120 mg/dL or 3.3–6.7 mmol/L) after 1 or 2 weeks of adjusting treatment, consider changing therapy to a four-injection regimen. Alternatively, if at diagnosis the patient agreed to try physiologic insulin start with Stage 4. The patient should have seen the Gestational Diabetes Master DecisionPath, and insulin therapies requiring an increased number of injections should have been discussed as a necessary option.

Stage 4 is an important modification in the dose timing of Stage 3 by omitting the morning N and adding a midday R or RA. This should improve the morning and midday post-prandial values, a problem generally found in GDM. This provides a more manageable approach for adjustments for midday meal related hyperglycemia.

The insulin action curves for Physiologic Insulin Stage 4 (see Chapter 3) produce a pattern that optimizes post-prandial glycemic control at every meal while adding bedtime long-acting insulin to meet both overnight and daytime basal insulin requirements.

Physiologic Insulin Stage 4/Start
R–R–R–N or G or RA–RA–RA–N or G

In order to omit the morning N recalculate the insulin dose as follows: drop the morning N and increase morning R or RA by 10 per cent. Next calculate the midday R or RA at 50 per cent of the original morning N. The midday dose may initially prove to be too high unless the individual consistently eats a large lunch. A more conservative dose of RA at 30 per cent of original morning N may be considered. Table 7.6 illustrates the recalculation based on 44 total units of insulin. This therapy will enable the patient to experiment with the dosage without experiencing mid-afternoon hypoglycemia. This, of course, assumes the pre-lunch blood glucose is within the target range. Maintain the same food plan and exercise regimen. Refer to the medical nutrition therapy section and recheck goals. When starting from diagnosis, begin with 0.1 U/kg of N at bedtime. Over the first five days raise the dose by 2 units each day. If fasting BG is less than 95 mg/dL (5.3 mmol/L) then hold at the current dose and begin to add R or RA before each meal. Start with 0.1 U/kg before the largest meal. Be prepared to add the same amount before each meal until the glucose targets are reached. Each injection can be increased by 2 units every second day. During the start phase do not exceed 1 U/kg. If 1 U/kg is reached consider referring the patient to a specialist.

Table 7.6 Example of conversion from Insulin Stage 3 to Physiologic Insulin Stage 4

	AM	Midday	PM	Bedtime
Stage 3	10R/20N	0	7R	7N
Stage 4	11RA	10RA	7RA	7N

Although some patients require as much as 1.5 U/Kg this increases the risk of hypoglycemia and thus needs to be administered under close supervision. Consider a short stay in the hospital if close surveillance can not be assured on an ambulatory basis or if 24 hour coverage is unavailable.

Physiologic Insulin Stage 4/Adjust
R–R–R–N or G or RA–RA–RA–N or G

Once the initial therapy is stabilized be prepared to make adjustments as the pregnancy progresses.

Generally, the patient will reach maximum dose by between the 30th and 32nd gestational week. However, there are always exceptions. Should adjustments be required they are usually related to fasting blood glucose (see Table 7.7). Recall that the bedtime N is usually the key insulin to consider. If the fasting level is below target (60 mg/dL or 3.3 mmol/L), reduce the N. If it is above target (95 mg/dL or 5.3 mmol/L), increase the amount of N. These adjustments are straightforward for the patient. If you suspect overnight hypoglycemia, have the patient test blood glucose at 2 or 3 AM. Since R or RA insulin is used in this regimen to cover each meal, post-prandial blood glucose levels should guide the changes. Since pinpointing the problem also will pinpoint the cause, begin by looking for some consistency. Since there are four insulin injections, finding the appropriate one to target and making incremental adjustments is fairly straightforward. Adjust one injection at a time. Once the problem is resolved, re-examine all glucose values and make further adjustments as needed. Self-monitoring of blood glucose is essential here since it is the only source of data. Be sure to increase testing if necessary, up to seven times per day.

Table 7.7 Physiologic Insulin Stage 4 Pattern Adjustment Guidelines (see Figure 7.11 for letter considerations)

Time	Pattern of BG in mg/dL (mmol/L) Pre-meal < 60 (3.3)	> 90 (5.0)	Post-meal < 90 (5.0)	2 hr > 120 (6.7) 1 hr > 140 (7.8)
AM	↓BT N or G (a,d)	↑BT N or G (a,n)	↓AM R or RA (b,k)	↑AM R or RA (f,j)
MIDDAY (MID)	↓AM R or RA (b,k)	↑AM R or RA (j,l)	↓MID R or RA (c,k)	↑MID R or RA (j,l)
PM	↓MID R or RA (c,k)	↑MID R or RA (j,m)	↓PM R or RA (k)	↑PM R or RA (j)
BEDTIME (BT)	↓PM R or RA (k)	↑PM R or RA (j)	–	–

Adjust insulin by 10% or 2 units, whichever is greater

Physiologic Insulin Stage 4/Maintain
R–R–R–N or G or RA–RA–RA–N or G

Many patients will benefit from this regimen and may achieve a level of glycemic control not possible with a three-injection regimen. Improvement should be rapid. Once the patient has stabilized with SMBG between 60 and 120 mg/dL (3.3 and 6.7 mmol/L), continue SMBG. Using exercise and the food plan to enhance stability is also an option at this point. Minor adjustments of 1–2 units in R or RA will often be required to maintain glycemic control due to increasing levels of human placental lactogen. By the 35th week, the amount of overnight N will likely remain unchanged. Make certain sufficient information is available from SMBG to ensure maintaining the treatment goals.

Pregestational (type 1 and type 2) diabetes treatment options

Women with either type 1 or type 2 diabetes need to be at near-normal levels of glycemia throughout their pregnancy. In general, women with type 1 diabetes will continue their current therapy if they are already in tight control or be placed on an intensive regimen (four injections or an insulin infusion pump). Follow the section on intensive insulin regimens in the chapter devoted to type 1 diabetes.

With regard to women with type 2 diabetes, in general they will follow the same regimen as for GDM. Medical nutrition therapy alone or in combination with glyburide or insulin are the options for treatment. Thus, women with type 2 diabetes that have achieved glycemic targets using medical nutrition therapy as monotherapy should continue this therapy. Women treated with oral agent(s) should be switched to glyburide or insulin therapy (Stage 3 or 4) immediately (see Chapter 4). (*Ideally they should be treated with either glyburide or insulin prior to pregnancy.*) Follow the GDM treatment guidelines for women with type 2 diabetes.

Fetal and maternal assessment

Because diabetes presents an increased risk for developing myriad fetal anomalies, SDM has established a comprehensive program for evaluation, monitoring, and intervention. For a woman with pregestational diabetes during the first trimester, screening for complications consists of evaluation at the 16th gestational week by amniocentesis for maternal α-fetoprotein. If elevated or decreased, a repeat test is completed. If the amniocentesis confirms existence of a congenital malformation or chromosomal abnormality, the patient should be provided with genetic counseling immediately. At the 20th gestational week, ultrasound examination is completed to rule out existence of sacral agenesis, and central nervous system (e.g. hydrocephalus) and cardiac (e.g. transposition of the great vessels) anomalies particular to diabetes.

For all patients with pregestational and gestational diabetes (independent of the trimester of diagnosis), evaluation for both macrosomic and small-for-gestational-age fetuses begins at the 28th gestational week. This consists of examination by ultrasound to calculate the femur/abdomen ratio, head/abdominal circumference ratio, and estimated fetal weight for a given gestational age. The measurements are repeated at 32nd to 33rd gestational week and the 37th gestational week. If the tests indicate macrosomic or intrauterine growth retardation (IUGR), immediately initiate intensive fetal surveillance. Simultaneously, begin intensification of the diabetes regimen to further improve metabolic control. The relationship between level of control and fetal growth is a U-shaped curve (see Figure 7.12).

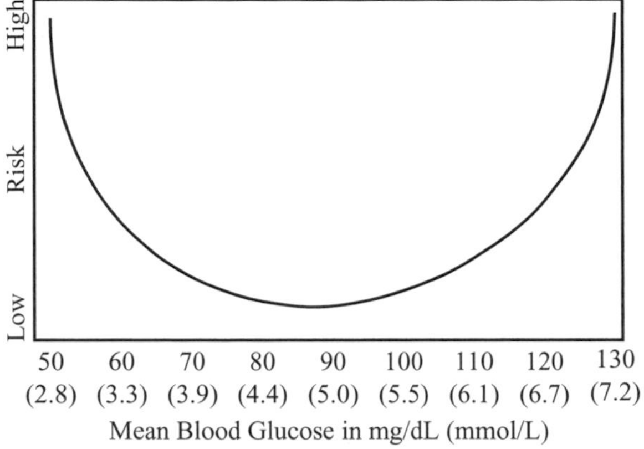

Figure 7.12 Blood glucose control and Fetal Development

Both prolonged hypoglycemia and hyperglycemia increase risk of adverse perinatal outcome. Hypoglycemia is associated with IUGR and hyperglycemia with LGA and macrosomic. Assessment for early delivery as a result of the presence of macrosomia is based on three factors:

- fetal lung maturity
- fetal measurements, biophysical profile, and velocity studies
- maternal metabolic control

Figure 7.13 lists specific points to cover in the postpartum visit. The main emphasis in maternal surveillance for gestational diabetes is on glycemic control. Additionally, careful evaluation of episodes of hyperglycemia and hypoglycemia is made through biweekly assessment of the electronic logbook produced from memory meter data. For both gestational and pregestational patients, special attention is placed on the early detection of pregnancy induced hypertension (pre-eclampsia) and polyhydramnios.

Postpartum Visit	
• Review weight change, SMBG since delivery • Review food plan if breast-feeding, modify as needed • Discuss risk factors for developing type 2 or GDM in future pregnancies	• Set follow-up plans for weight management, if needed, or refer to community resources

Figure 7.13 Postpartum evaluation

Behavioral issues and assessment

The discovery of diabetes in pregnancy often results in feelings of anxiety and guilt. Although the risk of adverse perinatal outcome is higher than in normal pregnancy, it can be reduced by co-operation between patient and provider. Sharing the Master DecisionPath is the first step to reducing anxiety. Setting short-term realistic therapeutic goals, along with directly addressing plans, will alleviate some of the anxiety. Because time is very limited, especially in gestational diabetes, consider referral to a psychologist or counselor if anxiety persists or dysfunctional behavior is observed.

Adherence assessment

Four diabetes related areas of adherence that can be readily assessed in the primary care setting include food plan, medication, SMBG, and exercise. Each area is approached in a similar manner. First, determine whether the patient understands the relationship between the behavior and diabetes. Second, determine whether the patient is prepared to set explicit short-term behavioral goals. Third, determine why the goals are not met; and fourth, be prepared to return to a previous step along this pathway if the current step is not completed.

DecisionPaths for assessing adherence to food plan, medication, and exercise regimens are located in the Appendix. They are based on the transtheoretical model of behavior change.[22] Adherence to a regimen of SMBG four to seven times per day is one of the more difficult areas for women with gestational diabetes. The Specific DecisionPath for assessing adherence to SMBG is shown in Figure 7.14. All of the adherence DecisionPaths begin with whether the patient understands the connection between the behavior and diabetes. It has been found that changing behavior without understanding why it is important to do so will most likely fail. Thus, providing the patient with specifics as to how food, exercise, medications, or SMBG are related to diabetes management and prevention of complications is critical. Next, determine specifically what the patient is willing to do. In most cases, any misunderstanding as to the importance of adhering to the prescribed regimen can be resolved through this systematic approach. The next step involves setting goals with the patient. Set simple, reasonable, and explicit short-term goals like "replace whole milk with skim milk," "increase walking by 10 minutes per day," or "add one more SMBG test per day before dinner." Setting impossible goals will assuredly result in failure. Next, determine whether the patient has met or is attempting to meet the goals. Be prepared to reset the goals and move back a step. As the behavior changes, negotiate new explicit goals. Always ask the patient to help set the new goal. There are, however, those patients for whom this approach will not work. Some patients are not ready to change their behaviors. Continued reinforcement for change, combined with education, will sometimes overcome this reluctance to modify behavior. If this is not effective, consider immediate referral to a behavioral expert (psychologist or counselor).

Psychological and social assessment

With the diagnosis of gestational diabetes or the realization of pregnancy in type 1 or type 2 diabetes, both psychological and social dysfunction may occur. This is often reflected in how the individual adjusts to changes in lifestyle brought about by pregnancy and diabetes. Initially, all concern focuses on the patient acquiring the

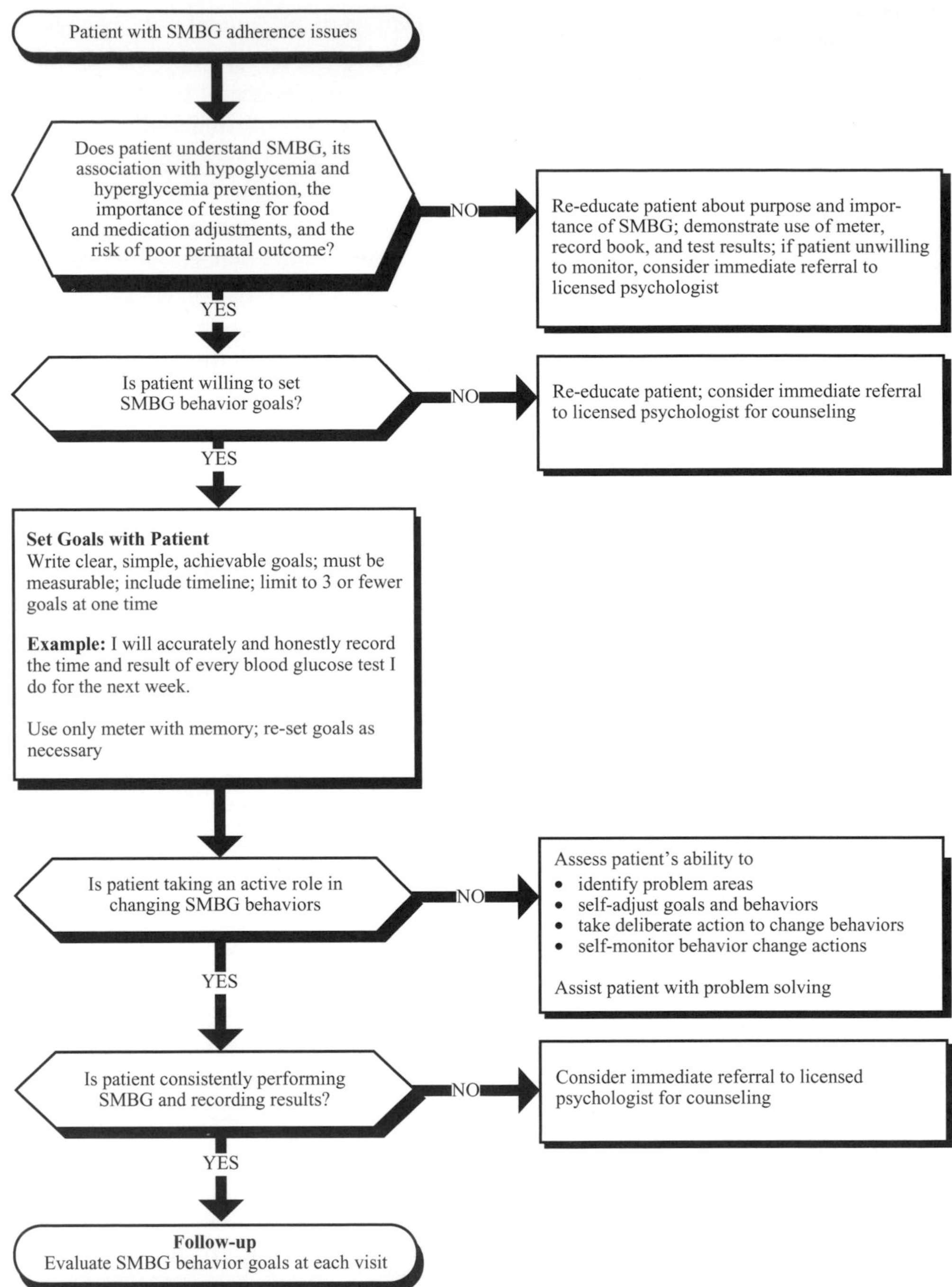

Figure 7.14 SMBG Adherence for Gestational Diabetes DecisionPath

knowledge and skills required for immediate survival and self-care. However, the patients' ability to acquire this new knowledge and skills is related to both psychological and social adjustment. Psychological factors, such as depression and anxiety, and social factors, such as conduct disorders, significantly interfere with acquiring self-care skills and accepting the seriousness of gestational diabetes and pregnancy (see Figure 7.15). If psychological and social adjustment prove dysfunctional, this is likely to be reflected in poor glycemic control. This, in turn, raises the risk of

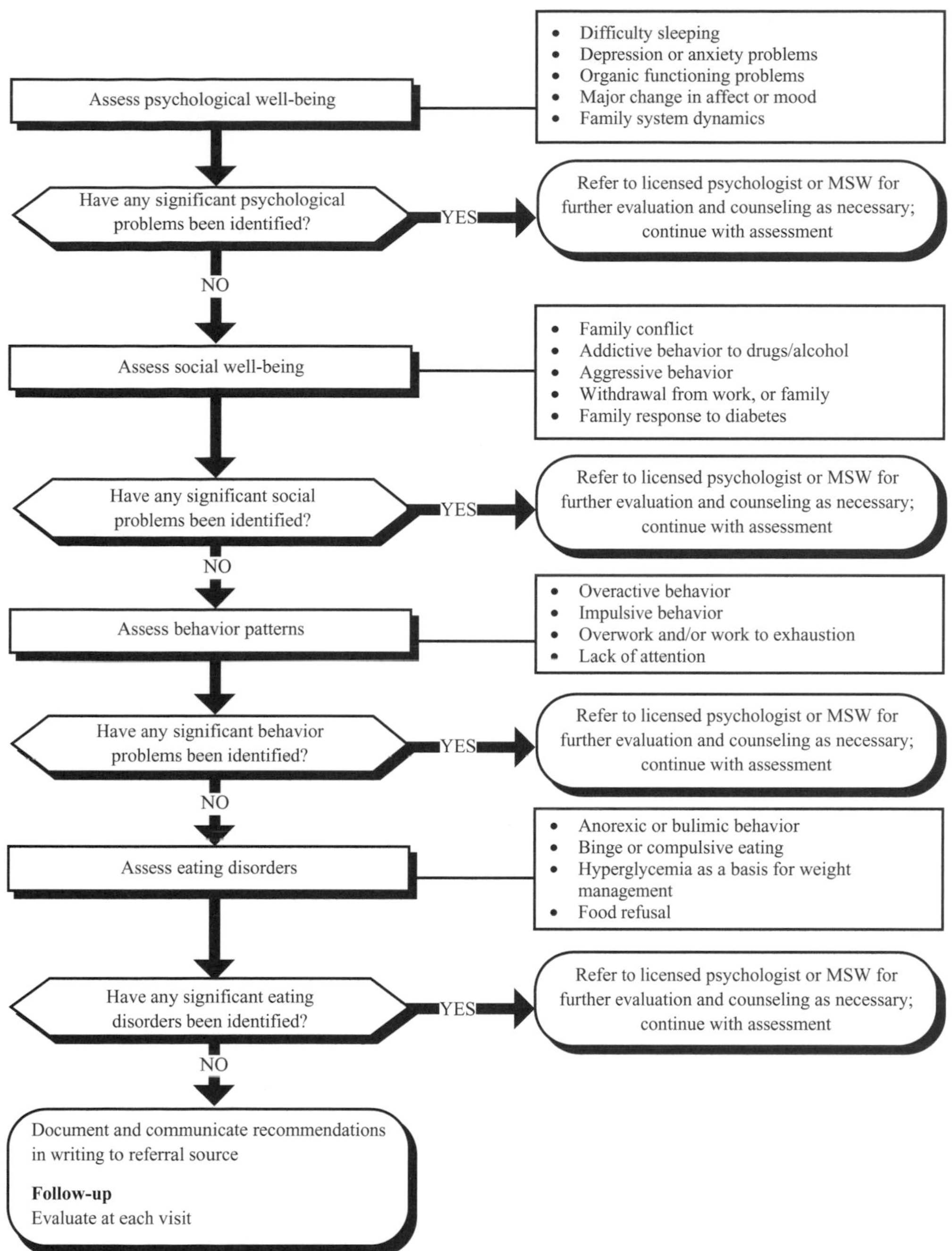

Figure 7.15 Psychological and Social Assessment DecisionPath

acute and chronic complications, which contributes further to the psychological and social dysfunction. To break this cycle, it is necessary to identify the earliest signs of dysfunction and to intervene. If there is any chance that this process might be occurring, physicians might refer the patient to a psychologist or social worker trained to detect the earliest symptoms of psychological or social dysfunction and to intervene before they result in destructive behaviors. Often one or two counseling sessions are required to detect underlying psychosocial problems and to effectively intervene.

Recognizing these early warning signs requires

a complete psychological and social profile. One approach to obtaining this information is to begin the patient encounter with the idea that diabetes will be co-managed by the patient and the physician (and team) and that the patient will be empowered to make decisions. Most patients begin interactions with physicians assuming the power to make all clinical decisions rests with the physician. For successful diabetes management co-empowerment of the patient with the healthcare team effectively brings the patient onto the healthcare team and ensures that the patient understands and assumes clinical care responsibilities. Co-empowerment recognizes that the patient and physician may have a different view of the seriousness of the disease, the responsibilities of each healthcare professional, and the expectations of the patient's performance. The individual with diabetes may feel the physician will make all decisions related to care and the patient should be passive. Alternatively, the physician may feel the patient should be the person to make daily decisions about diet, insulin, and exercise.

Co-empowerment is an agreement between the patient and health care team that delineates the responsibilities and expectations of each participant in care. It also established the DecisionPath all team members have agreed to follow. From a psychosocial perspective, it may be seen as a contract in which the patient spells out in detail his or her expectations and in which the healthcare professionals have an opportunity to determine how well those responsibilities and expectations fit with the diabetes management plan. It presents an opportunity to review behaviors that may be dysfunctional to the overall treatment goal.

References

1. Buchanan TA. Pregnancy in preexisting diabetes. In: *Diabetes in America* 2nd Ed, 1995: 719–733.
2. Benjamin E, Winters D, Mayfield J and Gohdes D. Diabetes in pregnancy in Zuni Indian women. *Diabetes Care* 1993; **16**: 1231–1235.
3. Coustan DR. Gestational diabetes. In: *Diabetes in America* 2nd Ed, 1995: 703–717.
4. O'Sullivan J and Mahan C. Criteria for the oral glucose tolerance test in pregnancy. *Diabetes* 1964; **13**: 278–285.
5. Mestman JH. Follow-up studies in women with gestational diabetes. In: Weiss P, Coustan D, eds. *Gestational Diabetes*. Vienna: Springer, 1988: 191.
6. O'Sullivan J and Mahan C. Diabetes subsequent to the birth of a large baby: a 16-year prospective study. *J Chronic Dis* 1980; **33**: 37–45.
7. Persson B, Edwall L, Hanson U, Nord E and Westgren M. Insulin sensitivity and insulin response in women with gestational diabetes mellitus. *Horm Metab Res* 1997; **29**(8): 393–397.
8. Kuhl C. Etiology and pathogenesis of gestational diabetes. *Diabetes Care* 1998; **21** (Suppl 2): B19–B26.
9. Goldenberg RL and Rouse DJ. Prevention of premature birth. *N Engl J Med* 1998; **339**: 313–320.
10. Peterson A, Peterson K, Mazze R *et al.* Glucose intolerance as a consequence of oral terbutaline treatment for preterm labor. *J Fam Pract* 1993; **36**: 25–31.
11. Mello G, Parretti E, Mecacci F *et al.* Glycemic thresholds in spontaneous abortion during the first trimester in pregnant women with insulin dependent diabetes. *Minerva Ginecol* 1997; **49**: 354–370.
12. Mironiuk M, Kietlinska Z, Jezierska-Kasprzyk K and Piekosz-Orzechowska B. A class of diabetes in mother, glycemic control in early pregnancy and occurrence of congenital malformations in newborn infants. *Clin Exp Obstet Gynecol* 1997; **24**: 193–197.
13. Weintrob N, Karp M and Hod M. Short- and long-range complications in offspring of diabetic mothers. *J Diabetes Complications* 1996; **10**: 294–301.
14. Langer O, Anyaegbunam A, Brustman L, Guidetti D, Levy J and Mazze R. Pregestational diabetes: insulin requirements throughout pregnancy. *Am J Obstet Gynecol* 1988; **159**: 616–621.
15. Piper JM, Field NT, Higby K, Elliot BD and Langer O. Maternal–fetal glucose metabolism and fetal growth retardation: is there an association? *J Reprod Med* 1996; **41**: 761–766.
16. Langer O. When diets fail: insulin and oral hypoglycemic agent as alternatives for the management of gestational diabetes mellitus. *J Matern Fetal Neonatal Med* 2002; **11**: 218–225.
17. O'Sullivan J, Mahan C, Charles D and Dandrow RV.

Screening criteria for high-risk gestational diabetic patients. *Am J Obstet Gynecol* 1973; **116**: 895–900.

18. Langer O. Maternal glycemic criteria for insulin therapy in gestational diabetes mellitus. *Diabetes Care* 1998; **21** (Suppl 2): B91–B96.
19. Langer O, Conway DL, Berkus MD, Xenakis EM and Gonzales O. A comparison of glyburide and insulin in women with gestational diabetes mellitus. *N Engl J Med* 2000; **343**: 1134–1138.
20. Jovanovic L, Ilic S, Pettitt DJ, Hugo K, Gutierrez M, Bowsher RR and Bastyr EJ. Metabolic and immunologic effects of insulin lispro in gestational diabetes. *Diabetes Care* 1999; **22**: 1422–1427.
21. Bhattacharyya A, Brown S, Hughes S and Vice PA. Insulin lispro and regular insulin in pregnancy. *QJM* 2001; **94**: 255–260.
22. Prochaska JO, Norcross JC and Diclemente CC. Changing for Good. New York: Avon, 1994.

PART THREE

INSULIN RESISTANCE AND DIABETES COMPLICATIONS

Overview

At some time most individuals with type 1 diabetes experience either an acute or chronic complication due to their disease. Therefore, the prevention, detection, and treatment of these complications are of major concern. Among acute complications, hypoglycemia and hyperglycemia occur most frequently. Extremely serious acute complications such as diabetic ketoacidosis occur less frequently, but become a clinical challenge for providers unfamiliar with proper treatment protocols. The management of microvascular and macrovascular complications associated with type 1 diabetes becomes of paramount importance, since these occur in more than 80 per cent of those with diabetes. Frequently, several of these co-morbidities are found in the same patient, making treatment decisions more complex, often requiring the assistance of a diabetes specialist. Confounding the presence of complications is the fivefold to eightfold greater risk of requiring hospitalization. Many of the complications of diabetes are preventable or at least their progress can be slowed. Poor glycemic control, hypertension and dyslipidemia are among the most prominent factors in the development and progression of type 1 diabetes associated complications.

Type 2 diabetes presents a somewhat different scenario. Many individuals who are at risk for development of type 2 diabetes already have the typical macrovascular and metabolic disorders (due to underlying insulin resistance) associated with pre-existing diabetes. As mentioned in previous chapters, hyperglycemia is closely associated with insulin resistance, which is associated with hypertension, dyslipidemia, and renal disease. There is increasing evidence that the latter disorders may occur in advance of type 2 diabetes. Thus, although most individuals with type 2 diabetes develop both microvascular and macrovascular disorders, they should not necessarily be considered as complications of type 2 diabetes. The one exception is the acute complication: hyperglycemic hyperosmolar syndrome HHS is a consequence of severe hyperglycemia in type 2 diabetes.

Gestational diabetes provides yet another scenario. Now believed to be closely associated with type 2 diabetes, the stresses of pregnancy may exacerbate some of the complications associated with underlying and untreated type 2 diabetes. Alternatively, these women, due to insulin resistance, may already have hypertension and/or dyslipidemia without underlying type 2 diabetes.

The following chapters describe the prevention, screening, and management of the microvascular and macrovascular diseases that are related to insulin resistance and/or diabetes. Once simply known as complications, we now know that they may occur in the person with diabetes or in advance of the development of overt diabetes. Since 95 per cent of all diabetes care occurs in the primary care setting, prevention of both acute and chronic co-morbidities should be the principal goal of treatment by primary care providers. Since the development of many of these diseases is slow and often without overt symptoms, frequent surveillance of high-risk patients is needed. Knowing the most current screening and diagnostic procedures optimizes prevention and promotes early intensive interventions, thus improving patient health.

Metabolic syndrome (insulin resistance syndrome) and complications

For more than three decades, it has been proposed that insulin resistance is at the core of the co-morbidities of type 2 diabetes, specifically hypertension, dyslipidemia, obesity, and renal disease. Metabolic syndrome is known by many names including Reaven's syndrome, syndrome X, insulin resistance syndrome, and dysmetabolic syndrome. The key to understanding the metabolic syndrome is the recognition that there may be a common pathway to these diseases that begins with a physiological state best described as reduced insulin sensitivity in insulin-sensitive tissues that is accompanied by high levels of circulating insulin (hyperinsulinemia). The exact nature of the relationship between insulin resistance and each of these co-morbid states will be discussed in the sections devoted to macrovascular and microvascular disease. It is important to note, from the outset, that much of what we understand about insulin resistance is still evolving.

Hospitalization overview

People with diabetes tend to be hospitalized most frequently for management of a chronic complication related to diabetes. However, they are also hospitalized for acute complications, such as diabetic ketoacidosis, and non-diabetes-related events. Special provisions are necessary and are discussed in Chapter 10.

8 Macrovascular Disease

While significant attention is focused on the microvascular complications associated with diabetes (nephropathy, neuropathy, and retinopathy), cardiovascular disease (CVD) remains at the forefront of co-morbidities to be prevented, detected, and treated in the individual with diabetes and or metabolic syndrome. Cardiovascular disease accounts for more than 86 per cent of all mortality in this population.[1] Clinical and epidemiologic studies have demonstrated a clear association between diabetes and CVD.[1]

Diabetes and the risk of cardiovascular disease

The Framingham Heart Study showed men and women with diabetes have a 2.4 times and 5.1 times greater risk of coronary heart disease, respectively, when compared with individuals without diabetes.[2] Subsequent studies have confirmed that, in the presence of diabetes, women have a greater risk of CVD than men. This finding is not completely understood. Results from the Strong Heart Study support the hypothesis that diabetes in women results in a greater negative impact on such CVD risk factors as hypertension and elevated cholesterol than in men.[3] Moreover, individuals with diabetes have significantly lower survival rates after myocardial infarction, compared with age and gender matched individuals without diabetes.[4] In addition to the established risk factors for CVD (family history, diabetes, hypertension, dyslipidemia, smoking, obesity, ethnicity), other diabetes related risk factors must be considered.

Poor glycemic control has been shown to be associated with increased CVD risk in several studies.[5,6] Supporting this is evidence that improved glycemic control reduces fasting triglyceride levels.[7] In the San Antonio Heart Study, individuals with type 2 diabetes were placed into quartiles on the basis of fasting plasma glucose levels. A more than fourfold increase in both CVD mortality and mortality from all causes was found in the quartile with the highest fasting plasma glucose when compared with the quartile with the lowest fasting plasma glucose.[8] The United Kingdom Prospective Diabetes Study demonstrated a 16 per cent reduction ($p = 0.052$) in risk for myocardial infarction in a cohort that maintained good glycemic control (HbA_{1c} of 7.0 per cent) compared with a cohort with average glycemic control (HbA_{1c} of 7.9 per cent). Thus, growing evidence supports improved glycemic control in the prevention of macrovascular disease.[9]

The risk of CVD increases with age in all

Staged Diabetes Management: A Systematic Approach (2nd Edition) R. S. Mazze, E. S. Strock, G. D. Simonson and R. M. Bergenstal
 ISBN: 0 470 86576 8

individuals. Duration of diabetes is an added independent risk factor. The Pittsburgh Epidemiology of Diabetes Complications Study demonstrated an association between the number of individuals with type 1 diabetes that died due to CVD and the duration of their disease.[10] Similar studies in type 2 diabetes are more difficult because the duration of the disease is less certain since many people have the disease for a number of years before they are diagnosed. Finally, the concomitant development of diabetic kidney disease and heart disease must not be overlooked. Microalbuminuria has been shown to be a predictor, or marker for, CVD in individuals with diabetes.[11]

Role of inflammation in macrovascular disease

The role of inflammation in the development of cardiovascular disease is an area of intense basic and clinical research.[12] Inflammation of the endothelium and atherosclerotic plaque is thought to occur through the deposition of oxidized low-density lipoprotein (LDL) in the arterial wall. The LDL deposition triggers a proinflammatory response through the depletion of nitric oxide and concomitant activation of numerous cytokine signaling pathways. Cytokines such as interleukin-6 and tumor necrosis factor α induce the release of C-reactive protein (CRP) by the liver. CRP is a non-specific marker of inflammation in the body that is positively correlated with body mass index and insulin resistance. The non-specificity is a drawback because several conditions unrelated to increased risk of cardiovascular disease may increase the level of CRP, including bacterial and/or viral infection, arthritis, and cancer. However, since it is currently not clinically feasible to directly measure inflammation in the vascular wall, indirect measures such as CRP have been used clinically to reflect vascular inflammation.

The clinical value of routine collection of CRP levels (and other markers of inflammation such as IL-6) in patients with or without classic risk factors for cardiovascular disease is currently debated. Those in favor of routine monitoring of CRP levels point to recent large prospective studies such as the Women's Health Study that show CRP is superior to LDL as a predictor of cardiovascular events.[13] Other studies clearly show that patients with increasing number and severity of cardiovascular related clinical syndromes (i.e. angina, myocardial infarction) have elevated CRP levels. Those in favor of routine CRP determinations would also point out that the new highly sensitive methodologies to measure CRP have made the test more readily available and accurate, especially in the sub-clinical range of 1–5 μg/mL. Detractors would argue that there are currently no clearly defined CRP criteria associated with a therapeutic intervention. Because of a lack in specificity and the high cost of the test, they argue against measuring CRP levels.

Despite the debate, a number of studies have identified well established therapies that reduce CRP levels. LDL reduction, daily aspirin therapy, insulin sensitizers (thiazolidinediones), ACE inhibitors, and fibrates have all been shown to reduce CRP levels. Recently, HMG-CoA reductase inhibitors (statins) have been shown to possess anti-inflammatory properties independent of LDL lowering.[14] While the debate over whether to routinely monitor CRP levels continues, the question to the clinician remains. Since Staged Diabetes Management relies on a "treat-to-target" approach, it does not recommend routine CRP determinations for all patients because of the current absence of a clearly defined CRP target. Individuals with diabetes and/or metabolic syndrome are already at increased cardiovascular risk, thus aggressive management of lipids and HTW should already be undertaken. CRP determinations should be considered in those patients at highest risk of cardiovascular disease. Note, that this recommendation may change as the role of markers of inflammation and potential treatment targets become clearer.

Prevention of cardiovascular disease in diabetes: importance of a multifactorial approach

Management of hyperglycemia, hypertension, and dyslipidemia is critical for the primary and secondary prevention of CVD in diabetes. While this may appear to be a daunting task, the impact of aggressive metabolic control on reducing the morbidity and morality due to CVD is significant. For example, in the Steno-2 Study, two groups of patients with type 2 diabetes and microalbuminuria (a strong predictor of future cardiovascular events) were studied for approximately 8 years.[15] One group of 80 patients were intensively treated with goals of $HbA_{1c} < 6.5$ per cent, BP < 130/80 mmHg, total cholesterol < 175 mg/dL (4.5 mmol/L) and triglycerides < 150 mg/dL (1.7 mmol/L). The second group was randomized to conventional treatment for hyperglycemia, hypertension, and dyslipidemia. The net result was a 50 per cent relative risk reduction and 20 per cent absolute risk reduction of cardiovascular events in the intensively treated group. Larger studies such as the Action to Control Cardiovascular Risk in Diabetes (ACCORD) trial are underway to address the relative importance of addressing each of these independent risk factors in type 2 diabetes.

Hypertension

Hypertension is found in nearly 60 million people in the United States.[16] Additionally, six million individuals are diagnosed with hypertension each year. Ten per cent of those with hypertension and those developing hypertension have existing diabetes. Of the remainder, as many as 80 per cent have metabolic syndrome. From the perspective of individuals with diabetes, approximately 60 per cent have hypertension. Like diabetes, hypertension has different prevalence rates due to ethnicity. For example, American Indians have a lower prevalence of hypertension than Caucasians, whereas African-Americans have a higher prevalence.[17,18]

For the most part, the etiology of essential hypertension is poorly understood, yet its association with cardiovascular disease has been known for decades. Studies have shown a statistically significant relationship between hypertension and the risk of stroke, myocardial infarction, and renal disease. Initially, the discovery of a link between hypertension and cardiovascular morbidity and mortality predated the discovery of antihypertensive drugs. Therefore, most studies compared hypertensive with normotensive age and gender matched subjects. These studies showed that survival was significantly more likely in those who were normotensive.[19] With the development of drug therapies, studies of whether treatment of the hypertensive patient would result in improved survival could be conducted. It was found that reduction in blood pressure to near-normal levels (< 130/80 mmHg for diabetes) significantly reduced the risk of life threatening cardiovascular disease.[19] Hypertension can be linked to two specific states: congestive heart failure and left-ventricular hypertrophy. Hypertension also directly affects the arterial vasculature expressed as macrovascular disease with specific emphasis on the coronary arteries.

Insulin resistance, hypertension, and cardiovascular disease

The pathway from insulin resistance development of cardiovascular disease is through such intermediaries as dyslipidemia, elevated blood pressure, inelastic arteries, inflammatory disease, and coagulation abnormalities. Obesity and hyperglycemia worsen and most probably accelerate these conditions. While the precise mechanism is subject to disagreement, the epidemiological data combined with the experimental data suggest that the mechanisms are multifactorial. For example, it is known that obese individuals have endothelial dysfunction characterized by a deactivation of the nitric oxide pathway. This is accompanied by a stiffening of vessel walls, which increase intra-arterial pressure. This is further compromised by hyperglycemia, which is known to interfere with normal endothelial function.

Diagnostic criterion

The current diagnostic criteria for hypertension in individuals with diabetes is a mean blood pressure $\geqslant$ 130/80 mmHg (with either systolic or diastolic BP meeting the criteria). Although the criterion for insulin resistance is yet to be determined, since both diabetes and insulin resistance place a higher than "normal" risk of CVD, there is no reason that the criterion should be different.

The development of hypertension in type 1 diabetes differs from type 2 diabetes. Blood pressure is usually normal at diagnosis and throughout the initial 7–15 years of type 1 diabetes. Hypertension often occurs concomitantly with the onset of diabetic kidney disease. In contrast, blood pressure is often elevated at the time of diagnosis of type 2 diabetes and is associated with underlying insulin resistance, obesity, nephropathy (often due to delayed diagnosis), and age. Many individuals with type 2 diabetes have isolated systolic hypertension, which may be a direct reflection on the progression of macrovascular disease. Individuals with type 2 diabetes and hypertension have three factors of clinical importance:

- reduced exercise ability
- abnormalities in ventricular filling
- abnormalities in contractile reserve

Treatment of hypertension in the individual with diabetes and/or insulin resistance is very important to prevent the development and progression of both microvascular and macrovascular disease (see Figure 8.1). The United Kingdom Prospective Diabetes Study (UKPDS)[20] demonstrated that statistically significant reductions in microvascular complications, cardiovascular events, strokes, and diabetes related mortality were found in the cohort with tight blood pressure control. While no similar study exists for individuals with metabolic syndrome without diabetes, there is no reason to believe the same intensive treatment would be less beneficial. The means to achieve blood pressure control in individuals with

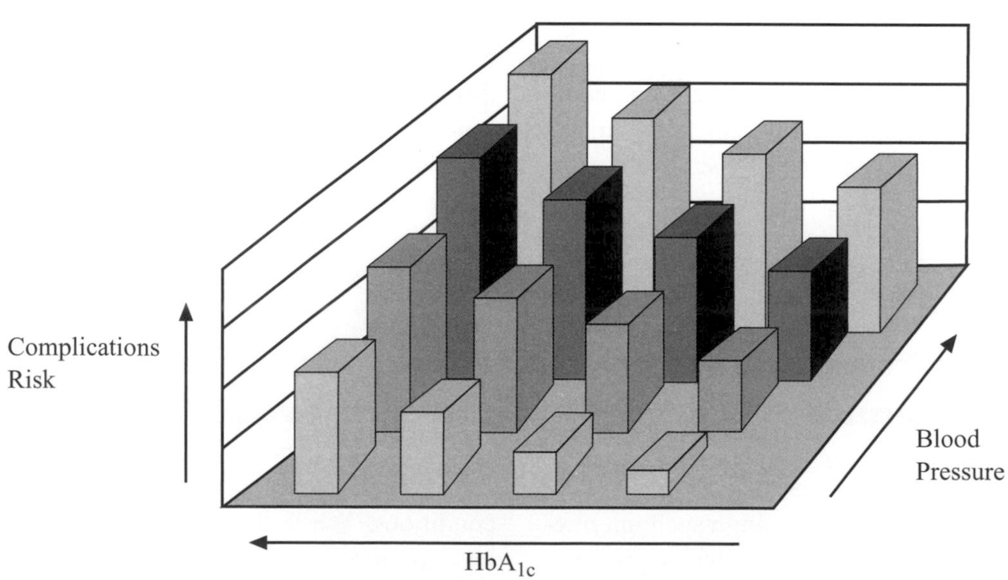

Figure 8.1 Relationship between diabetes complications, hypertension, and hyperglycemia in the UKPDS

diabetes and/or metabolic syndrome differs from people without these disorders. For example, ACE inhibitors or angiotensin II receptor blockers (ARBs) are recommended as the first-line blood pressure medication in patients with diabetes. Studies have shown the presence of a renal protective effect over and above the effect of lowering blood pressure on slowing the progression of diabetic kidney disease.[21,22,23] In addition, some pharmacologic agents normally used to treat hypertension may aggravate the treatment of diabetes. Close monitoring of blood glucose after the introduction of antihypertensive medication is recommended.

Dyslipidemia

Dyslipidemia is found in 80 million individuals, occurring annually as new cases in approximately six per cent of the United States population. Approximately 80 per cent of those with type 2 diabetes and/or metabolic syndrome are dyslipidemic. Generally, a much smaller proportion of individuals with type 1 diabetes have dyslipidemia. Dyslipidemia is a general term encompassing different abnormalities in lipid levels. Hyperlipidemia is defined as elevated levels of total cholesterol, triglyceride, and low-density lipoprotein (LDL). Other states of dyslipidemia are characterized by reduced levels of high-density lipoprotein (HDL) and may be found in combination with elevated levels of total cholesterol, triglyceride, and LDL. The relationship between dyslipidemia and atherosclerotic disease is through the formation of fatty deposits (plaque) in arterial walls, resulting in diminished circulation. Thus, it is not surprising that the risk of cardiovascular disease, similar to hypertension, shows a linear relationship with increasing serum cholesterol. Commonly associated with both hypertension and type 2 diabetes, dyslipidemia (specifically, hyperlipidemia) contributes to rapid progression of the complications found with both conditions. Type 2 diabetes and dyslipidemia may result in accelerated peripheral vascular disease combined with coronary artery disease and cerebrovascular disease.

Detection and treatment of hyperglycemia, hypertension, and dyslipidemia

Awaiting the clinical manifestations of insulin resistance, diabetes, hypertension, or dyslipidemia is counterproductive. It is unlikely that persistent hyperglycemia, hypertension, or dyslipidemia will be recognized by the patient, since their overt symptoms are also associated with aging and are slow to be recognized. Furthermore, it is unlikely that only one of these disorders exists. Therefore, whenever any one of these conditions is found, the recommendation is to screen for the others. For example, the risk of hypertension or dyslipidemia in the presence of pre-existing type 2 diabetes may reach 80 per cent. Both hypertension and dyslipidemia are well established risk factors for type 2 diabetes. Like diabetes, the risk of hypertension and dyslipidemia increases with age, positive family history, impaired glucose homeostasis (pre-diabetes), and obesity. Additionally, certain racial and ethnic groups may be at higher risk (African-Americans, Native Hawaiians and other Pacific Islanders, Asian-Americans and Hispanics).

The detection and treatment of these disorders is divided into three areas:

1. tests undertaken in a laboratory to make the diagnosis
2. steps necessary to monitor the condition or the abnormality (such as self-monitoring of blood pressure)
3. appropriate treatment for the current disorder

Optimally, prevention of diabetes, hypertension, and dyslipidemia is the goal. Primary prevention of type 2 diabetes, hypertension, and dyslipidemia should focus on modest weight reduction, regular physical activity, and smoking cessation. Secondary prevention focuses on early detection and rapid interventions to prevent the complications associated with these disorders. All three diseases are so closely associated that whenever one is present, the other two should be suspected. Tertiary prevention aims at reduction in the progression of complications through normalization of blood glucose, lipids, and blood pressure.

Note. While hypertension is predominant in type 2 diabetes and insulin resistance, it is also found in type 1 diabetes, often as an early sign of underlying kidney disease.

Practice guidelines: hypertension and dyslipidemia

The standards of care for hypertension and dyslipidemia for individuals with diabetes and or metabolic syndrome differ from those found in people without diabetes. These standards are summarized in this section and in Figure 8.2.

Diagnosis		
	Hypertension	Systolic BP $\geqslant$ 130 mmHg on 2 occasions and/or diastolic BP $\geqslant$ 80 mmHg on 2 occasions
	Dyslipidemia	Cholesterol $\geqslant$ 200 mg/dL (5.2 mmol/L); HDL $\leqslant$ 40 mg/dL (1.0 mmol/L); LDL $\geqslant$ 100 mg/dL (2.6 mmol/L); triglycerides $\geqslant$ 150 mg/dL (1.7 mmol/L)
Symptoms		Commom (classic): none Occasional (subtle): blurred vision, fatigue, infection
Risk Factors		• Obesity – BMI > 25 kg/m^2 (weight/height^2) and/or waist-to-hip ratio > 1.0 • Duration of diabetes • Positive family history • Nephropathy • Smoking • Insulin resistance syndrome • American Indian or Alaska Native; African-American; Asian; Native Hawaiian or other Pacific Islander; Hispanic
Treatment Options		Establish tight metabolic control (HbA$_{1c}$ $\leqslant$ 1.0 percentage point above upper limit of normal)
	Hypertension	Medical nutrition therapy alone, or in combination with pharmacologic agents (ACE inhibitors, angiotensin II receptor blockers, calcium channel blockers, α-blockers, diuretics, β-blockers)
	Dyslipidemia	Medical nutrition therapy and exercise; alone or in combination with pharmacologic agents (HMG CoA reductase inhibitors, fibric acid, bile acid sequestrants, nicotinic acid, cholesterol absorption inhibitor)
Targets		
	Hypertension	BP < 130/80 mmHg
	Dyslipidemia	Cholesterol < 200 mg/dL (5.2 mmol/L); HDL > 40 mg/dL (1.0 mmol/L); LDL < 100 mg/dL (2.6 mmol/L); triglycerides < 150 mg/dL (1.7 mmol/L)
Monitoring		Self-BP and SMBG daily while in adjust phase Self-monitored BP (SMBP)
Follow-up		
	Monthly	Office visit during adjust phase (weekly phone contact may be necessary)
	Every 3 Months	Evaluate hypoglycemia; weight or BMI (kg/m^2 = weight/height^2); medications; blood pressure; fasting lipid profile; urinalysis; SMBG data (clean and check meter); medical nutrition therapy; foot care; HbA$_{1c}$; smoking cessation counseling; aspirin therapy; SMBP
	Yearly (in addition to 3–4 month visit)	History and physical; annual screening for albuminuria; neurologic examination; eye examination with dilation; dental examination; diabetes and nutrition continuing education; complete foot examination (pulses, nerves, and inspection)

Figure 8.2 Hypertension and Dyslipidemia Practice Guidelines

Common clinical manifestations

Note. The most common of the clinical manifestations when these diseases occur in the same individual is obesity. Only when there is persistent hyperglycemia or persistent hypertension will the classic symptoms of these two disorders become apparent. Thus, careful surveillance, with recognition of the key risk groups, is the best method to detect these disorders.

Staged management of hypertension

Diagnosis of hypertension

Current standards for diagnosis of hypertension in individuals with diabetes and or metabolic syndrome are more stringent than those of the general population because of the high risk of macrovascular and microvascular disease associated with these disorders. Mean systolic blood pressure ⩾ 130 mmHg and/or diastolic blood pressure ⩾ 80 mmHg on two occasions is considered diagnostic for hypertension. Repeated measures of blood pressure in the office may be supplemented by at-home self-monitored blood pressure (SMBP). While previously used to detect white coat hypertension, SMBP has been shown to detect hypertension among patients believed to have normal BP when BP measurement is based only on the office visit.[24] Although home blood pressure monitors are readily available and have proven reliable and accurate, they are seldom used in practice. Several studies confirm that there is a great disparity between office measurement of BP and SMBP.[24,25,26] In one study, while office BP classified 80 per cent of the subjects as uncontrolled hypertension, SMBP identified 97 per cent of the subjects with uncontrolled hypertension. Another study found that 54 per cent of the patients had "white coat hypertension" and were "unnecessarily treated".[16] A third study reclassified 23 per cent of the stage 1 hypertensive patients as having "white coat hypertension" and 23 per cent of those with controlled hypertension as having uncontrolled hypertension.[11] Perhaps the most important finding is that among those with controlled hypertension (office BP < 130/80 mmHg), up to 93 per cent would have been reclassified as having uncontrolled hypertension if SMBP had been used in place of office BP determinations. These data are especially significant in light of the findings that elevated BP is linked to increased left ventricular hypertrophy (an early indicator of underlying cardiovascular disease) as well as to declining renal function.[27–29] One study concluded that "the use of SMBP provides an exceptional vantage point from which clinicians are able to obtain important clinical data that are not uniformly available during routine office visits."[24]

The DecisionPath for diagnosis of hypertension shown in Figure 8.3 notes that blood pressure measurement should be made after 5 minutes of rest with the patient in a seated position. It is important to use the same method each time so that the results are comparable. If the systolic pressure is ⩾ 130 mmHg and/or the diastolic is ⩾ 80 mmHg, repeat the measure in the same position with a resting interval of at least 2 minutes. If the values are between 130/80 and 180/100 mmHg, repeat the measure twice more within the next two weeks. If the values are ⩾ 180/100 mmHg at any time, the patient is considered severely hypertensive and should be given a complete medical evaluation and pharmacologic treatment should be initiated immediately. If the values remain between 130/80 and 180/100 mmHg on the first and subsequent visits, therapy should be initiated. For all patients, although not a requirement for diagnosis, consider using SMBP to confirm in office measurements. Two weeks of home monitoring, with four tests each day at various times should provide sufficient data to corroborate or refute office BP measurement. Research has shown that many patients with diabetes considered by office BP measurement to have controlled HTN, when measured by SMBP are found to have uncontrolled HTN.[24] If there is

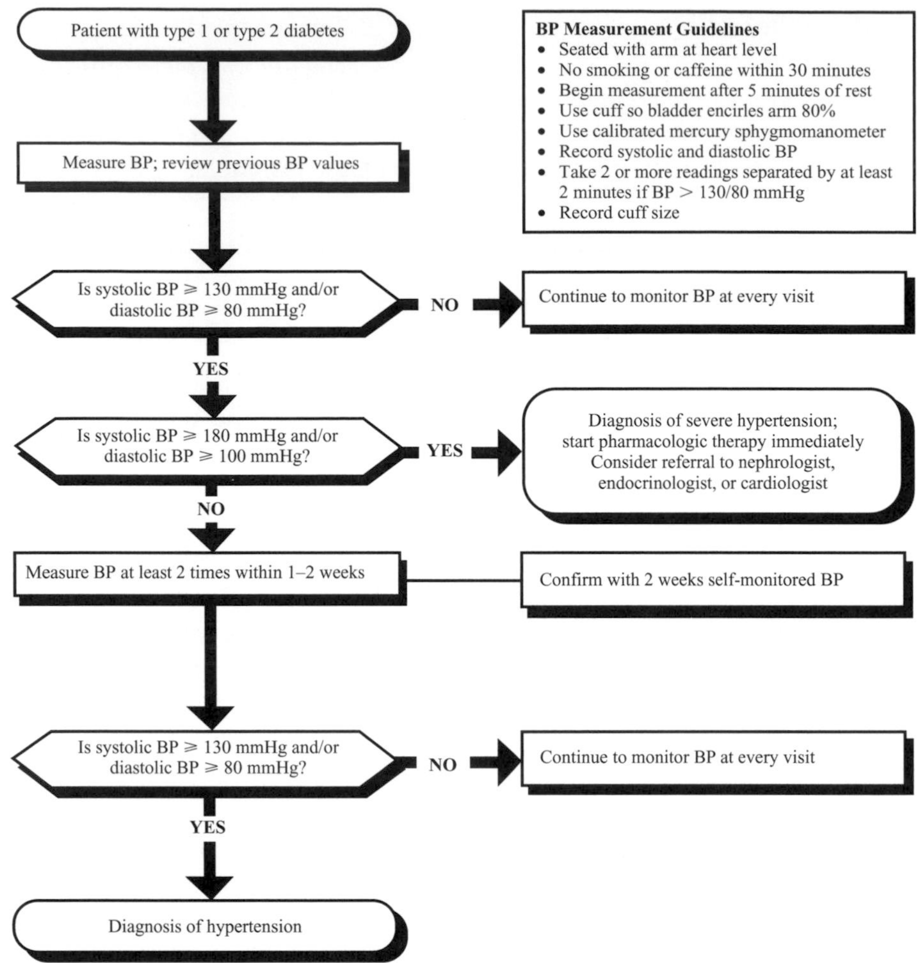

Figure 8.3 Hypertension Diagnosis DecisionPath

a substantial discrepancy between office BP and SMBP, consider 24 hour ambulatory monitoring.

Clinical manifestations of hypertension

The majority of patients with hypertension have no symptoms. Occasionally, some patients report headache, dizziness, or blurred vision. However, these symptoms are associated with many diseases and therefore cannot be used as a method of monitoring whether hypertension should be suspected. Given current estimates that 50 per cent of all adults are at risk for, or already have, hypertension, measuring BP at each office visit is a necessity. Particular racial and ethnic groups (e.g. African-Americans and Hispanics) are at significantly higher risk, as are those who are overweight, hyperglycemic, or hyperlipidemic, have a family history of hypertension, are over 50 years of age, or are smokers.

Determining the starting treatment for hypertension

Typically, hypertension management begins with alterations in caloric intake and composition, exercise, and changes in lifestyle, especially related to stress (see Table 8.1 and Figure 8.4). Specific to dietary changes is the elimination of significant amounts of salt. This is best accomplished through reduction in use of processed foods in conjunction with reduction in fats and

Table 8.1 Changes in diabetes therapy for hypertension

Condition	Medical nutrition therapy	Oral agent therapy	Insulin therapy (Type 1 and Type 2 Diabetes)
Mild hypertension 130/80 to < 160/95 mmHg	Modify food plan to reduce salt intake and increase exercise; consider oral agent therapy	Start combination oral agent therapy; modify salt intake	Intensify insulin therapy; modify salt intake
Moderate hypertension 160/95 to 180/105 mm Hg	Start oral agent therapy; reduce salt intake	Start insulin therapy	Consider referral to specialist
Severe hypertension > 180/105 mmHg	Consider insulin therapy	Start intensive insulin therapy	Refer to specialist

If the HbA_{1c} is > 1.0 percentage points above the upper limit of normal, a change in diabetes therapy is indicated.

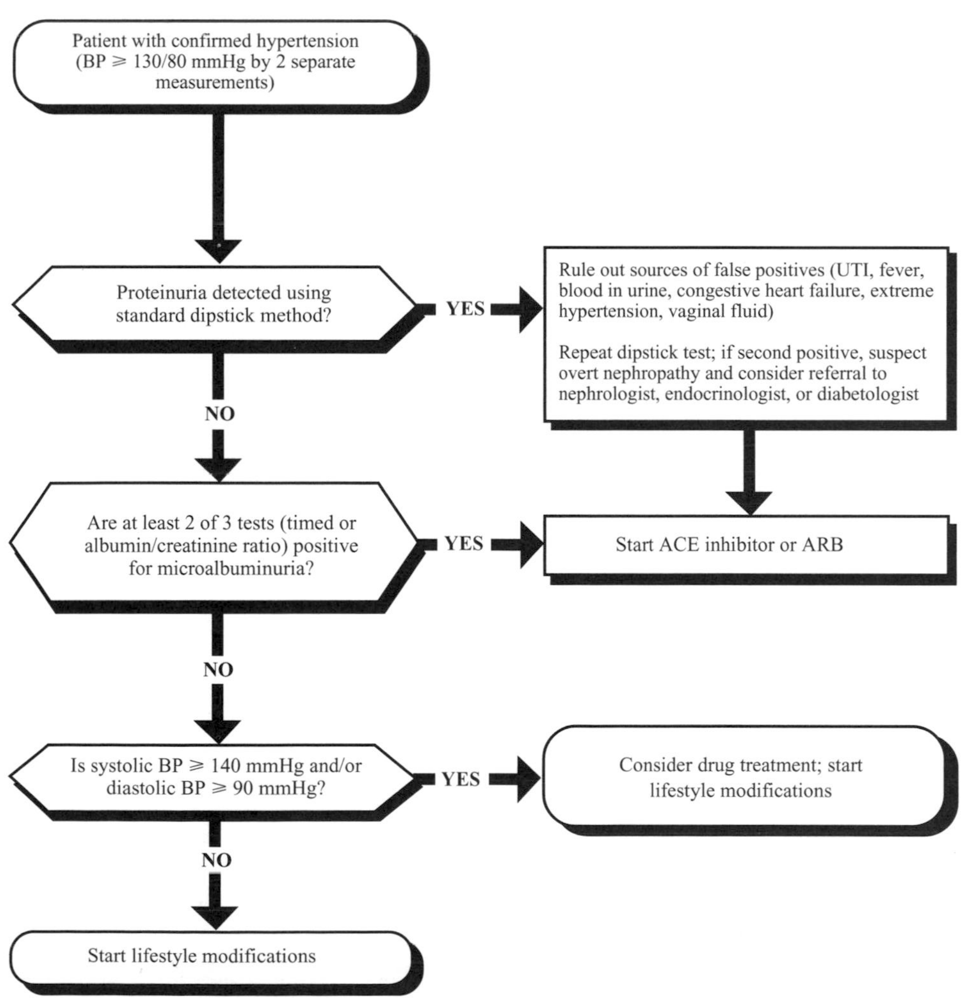

Figure 8.4 Hypertension/Start Treatment DecisionPath

modest weight reduction. Monitoring blood pressure at home and at work will provide necessary interim data to determine how well these steps are working. If these interventions fail, mono-drug therapy consisting of either an ACE inhibitor or ARB should be considered as first-line therapy. If one antihypertensive agent is insufficient to provide BP control, combination therapy should be considered. Additional antihypertensive agents should be added from one or more of the following classes: calcium channel blocker, β-blocker, α-blocker, or diuretics.

Currently there are several classifications of pharmacologic therapies from which to select. Choosing the appropriate lifestyle modifications and pharmacologic agent(s) requires careful attention to several factors:

1. severity of hypertension
   - level of blood pressure
   - duration of hypertension
2. associated complications
   - renal (albuminuria)
   - cardiac (congestive heart failure, previous MI)
   - retinal
3. presence of obesity
   - waist/hip ratio > 1
   - BMI > 30 kg/m^2
4. current composition of diet
   - sodium intake
   - fat intake

Keeping these factors in mind the choices are initially among:

- medical nutrition therapy – for mild hypertension
- angiotensin-converting enzyme (ACE) inhibitors
- angiotensin II receptor blockers (ARBs)
- diuretics (low-dose thiazides recommended)
- α-adrenergic receptor blockers
- β-adrenergic receptor blockers
- calcium channel blockers

Note. If hypertension and microalbuminuria are present the therapy of choice is an ACE inhibitor or ARB.

Low-dose thiazide diuretics (12.5–25 mg) are recommended in individuals with diabetes and/or metabolic syndrome to prevent deterioration of blood glucose and lipid levels. In addition, low-dose thiazides are especially effective in elderly patients. The results of the 8 year Antihypertensive and Lipid-Lowering Treatment to Prevent Heart Attack Trial (ALLHAT) that enrolled more than 33,000 people with hypertension and at least one other risk factor for CHD demonstrated that the thiazide diuretic chlorthalidone was equal or superior to the calcium channel blocker amolopdine or ACE inhibitor (lisinopril) in prevention of CHD and heart failure.[30] Approximately 36 per cent of the in patients in ALLHAT had type 2 diabetes. Sub-analysis of this high-risk group demonstrated that chlorthalidone was superior to lisinopril in most CVD endpoints and equal to lisinopril in terms of preventing development of end-stage renal disease. The United Kingdom Prospective Diabetes Study demonstrated that β-blockers are safe and effective in people with type 2 diabetes and should be used with caution in those with a history of severe hypoglycemia.[20]

In most instances, the detection of hypertension when type 1 or type 2 diabetes already exists will not require a change in diabetes therapy. The exception is when chlorpropamide is in use, as it may potentiate an antidiuretic hormone effect (water retention).

Selecting the appropriate therapy

Once hypertension has been confirmed, the next step is to determine whether there is underlying kidney disease (see Chapter 9). Proteinuria should be measured using the "dipstick" method. If positive for proteinuria, sources of false positives must be ruled out, including urinary tract infection, fever, blood in urine, congestive heart failure, extreme hypertension, and vaginal fluid contamination. Repeat the test. If positive again, start an ACE inhibitor immediately (unless contraindicated), and consider referral to a specialist (nephrologist or endocrinologist). If the test for proteinuria is negative, screening for microalbuminuria should be performed annually (see Chapter 9). If a patient has microalbuminuria, ACE inhibitor or ARB therapy should be initiated if there are no contraindications for use. If there is no indication of albuminuria and if the patient has blood pressure between 130/80 and 140/90 mmHg, changing both diet and activity should be the initial therapy. In general, however, drug therapy is recommended if blood pressure is > 140/90 mmHg.

Initiation of treatment requires a complete history and physical that should take into account potential for lifestyle modification. The target blood pressure for people with diabetes and/or metabolic syndrome is < 130/80 mmHg. This may be adjusted for the elderly or the presence of autonomic neuropathies. Referral to a registered dietitian to reinforce lifestyle changes is strongly recommended. Lifestyle modifications are also started on all patients placed on pharmacological therapies for their hypertension.

Lifestyle modification – medical nutrition therapy

For all individuals with diabetes and hypertension, changes in lifestyle will be necessary.

Six primary areas of change that are beneficial include:

- weight reduction or management
- increased physical activity
- reduction in dietary fats
- moderation in dietary sodium
- reduction in alcohol intake
- cessation of smoking

Many of these factors are interlinked. Clearly, changes in diet and exercise are important to emphasize since these reduce numerous risk factors at the same time (i.e. hypertension and hyperglycemia). Do not attempt to change everything at once. For most individuals with diabetes and or metabolic syndrome, the best results are achieved when only one or two modifiable lifestyle factors are addressed at one time. Refer patients to a dietitian (if possible) for a food plan that will result in modest weight loss and low sodium intake. Modest weight loss (4–5 kg) will not only improve blood pressure, but often will improve both lipid and glucose levels as well. Alcohol intake and smoking should be addressed. Level of dependence should be assessed and the appropriate therapy offered.

Start drug therapy

In general an ACE inhibitor or angiotensin II receptor blocker (ARB) should be used as the first-line pharmacologic agent in hypertensive patients with diabetes or metabolic syndrome (see Figure 8.5). Contraindications to ACE inhibitors include hyperkalemia, bilateral renal artery stenosis, and potential for drug interactions. Note that patients with impaired renal function (serum creatine > 2.5 mg/dL or 220 μmol/L) require significantly lower doses of ACE inhibitors to provide the same therapeutic response. If there are side effects (such as a cough), consider treating with an angiotensin II receptor blocker (losartan, valsartan). If angiotensin II receptor blockers are not an option, consider calcium channel blockers, low-dose thiazides, α-blockers, or β-blockers (see Figure 8.5 for considerations).

Initial follow-up should be twice weekly for 2–3 weeks to determine the reaction to the ACE inhibitor or ARB. If taking an ACE inhibitor, consider switching to an alternative antihypertensive drug if any of the following occur: hyperkalemia (K > 5), increased creatinine, cough, hypotension, rash, or leukopenia.

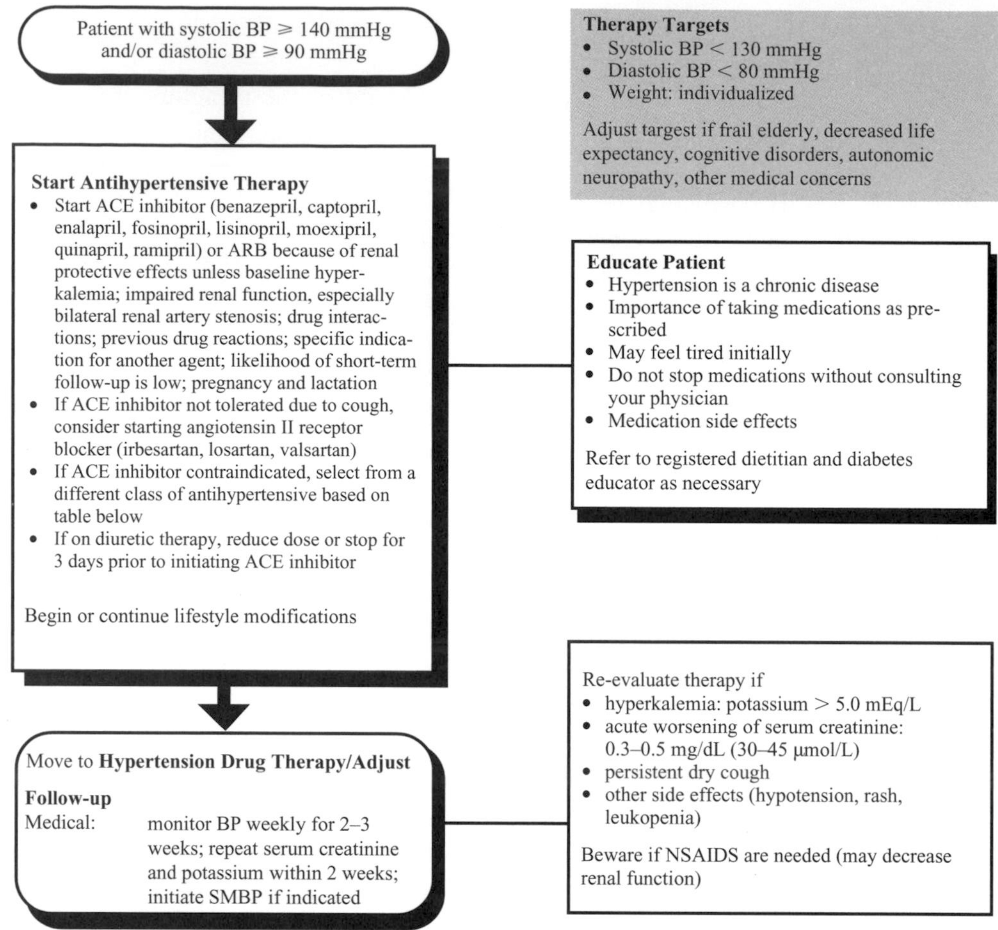

Treatment options when adding an additional antihypertensive medication, or when ACE inhibitors and/or angiotension II receptor blockers are contraindicated or unavailable

Drug class	Thiazide Diuretics	α-blockers	β-blockers	Calcium channel blockers
Drug names	Chlorthalidone hydrochlorothiazide (low dose thiazides, ≤ 25 mg/day are recommended)	Doxazosin, prazosin, terazosin	Acebutolol, atenolol, betaxolol, bisoprolol, metoprolol, nadolol, penbutolol, timolol	Amlodipine, diltiazem, isradipine, nifedipine, verapamil
Comments	No negative effects on BG or lipids with low-dose therapy, effective in elderly, less effective with renal insufficiency	Effective in combination therapy, neutral lipid effect, use with caution if orthostatic hypotension	Effective in patients with previous MI, use with caution with history of severe hypogycemia	Not recommended as a monotherapy, use in combination with other classes of antihypertensives.

Figure 8.5 Hypertension/Drug Therapy/Start DecisionPath

Adjust/maintain treatment

The adjust treatment phase is marked by the need to re-evaulate therapy because the target blood pressure has not been reached (see Figure 8.6). However, if the therapy has resulted in reaching the target blood pressure, the patient moves into the maintain phase. Continue to monitor the patient every 4 months. After 6 months to 1 year in the maintain phase, reduction in antihypertensive drug dose may be considered unless patient has microalbuminuria.

If the patient has not reached target blood pressure, assess overall adherence to the prescribed regimen. This should address changes in lifestyle as well as following the medication dose

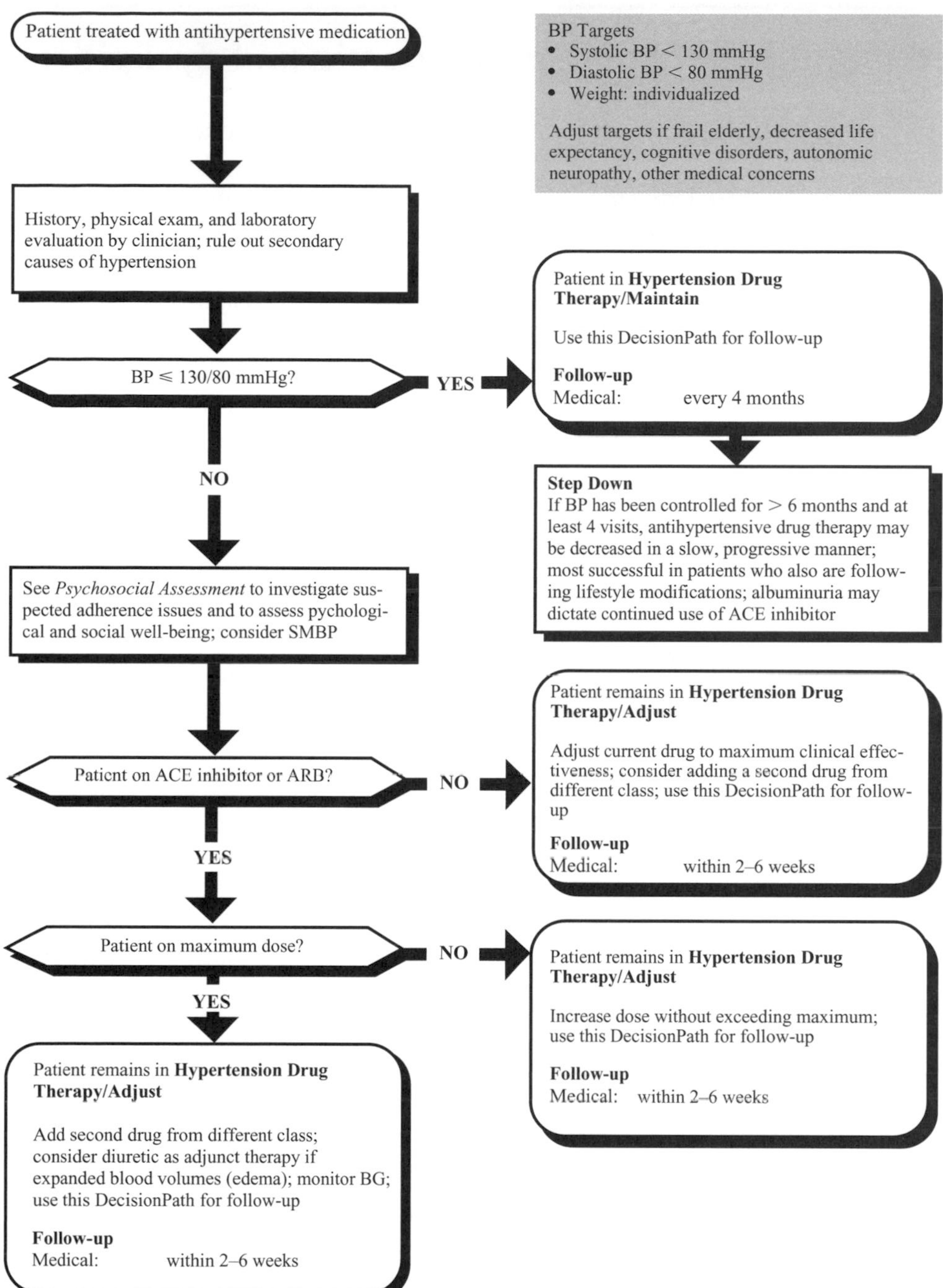

Figure 8.6 Hypertension Drug Therapy/Adjust DecisionPath

and timing. If the patient is adhering to the regimen, increase the dose of ACE inhibitor or ARB until the maximum dose is reached. If blood pressure is still not controlled, consider adding a second antihypertensive drug from another classification. If the second drug is not effective, consider a substitute drug from the same classification. If significant edema is present, low-dose thiazide diuretics may be added to enhance the antihypertensive properties of the initial drug. It is common for people with diabetes or metabolic syndrome to be taking three different antihypertensive drugs.

Staged management of hyperlipidemia and dyslipidemia

Diagnosis of hyperlipidemia/dyslipidemia

Lipid abnormalities are more likely to be found in individuals with type 2 diabetes and/or metabolic syndrome than in people with type 1 diabetes. Nevertheless, the standards are the same. Staged Diabetes Management supports the National Cholesterol Education Program (NCEP) guidelines for the detection of dyslipidemia in the presence of diabetes.[31] The diagnosis of dyslipidemia in individuals with diabetes includes one or more of the following:

- total cholesterol $\geqslant$ 200 mg/dL (5.2 mmol/L)
- LDL cholesterol $\geqslant$ 100 mg/dL (2.6 mmol/L)
- triglyceride level $\geqslant$ 150 mg/dL (1.7 mmol/L)
- HDL cholesterol $\leqslant$ 40 mg/dL (1.1 mmol/L)

Note – different conversion factors are used for cholesterol and triglyceride.

According to NCEP, diabetes is considered a CHD risk equivalent. Thus, the lipid goals for individuals with diabetes are the same as for individuals with documented CHD. For example, the goal of therapy for LDL cholesterol is to achieve a level $<$ 100 mg/dL (2.6 mmol/L). NCEP has recognized that very low levels of HDL ($<$ 40 mg/dL [1.1 mmol/L]) increase the risk of CHD. Conversely, high levels of HDL cholesterol ($>$ 60 mg/dL [1.7 mmol/L]) are considered cardioprotective.

Note. As with hypertension, the targets for people with metabolic syndrome and dyslipidemia should be the same as for those with diabetes. While the evidence for these targets is sparse, there is reason to believe that NCEP recommendations will be equally beneficial for people with metabolic syndrome.

Clinical manifestations of hyperlipidemia/dyslipidemia

Generally there are no signs of hyperlipidemia or dyslipidemia that would be readily recognized by the patient. The one exception is lipid deposits in the eye that may be associated with changes in vision. Changes in vision, however, are also associated with hyperglycemia and hypertension and therefore careful evaluation to determine the cause must be carried out. Therefore, it is important to maintain a program of careful surveillance using periodic fasting lipid profile determination, especially in those individuals at highest risk. Once again the combination of type 2 diabetes and/or metabolic syndrome, and obesity with a family history of hyperlipidemia, present the highest-risk group in which hyperlipidemia or dyslipidemia may be identified.

Determining the starting treatment for dyslipidemia

While the discovery of lipid abnormalities in people with hyperglycemia is common, its presentation may be different from that found in patients without diabetes. The key differences are:

- elevated triglyceride level
- low HDL cholesterol level
- small dense LDL cholesterol

These differences require that a fractionated lipid profile (total cholesterol, HDL cholesterol, and triglyceride) should be carried out. The "calculated" LDL should then be determined (see Figure 8.7).

As in the case of hypertension, treatment of lipid abnormalities usually will not require a change in diabetes therapy if the patient is maintaining HbA_{1c} within 1.0 percentage point of the upper limit of normal. In those patients with type 2 diabetes and/or metabolic syndrome treated by medical nutrition therapy only, some minor alterations in food plan (reduction in saturated fats) may be required with concomitant weight management. The selection of pharmacologic agents to combat hyperlipidemia and dyslipidemia raises

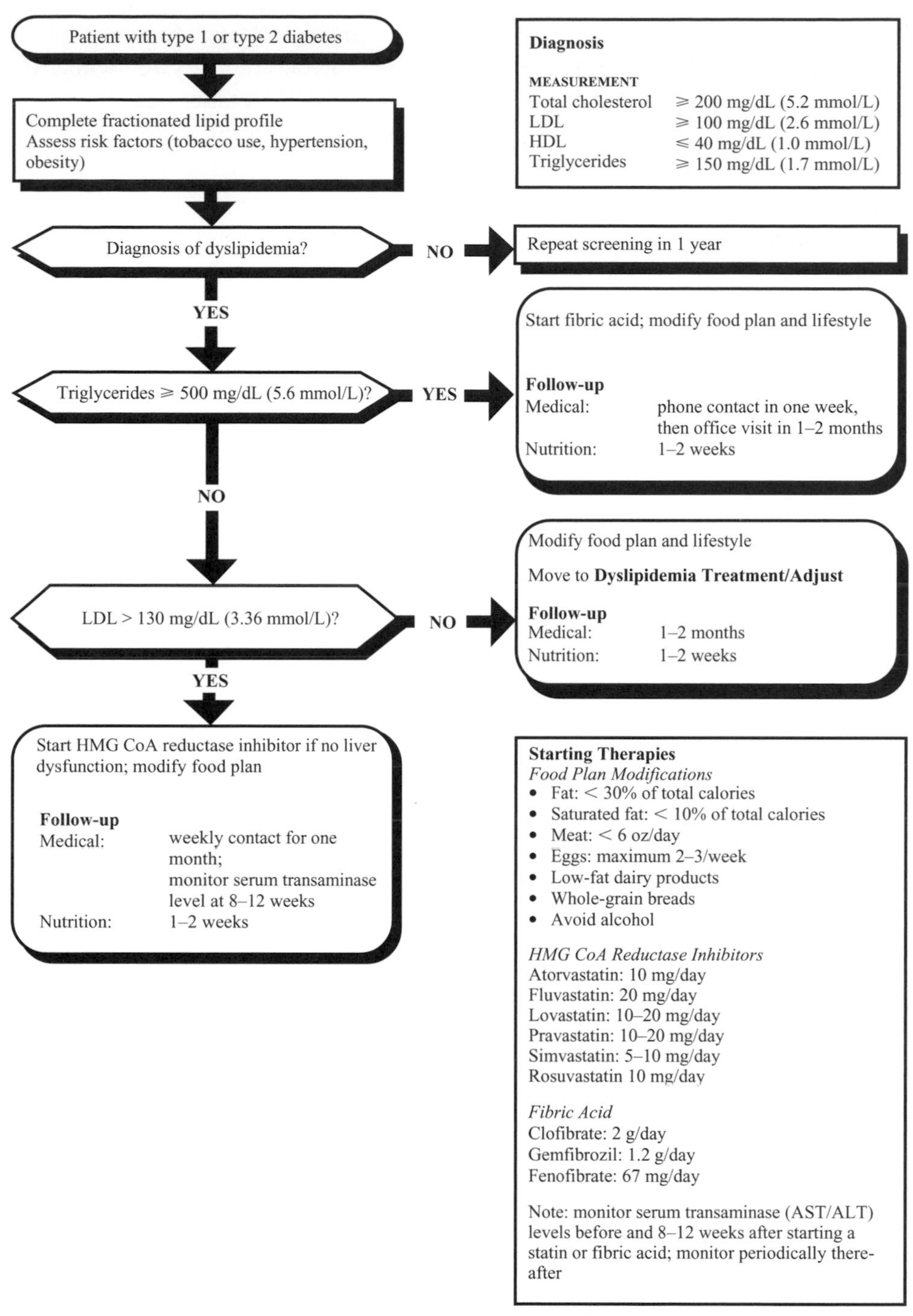

Figure 8.7 Dyslipidemia Diagnosis and Start Treatment DecisionPath

additional considerations, since some lipid lowering drugs are known to aggravate blood glucose control.

The current therapies are:

- medical nutrition therapy
- HMG-CoA reductase inhibitors (statins)
- fibric acid derivatives
- bile acid sequestrants
- nicotinic acid (note: may raise blood glucose level)

- cholesterol absorption inhibitors

Treating hyperglycemia

Hyperlipidemia or dyslipidemia in the presence of diabetes and/or metabolic syndrome requires certain precautions. In type 2 diabetes and/or metabolic syndrome, if blood glucose is well controlled by food planning and exercise alone then no modifications in this therapy will be necessary. However, when blood glucose is high ($HbA_{1c} > 1.0$ percentage point above normal) and there is hyperlipidemia, lowering blood glucose is important and may require moving to a pharmacological diabetes regimen, e.g. from food plan to oral agent or insulin. Similarly, in type 1 diabetes, if HbA_{1c} is not at target, more intensive blood glucose management is necessary (see Chapter 6). In terms of priorities, the first step is to determine the severity of the cholesterol level (see Table 8.2). Next, alter the treatment for diabetes if the $HbA_{1c} > 1.0$ percentage points above upper limit of normal.

Selecting the appropriate therapy

Staged Diabetes Management recommends the following strategy to select the appropriate starting therapy for dyslipidemia that is consistent with NCEP guidelines. Begin by evaluating the LDL cholesterol and triglyceride level. Lifestyle and dietary modifications are the primary therapies when both of the following conditions are met: LDL < 130 mg/dL (3.6 mmol/L) and triglyceride < 200 mg/dL (2.4 mmol/L). Both conditions are required. When LDL ⩾ 130 mg/dL (3.6 mmol/L) and/or triglyceride ⩾ 200 mg/dL (2.4 mmol/L) pharmacologic therapy, along with lifestyle and dietary modifications, is required to achieve lipid targets. Triglyceride levels ⩾ 500 mg/dL (5.6 mmol/L) take precedence over an elevated LDL level for the drug of first choice because of the risk for chylomiconemia syndrome and pancreatitis. Patients with severe hypertriglyceridemia (> 1000 mg/dL (11.3 mmol/L)) will require extremely low-fat diets, weight management, and a fibrate.

Lifestyle modification and dietary interventions

Significant changes in lifestyle will be necessary for all patients with dyslipidemia. As with hypertension, several areas of change are beneficial:

Table 8.2 Changes in diabetes therapy for dyslipidemia

Condition	Medical nutrition therapy	Oral agent therapy	Insulin therapy
Mild Dyslipidemia LDL cholesterol 100–130 mg/dL (2.6–3.4 mmol/L)	Modify food plan to < 30% of total calories from fat, increase exercise	Start combination therapy, modify food plan to < 30% of total calories from fat, increase exercise	Intensify insulin regimen, modify food plan to < 25% of total calories from fat, increase exercise
Moderate Dyslipidemia LDL cholesterol* 130–140 mg/dL (3.4–4.1 mmol/L)	Start oral agent therapy, modify food plan to < 25% of total calories from fat, increase exercise	Start insulin therapy, modify food plan to < 25% of total calories from fat, increase exerise	Consider referral to specialist, modify food plan to < 20% of total calories from fat, increase exercise
Severe Dyslipidemia LDL cholesterol* > 160 mg/dL (4.1 mmol/L)	Consider insulin therapy, modify food plan to < 20% of total calories from fat, increase exercise	Start intensive insulin therapy, modify food plan to < 20% of total calories from fat, increase exercise	Refer to specialist continue food plan modification to < 20% of total calories from fat, increase exercise

If the HbA_{1c} is > 1.0 percentage points above the upper limit of normal, change in diabetes therapy is indicated.
* Add pharmacologic agent and monitor blood glucose closely.

weight reduction, increased physical activity, reduction in alcohol intake, reduction in dietary fats, and moderation in dietary sodium. Many of these are interlinked. Clearly, alterations in diet and physical activity level are important to emphasize since they have an impact on lipids, hypertension, and hyperglycemia.

Medical nutrition therapy start treatment

The best results occur when alterations in food and exercise occur over time and are planned. Slow changes in behavior provide both immediate and long-term feedback. As in hypertension management and glycemic control, moderating food intake and increasing activity provide rapid positive feedback, often lowering lipid levels and reducing blood glucose and blood pressure. Replacement of high-calorie and high-fat foods and drinks with lower-calorie substitutes is beneficial. If this fails to improve lipids, reduction in food intake is often helpful. A 10–20 per cent reduction in meal size will lower total caloric intake by the same amount. If this fails to improve lipid levels, the restriction of food and drink should be attempted. This approach lists those foods, such as red meat, and drinks, such as whole fat milk, that are not acceptable. The goal should be caloric reduction by between 250 and 500 calories per day, which will result in a 2–4 lb (1–2 kg) per month weight loss. If increased exercise of 30 minutes per day, three times per week, is added, the patient may lose up to an additional 2 lb (1 kg) per month. Reduction in calories should be accompanied by modification in both fat and sodium intake. Since fat provides more than double the calories of equivalent quantity of carbohydrate or protein, further reduction in weight can be realized by replacing fat with carbohydrate and protein.

General recommendations include:

- fat at less than 30 per cent of total calories
- saturated fat less than seven per cent of total calories
- fat limited to monounsaturated and polyunsaturated (avoid animal fats)
- meat limit to 6 ounces per day (avoid high-fat products)
- dairy limit to low-fat variety
- eggs limit to 2–3 per week
- breads, whole-grain variety
- avoid alcohol if high triglyceride level

These recommended changes are for patients on medical nutrition therapy as a solo therapy or as part of the pharmacologic therapy.

Medical nutrition therapy adjust/maintain treatment

Improvement in the lipid levels should occur within 3 months of initiation of treatment and continue until normal levels of total cholesterol and LDL cholesterol are reached. Continued modification in diet and increase in activity level should be encouraged to maintain improved lipid levels. If improvement is not occurring, consider evaluation for adherence and introduction of pharmacologic therapy. Return to the Dyslipidemia Start DecisionPath (see Figure 8.7) to select the appropriate drug therapy and then follow the specific Adjust/Maintain DecisionPath (see Figure 8.8).

Start drug treatment

The choice of drugs is based on the nature of the lipid abnormality. In general, however, treatment for hyperglycemia takes precedence unless, as already noted, the lipid abnormality is severe. Thus, the drug to be avoided initially is nicotinic acid, which tends to aggravate blood glucose control. The one exception is the patient already treated with insulin. In this case, adjusting the insulin dose will counteract the hyperglycemic effect of nicotinic acid. In all cases, the lipid treatment should be targeted with the best drug for the particular abnormality.

Start all pharmacologic therapies at the minimum dose. If the LDL is $\geqslant 130$ mg/dL

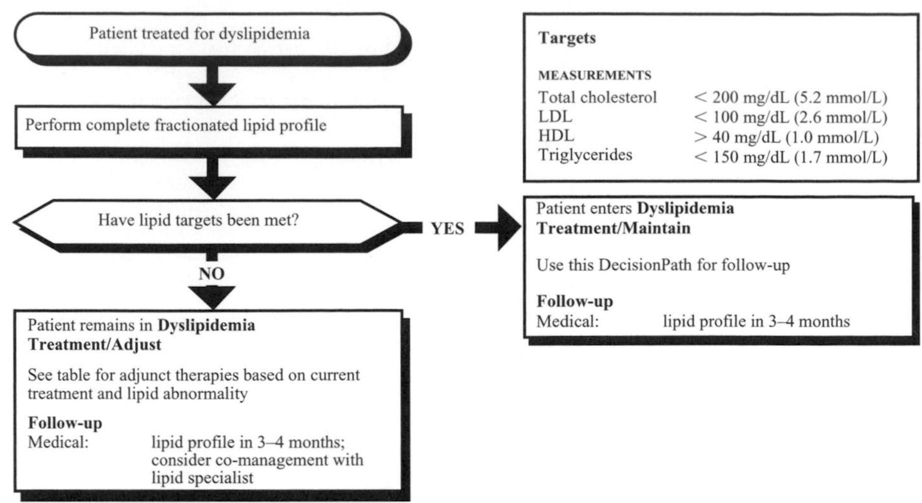

Changes in Therapy for Dyslipidemia

Current Treatment	Only LDL Above Target	Only Triglycerides Above Target	Both LDL and Triglycerides Above Target
Food plan	Start HMG CoA reductase inhibitor	Start fibric acid	If triglycerides > 500 mg/dL (5.6 mmol/L) start fibric acid; otherwise start a statin
HMG CoA reductase inhibitor (statin)	Adjust dose; if at maximum, add ezetimibe or bile acid sequestrant	Add fibric acid	Adjust dose; if at maximum and triglycerides < 400 mg/dL (4.5 mmol/L), add ezetimibe or bile acid sequestrant; otherwise refer to lipid specialist
Fibric acid	Start HMG CoA reductase inhibitor	If LDL > 100 mg/dL add atorvastatin or simvastatin; otherwise add nicotinic acid (may raise BG)	Consider adding atorvastatin or simvastatin

Drug Adjustment Guidelines

HMG CoA Reductase Inhibitors	START	CLINICALLY EFFECTIVE
Atorvastatin	10 mg/day	10–80 mg/day
Fluvastatin	20 mg/day	20–40 mg/day
Lovastatin	10–20 mg/day	20–80 mg/day
Pravastatin	10–20 mg/day	10–40 mg/day
Simvastatin	5–10 mg/day	5–40 mg/day
Rosuvastatin	10 mg/day	10–40 mg/day
Fibric Acid		
Clofibrate	1–2 g/day	2 g/day
Gemfibrozil	1.2 g/day	1.2 g/day
Fenofibrate (micronized)	67 mg/day	67–201 mg/day
Nicotinic Acid	1.5 g/day	3–4.5 g/day
Nicotinic Acid *(ext. release)*	500 mg/day	1–2 g/day
Bile Acid Sequestrants		
Cholestryamine	8 g/day	16–24 g/day
Colestipol	10 g/day	20–30 g/day
Colesevelam	2.5–3.8 g/day	2.5–3.8 g/day
Cholesterol Absorption Inhibitor		
Ezetimibe	10 mg/day	10 mg/day

Comments

Monitor serum transaminase (AST/ALT) levels before and 8–12 weeks after starting a statin or fibric acid; monitor periodically thereafter

When using a statin and fibric acid in combination therapy, monitor for myopathy (especially rhabdomolysis); ask about muscle weakness or tenderness; monitor plasma creatine kinase (CK) levels

Figure 8.8 Dyslipidemia Treatment/Adjust DecisionPath

(3.4 mmol/L), an HMG-CoA reductase inhibitor is recommended as long as the triglyceride level is < 500 mg/dL (5.6 mmol/L). For triglyceride levels $\geqslant 500$ mg/dL (5.6 mmol/L), independent of the LDL level, initiate fibric acid therapy. If nicotinic acid is selected as the initial therapy, titrate the dose slowly to avoid flushing. Initial patient contact should be weekly for 2–3 weeks to determine the reaction to the drug therapy. If an HMG-CoA reductase inhibitor is started, recheck liver profile in eight weeks. Consider referral to a registered dietitian and diabetes educator to reinforce lifestyle changes.

Adjust/maintain drug treatment

At the four month visit cholesterol, LDL, HDL, and triglyceride levels are measured to identify any current lipid abnormality (see Figure 8.8). If the therapy has resulted in reaching the target, the patient moves into the maintain phase. Continue to monitor the patient every 4–6 months. After 1 year in the maintain phase, reduction in drug therapy may be considered. If the patient has not reached target, first determine whether the lipid abnormality is the same as before. If it is the same, assess overall adherence to the prescribed regimen. This should address changes in lifestyle as well as whether the medication dose and timing are followed. Lifestyle changes should be reflected in alteration in diet, activity level, weight, and blood glucose levels. If the patient is on drug therapy and adhering to regimen, increase the initial drug until the maximum dose is reached. If the maximum dose is reached, consider adding the next drug category. If the first drug has been of some benefit, the second drug is added while the first drug is maintained at the current dose. If the first drug was of no apparent benefit, replace it with the next category drug.

Note. Should the the patient develop a different lipid abnormality or an additional abnormality follow the change in therapy for dyslipidemia protocol (Table 8.2).

Initial LDL abnormality

If there originally was an elevated LDL, at the four month follow-up the patient could have one of the following conditions:

1. all lipid levels are normal;
2. continued elevated LDL;
3. LDL improved but now triglyceride is elevated ($>$ 400 mg/dL [4.5 mmol/L]);
4. both LDL and triglyceride are abnormal.

If the LDL abnormality remains the principal concern, HMG-CoA reductase inhibitor should be increased until the maximum dose is reached. At this point, if there is still insufficient improvement, a bile acid sequestrant or cholesterol absorption inhibitor (ezetimibe) should be added. If there is still no improvement, nicotinic acid may be considered; however, blood glucose must be monitored and modification of the diabetes regimen may be required. If the LDL is being managed and triglyceride levels are now abnormal, fibric acid is added at starting dose. When both LDL and triglyceride levels are high, the LDL lowering drug should be increased and fibric acid initiated. Continue this until the maximum dose is reached or normal levels are restored. In the event that the therapies are not succeeding, consider referral to a specialist in lipid disorders.

Initial triglyceride abnormality

If the patient originally had an elevated triglyceride level, at the four month follow-up one of the following conditions might be present:

1. continued elevated triglyceride;
2. triglyceride level improved but now has elevated LDL as well;
3. abnormal LDL and triglyceride;
4. all values normal.

If the triglyceride abnormality remains the principal concern, fibric acid should be increased until the maximum dose is reached. At that point, if there is still insufficient improvement, add nicotinic acid (however, blood glucose should be followed and medications adjusted). If the triglyceride level is being managed and LDL is now abnormal, HMG-CoA reductase is added at minimum dose. Whenever HMG-CoA reductase and fibric acid are used together, the risk of myopathy is increased. Ask the patient to report muscle weakness or tenderness. When both LDL and triglyceride levels are high, the triglyceride lowering drug should be increased and HMG-CoA reductase initiated. Continue this until the maximum dose is reached for both agents or normal levels are restored.

Note. In the event that the therapies are not succeeding, consider referral to a lipid specialist.

Initial LDL/triglyceride abnormality

If there originally was an elevated LDL and abnormal triglyceride level, at the four month follow-up one of the following conditions might be present:

1. continued elevated LDL/triglyceride;
2. LDL improved but now has elevated triglyceride (> 400 mg/dL or 4.5 mmol/L) as well;
3. triglyceride level improved, LDL still abnormal;
4. all values are normal.

Maintain the current therapy when there is improvement. If there is no improvement, continue to adjust the drug until the maximum dose is reached. Change the category of drug if the initial therapy fails.

Selecting the appropriate therapy for hypertension and dyslipidemia

Many of the drug therapies and all of the dietary changes benefit more than one of the abnormalities. Medical nutrition therapy for hypertension is identical to that for diabetes or insulin resistance. Further modifications of fat intake due to dyslipidemia would benefit both hyperglycemia and hypertension. Reduction in blood glucose levels to near normal will contribute to improved lipid levels, independent of the type of therapy (medical nutrition, oral agent, or insulin).

Additional therapeutic options for prevention and treatment of cardiovascular disease

Recently, adjunctive therapies have been introduced for the primary and secondary prevention of CVD in individuals with diabetes (and for people with metabolic syndrome as well). Some of these therapies are highly recommended as part of Staged Diabetes Management (i.e. aspirin therapy) based on evidence from numerous clinical studies, while others are less well investigated and accepted (i.e. folate supplementation). Ultimately, it is up to the provider to weigh the possible benefits and risks before initiating any of these therapies.

Aspirin therapy

Numerous primary and secondary prevention trials have demonstrated the ability of aspirin therapy to offer significant protection from myocardial infarction, stroke, and mortality due to cardiovascular events.[32] Aspirin blocks the synthesis of thromboxane, a potent vasoconstrictor and stimulator of platelet aggregation. Because of the overwhelming evidence in support of using aspirin therapy to prevent cardiovascular events, SDM recommends aspirin therapy for all individuals greater than 30 years of age. While no current studies in individuals with diabetes and/or metabolic syndrome have established the appropriate dose for primary or secondary prevention of CVD, SDM recommends a daily dose of 325 mg of aspirin. Enteric-coated tablets should be considered to minimize gastrointestinal side effects. Consider lower-dose aspirin therapy (81–162 mg qd) if patient experiences minor gastrointestinal upset (stomach pain, heartburn, nausea/vomiting). Contraindications for aspirin therapy include anticoagulant therapy (warfarin) or other antiplatelet therapy (ticlopidine), allergy to salicylates, severe liver disease, and bleeding disorders.

Hormone replacement therapy

Hormone replacement therapy, which includes estrogen or combined progestin and estrogen, is commonly used to ameliorate conditions associated with menopause (hot flashes, vaginal dryness, and osteoporosis). Several observational clinical studies have shown a strong association between hormone replacement therapy and reduced morbidity and mortality due to CVD in postmenopausal women. This would appear to be of clinical importance to women with diabetes because they experience a significantly higher rate of CVD than women without the disease. However, in two large randomized clinical trials (Heart and Estrogen/Progestin Replacement Study and Women's Health Initiative) no long-term cardiovascular benefit was demonstrated in subgroup analysis of women in these studies with diabetes.[33,34] Thus, SDM recommends that the decision to initiate hormone replacement therapy for post-menopausal women should not be based on purported protection against CVD and must be weighed against the modest increased risk of endometrial carcinoma and breast cancer found associated with long-term estrogen supplementation. Contraindications for hormone therapy replacement include pregnancy, known or suspected breast cancer, known or suspected estrogen dependent neoplasia, abnormal vaginal bleeding, thrombophlebitis, or thromboembolic disease.

Nutritional therapies for cardiovascular disease

Antioxidant supplementation

Vitamins C and E and β-carotene serve as antioxidants in the body by scavenging free radicals that are responsible for catalyzing the oxidation of many cellular components. While the relationship between antioxidant therapy and coronary heart disease is not clearly delineated, it is thought to involve the inhibition of oxidation of LDL-C. Oxidation of LDL-C appears to be required before it can be taken up by macrophages in the arterial wall, leading to atheroma. People with diabetes have enhanced susceptibility to LDL-C oxidation, which may be one of the factors explaining the increased risk of CVD in these individuals. Since large placebo controlled studies have failed to demonstrate the CVD benefit of high-dose vitamin E,[18] SDM recommends that patients avoid-special supplements of vitamin E; rather, a daily multivitamin should be considered.

Folate supplementation

Folate, and to a lesser extent vitamins B6 and B12, have been suggested to be effective in preventing CVD because of their ability to lower homocysteine levels. Homocysteine is an amino acid that is formed by the metabolism of methionine in the liver. Folate, vitamin B6, and vitamin B12 are critical for the metabolic conversion of homocysteine into other amino acids and have been shown to be effective at reducing homocysteine levels. Elevated homocysteine levels have been shown to be an independent risk factor for coronary artery disease.[35] Currently, SDM does not recommend determining homocysteine levels on a routine basis. Determining homocysteine levels should be considered primarily for patients with established CVD in the absence of other risk factors. If homocysteine levels are elevated (above normal laboratory reference range), folate supplementation of 0.4–1 mg per day is recommended. Folate supplementation is not recommended for the prevention of CVD unless elevated homocysteine levels have been documented. Homocysteine levels should be determined after 8–12 weeks of folate supplementation to ascertain the effectiveness of therapy.

Fish oil therapy

Omega-3 fatty acids that are found in fish oil have been shown to be an effective alternative to fibrates and niacin for treating hypertriglyceridemia. Omega-3 fatty acids reduce triglyceride levels by decreasing the production of VLDL triglycerides in the liver. A meta-analysis of 26 clinical studies demonstrated that fish oil effectively lowers triglyceride levels by up to 30 per cent with no significant change in HbA_{1c}.[36] Fatty (non-farm raised) fish are high in the omega-3 fatty acids eicosapentaenoic acid (EPA) and docosahexaenoic acid (DHA). The American Heart Association recommends that patients without documented CHD eat fatty fish (lake trout, sea salmon, albacore tuna) at least twice per week because sufficient epidemiological and clinical data exist to support their role in reducing the risk of cardiovascular disease.[37] It is important to consider that certain fatty fish may have high levels of mercury and other contaminants. In patients with documented CHD, increased consumption of fatty fish and/or supplementation in order to achieve 1 g of EPA and DHA/day is recommended. In patients with isolated hypertriglyceridemia ($>$ 200–400 mg/dL or 2.3–4.5 mmol/L), further supplementation of EPA and DHA to 2–4 g/day may be considered to lower triglyceride levels.

References

1. Wingard DL and Barrett-Connor EL. Heart disease and diabetes. In *Diabetes in America*. 1995 NIH publication no 95-1468, pp 429–448.
2. Kannel WB. Lipids, diabetes, and coronary heart disease: insights from the Framingham Study. *Am Heart J* 1985; **110**: 1100–1107.
3. Howard BV, Cowan LD, Go O, *et al*. Adverse effects of diabetes on multiple cardiovascular disease risk factors in women: the Strong Heart Study. *Diabetes Care* 1998; **21**: 1258–1265.
4. Chun BY, Dobson AJ and Heller RF. The impact of diabetes on survival among patients with first myocardial infarction. *Diabetes Care* 1997; **20**: 704–708.
5. Kuusisto J, Mykkanen L, Pyorala K and Laakso M. NIDDM and its metabolic control predict coronary heart disease in elderly subjects. *Diabetes* 1994; **43**: 960–967.
6. Klein R. Hyperglycemia and microvascular and macrovascular disease in diabetes. *Diabetes Care* 1995; **18**: 258–268.
7. Alberti G, Mazze R, eds. Frontiers in Diabetes Research: Current Trends in Non-Insulin Dependent Diabetes Mellitus. Amsterdam: *Excerta Medica*, 1989.
8. Wei M, Gaskill SP, Haffner SM and Stern MP. Effects of diabetes and level of glycemia on all-cause and cardiovascular mortality. The San Antonio Heart Study. *Diabetes Care* 1998; **21**(7): 1168–1172.
9. UK Prospective Diabetes Study Group. Intensive blood-glucose control with sulphonylureas or insulin compared with conventional treatment and risk of complications in patients with type 2 diabetes (UKPDS 33). *Lancet* 1998; **352**: 838–853.
10. Orchard TJ, Dorman JS, Maser RE, *et al*. Factors associated with avoidance of severe complications after 25 yr of IDDM: Pittsburgh Epidemiology of Diabetes Complications Study I. *Diabetes Care* 1990; **13**: 741–747.
11. Neil A, Hawkins M, Potok M, *et al*. A prospective population-based study of microalbuminuria as a predictor of mortality in NIDDM. *Diabetes Care* 1993; **16**: 996–1003.
12. Dandona P. Endothelium, inflammation and diabetes. *Curr Diab Rep* 2002; **2**: 311–315.
13. Ridker PM, Rifai N, Rose L, *et al*. Comparison of C-reactive protein and low-density lipoprotein cholesterol levels in the prediction of first cardiovascular events. *N Engl J Med* 2002; **347**: 1557–1565.
14. Kinlay S and Selwyn AP. Effects of statins on inflammation in patients with acute and chronic coronary syndromes. *Am J Card* 2003; **91**: 9B–13B.
15. Gaede P, Vedel P, Larsen N, Jensen G, Parving HH and Pedersen O. Multifactorial intervention and cardiovascular disease in patients with type 2 diabetes. *N Engl J Med* 2003; **348**: 383–393.
16. He J and Whelton PK. Epidemiology and prevention of hypertension. *Med Clin North Am* 1997; **81**: 1078–1097.

17. Gohdes D, Kaufman S and Valway S. Diabetes in American Indians: an overview. *Diabetes Care* 1993; **16**: 239–243.
18. Flack JM, Ferdinand KC and Nasser SA. Epidemiology of hypertension and cardiovascular disease in African Americans. *J Clin Hypertens (Greenwich)* 2003; **5** (Suppl 1): 5–11.
19. Ferriss JB. The causes of raised blood pressure in insulin-dependent and non-insulin-dependent diabetes. *J Hum Hypertens* 1991; **5**: 245–254
20. UK Prospective Diabetes Study Group. Tight blood pressure control and risk of macrovascular and microvascular complications in type 2 diabetes: UKPDS 38. *Br Med J* 1998; **317**: 703–726.
21. Lewis EJ, Hunsicker LG, Bain RP and Rohde RD. The effect of angiotensin-converting-enzyme inhibition on diabetic nephropathy: the Collaborative Study Group. *N Engl J Med* 1993; **329**: 1456–1462.
22. Parving HH, Lehnert H, Brochner-Mortensen J, Gomis R, Andersen S and Arner P. The effect of irbesartan on the development of diabetic nephropathy in patients with type 2 diabetes. *N Engl J Med* 2001; **345**: 870–878.
23. Lewis EJ, Hunsicker LG, Clarke WR, *et al.* Renoprotective effect of the angiotensin-receptor antagonist irbesartan in patients with type 2 diabetes. *N Engl J Med.* 2001; **345**: 851–860.
24. Mazze RS, Simonson GD, Robinson RL, Kendall DM, Idrogo MA, Adlis SA, Boyce KS, Dunne CJ, Anderson RL and Bergenstal RM. Characterizing blood pressure in individuals with type 2 diabetes: the relationship between clinic self-monitored blood pressure. *Diabet Med* 2003; **20**: 752–757.
25. Jain A and Krakoff LR. Effect of recorded home blood pressure measurements on the staging of hypertensive patients. *Blood Press Monit* 2002; **7**: 157–161.
26. Masding MG, Jones JR, Bartley E and Sandeman DD. Assessment of blood pressure in patients with Type 2 diabetes: comparison between home blood pressure monitoring, clinic blood pressure measurement and 24-h ambulatory blood pressure monitoring. *Diabet Med* 2001; **8**: 431–437.
27. Mion Jr D, Pierin AMG, Lima JC, *et al.* Home blood pressure correlates better with left ventricular mass index than clinic and ambulatory blood pressure measurement. 19th Scientific Meeting of the International Society of Hypertension, 2002, Prague.
28. Lou LM, Gimeno JA, Gomez Sanchez R, *et al.* Comparison of clinical arterial blood pressure, home-arterial blood pressure measurement and ambulatory arterial pressure monitoring in patients with type II diabetes mellitus and diabetic nephropathy. *Nefrologia* 2002; **22**(2): 179–189.
29. Suzuki H, Nakamoto H, Okada H, Sugahara S and Kanno Y. Self-measured systolic blood pressure in the morning is a strong indicator of decline of renal function in hypertensive patients with non-diabetic chronic renal insufficiency. *Clin Exp Hypertens* 2002; **24**(4): 249–260.
30. ALLHAT Collaborative Research Group. Major outcomes in high-risk hypertensive patients randomized to angiotensin-converting enzyme inhibitor or calcium channel blocker vs diuretic. The Antihypertensive and Lipid-Lowering Treatment to Prevent Heart Attack Trial (ALLHAT). *JAMA* 2002; **288**: 2981–2997.
31. NCEP Expert Panel. *Third Report of the National Cholesterol Education Program (NCEP) Expert Panel on Detection, Evaluation and Treatment of High Blood Cholesterol in Adults (Adult Treatment Panel III)*. National Institutes of Health Pub. No. 01-3670, 2001.
32. Colwell JA. Aspirin therapy in diabetes. *Diabetes Care* 1997; **20**: 1768–1771.
33. Rossouw JE, Anderson GL, Prentice RL, *et al.* Risks and benefits of estrogen plus progestin in healthy postmenopausal women: principal results from the Women's Health Initiative randomized controlled trial. *JAMA* 2002; **288**: 321–333.
34. Grady D, Herrington D, Bittner V, *et al.* Cardiovascular disease outcomes during 6–8 years of hormone therapy: Heart and Estrogen/Progestin Replacement Study follow-up (HERS II). *JAMA* 2002; **288**: 49–57.
35. Stampfer MJ, Malinow MR, Willett WC, *et al.* A prospective study of plasma homocyst(e)ine and risk of myocardial infarction in US physicians. *JAMA* 1992; **268**: 878–881.
36. Friedberg CE, Janssen MJ, Heine RJ and Grobbee DE. Fish oil and glycemic control in diabetes: a meta-analysis. *Diabetes Care* 1998; **21**: 494–500.
37. *AHA Scientific Statement: Fish Consumption, Fish Oil, Omega-3 Fatty Acids and Cardiovascular Disease*, 71-0241 Circulation 2002; **106**: 2747–2757.

Gabay C and Kushner I. Acute-phase proteins and other systemic responses to inflammation. *N Engl J Med* 1999; **340**: 448–454.

Heinecke JW. Clinical trials of vitamin E in coronary artery disease: is it time to reconsider the low-density lipoprotein oxidation hypothesis. *Curr Atheroscler Rep* 2003; **5**: 83–87.

9 Microvascular Complications

Detection and treatment of diabetic nephropathy

Recent evidence suggest that renal disease may precede diabetes, or it may occur as a result of persistent hyperglycemia. Generally termed diabetic nephropathy, to distinguish it from other forms of nephropathy (such as IgA nephropathy), it is a serious co-morbidity of diabetes mellitus and is the leading cause of end-stage renal disease. The purpose of this section is to clarify the relationship between diabetic nephropathy, blood glucose, and blood pressure. In addition, the current standards of care for assessing, diagnosing, and treating diabetic nephropathy are outlined. The key points are:

- screening and early detection of diabetic nephropathy is critical
- management of hypertension and hyperglycemia will dramatically slow the onset and progression of diabetic nephropathy

The interrelationship between the progression of diabetic nephropathy and hypertension has been known for many years.[1,2] Hyperglycemia and, to a lesser extent, dyslipidemia have been identified as risk factors for diabetic nephropathy and have been implicated in its pathogenesis.[3,4] Therefore, treatment to prevent or slow the progression of diabetic nephropathy is based on the management of hyperglycemia, hypertension, and dyslipidemia. Chapters 4–6 provide DecisionPaths for management of type 2 and type 1 diabetes in detail. Chapter 8 discusses the treatment of hypertension and dyslipidemia for individuals with diabetes or metabolic syndrome.

The current impact of diabetic nephropathy

As many as one million people with diabetes in the United States may have kidney disease. Nephropathy is a serious complication of diabetes and is the leading cause of end-stage renal disease (ESRD). More than 40 per cent of individuals with type 1 diabetes (~300 000) will progress to overt diabetic nephropathy within 20 years of diagnosis.[5] It is quite rare for individuals with type 1 diabetes to develop overt diabetic nephropathy within five years of diagnosis, during what is often referred to as the "silent" period. Approximately 10 per cent of people with type 2 diabetes (~800 000) develop overt diabetic nephropathy; however, studies indicate that when the duration of diabetes exceeds 25 years, the percentage of individuals with type 2 diabetes that develop overt nephropathy is the same as that with type 1 diabetes.[5] Most individuals diagnosed with overt nephropathy will proceed to ESRD and

Staged Diabetes Management: A Systematic Approach (2nd Edition) R. S. Mazze, E. S. Strock, G. D. Simonson and R. M. Bergenstal
 ISBN: 0 470 86576 8

require dialysis (or a kidney transplant). In the United States 45 per cent of patients with ESRD have diabetes, and, of these, approximately 60 per cent have type 2 diabetes and 40 per cent have type 1 diabetes.[14] The incidence of diabetic ESRD has risen exponentially over the past decade, primarily due to the increasing number of individuals with type 2 diabetes progressing to ESRD. Not surprisingly, groups at highest risk for diabetes also have the highest prevalence of ESRD. African-Americans and American Indians are at particular risk. They have a three-fold greater chance of developing ESRD compared with Caucasians.[14]

Pathogenesis and stages of diabetic nephropathy

Diabetic nephropathy results from the formation of lesions in the kidney. The underlying pathogenesis of diabetic nephropathy is still not clearly understood, but involves a combination of HTN, hyperglycemia, and proteinuria. Diabetic nephropathy is characterized by distinct morphologic and biochemical changes in the kidney that coincide with the onset and progression of renal disease. Enlargement of the mesangium, a membrane composed of mesangial cells and extracellular matrix supporting the glomerular capillary loops, is one of the most prominent morphologic changes. Elevated glucose levels have been shown to increase the production of collagen, fibronectin, and laminin in the mesangial extracellular matrix, resulting in a significant thickening of the mesangial basement membrane.[6,7] This thickening compresses the glomerular capillaries, altering intraglomerular hemodynamics. Other changes include a dramatic loss in capillary surface area and decreased levels of heparin sulfate in the extracellular matrix.

Diabetic nephropathy progresses through distinct stages characterized by the amount of albumin "spilled" into the urine. The earliest stage, incipient diabetic nephropathy, is characterized by low levels of albumin in the urine (referred to as microalbuminuria). Studies have shown that microalbuminuria is the best predictor of the progression to the next stage, called overt diabetic nephropathy.[8] Not only does albumin serve as a marker of the progression of diabetic nephropathy, but it appears to directly damage the glomerulus. The progression from incipient to overt diabetic nephropathy normally takes many years. Approximately 80 per cent of patients with microalbuminuria progress to overt diabetic nephropathy (proteinuria). Overt diabetic nephropathy is characterized by macroalbuminuria, which can be detected with the standard urinalysis "dipstick" test for proteinuria. As diabetic nephropathy progresses, renal insufficiency ensues, leading to elevated serum creatinine levels. Normally, renal failure or ESRD develops in 3–15 years after the development of overt diabetic nephropathy. End-stage renal disease is marked by severe proteinuria and azotemia, a condition caused by high levels of urea and creatinine in the bloodstream. At this point renal replacement therapies (dialysis) are begun and kidney transplantation is considered. Although, at this juncture, dialysis and/or kidney transplants are the only solutions for diabetic nephropathy, they are not ideal because of the associated high mortality of patients undergoing these therapies.

Hyperglycemia and diabetic nephropathy

The Diabetes Control and Complications Trial[3] showed that the maintenance of near euglycemia in type 1 diabetes drastically reduces the frequency and severity of kidney disease. Intensive metabolic control resulted in a 39 per cent risk reduction in microalbuminuria in the primary prevention cohort and a 54 per cent risk reduction in the occurrence of macroalbuminuria in the secondary intervention cohort (participants with microalbuminuria at the start of the study). A similar reduction in risk was found in the United Kingdom Prospective Diabetes Study for type 2 diabetes patients undergoing intensive management.[9] Other studies have also shown the predictive nature of elevated glucose levels, making it one of the major risk factors for microalbuminuria and macroalbuminuria.[7,10] Thus, maintenance of near-normal blood glucose levels clearly is imperative for the prevention of diabetic nephropathy or to slow the progression of the disease.

Hypertension, dyslipidemia, and diabetic nephropathy

The causes of hypertension in individuals with type 1 diabetes are generally different from those in patients with type 2 diabetes. In type 1 diabetes, hypertension is often associated with underlying renal disease. In type 2 diabetes, obesity and insulin resistance (even in the absence of renal disease) are thought to be the critical link. Nevertheless, hypertension has been a principal factor for both the onset and progression of diabetic kidney disease in both type 1 and type 2 diabetes. Research by the Microalbuminuria Collaborative Study Group[11] indicates that increases in blood pressure occur concurrent with rising urinary albumin levels. This takes place even when albumin levels are within the normal range (albumin/creatinine ratio < 30 mg/g, < 30 mg albumin/24 hours, or albumin excretion rate < 20 µg/min). Hypertension may play a role in the pathogenesis of diabetic nephropathy, thus aggressive treatment of hypertension is critical for its prevention.

Dyslipidemia is often associated with albuminuria in diabetes. Elevated levels of total cholesterol, and LDL, triglycerides, and reduced HDL levels, appear to be risk factors for the development of diabetic nephropathy. The precise role of dyslipidemia in the onset and progression of diabetic nephropathy is not fully understood. However, treatment of dyslipidemia is an important facet of care for those with diabetic nephropathy.

Renal disease, type 2 diabetes, and metabolic syndrome

Does renal disease precede diabetes? Increasingly this question is being asked by researchers interested in determining the etiology of renal failure in persons with type 2 diabetes. Thought to be a consequence of diabetes, renal disease is now considered to be part of a metabolic syndrome that encompasses several inter-related disorders: hypertension, dyslipidemia, hyperglycemia, and obesity. Does it matter whether renal disease is a consequence of, co-morbidity with, or precursor to diabetes? The answer is that it matters only if clinical decisions rely on the sequence of disorders. The SDM approach is, in the presence of any of these co-morbidities, to screen for the others.

Diabetic nephropathy practice guidelines

The standards of care for kidney disease and hypertension in type 1 and type 2 diabetes differ slightly from those for individuals without diabetes. These standards are summarized in the practice guidelines (see Figure 9.1) and in this section.

Common clinical manifestations

While there are no specific clinical signs of underlying kidney disease, there are risk factors that should invoke a concern for diabetic nephropathy. Poor glycemic control, hypertension, retinopathy, elevated LDL cholesterol, and duration of diabetes greater than 5 years are all predictors of diabetic nephropathy.

Screening and diagnosis of diabetic nephropathy

In general, the diagnosis of diabetic nephropathy relies on persistent elevated albumin levels in the urine. Abnormal glomerular filtration rate (GFR) is another indicator, but this information is often not available. All newly diagnosed patients with diabetes should initially be screened for proteinuria using a standard dipstick test (see Figure 9.2). Clinicians need to be cognizant of and evaluate for potential contamination or conditions at the time of specimen collection that can affect albumin levels in the urine. These include urinary tract infections, poor glycemic control, fever, blood in the urine, congestive heart failure, extreme hypertension, and vaginal fluid contamination. Any of

Diagnosis

Incipient Diabetic Nephropathy
Persistent microalbuminuria (on at least 2 out of 3 occasions)
Random urine collection 30–300 mg albumin/g creatinine
24 hour urine collection 30–300 mg albumin/24 hours
Time urine collection 20–200 μg albumin/minute

Overt Diabetic Nephropathy
Macroalbuminuria (proteinuria indicated by a positive dipstick test)
Random urine collection > 300 mg albumin/g creatinine
24 hour urine collection > 300 mg albumin/24 hr
Time urine collection > 200 μg albumin/minute
Note: albumin/creatinine ratio not sensitive when urine protein > 2–3 g/24 hours

Hypertension
Systolic BP ⩾ 130 mmHg on 2 occasions or diastolic BP ⩾ 80 mmHg on 2 occasions

Glomerular Disease
Evidence includes mesangial cell matrix expansion, increased basement membranethickness, and loss of glomerular capillary surface area

Risk Factors

- HbA_{1c} > 2 percentage points above limit of normal
- Family history of hypertension and/or dyslipidemia
- Sibling with diabetic nephropathy
- Duration of diabetes > 5 years
- Smoking
- American Indian or Alaska Native; African-American; Asian; Native Hawaiian or other Pacific Islander; Hispanic

Treatment Options

Hypertension Medical nutrition therapy; ACE inhibitors; calcium channel blockers; α-blockers; diuretics; β-blockers

Dyslipidemia Medical nutrition therapy; HMG CoA reductase inhibitors; bile acid sequestrants; fibric acid; cholestorol absorption inhibitors

Hyperglycemia Medical nutrition therapy; oral agents; insulin

Targets

BP < 130/80 mmHg if renal disease <120/75 mmHg; glomerular filtration rate (GFR) decrease < 0.2 ml/minute/month acceptable; HbA_{1c} within 1.0 percentage point of uppper limit of normal

Monitoring

SMBP and SMBG daily while adjusting treatment

Follow-up

If no nephropathy present, screen annually for albuminuria
Nephropathy present, see below

Monthly Office visit during adjust phase (weekly phone contact may be necessary)

Every 3 Months Urinalysis with dipstick test for proteinuria; determine HbA_{1c}

Yearly (in addition to 3-4 month visit) Albuminuria screening should be performed annually in all adults and in all post-pubertal patients with at least 5 years duration of diabetes. Serum creatinine and blood urea nitrogen (BUN) annually in patients with albuminuria. If macroalbuminuria present, consult with endocrinologist, diabetologist, or nephrologist.

Figure 9.1 Diabetic Nephropathy Practice Guidelines

these situations or conditions can increase albumin levels. The dipstick test for proteinuria is inadequate for making a diagnosis of incipient diabetic nephropathy, characterized by microalbuminuria, because the test is not sensitive enough to detect low levels of albumin. Thus, all negative protein dipsticks must be followed by a laboratory test for microalbuminuria.

Staged Diabetes Management recommends that a random urine sample be used for albuminuria screening because of sensitivity, convenience to the patient and ease of sample collection. To account for variability in the concentration of solutes and in the time of specimen collection, all random urine collection tests for albuminuria should be adjusted with urine creatinine. Table 9.1 provides the ranges for normal, microalbuminuria, and macroalbuminuria for the three most

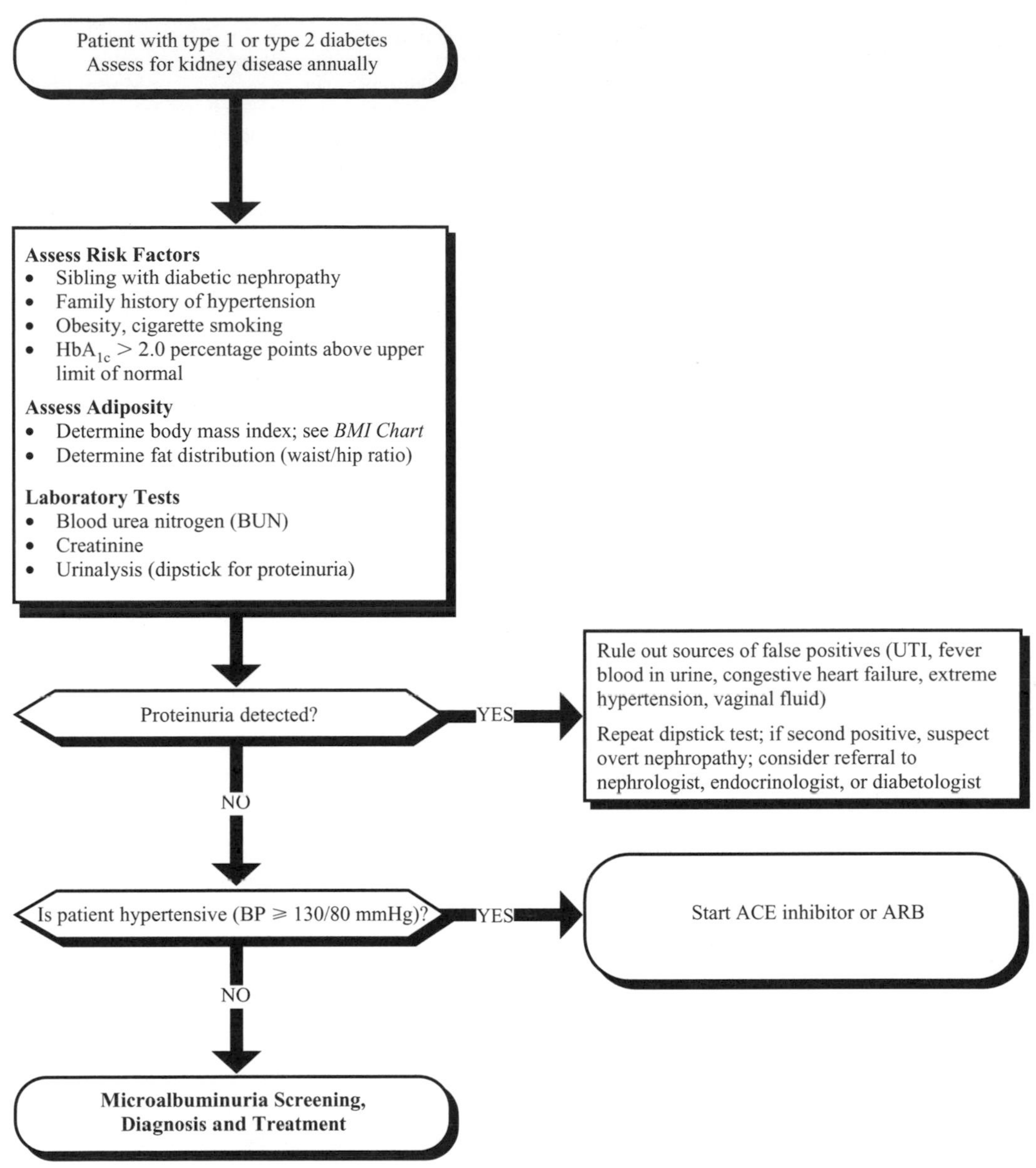

Figure 9.2 Kidney Disease Assessment DecisionPath

common laboratory tests. Because of inherent day-to-day variability in urine albumin levels, diagnosis requires that at least two out of three tests be positive in order to make the diagnosis of microalbuminuria. Twenty-four hour urine collection used to be considered the "gold standard" for albuminuria screening. This test may be used for screening and diagnosis of albuminuria, but due to patient inconvenience and concerns over accuracy of sample collection (i.e. missed collection) it is neither recommended nor required.

In many cases, the presence of incipient or overt diabetic nephropathy is associated with underlying hypertension (see Figure 9.3). The increase in blood pressure is a response to the renal disease but may also be part of the pathogenesis of diabetic nephropathy. The majority of patients have no symptoms, but occasionally headache, dizziness, or blurred vision is reported. Risk factors for hypertension include obesity, visceral adiposity, insulin resistance manifested as hyperinsulinemia, hyperlipidemia, family history of hypertension, lack of exercise, smoking, and age greater than 50. African-Americans and Hispanics

Table 9.1 Diagnosis of albuminuria[12]

Test	Normal	Microalbuminuria	Macroalbuminuria
Random urine	< 30 mg/g creatinine	30–300 mg/g creatinine	> 300 mg/g creatinine
24 hour urine	< 30 mg/24 hour	30–300 mg/24 hour	> 300 mg/24 hour
Overnight urine	< 20 μg/min	20–200 μg/min	> 200 μg/min

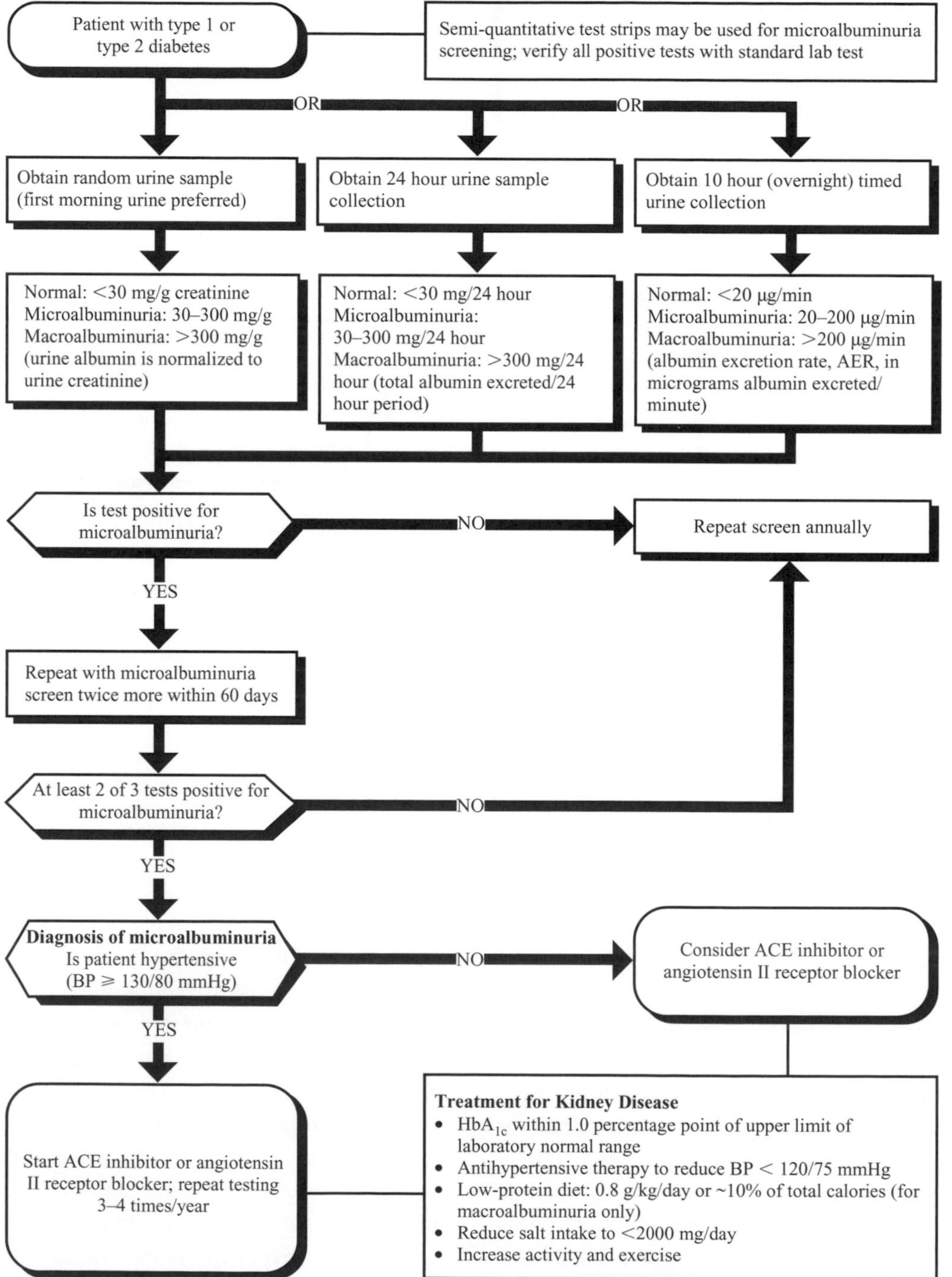

Figure 9.3 Microalbuminuria Screening, Diagnosis and Treatment

form particular groups at high risk for hypertension. As part of good diabetes management, blood pressure needs to be monitored at every visit. Any evidence of hypertension should be treated aggressively.

Glomerular filtration rate. The determination of the glomerular filtration rate (GFR) is an alternative and complementary diagnostic measurement of kidney function. While not a routine test, GFR is often used in clinical studies to detect and monitor the progression of diabetic nephropathy. At the time of diagnosis of type 1 diabetes, the GFR is normally elevated because of glucose induced hyperfiltration, osmotic effects, and increased blood pressure. The GFR of newly diagnosed patients with type 2 diabetes is variable.

Glomerular filtration rate is commonly measured by following the urinary clearance of radioactively labeled compounds. Inulin, a naturally occurring polysaccharide, is available for a nonradioactive determination of GFR, but this test is not widely available. Normal reduction in GFR in the general population is less than 0.03 ml/min/month; an acceptable limit in patients with diabetes is less than 0.2 ml/min/month.

Creatinine clearance. The determination of creatinine clearance provides a means to test kidney function and is considered an indicator of GFR. Creatinine is generated in muscle from the spontaneous cyclization of creatine into creatinine, which is subsequently released into the bloodstream and excreted via the kidneys. This endogenous source of creatinine is directly proportionate to muscle mass and varies with age and sex. However, in the absence of renal disease, the clearance of creatinine is relatively constant in any one individual. Creatinine clearance is calculated from measurements of creatinine in the urine or serum. For males under age 40, the normal reference interval for urine creatinine clearance is 90–140 mL/min/1.73 m^2; for females under age 40, it is 80–125 mL/min/1.73 m^2.[13] Creatinine clearance decreases by 5–8 per cent every decade after age 40. Often, only the serum (or plasma) creatinine level is measured. The normal reference interval for serum (or plasma) creatinine is 0.8–1.5 mg/dL (70–130 μmol/L). In contrast to the GFR, at the time of diagnosis of type 1 diabetes, the serum creatinine levels are often quite low (~0.8 mg/dL or 70 μmol/L) because of glomerular hyperfiltration. Patients with incipient or overt diabetic nephropathy usually maintain serum creatinine levels in the normal reference range. As the diabetic nephropathy progresses to end-stage renal failure, there is a corresponding rise in the serum creatinine to $>$ 2.0 mg/dL (180 μmol/L). This increase continues to $>$ 10 mg/dL (880 μmol/L), signaling a total shutdown of kidney function.

Treatment of diabetic nephropathy

Diabetic nephropathy cannot be cured. However, evidence has been accumulating that the onset of diabetic nephropathy can be delayed and its progression retarded. Near-normal glycemic control and the aggressive treatment of hypertension are the two most important treatment options available for the management of diabetic nephropathy. Chapters 4–6 provide guidelines for achieving and maintaining metabolic control in individuals with diabetes. The maintenance of near euglycemia (HbA_{1c} within one percentage point of the upper limit of normal) is of paramount importance for those diagnosed with diabetic nephropathy. Table 9.2 details recommended therapy changes for patients with diabetes, nephropathy, and an $HbA_{1c} > 1.0$ percentage points above the upper limit of normal.

Serum creatinine levels are an important consideration in diabetes oral agent selection. Table 9.3 provides guidelines for selecting the appropriate oral agent.

Treatment of hypertension. Aggressive treatment of hypertension is essential in delaying the onset and slowing the progression of diabetic nephropathy. Practice guidelines and DecisionPaths, located in Chapter 8, have been formulated for the assessment, diagnosis, and treatment

Table 9.2 Recommended changes in diabetes therapy for nephropathy

Current therapeutic stage*	Therapy changes for incipient nephropathy	Therapy changes for overt nephropathy
Type 2 diabetes: medical nutrition therapy stage	Start oral agent therapy,** reduce salt intake to < 2400 mg/day	Start insulin therapy; modify protein intake; restrict salt intake to < 2000 mg/day
Type 2 diabetes: oral agent stage	Start insulin therapy; reduce salt intake to < 2400 mg/day	Start intensive insulin therapy; modify protein intake; restrict salt intake to < 2000 mg/day
Type 1 and type 2 diabetes: any insulin stage	Intensify insulin therapy; reduce salt intake to < 2400 mg/day	Intensify insulin therapy, consider referral to specialist; modify protein intake; restrict salt intake to < 2000 mg/day

* If the HbA_{1c} is > 1.0 percentage points above the upper limit of normal, a change in diabetes therapy is indicated.
** Avoid any oral agent contraindicated when kidney disease is present.

Table 9.3 Oral agent selection in the presence of diabetic nephropathy

Serum creatinine	Oral agent
> 2.0 mg/dL (> 180 μmol/L)	Meglitinide or thiazolidinedione
1.4–2.0 mg/dL (120–180 μmol/L)	α-glucosidase inhibitor, meglitinide, sulfonylurea, or thiazolidinedione
< 1.4 mg/dL (< 120 μmol/L)	All oral agents

of hypertension. Briefly, hypertension management begins with appropriate medical nutrition therapy along with changes in lifestyle. Specific dietary changes include reduction of sodium in the diet by limiting the use of processed foods, and limiting alcohol intake. Lifestyle changes include increased activity/exercise and smoking cessation. Monitoring blood pressure at home and at work may provide necessary interim data to determine how well lifestyle changes are working.

If medical nutrition therapy is not sufficient for blood pressure control, mono-drug therapy with an angiotensin converting enzyme (ACE) inhibitor or angiotensin II receptor blocker (ARB) should be initiated. Both ACE inhibitors and ARB blockers have been shown in large prospective clinical research studies to slow the progression of nephropathy.[15–17] If patients experience side effects (cough) while taking an ACE inhibitor, consider switching to an angiotensin II receptor blocker. If ACE inhibitor or ARB therapy alone is not sufficient to reduce blood pressure, other antihypertensive drugs, including calcium channel blockers, β-blockers, diuretics, or α-blockers should be added (see Chapter 8). It is important to note that the recently published Antihypertensive and Lipid-Lowering Treatment to Prevent Heart Attack Trial (ALLHAT)[18] demonstrated that no significant differences were noted between the diuretic chlorthalidione and ACE inhibitor lisinopril in incidence of ESRD. Thus, thiazide diuretics should be considered in combination with ACE inhibitor/ARB therapy or if contraindications preclude the use of these two classes of antihypertensive medications. Recently, small studies testing the effect of dual blockade of the renin–angiotensin system have been conducted to look at potential benefits of using an ACE inhibitor and ARB in combination.

Treatment of dyslipidemia. Dyslipidemia is often associated with incipient diabetic nephropathy. In particular, elevated LDL and triglyceride levels are predictors of microalbuminuria. Dyslipidemia should be treated aggressively (see Chapter 8). Recommendations call for increased physical activity and less than 30 per cent of total caloric intake from fat (<10 per cent saturated fat). If food plan, exercise, and lifestyle modifications are not sufficient to achieve near-normal lipid levels, pharmacologic agents that improve lipid levels should be initiated. HMG-CoA reductase inhibitors, fibric acid derivatives (fenofibrate and gemfibrozil), and bile acid binding resins (colestipol and cholestyramine) are all viable therapeutic options for the treatment of dyslipidemia in the presence of diabetes. Nicotinic acid should be used with caution because of its tendency to aggravate blood glucose control.

Modifications in dietary protein. Diets low in protein have been shown to have renal protective effects and to slow the progression of overt diabetic nephropathy (macroalbuminuria) in animal studies and in human studies with small cohorts. To date, no conclusive evidence has shown that low-protein diets slow the progression from incipient diabetic nephropathy (microalbuminuria) to overt diabetic nephropathy. It is hypothesized that excess protein in the diet causes glomerular hyperfiltration, renal vasodilatation, and changes in intraglomerular pressure, all of which are associated with proteinuria. The American Diabetes Association[12] recommends a protein dietary intake of 0.8 g/kg body weight per day, or ~10 per cent of total caloric intake, for individuals with macroalbuminuria (overt nephropathy). Further reduction of protein intake to 0.6 g/kg body weight per day may be considered for patients with rapidly declining GFRs. Preliminary evidence suggests that the protein source, plant versus animal, may play an important role in the observed renal protective effect of a low-protein diet. Vegetable protein may be more beneficial and animal protein more harmful. More studies are required before any conclusions can be drawn.

Detection and treatment of eye complications

Retinopathy, cataracts, and glaucoma are serious complications of diabetes. Diabetic retinopathy is the leading cause of non-injury-related blindness in the United States and is responsible for reduced visual acuity. The purpose of this section is to detail the relationship between diabetic eye complications and hyperglycemia, outline the current standards of care for assessing, diagnosing, and treating diabetic retinopathy, and set the criteria and timelines for referring patients to eye-care specialists. The key points are:

- screening and early detection of diabetic retinopathy are critical
- when properly detected and treated, management of hyperglycemia and hypertension (and to a lesser extent dyslipidemia) will dramatically slow the onset and progression of diabetic retinopathy

The progression of diabetic retinopathy as a consequence of hyperglycemia in type 1 diabetes has been established for several years.[1,2] The association of hypertension and diabetic retinopathy in type 2 diabetes was shown in the United Kingdom Prospective Diabetes Study.[15] Patients in the "tight" hypertension control cohort had a 34 per cent reduction in progression of diabetic retinopathy versus the "less tight" hypertension control group. The association of dyslipidemia with the pathogenesis of diabetic retinopathy remains unclear, but is thought to be a risk factor for its development. Current diabetes care to prevent the onset of diabetic retinopathy, or to slow its progression, is based primarily on early detection through routine screening and intensive management of hyperglycemia and hypertension.

Staged Diabetes Management addresses these issues by providing a systematic approach to the prevention, detection, and initial management of diabetic retinopathy along with DecisionPaths with guidelines for referral of patients with diabetic retinopathy to eye-care specialists.

The current impact of diabetes related eye complications

Diabetes is the leading cause of legal blindness (best corrected visual acuity of 20/200 or worse in the better eye) in people age 20–74.[3] Approximately 12 per cent of all individuals with type 1 diabetes with duration of diabetes more than 30 years are legally blind, and an overwhelming majority of individuals with type 2 diabetes with duration of disease more than 15 years have some type of diabetes related eye complication.[2] Retinopathy, cataracts, and glaucoma comprise the three primary diabetes related eye complications. Alone, or in combination, they may all lead to legal blindness. Of principal concern for patients with diabetes is retinopathy, characterized by changes in the vascularization of the retina. Diabetic retinopathy is either totally or at least partially responsible for approximately 85 per cent of legal blindness (sufficiently impaired vision to make driving and other routine activities impossible) in these individuals. Glaucoma and cataracts are the primary causes of legal blindness in individuals with type 2 diabetes, with diabetic retinopathy becoming a greater concern as the mean age of diagnosis is occurring at a younger age.

Types of eye complication diabetic retinopathy

Diabetic retinopathy is the major ocular complication associated with diabetes. The pathogenesis of diabetic retinopathy is still unclear. Persistent hyperglycemia has been implicated in the onset and progression of diabetic retinopathy, but the precise role of elevated glucose has yet to be elucidated. Diabetic retinopathy actually encompasses a range of retinal abnormalities that have been staged in accordance to the severity of retinal damage.

The first stage is early nonproliferative diabetic retinopathy (NPDR) and is characterized by retinal microaneurysms, dot and blot hemorrhages, hard lipid exudates, and macular edema. The next stage is called moderate to severe NPDR and is characterized by cotton wool spots (soft exudates indicating localized arteriolar closing), venous abnormalities, and intraretinal microvascular abnormalities (dilated capillaries in ischemic areas of the retina).

The most severe stage is called proliferative diabetic retinopathy (PDR). This stage is characterized by the development of neovascularization. The new blood vessels that develop to supply blood flow to the retina are fragile and subject to rupture. New blood vessels are classified into two distinct categories based on the site of formation. New vessels on the disk (NVD), located on the optic nerve head, and new vessels elsewhere (NVE) are at a greater risk of rupture. The extent and location of the new vessels and the presence of preretinal or vitreous hemorrhages determine the severity of proliferative retinopathy. Extensive NVD (> 1/3 disk diameter) and/or NVE with accompanying vitreous bleeding is considered high risk for visual loss.

The various mechanisms of vision impairment associated with diabetic retinopathy are well established. Central vision impairment usually involves macular edema, a condition in which the retina swells due to the leakage of tissue fluid and lipoproteins from abnormal retinal vasculature. Macular edema accounts for a significant amount of vision impairment in the diabetes population. Vision impairment can also result when strands of fibrous tissue accompanying neovascularization cause a distortion of the retina. If the formation of new vessels continues unabated, the strands of fibrous tissue begin to produce tractional forces, eventually leading to tractional retinal detachment. Vision is lost if tractional retinal detachment involves the macula. Partial loss of vision may occur if the detachment occurs at the retinal periphery. Another cause of visual impairment is formation of new blood vessels, characteristic of proliferative diabetic retinopathy. This may result in vitreous hemorrhage. The gel-like vitreous becomes cloudy with the resultant visual impairment proportionate to the severity of hemorrhage.

Cataracts

Cataracts result from the opacification of the crystalline lens. The opacification of the lens results in diminished visual acuity. Surgery is generally required to correct this condition. Cataracts in individuals with or without diabetes (senile cataracts) are morphologically similar, but recent evidence suggests that they differ biochemically. Research suggests that high glucose levels induce nonenzymatic glycation and browning of lens crystallins (by the same mechanism responsible for glycosylation of hemoglobin), leading to opacification of the lens in the senile-like diabetic cataract.[4,5] Senile cataracts in individuals without diabetes do not contain aberrantly glycated lens crystallins. Moreover, increased lens sorbitol, from the conversion of glucose into sorbitol by aldose reductase, has been implicated in the formation of cataracts in animal models of diabetes.[6] Whether sorbitol plays a role in the formation of cataracts in humans is still unresolved. A second type of cataract, called "snowflake" occasionally develops in untreated or poorly controlled patients with type 1 diabetes. These cataracts normally disappear once near-normal glycemic control is established.

Glaucoma

Two forms of glaucoma (primary and secondary) occur most often in individuals with diabetes. Primary open angle glaucoma is characterized by elevated intraocular pressure that may lead to optic nerve damage and subsequent loss of visual field and central vision. Diabetes has often been noted as a risk factor for primary open angle glaucoma, but the relationship has not been corroborated in all studies. Neovascular glaucoma (rubeosis) is a secondary form of glaucoma resulting in the development of abnormal new vessels on the iris that obstruct the outflow channels of the eye, causing an increase in intraocular pressure. This form of glaucoma is often painful and results in loss of the eye. It is associated with severe abnormal ischemia and proliferative retinopathy.

Hyperglycemia and diabetic retinopathy

Intensive metabolic control ($HbA_{1c} \sim 7$ per cent) in the nine year Diabetes Control and Complications Trial[7] resulted in a 76 per cent reduction in the risk of developing retinopathy in patients with type 1 diabetes and slowed the progression of retinopathy. The earlier Kroc Study[8,9] comparing conventional insulin therapy with intensive insulin therapy showed no significant improvement in slowing the progression of nonproliferative diabetic retinopathy over a 1–2 year period. This observation was also noted during the first two years of the Diabetes Control and Complications Trial, reinforcing the concept that long-term, not short-term, near normalization of blood glucose is critical for slowing the progression of diabetic retinopathy. The United Kingdom Prospective Diabetes Study Group[10] demonstrated the benefit of improved glycemic control in reducing the risk of diabetic retinopathy in individuals with type 2 diabetes. In addition, epidemiologic data are strongly supportive of a positive correlation between blood glucose level and risk of diabetic retinopathy in patients with type 2 diabetes. Thus, maintenance of normal blood glucose levels is imperative for the prevention of diabetic retinopathy in both types of diabetes.

Typically, individuals with undiagnosed diabetes or with poorly controlled diabetes experience blurred vision due to changes in blood glucose level. Episodic hyperglycemia alters the metabolism of glucose in the eye, leading to changes in the shape of the lens. These changes may modify visual acuity, thus making fluctuations in vision a warning sign of diabetes. Persistent hyperglycemia, in contrast, leads to the more serious long-term complications associated with diabetic retinopathy. The Wisconsin Epidemiologic Study of

Diabetic Retinopathy (WESDR) demonstrated a clear positive correlation between the level of glycosylated hemoglobin and the incidence of diabetic retinopathy.[11] This study also showed that the establishment of near-normal glycemic control was associated with a significant risk reduction in the progression of nonproliferative diabetic retinopathy to the more severe proliferative diabetic retinopathy.

How elevated glucose levels induce the onset and progression of diabetic retinopathy is still uncertain. It was once believed that excess glucose is converted into sorbitol, a metabolite strongly implicated in the pathogenesis of diabetic neuropathy. Sorbitol is converted by aldose reductase in the polyol pathway. It has been suggested that the accumulation of sorbitol may lead to diabetic retinopathy.[6] More recent reports seem to indicate that excess sorbitol in the eye may not be the major factor in the pathogenesis of diabetic retinopathy because treatment with aldose reductase inhibitors has no effect on the formation of microaneurysms or neovascularization characteristics of diabetic retinopathy. More research is required to clarify the role of sorbitol in diabetic retinopathy.

Hypertension, dyslipidemia, and diabetic retinopathy

Hypertension has been suggested to play a role in the development and progression of diabetic retinopathy. Increased blood flow due to high blood pressure is hypothesized to damage the retinal capillary beds. Many studies have been undertaken to establish the relationship between hypertension and diabetic retinopathy, but the results are not consistent, nor are they conclusive. The United Kingdom Diabetes Prospective Diabetes Study (UKPDS) demonstrated that the cohort randomized to the "tight" blood pressure control group had a 34 per cent reduction in progression of retinopathy versus the "less-tight" blood pressure control group.[15] However, the Appropriate Blood Pressure Control in Diabetes Trial showed no significant difference in progression of diabetic retinopathy between the tight-control blood pressure cohort and the moderate blood pressure control group.[16] Like hypertension, the association of serum lipids with the pathogenesis of diabetic retinopathy remains unclear. Dyslipidemia, especially elevated triglycerides and LDL cholesterol, was found to be associated with increased risk of forming hard (lipid) exudates in the Early Treatment of Diabetic Retinopathy Study (ETDRS).[12] These hard exudates are often found in the macular region and are associated with macular edema.

Diabetic retinopathy practice guidelines

The standards of care for diabetic retinopathy are summarized in the practice guidelines shown in Figure 9.4. Diagnostic criteria are provided for classifying the severity of diabetic retinopathy. Treatment options and therapeutic targets are clearly delineated. Appropriate guidelines for monitoring and follow-up are established based on the classification of diabetic retinopathy.

Common clinical manifestations

The problem facing the clinician is that there is often no loss of visual acuity or pain to signal the start or progression of diabetic retinal disease. Even when proliferative retinopathy with clinically significant macular edema is present and threatening vision, the patient may be asymptomatic. However, there are risk factors that should invoke screening for diabetic retinopathy. Blurred vision, $HbA_{1c} > 2.0$ percentage points above upper limit of normal, hypertension, albuminuria, and duration of diabetes ($>$ 5 years) are predictors of diabetic retinopathy.

Screening and diagnosis of diabetic retinopathy

The clinician assumes a critical role in the early detection of diabetic retinopathy. While the majority of patients have access to an eye care specialist for the annual dilated eye examination, in certain situations the dilated eye examination may have to be performed by a non-specialist.

Diagnosis	
Early Nonproliferative Diabetic Retinopathy (NPDR)	Microaneurysms; dot hemorrhages; sparse blot hemorrhages; hard (lipid) exudates
Moderate to Severe NPDR (preproliferative)	Macular edema; cotton wool spots; venous abnormalities; intraretinal microvascular abnormalities (IRMA); venous dilation
Proliferative Diabetic Retinopathy (PDR)	New vessels on the disk (NVD); new vessels elsewhere (NVE); retinal detachment
Risk Factors	• Persistent hyperglycemia • Age (risk increases with age) • Duration of diabetes (> 5 years) • Albuminuria • Hypertension • American Indian or Alaska Native; African-American; Asian; Native Hawaiian or other Pacific Islander; Hispanic
Treatment Options	Note: refer to retinal specialist experienced in diabetic retinopathy
NPDR	Enforce tight metabolic control Hyperglycemia: medical nutrition therapy, pharmacologic agents; adjustments in insulin therapy or oral agents; increase SMBG frequency
PDR	Panretinal photocoagulation, small laser burns (~500 μ) outside venous arcades in mid-periphery of retina to prevent further neovascularization
Severe PDR	Vitrectomy to remove vitreous humor, cut fibrous traction bands, and repair retinal detachments
Macular Edema	Focal photocoagulation, very small laser burns (~50–100 μ) to leaking microaneurysms and areas of ischemia in the macular region
Targets	Near euglycemia ($HbA_{1c} \leq 1.0$ percentage point above upper limit of normal) Improved vision; prevention or slowing progression of retinopathy BP < 130/80 mmHg
Monitoring	Encourage patient to report diminished visual acuity; blurred vision; other eye-related problems
Follow-up	For patients with retinopathy
Yearly	Type 1: annual dilated opthalmoscope examinations beginning 3–5 years after diagnosis once child is 10 years old. Type 2: if never screened, screen now and annual screening thereafter; consider screening patients in poor control and/or with albuminuria every 6 months During pregnancy: dilated eye exam prior to conception and during first trimester and monthly thereafter for all women with pre-existing diabetes (not GDM)

Figure 9.4 Diabetic Retinopathy Practice Guidelines

Thus, the Diabetic Retinopathy Screening and Diagnosis DecisionPath (see Figure 9.5), along with the retinal photographs (see Photos 9.1–9.12) showing the various stages of diabetic retinopathy, are intended to assist in screening for diabetic retinopathy, making the appropriate diagnosis of diabetic retinopathy, and providing guidelines for referral to an ophthalmologist. Screening for diabetic retinopathy should be performed using monocular ophthalmoscope examination with a dilated pupil. The risk of inducing narrow-angle glaucoma when dilating the pupil is rare in

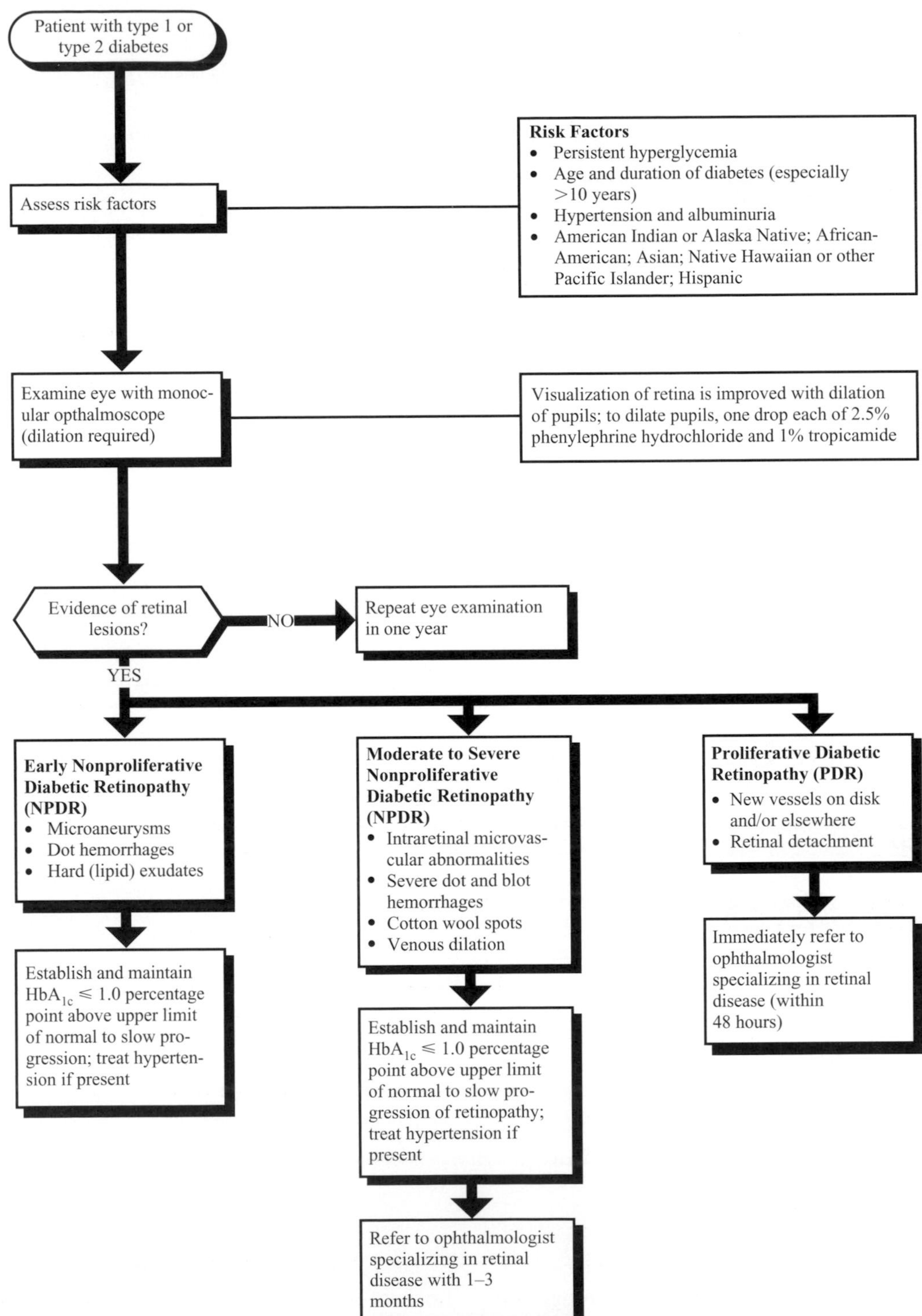

Figure 9.5 Diabetic Retinopathy Screening and Diagnosis DecisionPath

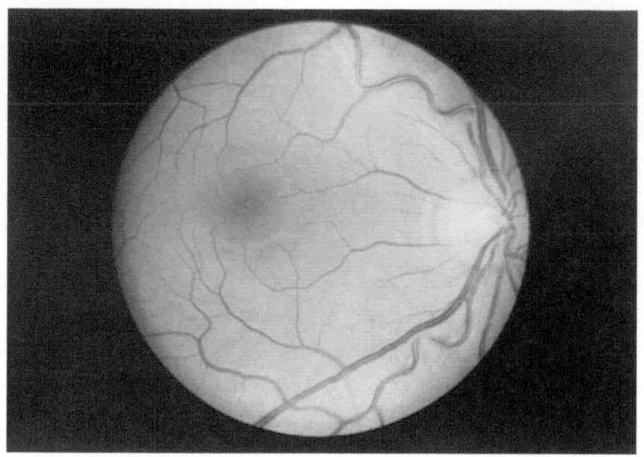

Photo 9.1 Normal optic nerve and retina. The reddish area to the left of center is the macula (the center of vision). The branching red lines are the blood vessels of the retina. Loss of vision from diabetes is a result of changes in the circulation within the retina

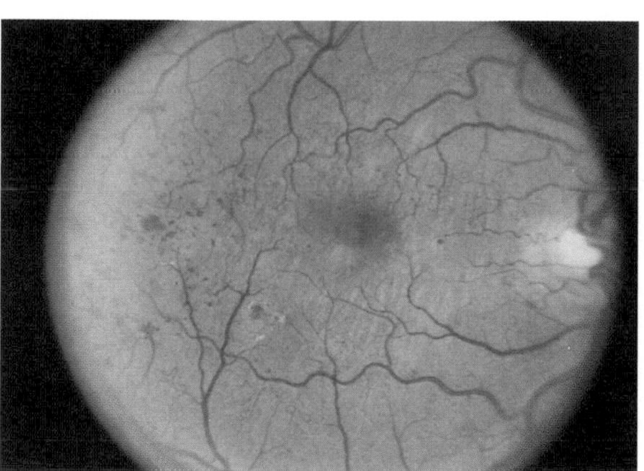

Photo 9.2 Early signs of diabetic retinopathy. The small red dots are microaneurysms, or bulges, in the blood vessel wall. The larger red areas are hemorrhages within the retina and the small yellow dots are tiny fat deposits

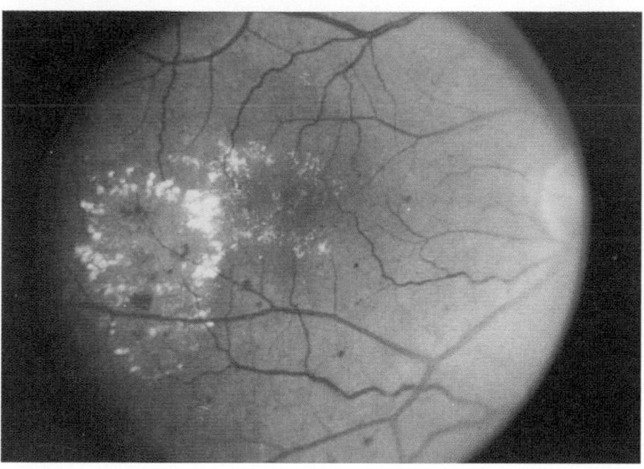

Photo 9.3 Early nonproliferative diabetic retinopathy. Clusters of small red dots are in and around the macula. The red dots are microaneurysms, which leak fluid into the retina. The bright yellow areas are regions of fatty deposits within the retina

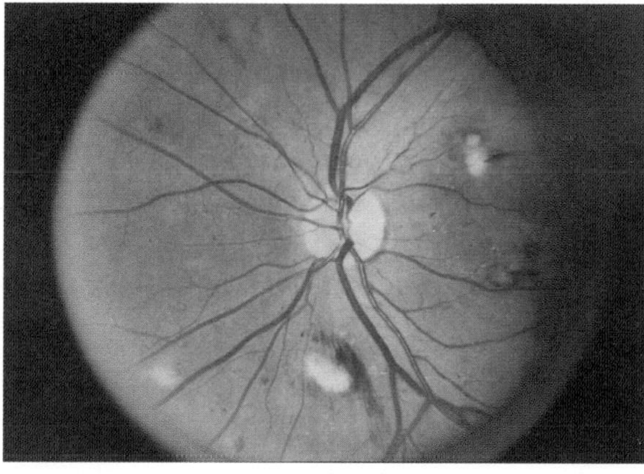

Photo 9.4 Moderate nonproliferative diabetic retinopathy. Both red and white patches are within the retina. The small red dots are microaneurysms; the larger red patches are hemorrhages within the retina. The white patches or "cottonwool" spots are areas of poor circulation within the retina

patients under the age of 40. In the presence of symptoms of acute narrow-angle glaucoma the patient should be immediately referred to an ophthalmologist. These symptoms include red and painful eye, corneal edema (characterized by loss of smooth light reflex from the cornea), and a mid-dilated pupil. Providers that are not comfortable performing dilated eye examination may want to consider referring patients to an eye-care specialist for routine screening.

The clinical presentation of lesions representative of the primary stages used for diagnosis of diabetic retinopathy appear in Table 9.4. This table should serve as a guide to make the diagnosis of diabetic retinopathy and should assist in the referral of patients to an eye-care specialist. Referring a patient to an ophthalmologist

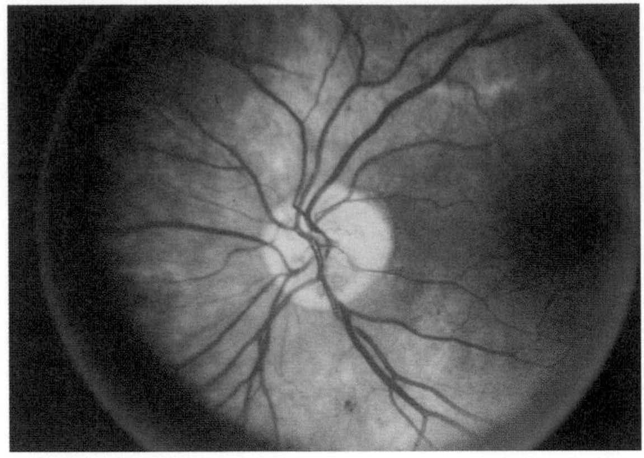

Photo 9.5 Proliferative diabetic retinopathy. The optic nerve and the surrounding retina. Fine new vessels can be seen growing on the surface of the optic nerve. These regions of "neovascularization" may rupture or burst, causing extensive bleeding within the eye. Laser treatment is helpful to treat this condition

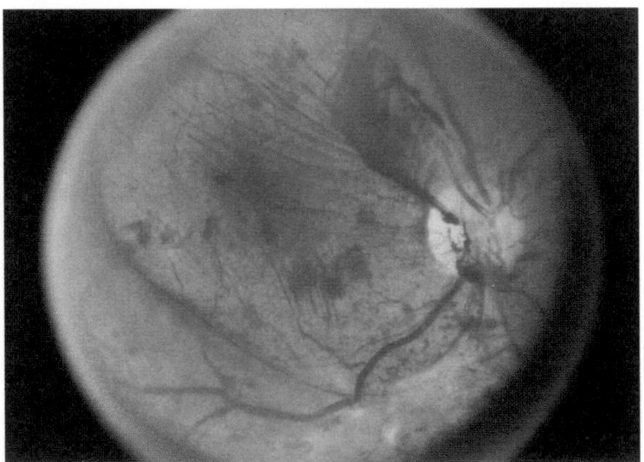

Photo 9.6 Neovascularization. An advanced stage of neovascularization (new blood vessel formation) combined with extensive hemorrhage and distortion of the retina. The retina becomes distorted from scar tissue associated with new vessel formation

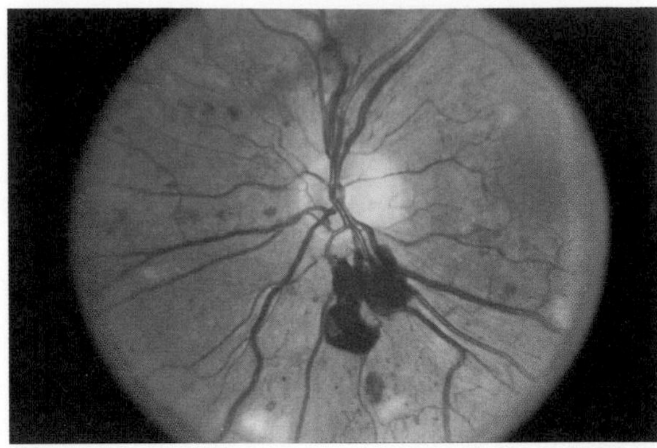

Photo 9.7 Severe proliferative diabetic retinopathy. There are many phases of retinal hemorrhage associated with diabetes. The small red blotches are points of retinal hemorrhage. The light patches are areas of poor circulation within the retina. The large red area just below the optic nerve is a localized area where bleeding into the vitreous has occurred. The diffuse red patches below the optic nerve show blood within the vitreous

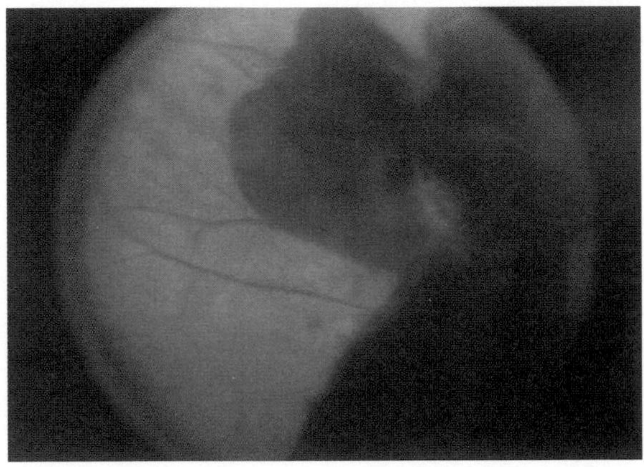

Photo 9.8 Vitreous hemorrhage. Extensive vitreous hemorrhage from new blood vessels growing on the surface of the retina. The retina is clouded by the extensive hemorrhage resulting in impaired vision. This is the most common cause of severe blindness in diabetes. Laser treatment cannot be used after such extensive hemorrhage has occurred

specializing in retinal disease is warranted for the following situations:

- presence of hard (lipid) exudates around the macula (indicative of macular edema)
- presence of any of the lesions characteristic of nonproliferative or proliferative diabetic retinopathy (see Table 9.4)
- vitreous or preretinal hemorrhage
- blurry vision that does not correct itself after 1–2 days or that is not associated with dramatic blood glucose fluctuations

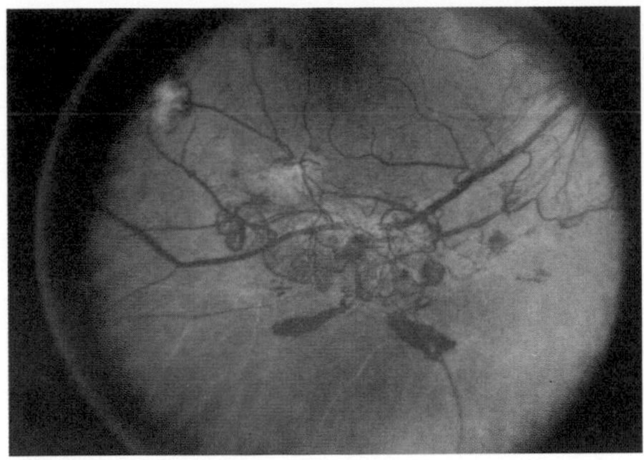

Photo 9.9 Proliferaton of blood vessels. Growth of blood vessels along the retinal surface are just below the center of vision. Regions of hemorrhage are shown below the center of vision. Laser treatment is efffective for eliminating these proliferating blood vessels and stopping the bleeding

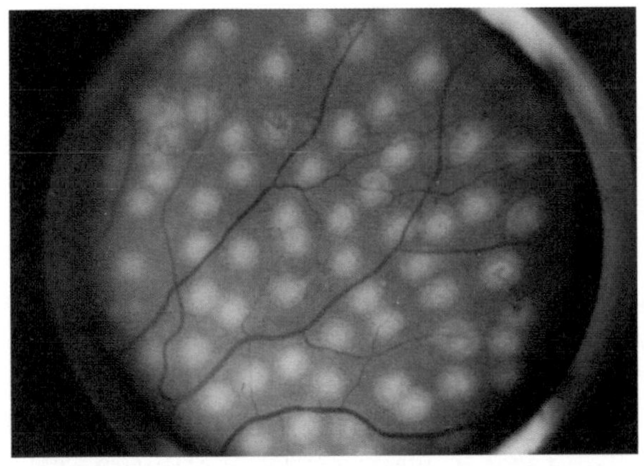

Photo 9.10 Laser photocoagulation therapy. Laser treatment scattered throughout the peripheral retina. This type of laser treatment does not affect central vision, but may affect peripheral vision, which is most noticeable at night

- sudden loss of vision (may be due to retinal detachment)
- dramatic changes in field of vision (flashing lights, spots, cobwebs)

It is important to verify that the patient is examined by the eye specialist and that the patient performs the recommended follow-up.

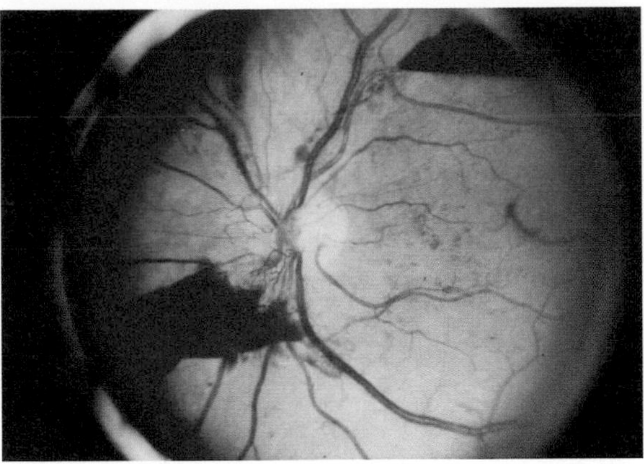

Photo 9.11 Before laser photocoagulation therapy. Active growing blood vessels with some vitreous hemorrhage. This patient needs to be treated with laser photocoagulation

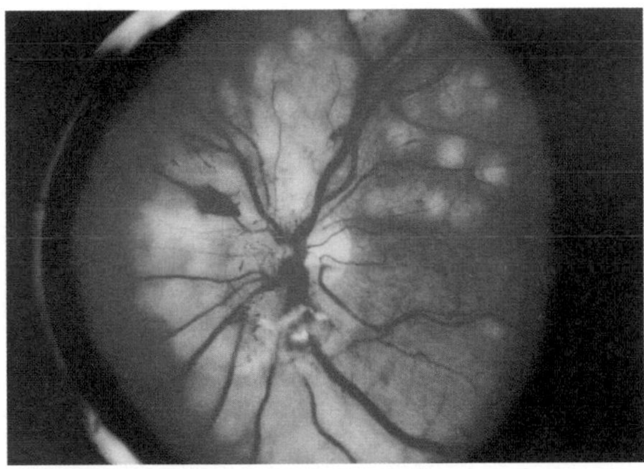

Photo 9.12 After photocoagulation therapy. The retina of the same patient as shown in Photo 9.11 four months after laser photocoagulation treatment. The hemorrhages have disappeared and the growth of new blood vessels has slowed dramatically. This type of laser treatment can save good central vision

Treatment of diabetic retinopathy

The strategies for treating NPDR, macular edema, and PDR are described below.

Nonproliferative diabetic retinopathy. Once diagnosed, early NPDR is not directly treated *per se*; rather, the risk factors associated with its progression to more severe forms of the disease

Table 9.4

Stage	Lesion	Clinical Presentation
Early Nonproliferative Diabetic Retinopathy (NPDN)	Microaneurysms (see Photo 9.2)	Small red dots, often in a punctate pattern.
	Dot and blot hemorrhages (see Photo 9.2 and 9.4)	Red round or blot shaped in the inner nuclear layer, or flame shaped in the nerve fiber layer.
	Hard (lipid exudates (see Photo 9.3)	Yellowish specks or patches of lipid-serum protein mixture.
Moderate to Severe NPDR	Cotton wool spots (soft exudates) (see Photo 9.4)	White spots or patches of swelling axoplasm and organelles of nerve fibers indicative of localized retinal ischemia.
	Venous abnormalities	Beads and loops of retinal veins.
	Intraretinal microvascular abnormalities (IRMA)	Loops of fine vessels stemming from either major arteries or veins.
Proliferative Diabetic Retinopathy (PDR)	Neovascularization of the disc (NVD) (see Photo 9.5 and 9.9)	Large bundles of new vessels on the optic nerve head.
	Neovascularization elsewhere (NVE) (see Photo 9.6)	Large bundles of new vessels on the periphery of the retina.
	Vitreous hemorrhage (see Photo 9.8)	Vitreous is cloudy or opaque and often with a reddish hue.
	Tractional retinal detachment	Loss of vision if the macula is detached.
Macular Edema	Retinal swelling around macula	Difficult to diagnoses with ophthalmoscope, but a ring of hard exudate around the macular region is a common inidication.

are treated. The key issues in the management of background diabetic eye disease are obtaining and maintaining glycemic and blood pressure control and regular monitoring of retinas for early detection of possible progression to the more serious stages of diabetic retinopathy. Staged Diabetes Management provides DecisionPaths for obtaining and maintaining metabolic control for type 2 and type 1 diabetes (see Chapters 4–6). The maintenance of near euglycemia is of paramount importance for individuals with mild nonproliferative diabetic retinopathy.

Aggressive treatment of high blood pressure to a target of ≤130/80 mmHg, appears to be beneficial because it is a risk factor for macular edema. DecisionPaths have been formulated for the assessment, diagnosis, and treatment of hypertension (see Chapter 8). Briefly, hypertension management begins with alterations in food plan, exercise, and changes in lifestyle, especially related to stress. Specific to dietary changes has been the elimination of significant amounts of salt. This is best accomplished through reduction in use of processed foods. Monitoring blood pressure at home and at work may provide necessary interim data to determine how well these steps are working. If these interventions fail, mono-drug therapy consisting of angiotensin converting enzyme (ACE) inhibitors or angiotensin II receptor blockers (ARB) should be initiated. If this therapy is not efficacious, other options include calcium channel blockers, β-blockers, diuretics, or α-blockers. Monitoring blood pressure is necessary. If one drug fails, another may be tried or a combination of antihypertensive agents may be prescribed. Note that management of hypertension in patients with type 2 diabetes often requires two or more classes of antihypertensive agents.

Macular edema. Macular edema is treated by focal laser photocoagulation. The goal of this treatment is to maintain or improve visual acuity. Leaking blood vessels and microaneurysms, which cause the retinal swelling in the region around the macula, are identified with fluorescein angiography. This technique involves the injection of fluorescein, a fluorescent dye, into a vein, followed by sequential photographs of the retina to identify the location of leaking vessels. A focal argon laser is used to make small burns at the site of leaking vessels in the macular region. The large and statistically powerful Early Treatment Diabetic Retinopathy Study[12] concluded that focal laser photocoagulation reduces the rate of visual loss due to macular edema by approximately 50 per cent .

Proliferative diabetic retinopathy. Proliferative diabetic retinopathy (PDR), the more severe form of diabetic retinopathy, is treated with panretinal photocoagulation. This procedure is common for treating proliferative diabetic retinopathy and severe NPDR with high-risk characteristics:

- new vessels on the disk (NVDs) greater than 25 per cent of the optic disk region
- any NVD with evidence of hemorrhage
- large areas of new vessels elsewhere (NVEs) with evidence of vitreous hemorrhage

Standard panretinal photocoagulation consists of making approximately 1500 small laser burns around the entire midperipheral retina, well away from the macular region. The laser burns may stop further neovascular growth and lead to regression of established new vessels, thus eliminating further complications associated with neovascularization. The ETDRS[12] showed that this procedure is effective for preventing further vision loss, but normally does not improve already diminished visual acuity.

Vitrectomy. Pars plana vitrectomy is a surgical procedure normally reserved for cases of severe PDR characterized by non-resolving hemorrhaging NVD and NVE clouding the otherwise clear vitreous filling the central portion of the eye. In addition, the new blood vessels are prone to cause tractional retinal detachments. Vitrectomy corrects these problems by replacing the blood-filled vitreous gel with a clear solution, cutting the fibrous traction bands, and in some instances directly repairing retinal detachment. Since vitrectomy is used only for severe cases of PDR, restoration of normal visual acuity may not be achieved. However, modest improvements in vision are often obtained. Vitrectomy is often delayed in patients with diabetes because vitreous hemorrhages sometimes correct themselves with time. The Diabetic Retinopathy Vitrectomy Study Research Group[13,14] showed, however, that the probability of recovering visual acuity of 20/40 or better was significantly increased in type 1 diabetes when vitrectomy was performed within the first few months of severe vitreous hemorrhage versus conventional treatment, which consists of waiting for 1 year before performing the surgery.

Note. The more serious complication of retinal detachment involving the macular region requires immediate vitrectomy by an ophthalmologist specializing in retinal problems.

Aspirin and diabetic eye complications. Aspirin has been hypothesized to be associated with slowing the progression of diabetic retinopathy. The ETDRS[12] addressed this and found:

- aspirin did not alter the progression to severe proliferative diabetic retinopathy
- aspirin did not reduce the risk of loss of visual acuity
- the incidence of vitreous hemorrhage did not change with aspirin therapy

These results clearly indicate that aspirin does not provide any ocular protective benefits, yet it is not contraindicated in patients with diabetes, especially those taking low doses of aspirin for prevention of cardiovascular events.[17]

SMBG and insulin injections for the visually impaired. The importance of intensive therapy to prevent further loss of visual acuity cannot be stated strongly enough, especially in patients with diabetes related visual impairment. Self-monitored blood glucose (SMBG) is a critical aspect of maintaining proper metabolic control, but can be a daunting task for the visually impaired. Easy to read glucose meters with large display screens are available. In addition, meters can be adapted with specially designed hand guidance platforms to assist the placement of blood samples and retrofitted with add-on voice modules that provide audible blood glucose results. Insulin requiring, visually impaired patients are quite capable of administering their own insulin using insulin pens. Insulin pens are available from several manufacturers and are a very effective means for administering insulin in patients with visual impairment.

Detection and treatment of diabetic neuropathy

Neuropathy often occurs early in the natural history of both type 1 and type 2 diabetes. The purpose of this section is to show the relationship between diabetic neuropathy and blood glucose and to present DecisionPaths that will help identify neuropathies and initiate appropriate treatments. Poor metabolic control can accelerate the onset and progression of diabetic neuropathy. However, when properly detected and treated, management of hyperglycemia will dramatically reduce the risk of onset and progression of diabetic neuropathy. A practice guideline and DecisionPaths containing the current standards of care for assessing, diagnosing, and treating diabetic neuropathy are provided. Diabetic neuropathy encompasses a wide variety of complications associated with diabetes. The main objective of this section is to describe the various forms of diabetic neuropathy, ranging from diffuse polyneuropathies to very specific focal neuropathies, and to detail their diagnosis and treatment.

The current impact of diabetic neuropathy

Diabetic neuropathies occur in equal proportions in individuals with type 1 and type 2 diabetes.[1] At the diagnosis of type 1 diabetes there are usually no neuropathic symptoms. In contrast, at the diagnosis of type 2 diabetes one of the presenting complaints is often diffuse pain or numbness due to an underlying neuropathy. These patients may have undiagnosed diabetes for several years. The pathogenesis of the diffuse and focal neuropathies can be directly attributed to several interrelated factors: persistent hyperglycemia, hypertension, hypercholesterolemia, and occasionally nutritional deficiencies. Recent evidence suggests that 60–70 per cent of all people with diabetes are affected by at least one form of diabetic neuropathy.[1]

Types of diabetic neuropathy

Diabetic neuropathies are classified into two broad categories: diffuse and focal. These two categories have entirely different clinical characteristics.

Diffuse neuropathy

Diffuse neuropathies are the most common type of diabetic neuropathy and tend to be progressive. They are subdivided further into distal symmetrical sensorimotor polyneuropathy (DSSP) and autonomic neuropathy. Approximately 30 per cent of individuals with diabetes have DSSP. The presenting complaint is typically mild to moderate "pins and needles" neuropathic paresthesia and dysesthesia (contact paresthesia) in the most distal extremities. In some instances, patients will present with a severe stabbing or tearing pain that is more pronounced at night. In addition, symptoms such as numbness in the distal extremities may gradually develop. However, often there are no symptoms of DSSP.

Autonomic neuropathy affects many different organ systems innervated by the autonomic nervous system. Organs and organ systems affected by autonomic neuropathy that produce clinical signs and symptoms include the cardiovascular system, gastrointestinal tract, genitourinary tract, sudomotor, adrenal gland, and iris. The prevalence of autonomic neuropathy is much lower than that of DSSP, affecting approximately 5 per cent of all individuals with diabetes.

Focal neuropathy.

In contrast, focal neuropathy may result from a lesion in a single major nerve branch or root. The onset of focal neuropathy is usually sudden and the symptoms normally subside in 1 or 2 months. Lesions in the third and/or sixth cranial nerves may result in cranial neuropathy, which is characterized by nerve palsies (Bell's palsy) and localized pain behind the eye. Femoral neuropathy (diabetic amyotrophy) often affects older individuals with type 2 diabetes and results in pain and weakening of the muscles in the thigh and buttocks. Diabetic radiculopathy, resulting from lesions in nerve roots, causes root pain primarily in the trunk. In addition, focal neuropathy can be induced by nerve entrapment. Carpal tunnel syndrome, which involves the entrapment and compression of the median nerve in the wrist, affects many people with diabetes.

Hyperglycemia and diabetic neuropathy

Results of the DCCT for type 1 diabetes show reduction of blood glucose with intensive insulin therapy reduces the risk of developing neuropathy by 69 per cent in patients without neuropathy.[2] Even for those patients entering the trial with sub clinical neuropathy, intensive therapy ($HbA_{1c} \sim 7$ per cent) resulted in a 57 per cent reduction in the risk of developing clinical neuropathy within five years. What mechanism(s) are responsible for hyperglycemic induction of nerve damage? Several are currently hypothesized to be involved in the pathogenesis of diabetic neuropathy. The polyol pathway, aberrant protein glycation, oxidative stress, and reduction in essential fatty acids are all areas currently being studied for an association with diabetic neuropathy.[3,4]

The pathogenesis of diabetic neuropathy is very complex and many factors contribute to this common complication of diabetes. While a complete description of pathophysiology is beyond the scope of this textbook, a brief review is in order. Hyperglycemia is thought to be a primary factor in the pathogenesis of diabetic neuropathy. It directly affects the polyol pathway.[5] In this pathway, glucose is converted into sorbitol by aldose reductase, with subsequent conversion of sorbitol into fructose by sorbitol dehydrogenase. Persistent hyperglycemia increases the flux of glucose through the pathway, resulting in elevated intracellular accumulation of sorbitol in the nerve. High levels of sorbitol are hypothesized to cause localized osmotic damage to the myelin sheath, reducing nerve conduction, and slowing the entry of myo-inositol into the nerve. Myo-inositol depletion correlates well with reduced nerve conduction velocity in experimental models of diabetes.

Several clinical trials are underway to reverse the etiology of diabetic neuropathy. One major effort is to determine the efficacy of aldose reductase inhibitors in preventing, or slowing, the progression of diabetic neuropathy. A second area of concentration is the formation of advanced glycosylation end products (AGEs) in the nerve. AGEs initiate a cascade of events, which result in nerve dysfunction. Support for the role of AGEs in nerve dysfunction comes from some studies of aminoguanidine (a compound that prevents the formation of AGEs) in animal models of diabetic neuropathy. Aminoguanidine improved motor nerve conduction and nerve action amplitude. A third area is microvascular insufficiency, which reduces the availability of key growth factors (NGF, IGF, insulin) to be supplied to the nerve, leading to structural nerve damage.

Diabetic neuropathy practice guidelines

The standards of care for diabetic neuropathy in type 1 and type 2 diabetes differ slightly from those neuropathies that occur in individuals without diabetes. The standards are summarized in the practice guideline (Figure 9.6) and in this section. Diabetic neuropathy related foot complications are addressed in the "Detection and Treatment of Foot Complications" section later in this chapter.

Diagnosis

Diffuse Neuropathies — Type 1 (at time of diagnosis): paresthesia and burning pains in legs and feet; symptoms usually disappear with insulin therapy (glycomic control)

Distal symmetrical Sensorimotor Polyneuropathy — Type 1 and type 2 (long-term): paresthesia and dysesthesia ("pins and needles") in distal extremities, diminished thermal discrimination; numbness; loss of motor control resulting in ataxic gait; unsteadiness

Autonomic Neuropathy — Cardiovascular: persistent tachycardia; reduced beat-to-beat variation on deep respiration; orthostatic hypotension; predisposition to painless myocardial infarction

Gastrointestinal: delayed gastric emptying (gastroparesis) causing early satiety/nausea/anorexia/vomiting; esophageal dysmotility; diabetic diarrhea; diabetic constipation

Genitourinary: atonic bladder paresis resulting in bladder infection; erectile dysfunction; retrograde ejaculation causing infertility; vaginal dryness

Sudomotor: gustatory sweating; decreased sweating in lower extremities

Adrenal: reduced hypoglycemia awareness

Iris: poor night vision; pinpoint pupils (no dilation with change in light)

Focal Neuropathies

Cranial Neuropathy — 3rd and 6th cranial nerve palsies causing sudden diplopia (double vision), strabismus, isolated pain behind eye; Bell's palsy

Diabetic Radiculopathy — Abdominal and/or thoracic pain due to nerve root lesions

Femoral Neuropathy — Often seen in older type 2 patients; pain followed by gradual weakening and atrophy of muscles in thigh and buttocks (diabetic amyotrophy)

Nerve Entrapment — Carpal tunnel syndrome involving median nerve in wrist; foot drop from entrapment of lateral popliteal nerve; tarsal tunnel syndrome

Risk Factors

Persistent hyperglycemia; $HbA_{1c} > 2$ percentage points above upper limit of normal; hypertension; hypercholesterolemia; duration of diabetes

Treatment Options

Good metabolic control; drug therapy when indicated; routine screening and patient education are critical

Diffuse Neuropathies

Distal Symmetrical Sensorimotor Polyneuropathy — Treat pain with standard analgesics, avoid narcotics; treat localized pain with topical Capsaicin; tricyclic antidepressants (amitriptyline, imipramine, desipramine, venlafaxine), anticonvulsants (carbamazepine, gabapentin, phenytoin), antiarrhythmic drug Mexilitene (oral lidocaine) may be effective

Autonomic Neuropathy — Orthostatic hyoptension: consider reducting or discontinuing antihypertensive medication for symptomatic orthostatic hypotension; use Fludrocortisone with caution, may precipitate CHF; may use elastic stockings/abdominal binders; increase salt; elevate head at night

Painless myocardial ischemia: consider imaging stress test

Gastroparesis: encourage frequent small meals, eythromycin, or dopamine antagonists (metoclopramide) may be effective

Diabetic diarrhea: treat with broad spectrum antibiotics (tetracycline) and bile salt sequestrants (cholestryramine)

Episodic diabetic constipation: treat with stool softeners and laxatives; severe cases may require pro-kinetic agents (metoclopramide)

Genitourinary: encourage regular bladder emptying; treat UTI as required; treat vaginal dryness with estrogen cream

Psychogenic erectile impotence (normal nocturnal erections): refer to psychologist

Organic impotence/retrograde ejaculations: sildenafil citrate vardenafil, tadalafil; vacuum devices with elastic constrictors to maintain erection; injection of vasoactive drugs (prostaglandin, alprostadil) into the corpus cavernosum; surgical implantation of penile prosthetics; referral to urologist is advised

Focal Neuropathies — Symptomatic palliation until symptoms disappear, usually 1–2 months

Targets	Near euglycemia ($HbA_{1c} \leq 1.0$ percentage point above uppper limit of normal) to prevent onset of clinical neuropathy and/or slow progression
Monitoring	Encourage patients to record pain and note intensity, duration, and time of day
Follow-up	With or without neuropathy
Monthly	Office visit during adjust phase (more frequently if changing medication)
Every 3–4 Months	Office visit during maintain phase (re-assess symptoms)
Yearly	Clinical evidence of diabetic neuropathy rarely is present in type 1 patients within 5 years of diagnosis (except paresthesia and burning sensations at time of diagnosis)
	Annual neurological screening with neurological history and neurological examination including sensory, motor, reflex, and autonomic responses; complete foot examination (pulses, nerves, and inspection)

Figure 9.6 Neuropathy Practice Guidelines

Common clinical manifestations

The common clinical manifestations of diabetic neuropathy are quite diverse and vary substantially from patient to patient. By far the most common form of diabetic neuropathy is DSSP, resulting from the loss of normal large and small nerve fiber conduction. Diminished light touch and thermal perception along with "pins and needles" sensations are common. In addition, numbness without clinical signs or symptoms is quite common. Autonomic neuropathies are not as common, but are very troubling for the individual with diabetes. Gastroparesis, alternating bouts of diarrhea and constipation, orthostatic hypotension, erectile dysfunction, and vaginal dryness are among the conditions found in individuals with diabetes with autonomic neuropathies.

Screening and diagnosis of diabetic neuropathy

Assessment for diabetic neuropathy should be performed at every visit (see Figure 9.7). Distal symmetric sensorimotor polyneuropathy is the most common neuropathy found in individuals with diabetes, occurring with approximately the same frequency in both type 1 and type 2 patients. Sensory perception is typically affected, but alteration of motor nerve function can also lead to ambulatory problems. This form of neuropathy presents with several distinguishing symptoms: (1) paresthesia and dysesthesia (resulting from progressive damage to large and small nerve fibers) and (2) "pins and needles" pain (starting in the most distal parts of the hands and feet, working proximally as the neuropathy progresses). Numbness without any significant clinical signs or symptoms is also common. Additionally, diminished thermal sensation normally accompanies DSSP. As this form of neuropathy progresses, the pain can become more severe, with patients complaining of acute pain that becomes more pronounced at night.

Autonomic neuropathy is not as common as DSSP, with a prevalence of serious cases in approximately 5–10 per cent of patients with diabetes. However, it often appears concomitantly with other neuropathies and accounts for several serious co-morbidities. The organs and organ systems most commonly affected are the cardiovascular system, gastrointestinal tract, genitourinary tract, sudomotor, adrenal gland, and iris. Autonomic neuropathy of the cardiovascular reflexes is manifested in orthostatic hypotension, persistent tachycardia, and reduced beat-to-beat variation on deep respiration. Autonomic neuropathy of the gastrointestinal tract causes delayed gastric emptying (gastroparesis), resulting in early satiety, nausea, and vomiting. Periodic diarrhea, often followed by diabetic constipation, is one of the most common symptoms of autonomic

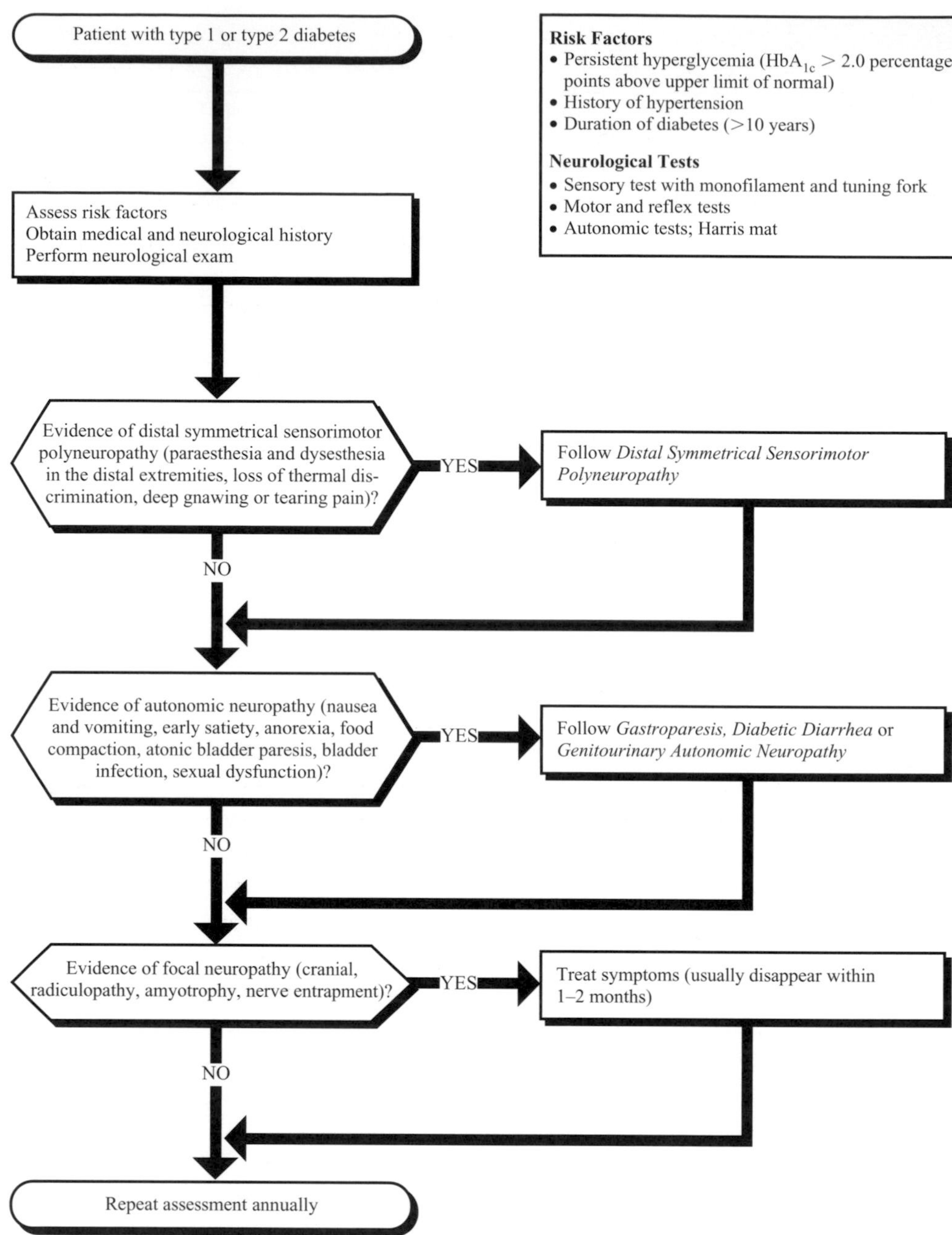

Figure 9.7 Neuropathy Assessment and Diagnosis DecisionPath

neuropathy. Autonomic neuropathy of the genitourinary tract results in atonic bladder paresis, leading to urinary tract infections. In addition, erectile dysfunction, retrograde ejaculations, and vaginal dryness are commonly found in patients with neuropathy of the genitourinary tract. Hypoglycemia unawareness due to adrenal involvement and gustatory sweating induced by hot or spicy foods results from sudomotor abnormalities.

Lesions to specific nerves cause focal neuropathies, and unlike DSSP symptoms normally arise suddenly. Palsies of cranial nerves may result in diplopia and strabismus (eyes not able to obtain binocular vision). Bell's palsy, characterized by distortion of one side of the face, is more common in individuals with diabetes. Carpal tunnel syndrome, tarsal tunnel syndrome, and foot drop are all focal neuropathies resulting from nerve entrapment.

Treatment of diabetic neuropathy

The most important aspect in the treatment and/or prevention of diabetic neuropathy is the establishment and maintenance of near euglycemia. Results from the DCCT[2] indicate that in type 1 diabetes intensive insulin therapy resulted in a 69 per cent reduction in the risk of developing diabetic neuropathy. Other studies have shown that intensive glucose control (in both type 1 and type 2 diabetes) relieves some of the pain associated with diabetic neuropathy. Staged Diabetes Management provides DecisionPaths for obtaining and maintaining metabolic control for individuals with diabetes (see Chapters 4–6). The maintenance of near euglycemia is important for all individuals with diabetes, especially for those with diabetic neuropathy.

Distal symmetric sensorimotor polyneuropathy. Begin with standard analgesics (acetaminophen, ibuprofen, and aspirin) and other comfort measures to treat mild pain (see Figure 9.8). Topical creams containing capsaicin can be used to treat localized mild to severe pain by applying three to four times per day for several weeks. Pain may initially worsen with capsaicin therapy and it may take several days before there is noticeable pain relief. Narcotic analgesics (oxycodone, oral morphine) should be utilized as a last resort for only the most severe pain. Tricyclic antidepressants, anticonvulsants, and antiarrythmics can be used as shown in Table 9.5 to manage pain in patients with acute painful diabetic neuropathy.[6–8] Use these pharmacologic agents with caution. Consult with a specialist if necessary. Currently, aldose reductase inhibitors and new classes of antidepressants and anticonvulsants are being studied in clinical trials to ascertain their ability to diminish acute pain from diabetic neuropathy.

Orthostatic hypotension. Manage orthostatic hypotension by discontinuing or reducing the dose of antihypertensive drugs. It is important to monitor for hypertension during alterations in dose. Pharmacologic intervention may include the use of fludrocortisone; however, this drug should be used with caution because it may precipitate congestive heart failure due to sodium and water retention. In addition, elastic stockings and abdominal binders may be tried along with increased salt and mineralocorticoids. Elevation of the head at night may provide some benefit as well.

Gastroparesis. To manage periodic mild gastroparesis encourage frequent, smaller meals and eliminate high-fat and carbonated beverages (see Figure 9.9).[9] Moderate to severe gastroparesis can be treated with the dopamine receptor antagonist metoclopramide, which may be helpful at accelerating gastric emptying when given (10 mg) 30 minutes prior to each meal and before going to bed. Erythromycin (250 mg tid) has been shown to stimulate gastrointestinal motility through its inherent motilin receptor agonist activity.[10]

Diabetic diarrhea and diabetic constipation. To treat diabetic diarrhea, a common complication, use standard over-the-counter antidiarrhea medications (loperamide and diphenoxylate). Bacterial colonization in the bowel is responsible for some cases of diabetic diarrhea. In these instances, a 10–14 day course of broad-spectrum antibiotics such as tetracycline and cephalosporin should rid the bowel of these colonies.[11] The establishment and maintenance of good metabolic control are also important aspects of treatment and prevention of diabetic diarrhea. Other drug interventions have also been shown to be effective (see Figure 9.10). Clonidine, an A2-adrenergic receptor agonist promotes fluid and electrolyte absorption in the gastrointestinal

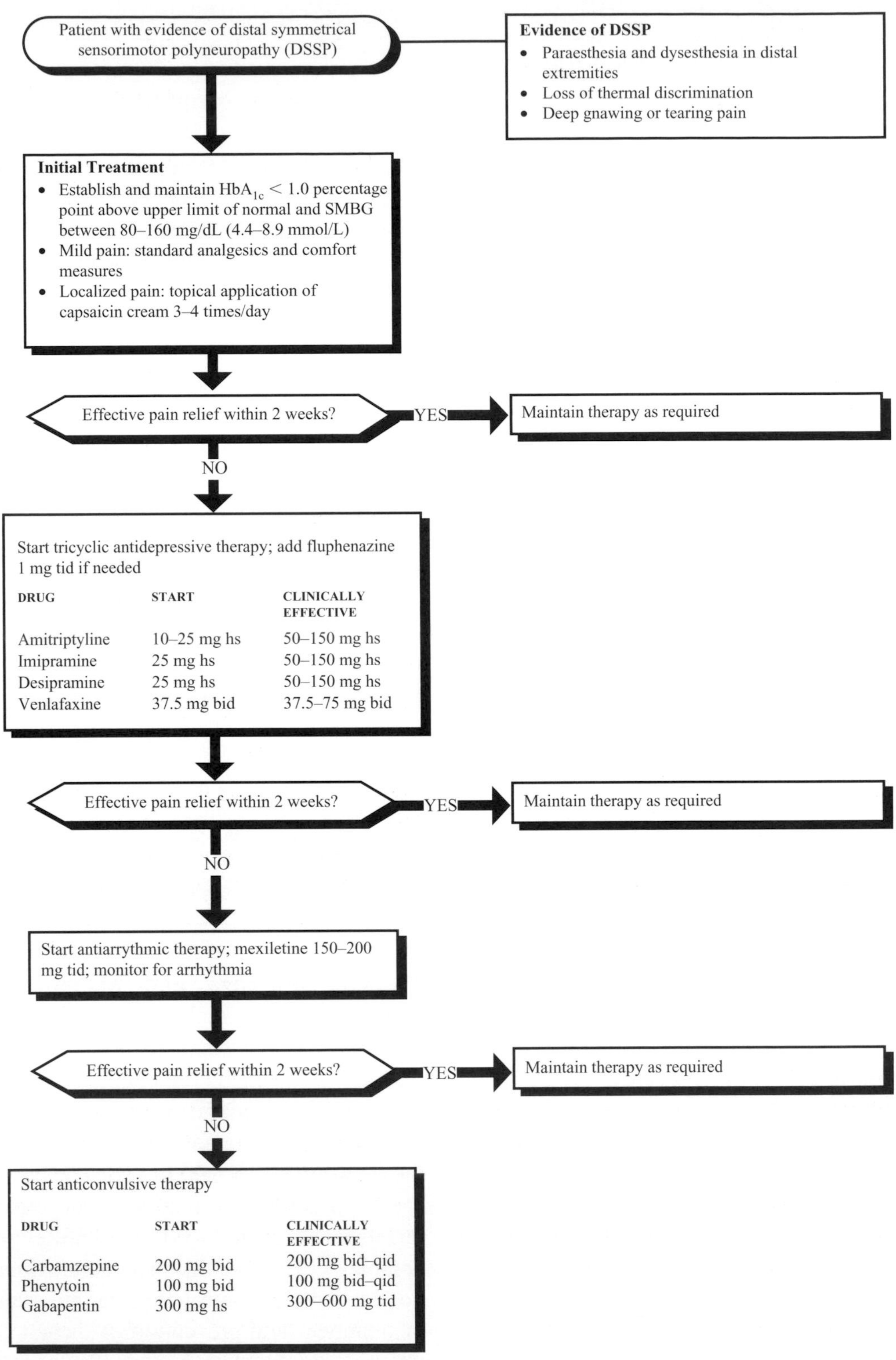

Figure 9.8 Distal Symmetrical Sensorimotor Polyneuropathy

Table 9.5 Drugs used to manage pain associated with diabetic neuropathy

Drug	Class	Starting Dose	Clinically effective dose	Comment
Amitriptyline, Desipramine Imipramine	Tricyclic antidepressant	10–25 mg hs	50–150 mg bedtime (hs)	Blocks uptake of nor-epinephrine and/or serotonin
Venlafaxine	Antidepressant	37.5 mg bid	37.5–75 mg bid	Blocks uptake of serotonin and norepinephrine; do not use in combination with monoamine oxidase inhibitors
Fluphenazine	Phenothiazine derivative	1 mg tid	1 mg tid	Sometimes used in combination with tricyclics
Carbamazepine	Anticonvulsant	200 mg bid	200 mg bid to qid	Unknown action, associated with aplastic anemia and agranulocytosis
Gabapentin	Anticonvulsant	300 mg hs	300–600 mg tid	Unknown action
Phenytoin	Anticonvulsant	100 mg bid	100 mg bid to tid	Promotes sodium efflux from neurons
Mexiletine	Antiarrythmic	150–200 mg tid	150–200 mg tid	Blocks sodium channels. Must monitor for arrhythmia

Abbreviations used for dosing; hs = bedtime, bid = twice day dressing, tid = three times/day, qid = four times/day

tract.[12] The starting dose of clonidine is 0.1 mg bid, with clinically effective doses up to 0.6 mg bid. Side effects associated with clonidine include orthostatic hypotension and increased gastric emptying. Somatostatin inhibits water loss from the gastrointestinal tract, making it another viable therapeutic option. Octreotide is a somatostatin analogue that is injected subcutaneously (50–75 μg) twice per day.[13]

In addition, bile acid sequestrants (cholestyramine resin bars) are sometimes prescribed because they effectively remove bile acids from the enterohepatic circulation. Free bile acids have been shown to disrupt the gastrointestinal tract, leading to diarrhea. Often, diabetic diarrhea is associated with fecal incontinence. Non-surgical treatment of this condition is accomplished using biofeedback techniques. Patients with moderate to severe fecal incontinence should be referred to a gastroenterologist with experience treating this condition. Paradoxically, diabetic diarrhea often leads to constipation, which can be treated with over-the-counter laxatives and stool softeners. Increasing intake of high fiber foods (bran, fruits, and vegetables) along with adequate hydration is important to prevent constipation. Prokinetic agents (metoclopramide and bethanechol) used for the treatment of diabetic gastroparesis also may be used to treat serious cases of chronic constipation.[14]

Treatment of genitourinary autonomic neuropathy. To manage autonomic neuropathies affecting the genitourinary tract, establish and maintain tight glycemic control. In addition, regular bladder emptying aided by abdominal compression is recommended to prevent urinary tract infections (UTIs). If present, treat any UTI as required. A referral to an urologist should be considered if more than two UTIs in male patients and three UTIs in female patients occur within a period of 6–9 months.

Erectile dysfunction is common in males and

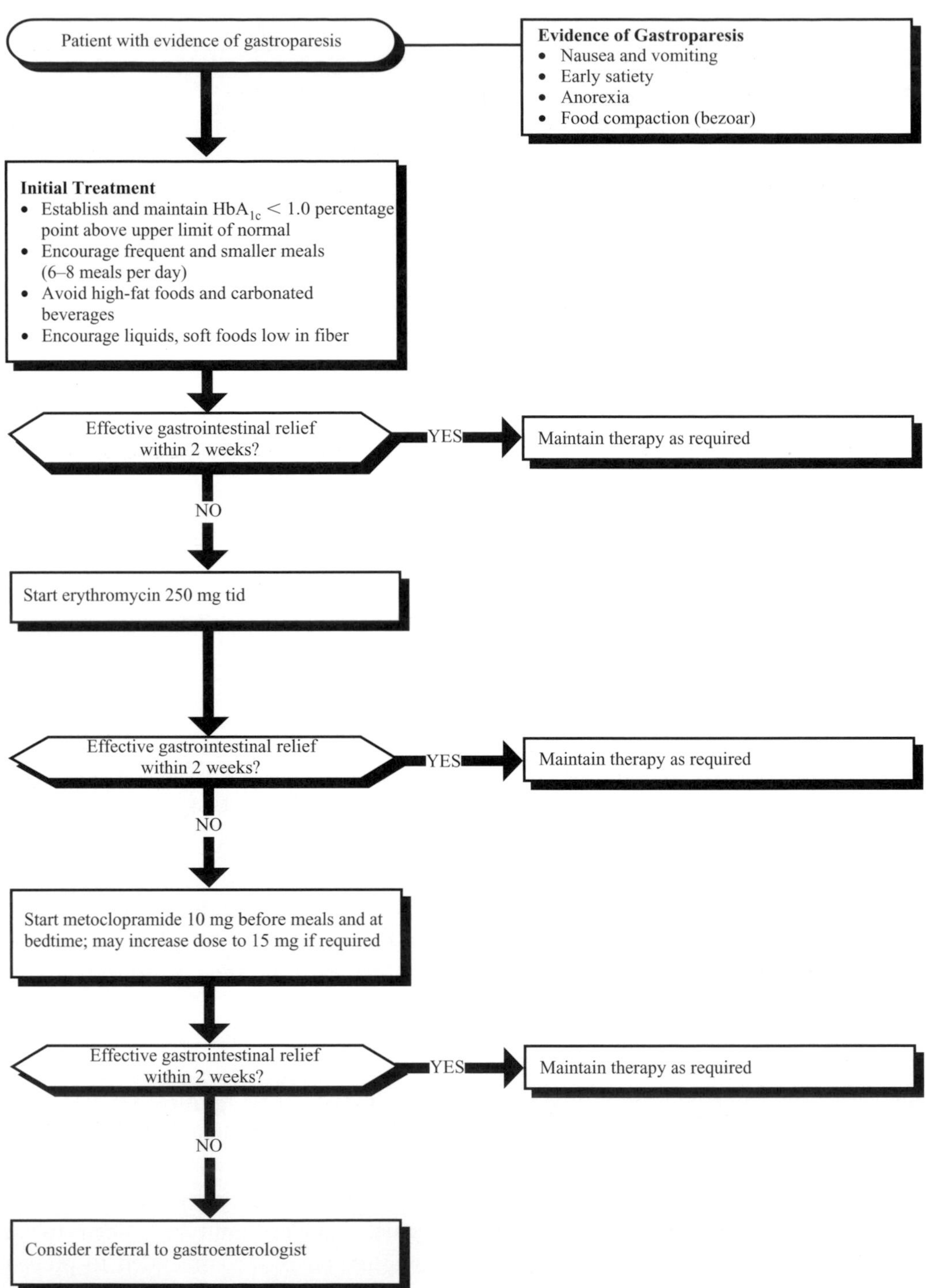

Figure 9.9 Gastroparesis DecisionPath

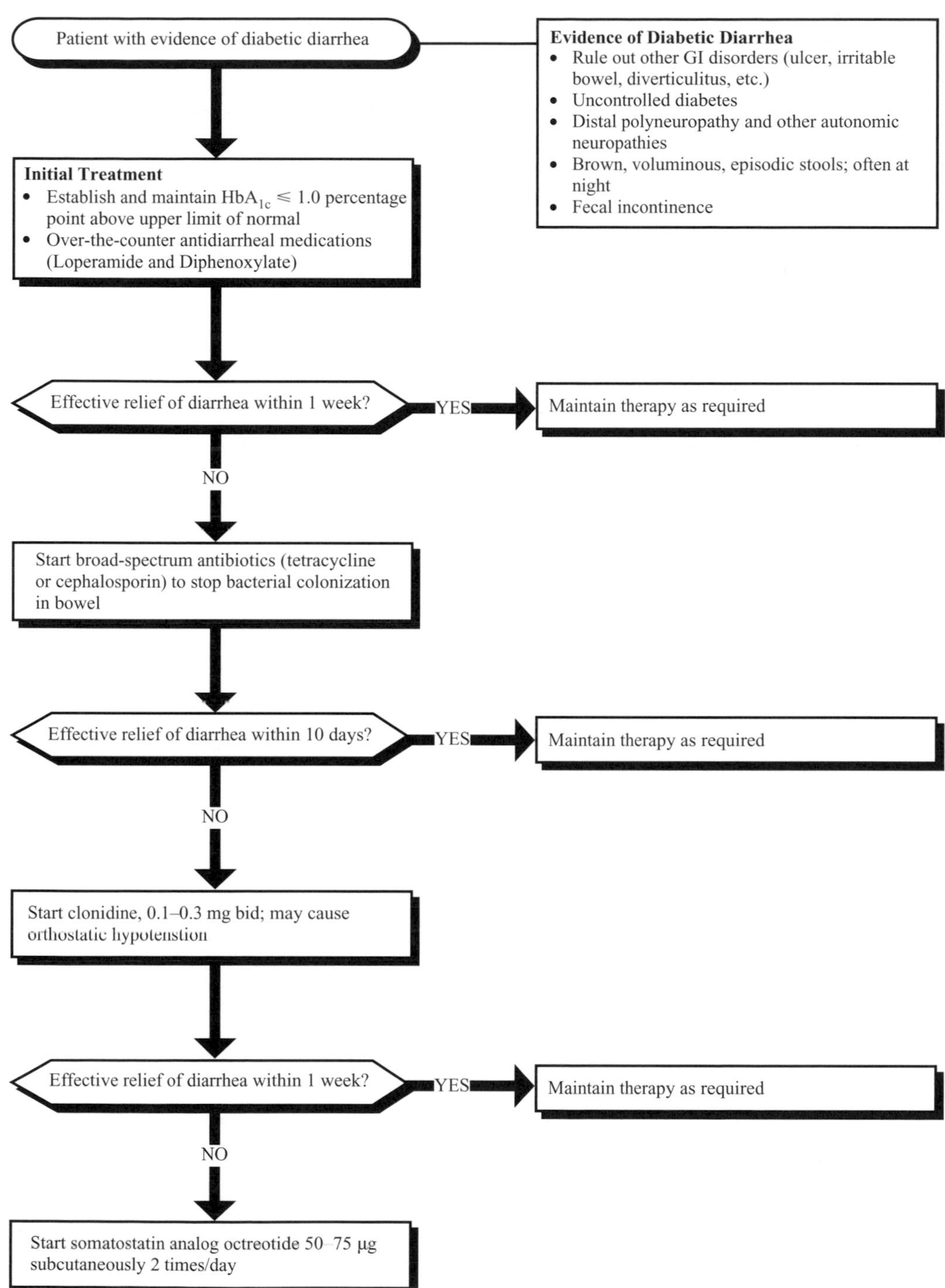

Figure 9.10 Diabetic Diarrhea DecisionPath

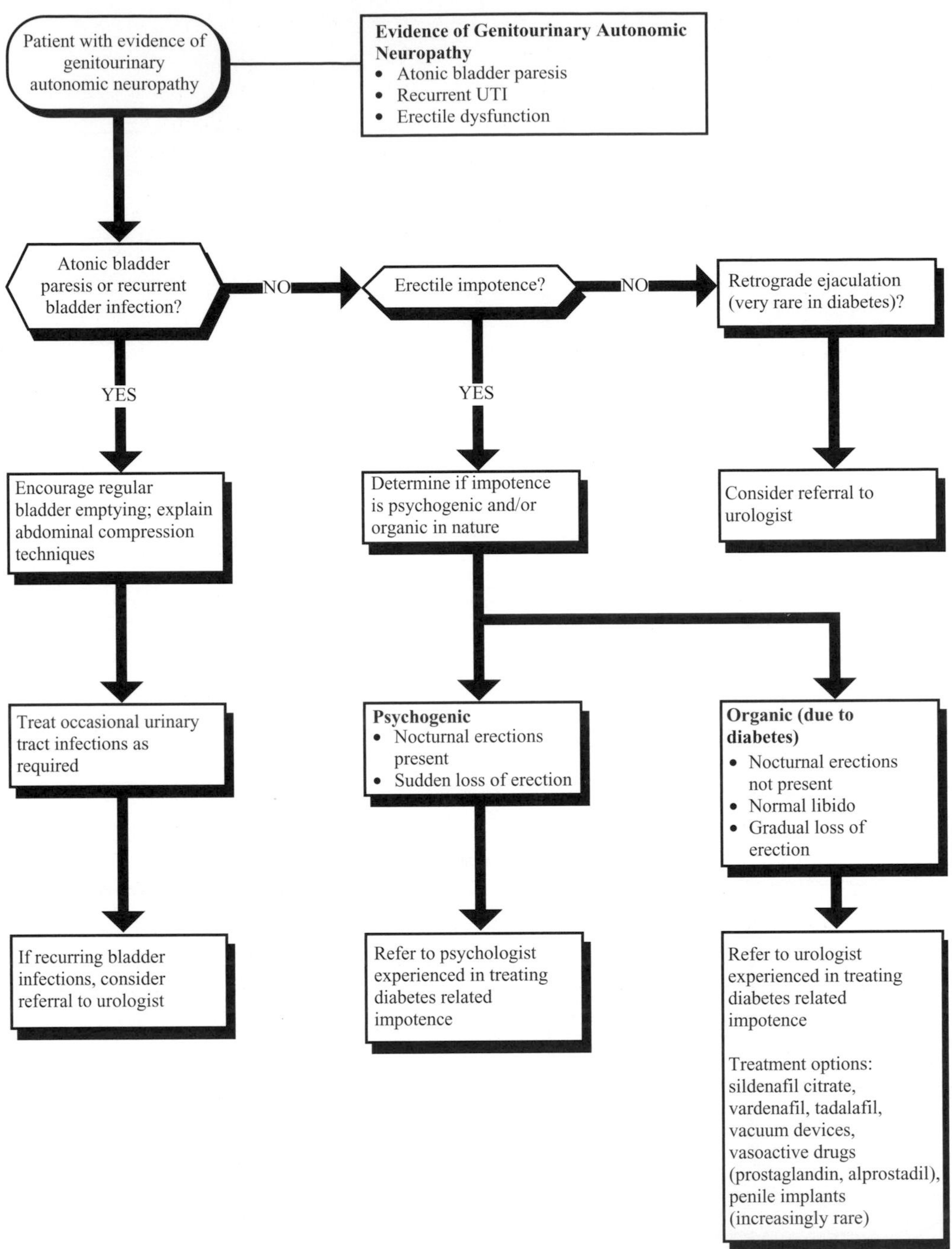

Figure 9.11 Genitourinary Autonomic Neuropathy DecisionPath

may be due to psychogenic or organic causes (resulting from autonomic neuropathy). The underlying cause of the erectile dysfunction must be determined before any therapy is initiated; referral to a psychologist with experience in treating impotence is recommended in cases psychogenic in nature (see Figure 9.11). Normal nocturnal erections and decreased libido suggest a psychogenic cause. Common options for the treatment of diabetic organic erectile impotence include sildenafil citrate, vardenafil, tadalafil vacuum devices with constrictors to maintain erection or the injection of vasoactive drugs (prostaglandins) into the corpus cavernosum to stimulate erection. The consequence of using this procedure is a long-lasting erection. In addition, surgical implantation of penile prosthetics is also a viable option but is becoming an increasingly rare procedure.

In many cases both psychological and physiological factors lead to impotence. Relying on a team approach, utilizing a specialist in impotence, is advisable. Female patients with diabetes may suffer from vaginal dryness, which can be treated with non-prescription lubricants or estrogen containing vaginal creams.

Co-morbidities

Patients with one neuropathy should be suspected of having other neuropathies as well. Additionally, patients with any neuropathy should be considered at risk for other complications, especially vascular and foot disease. Surveillance is necessary when any complication is detected. In general, maintaining near-normal blood glucose levels is beneficial in the presence of any of the complications associated with diabetes and may prevent their progression.

Detection and treatment of foot complications

The practice guidelines for diabetic foot care management are designed to promote consistent quality diabetic foot care with resources typically available in primary-care settings. The guidelines are divided into progressive stages that follow primary, secondary, and tertiary prevention as well as primary care. Intensive management of highly complex foot disease should be referred to specialists. Algorithms are provided to facilitate clinical decision-making.

Lower-extremity amputation (LEA) is a common problem in diabetes. The focus of most comprehensive diabetes treatment programs is to reduce the frequency of this outcome. Clinics that offer patient education, palliative skin and nail care, access to protective footwear, and aggressive management of plantar ulcers have demonstrated that the majority of diabetes related amputations are preventable.[1] The challenge is to offer these services in an appropriate and timely manner, and on a consistent basis.

Pathogenesis of diabetic foot disease

The path from diabetes to foot disease involves several factors including abnormal blood flow due to vascular disease, immune system suppression, and structural deformities and neuropathy. Large, medium, and small blood vessel disease, present in many individuals with diabetes, contributes to abnormal blood flow. Together, these vessel diseases reduce and impede blood flow to the skin, primarily in distal body points. Diabetic neuropathies, both peripheral and autonomic, contribute to a breakdown in the pain feedback loop that signals the presence of injury or infection. Peripheral diabetic neuropathy causes loss of sensation and an insensate foot, leading to painless trauma, ulceration, infection, and ultimately gangrene and LEA. Motor nerves may also be affected by peripheral neuropathy, leading to an imbalance of the interosseous muscles and hammer toes. These deformities make the tips and tops of the toes vulnerable to ulceration. Autonomic neuropathy may result in decreased perspiration leading to dry and cracked skin. Cracks in the skin are portals of entry for bacteria and infection. Added to these factors are the normal physical stresses (weight, pressure, and trauma) on the foot that result in injury. These multiple factors lead to an impaired ability to detect injury and infection. If treated incorrectly or too late, the infection may progress to gangrene and ultimately to an amputation of the toe, foot or, in some cases, the lower extremity. The ability to "fight off" the infection is closely related to glycemic control, because elevated blood glucose levels impair leukocyte function. Infections usually develop independent of the cause of the initial injury, trauma, or pressure. The most common infecting organisms are staphylococci and streptococci. Gram-negative bacteria and anaerobic infections are also common. If treated early, they may succumb to antibiotic therapy. Treated too late they result in a cascade of events beginning with superficial skin discoloration, moving on to an inactive ulcer then to an active ulcer and finally to a deep ulcer. Severity of disease can occur rapidly and may result in gangrene. Control of blood glucose to near-normal levels is extremely important.

Diabetic foot management practice guidelines

The standards of care for diabetic foot management are summarized in the practice guidelines shown in Figure 9.12. Diagnostic criteria are provided for classifying the patient's foot along with risk factors to be considered when performing a foot assessment. Staged Diabetes Management has developed a unique system for classifying feet based on the patient's history of foot complications, presence of any foot abnormalities, and size of foot ulcers. In addition, treatment options and therapeutic targets are clearly delineated. Appropriate guidelines for monitoring and follow-up are established based on the severity of the foot disease.

Common clinical manifestations

Patients may present with foot deformities, including claw or hammer toes, bony prominence, and or Charcot's foot. Loss of vibratory sensation is an early warning sign of loss of sensation in the foot. Loss of sensation to the 10 g, 5.07 monofilament is a warning sign that sensory protection has been lost. Simple to complex foot ulcers may be found which require aggressive treatment and follow-up.

Screening and diagnosis of foot complications

At each visit feet should be inspected (including between toes) for acute problems and a monofilament test performed (see Figure 9.13). A complete history and examination should be performed annually. This examination should include:

- vibratory sensation with 128 Hertz tuning fork or monofilament testing
- inspection for deformity
- inspection of shoes inside and out
- doppler measurement of pulses

Testing with the Semmes-Weinstein 10 g, 5.07 monofilament is an extremely important part of the assessment of each foot by providing a simple, noninvasive test for sensory neuropathy (see Photos 9.13–9.16). Show patients the monofilament and let them touch it so they are not afraid it will hurt. Ask patients to close their eyes and press the tip of the 10 g, 5.07 monofilament against the skin until it bends for 1 to 2 seconds, indicating that a 10 g force has been applied (avoid brushing the monofilament across the skin). Document results in the patient's chart. Patients who cannot feel the monofilament have a loss of protective sensation and are considered at risk for ulceration after even slight injury. Patients must be educated on the prevention of foot complications and their inability to sense pain (especially caused by cuts, blisters, abrasions, and poorly fitting shoes). Semmes-Weinstein 10 g, 5.07 monofilaments are readily available from several manufacturers. Check the patient's footwear to make sure it is well fitting and appropriate for the patient. Examine the inside of the shoe for small objects (rocks, keys, buttons) that the patient may not be able to feel.

While the use of the 10 g, 5.07 monofilament is considered the standard for screening for foot neuropathy; another option is the use of the low-pitched tuning fork (128 Hz) to screen for the presence or absence of vibratory sensation in the foot. Loss of vibratory sensation usually preceeds the loss of protective sensation (measured using the 10 g, 5.07 monofilament) allowing for the detection of earlier stages of neuropathy. Proper tuning fork testing is as follows: the patient is first taught the difference between pressure from applying the tuning fork and vibration. The tuning

Diagnosis	
Low-Risk Normal Foot	Normal foot, no ulcer; sensate to 10 g, 5.07 monofilament; no deformities; no history of ulcer or amputation
High-Risk Abnormal Foot	Abnormal foot, no active ulcer; insensate to 10 g, 5.07 monofilament; deformities; history of ulcer; amputation
High-Risk Simple Ulcer	Active ulcer, superficial involvement; ulcer < 2 cm wide and < 0.5 cm deep; no infection; vascular status intact; no systemic symptoms
High-Risk Complex Ulcer	Active ulcer, extensive involvement; ulcer $\geqslant 2$ cm wide and/or $\geqslant 0.5$ cm deep; infection; hyperglycemia; vascular disease; systemic symptoms present

Risk Factors

- Previous amputation
- Previous ulcers
- Foot deformities
- Age (>40 years)
- Persistent hyperglycemia ($HbA_{1c} > 1.0$ percentage point above upper limit of normal)
- Duration of diabetes (>5 years)
- Male

Treatment Options	
Low-Risk Normal Foot	Patient preventative care; educate and refer for risk reduction such as intensified diabetes management, tobacco cessation, and other behavioral changes
High-Risk Abnormal Foot	Patient education; protective footwear; non-invasive vascular evaluation (vascular lab); treatment if required
High-Risk Simple Ulcer	Outpatient wound care 2–3 times/week until ulcer healed; frequent follow-up to prevent recurrence; patient education; protective footwear; appropriate referral
High-Risk Complex Ulcer	Inpatient wound care; revascularization or minor amputation if needed; appropriate referral
Targets	$HbA_{1c} \leqslant 1.0$ percentage point above upper limit of normal, with frequent SMBG, prevention of foot disease; complete healing of ulcer and prevention of recurrence
Monitoring	Self-care: daily foot inspection; record all foot-related symptoms Inpatient: daily foot inspection by provider
Follow-up	**Patients with foot disease**
Daily	For inpatient management of complex ulcer, monitor BG
2–3 Times Per Week	For outpatient management of simple ulcer, measure BG at each visit
Monthly	Once stabilized, re-inspect foot each visit (up to 6 months) to prevent recurrence; HbA_{1c} each visit
	Patients with no foot disease
Every 3–4 months	Complete foot examination; HbA_{1c} each visit
Yearly	For low-risk feet, complete foot examination (pusles, nerves, and inspection)

Figure 9.12 Diabetic foot management Practice Guidelines

fork is placed on the patient's distal interphalangeal (DIP) joint on the first finger of the hand when it is not vibrating to demonstrate the concept of pressure followed by application to the same joint with the tuning fork vibrating. The patient is then asked to close their eyes and the vibrating tuning fork is applied to the DIP joint of the unsupported great toe. The patient is instructed to inform the tester when they stop feeling the vibration from the tuning fork. The

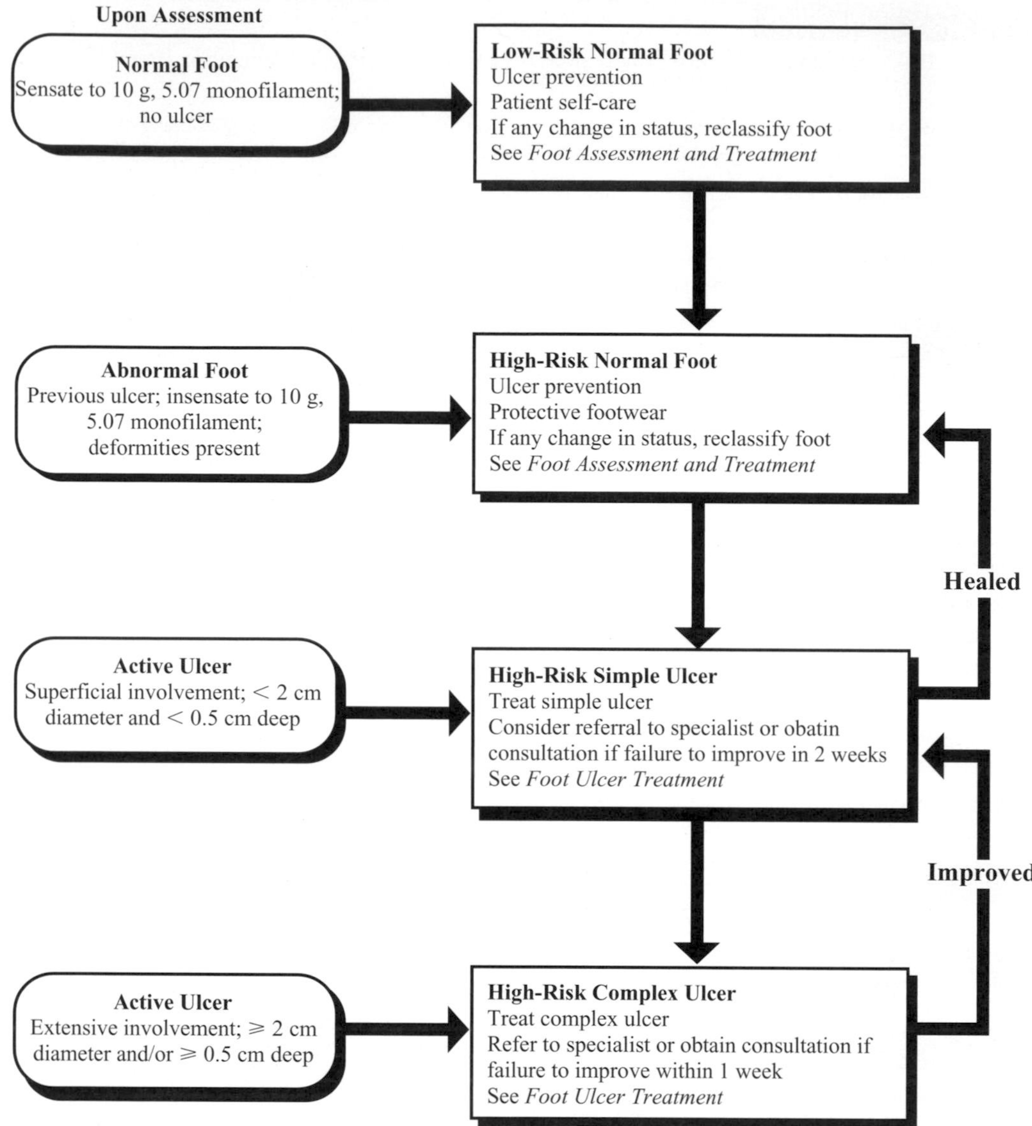

Figure 9.13 Diabetic Foot Master DecisionPath

tuning fork is then placed on the DIP joint on the first finger of the tester and the time until they stop feeling vibration is measured. Note, if the tester has neuropathy, the patient may serve as his or her own control and the vibrating tuning fork may be placed on the DIP joint of the patient's first finger. If the tester (or patient) feels the vibration for less than 10 seconds, the patient is considered to have normal vibration sensation. If the tester (or patient) feels the vibration for 10 seconds or longer the patient has reduced vibration sensation and the patient should be tested using the 10 g, 5.07 monofilament for loss of protective sensation. In some patients the vibratory sensation is completely absent and will require monofilament testing for loss of protective sensation. Repeat tuning fork testing on the other foot

Based on the presence or absence of high-risk findings, patients are assigned to low- or high-prevention stages. Low-risk patients receive patient education directed at maintaining their low-risk status. High-risk individuals without ulcers receive protective footwear in addition to patient education. High-risk patients with ulcer receive immediate treatment. If a patient is found to have an ulcer on the first assessment, a more extensive

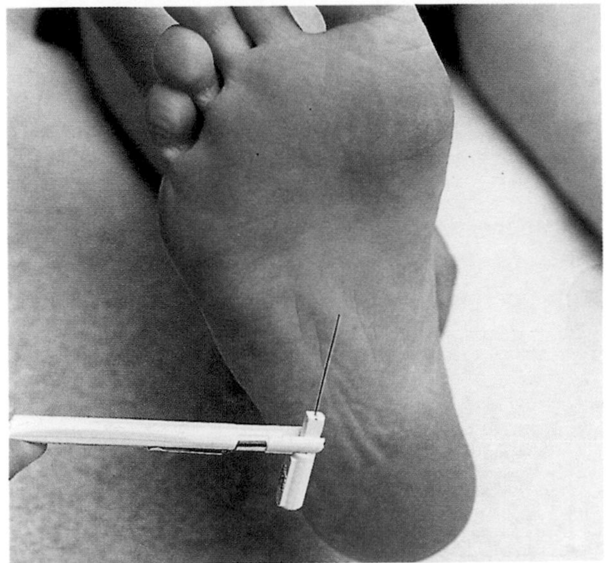

Photo 9.13 Foot examination; example of 10 g, 5.07 monofilament

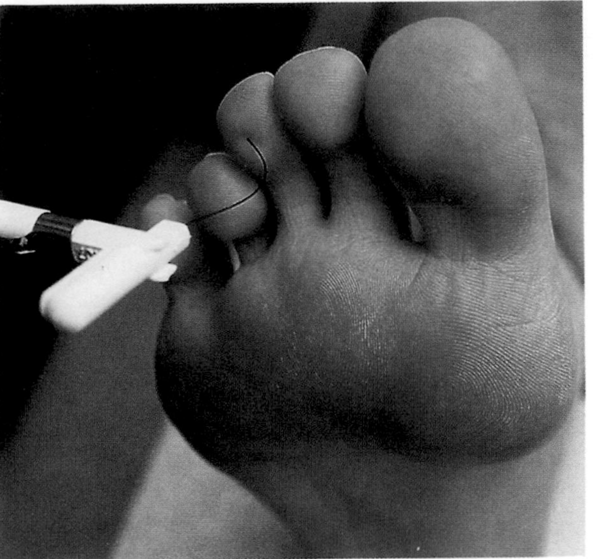

Photo 9.14 Foot examination; toe sensation

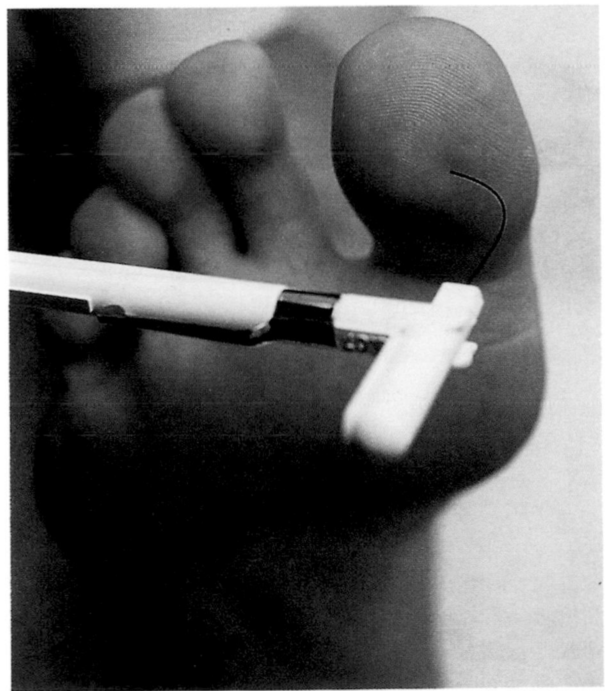

Photo 9.15 Foot examination; demonstration of appropriate use of 10 g, 5.07 monofiliament

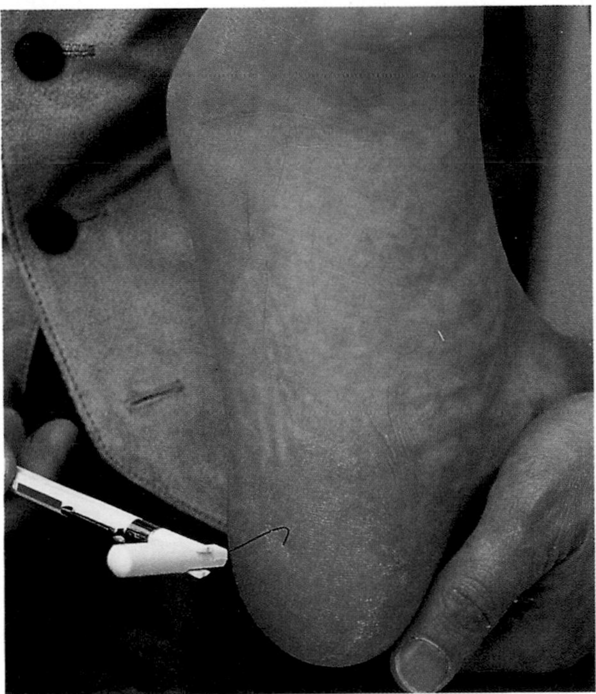

Photo 9.16 Foot examination; heel sensation

evaluation is performed during that visit. Patients with small ulcers and no complicating factors are candidates for intensive outpatient management. Patients with large ulcers and/or with complicating factors (i.e. sepsis, hyperglycemia, impaired blood flow) are staged to hospital care.

The next section details guidelines for each stage. They include a brief description of the stage, the entry criteria, the baseline assessment and diagnosis, therapeutic interventions, and stabilization goals. These guidelines are also summarized in Figures 9.13 and 9.14.

Low-risk normal foot

A patient with diabetes is considered to have "low-risk feet" (see Photo 9.17 p. 360) if neuropathy, peripheral vascular disease, and history of lower-limb amputation and/or plantar ulcer are

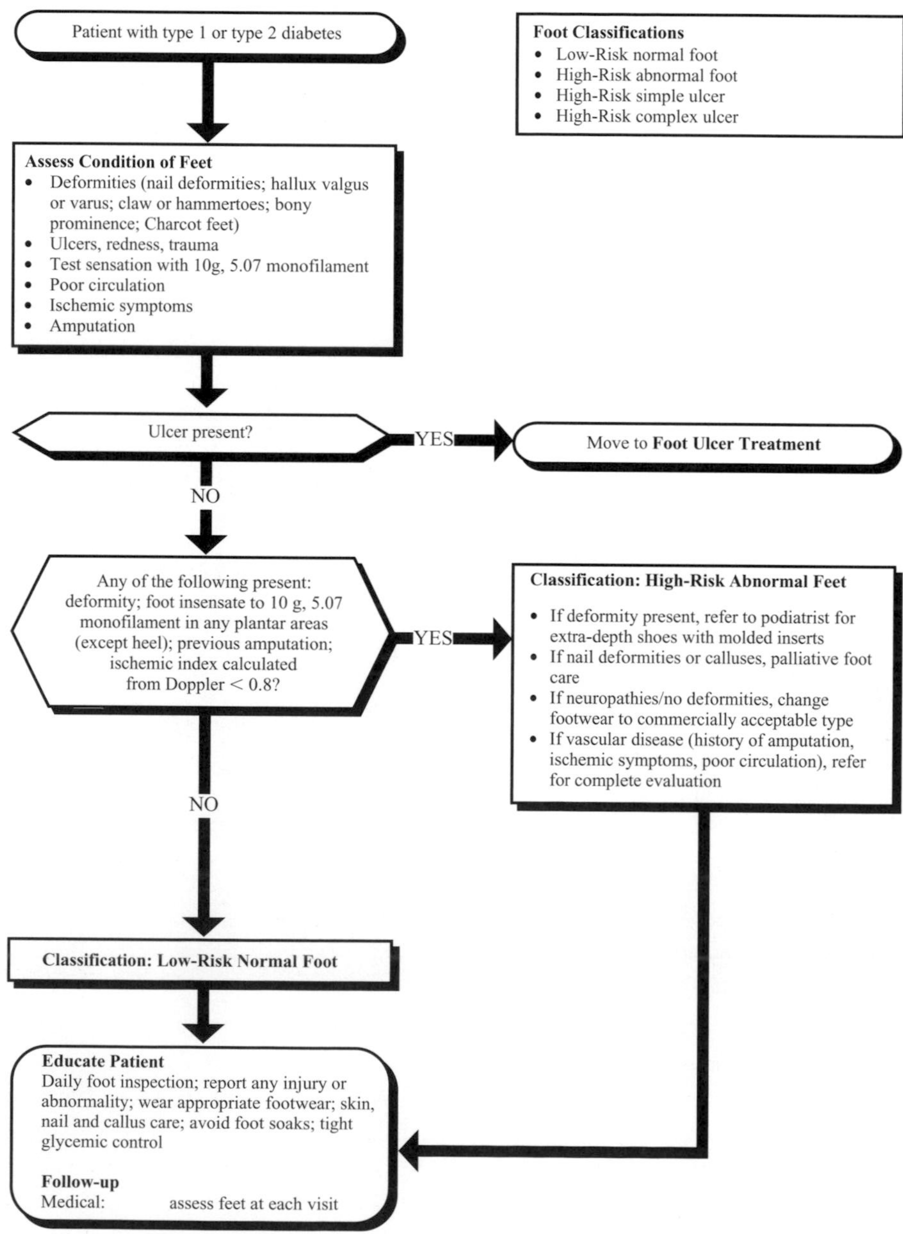

Figure 9.14 Foot Assessment and Treatment DecisionPath

absent. The low-risk normal foot category represents approximately 70 per cent of people with diabetes. The treatment goal for patients with low-risk feet is designed to prevent the development of foot disease by addressing modifiable risk factors that increase the likelihood of developing a foot complication (e.g. poor glycemic control, inappropriate footwear, foot injury) and to promote healthy foot care habits. Foot self-care education, including referral for risk factor reduction, is the essential intervention for achieving these therapeutic goals. Minimally, a yearly complete foot examinations is required to verify that patients with "low-risk feet" have not progressed to having "high-risk feet".

Entry criteria. Patients are considered to be at "low risk" if they have all of the following:

- sensation to the 10 g, 5.07 monofilament in all plantar areas tested, except the heel
- no foot deformities (hallux valgus or varus, claw or hammer toes, bony prominence, or Charcot foot)
- palpable pulses (dorsalis pedis or posterior tibial) on both feet
- an ankle brachial index (ABI) calculated from ankle/arm Doppler blood pressures measurements > 0.80
- no current or prior lower extremity amputation(s) or ulcer(s)

Baseline assessment. Shoes and socks should be removed to inspect feet for acute problems at each clinic visit. The presence of ulcers, redness, pain, trauma, infection, and nail deformity should be recorded. A complete foot examination should be performed annually and include monofilament testing, and observation for deformities. Perform a simple noninvasive vascular assessment such as a qualitative pulse check and/or an ankle brachial index (ABI) obtained by Doppler. The patient should be interviewed and medical records reviewed for a history of plantar ulceration or lower-extremity amputation. Results of the examination should be documented in the medical record. Since diabetic neuropathy is closely associated with foot disease, the history should include alcohol abuse, smoking, and level of glycemic control. These risk factors are modifiable and should be addressed as part of diabetes care. Similarly, poor glycemic control ($HbA_{1c} \geqslant 2.0$ percentage points above the upper limit of normal) should be vigorously treated (see Chapters 4–6).

Therapeutic interventions for low-risk normal foot. Self-care patient education is the principal intervention and can be offered as part of a formal structured curriculum or integrated into routine diabetes clinic visits. Assess the patient's current foot care and footwear practices, health beliefs, and support and barriers to care. Take advantage of "teachable moments" by demonstrating educational principles when shoes are removed for foot inspection or during monofilament examinations. Consider including family members and/or a friend in the education process, especially if visual or physical disability limits the patient in adequately performing self-care. The content of the instruction should include:

- daily foot inspection
- prompt reporting of acute problems to the primary care provider
- use of appropriate footwear
- appropriate skin, nail, and callus care
- smoking cessation
- avoidance of foot soaks and caustic agents
- maintenance of acceptable metabolic control

Education should be presented at the yearly foot examination and reinforced during clinic visit foot inspections. Self-care practices and footwear use should be assessed at subsequent annual foot examinations. Patients who demonstrate limited or poor understanding of self-care practices should be reassessed and receive education at the next scheduled clinic visit. Patients should be offered advice on treatments for modifiable risk factors. Patients who express interest should be referred to available programs.

Medical assistants and nursing staff should be involved in foot complication prevention by asking patients to remove shoes and socks at every visit to provide a visual reminder for the provider and reduce time for inspection/examination. Many organizations have provided foot care training for these health professionals and they become responsible for foot inspections and examinations. Evidence of foot problems (ulcers, deformities, insensitivity) are then reported to the provider.

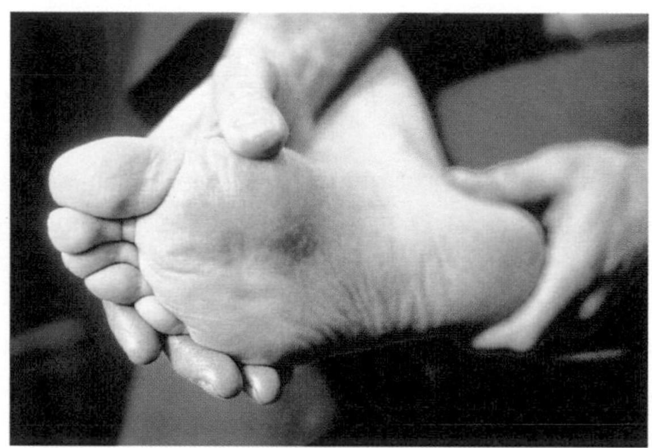

Photo 9.17 Low-risk normal foot

Maintain goal. A patient is stabilized when foot self-care demonstrated at follow-up visits is appropriate, i.e., skin hygiene, nail care, footwear, and health-seeking behaviors in response to self-identified problems. Understanding and self-care skills are reassessed and reinforced during annual diabetic foot examinations. The status of referrals for risk factor modification should be checked periodically. Patients remain in this category unless high-risk factors develop.

High-risk abnormal foot

The high-risk abnormal foot category includes patients with diabetes who are at "high risk" (see Photo 9.18) for amputation because of the presence of neuropathy, peripheral vascular disease, or a history of LEA or ulcer. This group represents approximately 25 per cent of people with diabetes. The therapeutic goal for this stage is secondary prevention or to prevent the development of ulcers, minor trauma, and infection that

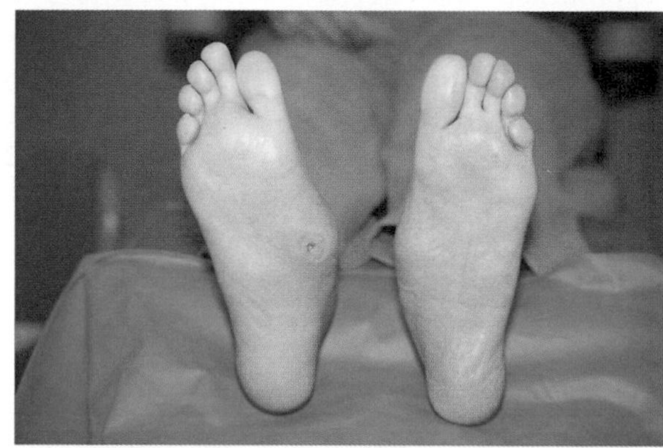

Photo 9.18 High-risk abnormal foot

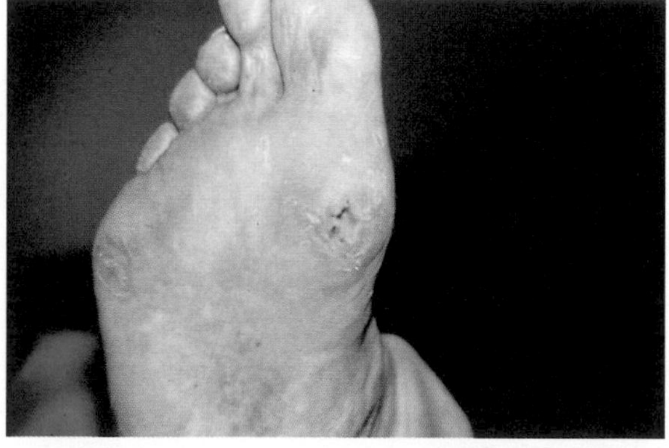

Photo 9.19 High-risk foot with simple ulcer

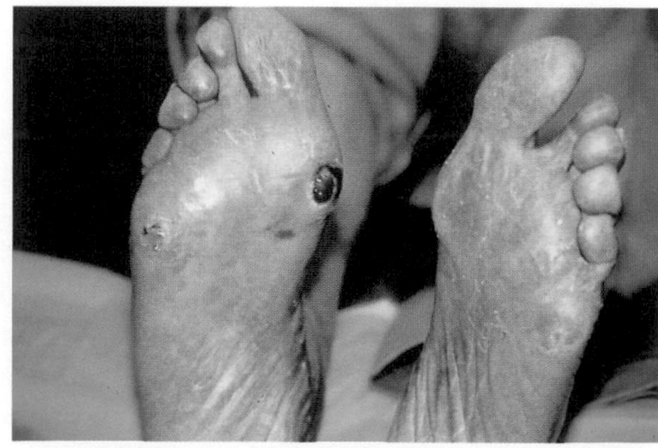

Photo 9.20 High-risk foot with complex ulcer

can lead to amputation. To meet this goal, therapeutic interventions for patients with high-risk feet include self-care education, podiatric care, and protective footwear.

Entry criteria. Patients are considered to be at "high risk" with abnormal feet if they have no active ulcer and any of the following:

- insensitivity to the 10 g, 5.07 monofilament in any plantar areas tested, except calluses and the heel
- foot deformity(ies) (hallux valgus or varus, claw or hammer toes, bony prominence, or Charcot foot)
- absent pulses (dorsalis pedis or posterior tibial) on either feet
- an ankle branchial index calculated from ankle/
arm Doppler blood pressures measurements < 0.80
- a history of lower extremity amputation(s) or ulcer(s)

Baseline assessment. Foot inspections at each clinic visit, a complete foot examination annually, and an assessment of treatable risk factors should be performed and documented as outlined for the low-risk normal foot.

Therapeutic interventions for high-risk abnormal foot. The following services should be offered as part of an individualized care plan.

1. All patients should receive foot self-care patient education as outlined above for patients with low-risk normal feet. In addition, the content should include principles of footwear selection. Self-care practices should be re-evaluated at follow-up visits every 1–6 months. Patients with limited understanding should be reinstructed and family members educated to assist in patient self-care.

2. For patients with minor nail deformities and calluses, offer palliative foot care as needed (usually every 1–2 months). Refer patients with severe nail deformities to a podiatrist. Calluses and nail deformities need to be treated prior to shoe fitting.

3. For patients with neuropathy and no deformity, encourage the purchase of an acceptable commercially available shoe of the patient's own choosing. Running shoes reduce the rate of callus build-up. Staff may wish to inventory local shoe retailers for acceptable shoes and provide a list with prices to patients as a guide. Some of these shoes may have padded non-slip liners or inserts. For those shoes that do not, provide a nylon covered shoe insert. After the shoe fitting, arrange for a follow-up in the clinic at 1 month and then every 6 months to assess use and condition of footwear.

4. For patients with deformity with or without neuropathy, prescribe extra-depth shoes with molded inserts. Alternatively, some patients with severe deformities may require molded shoes. Patients should be referred to a contract pedorthist for insert and shoe fitting. After the shoe fitting, arrange for follow-up at 1 month and then every 3–4 months to assess use and condition of footwear.

5. Refer selected patients at high risk for vascular disease for definitive evaluation and treatment. High-risk patients may include those with the following:

   - history of an amputation with prior vascular evaluation
   - ischemic symptoms such as claudication or rest pain
   - failure to heal despite aggressive therapy

Because many patients with peripheral vascular disease have cardiovascular and cerebrovascular disease, selection of a patient for vascular assessment/treatment requires clinical judgment of the risk/benefit ratio. Contrast materials used during arteriography for definitive diagnosis can have significant adverse effects on renal function among those patients with pre-existing diabetic kidney disease.

Patients with alcohol abuse should be referred to an alcohol treatment program. Patients who abuse tobacco should be educated and referred to a smoking cessation program. Use opportunities to stress the importance of metabolic control in preventing progression of risk factors.

Maintain goal. Patients are considered stabilized when they demonstrate foot self-care practices and utilization of prescribed footwear. A tracking system, such as a diabetes registry with a high-risk foot "field," can be used to enhance patient follow-up. A regularly scheduled high-risk foot clinic may improve access for patients who need frequent follow-up. Patients who develop plantar ulcers are treated in accordance with guidelines outlined for high-risk simple ulcer and high-risk complex ulcer.

High-risk simple ulcer

Patients in the high-risk simple ulcer category (see Photo 9.19) include those with a small, superficial ulcer and no complicating features (peripheral vascular disease, infections, etc.). This stage represents approximately 2–3 per cent of people with diabetes. The therapeutic goal is tertiary prevention, or complete healing of the ulcer. To meet this goal, therapeutic interventions focus on aggressive wound care (see Figure 9.15). Management usually can be performed in the outpatient setting. Selected patients may require hospitalization to optimize adherence to the treatment regimen.

Entry criteria. Patients who are treated in accordance with the high-risk simple ulcer guidelines include those with any of the following findings:

- The ulcer is < 2 cm in diameter and < 0.5 cm deep.
- Cellulitis is limited to a 2 cm margin and there is no ascending infection.
- Temperature is < 38°C (100.5 °F).
- White blood count is $< 12\,000$.
- There is no deep space infection such as abscess, osteomyelitis, gangrene, and a sinus tract.
- Pulses are present, ankle brachial index is > 0.8, and ischemic symptoms are absent.

Baseline assessment. When a plantar ulcer is identified, a careful inspection of the foot must be performed. Debridement must be done and the size and depth measured and documented for follow-up comparison. Using a blunt metal instrument, probe the wound, looking for involvement below the subcutaneous tissue or sinus tracks. Note evidence of extensive infection such as gangrene, lymphadenitis, osteomyelitis, or abscess. A plain film X-ray should be completed if a foreign body, gas gangrene, or osteomyelitis is suspected. Obtain vital signs and a white blood cell count (WBC) to assess for systemic involvement. Note that patients with significant infection may be afebrile and have normal WBC. Assess patient's alcohol use pattern and record tobacco use history. Check lower-extremity pulses, calculate ankle brachial index (ABI) from Doppler measurements, and determine digital pressure. Assess and document patient education needs for foot and wound care. Assess social support and transportation needs (consider contacting public health nurse or home health nursing staff).

Therapeutic interventions for high-risk simple ulcer. (See Photo 9.19 on page 360)

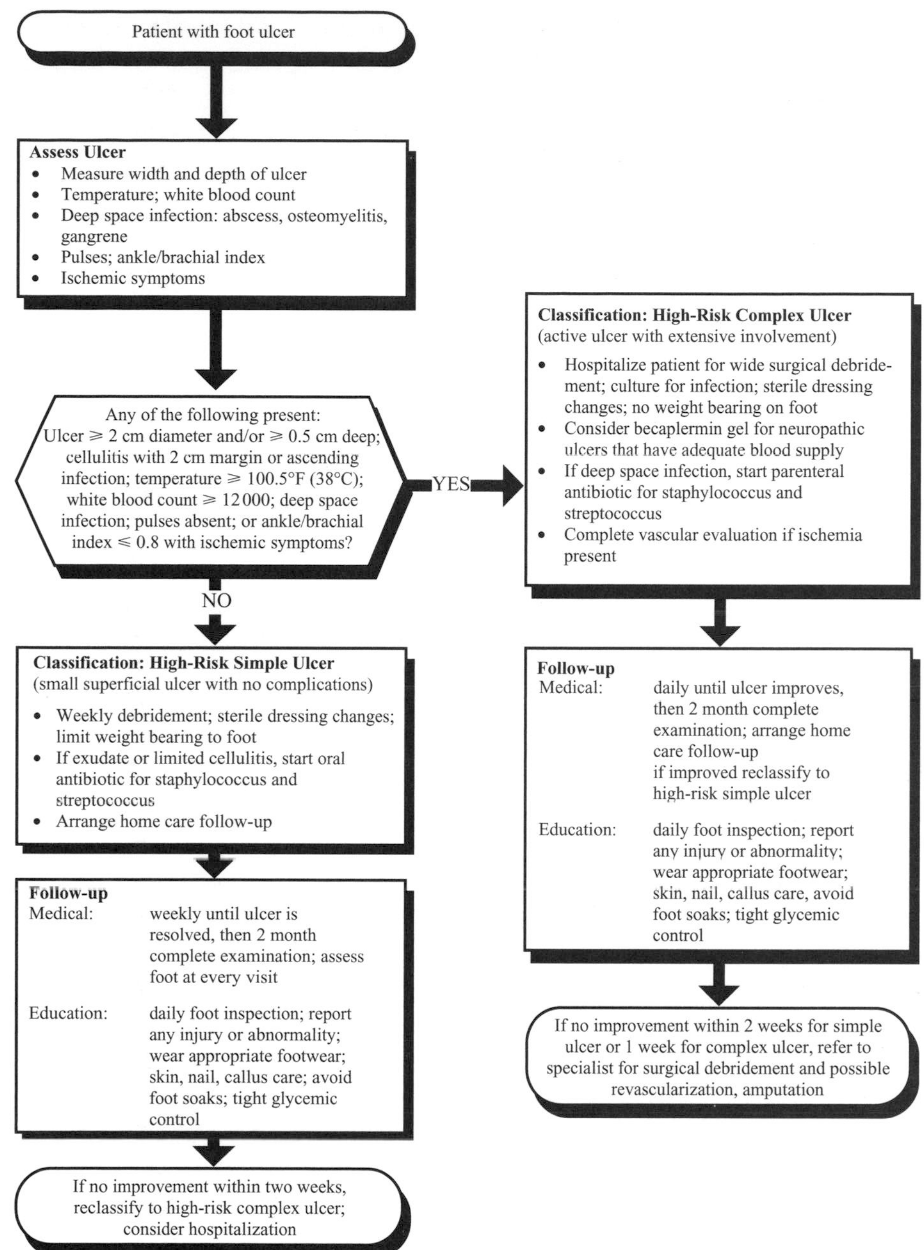

Figure 9.15 Foot Ulcer Treatment DecisionPath

Outpatient treatment should include the following.

- Debridement every week in clinic (preferably by the same provider). Document ulcer size to facilitate future assessment of wound healing.
- Limit weight bearing (bed rest, wheelchair, crutches, and/or contact cast).
- Sterile dressing changes every day: topical antibiotics, consider an available hydrocolloid for suppurative wounds. Avoid toxic agents (no betadine, H_2O_2, acetic acid, or Dakin's solution).
- Use oral antibiotics that cover staphylococcus and streptococcus infections for 2–4 weeks if an exudate or limited cellulitis is present.

(Studies have shown that more than 90 per cent of limited diabetic foot infections respond to oral cephalexin or clindamycin, even though most are mixed infections.) Consider adding metronidazole to cover anaerobic infections if peri-wound erythema persists after 2 weeks of the initial antibiotic therapy.

- Patient education to reinforce the care plan.
- Home care follow-up every 1–3 days by a public health nurse to assess adherence to care plan until healing is accomplished.
- Medical follow-up every week in clinic to monitor healing and modify care plan until healing is accomplished.

For patients whose alcohol use pattern may aggravate wound healing or self-care practices, initiate a referral to an alcohol treatment program. Consider hospitalization to supervise care Patients who use tobacco should be educated and referred to a smoking cessation program. Consider hospitalization for patients with limited ability to adhere to self-care practices, poor visual acuity, insufficient social support, and inability to minimize weight bearing.

Maintain goal. A patient is stable when the ulcer heals. Future management should follow guidelines for the high-risk abnormal foot. Ulcers that are non-responsive to therapy (worse at any time or not improved after 2 weeks) become complicated ulcers and are managed according to guidelines for high-risk complex ulcer.

High-risk complex ulcer

Patients in with a high-risk complex ulcer (see Photo 9–20 p. 360) have large ulcers and/or have complicating factors. This represents approximately 1–2 per cent of people with diabetes. The therapeutic goal for patients with complicated ulcers is to reduce the size of the wound and eventually complete healing of the wound (see Figure 9.15). To meet this goal, interventions focus on hospitalization and surgical consultation for wide surgical debridement, aggressive wound care, and re-vascularization if indicated. Amputation is limited to nonviable tissue and considered only as a last resort.

Entry criteria. Patients included in the high-risk complex ulcer category are those with any of the following findings:

- an ulcer $\geqslant 2$ cm in diameter and/or $\geqslant 0.5$ cm deep
- cellulitis with a margin > 2 cm or the presence of ascending infection
- temperature 38 °C (100.5 °F)
- white blood count $> 12\,000$
- presence of deep space infection such as abscess, osteomyelitis, gangrene, or a sinus tract
- absent pulses, an ankle brachial index < 0.8, or the presence of ischemic symptoms
- patients with simple ulcers that fail to improve after 2 weeks of management

Baseline assessment. When a plantar ulcer is identified, a careful inspection of the foot must be performed. Debridement must occur, with removal of all necrotic material and eschars. Do aerobic and anaerobic cultures. The size and depth must be measured in centimeters and documented for follow-up comparison. Using a blunt metal instrument, probe the wound looking for involvement below the subcutaneous tissue, or sinus tracts. If the probe reaches the bone, suspect osteomyelitis. Note evidence of extensive infection such as gangrene, lymphadenitis, osteomyelitis, or abscess. A plain film X-ray should be done to determine whether a foreign body, gas gangrene, or osteomyelitis is present. Obtain vital signs, WBC, and ESR to assess for systemic involvement (although they may remain normal even with complex ulcers). Assess patient's alcohol use pattern and record tobacco use history. Check lower-extremity pulses, calculate ABI from Doppler measurements and digital pressure. Assess and document overall glycemic control and patient education needs for foot and wound care. Assess social support and transportation needs (consider contacting a public health nurse).

Therapeutic intervention for high-risk complex ulcer. All patients with a high-risk complex ulcer should be hospitalized. A consulting surgeon, wound care specialist or podiatrist knowledgeable in wound care should direct patient care. However, the primary care provider can deliver much of the care.

Inpatient care. Inpatient hospital care (see Chapter 10) should include the following:

- Wide surgical debridement including cultures of excised tissue/bone suspicious for infection (aerobic and anaerobic).
- Post-operative sterile dressing changes every day: topical antibiotics, consider an available hydrocolloid for suppurative wounds. Avoid toxic agents (no betadine, H_2O_2, acetic acid, Dakin's solution).
- Strict enforcement of non-weight bearing status on the affected limb.
- Optimized metabolic control.
- If deep space infection or cellulitis is present, treatment with parenteral antibiotics should be initiated. Provide broad-spectrum coverage until selection can be guided by culture results. Switch to appropriate oral antibiotic when systemic symptoms abate and the infection nears resolution.
- Patients with signs or symptoms of ischemia should proceed to definitive vascular evaluation and treatment. This includes patients with claudication or rest pain, abnormal findings on noninvasive vascular examinations, gangrene, or blue toe(s). Because many patients with diabetes have peripheral vascular disease, cardiovascular, and cerebrovascular disease, selection of a patient for vascular assessment and treatment requires clinical judgment of the risk/benefit ratio. Contrast materials used during arteriography for definitive diagnosis can have significant adverse effects on renal function among those patients with pre-existing diabetic kidney disease.
- Patient education to promote required self-care practices following hospital discharge.
- Communication with the primary-care provider for subsequent outpatient wound care.
- Therapeutic shoes to prevent reoccurrence of ulcer.

Stabilization. A patient is stabilized when the wound size is decreased, infection is controlled, and vascular supply is sufficiently improved to promote wound healing according to the guidelines for high-risk simple ulcer. Amputation should be considered after other treatments have failed. The goal is to preserve as much of the limb as possible. Post-amputation patients are managed according to guidelines for high-risk complex ulcer.

Detection and treatment of dermatological, connective tissue, and oral complications

Surveillance for complications of diabetes involving the skin, joints, and mouth are often overlooked in the management of individuals with diabetes. The following section outlines the criteria for diagnosis and treatment of these common complications of diabetes.

Dermatological complications

Dermatological complications associated with diabetes are fairly common, but often go undiagnosed. A recent study of individuals with longstanding diabetes revealed that 71 per cent of the study participants had at least one cutaneous complication associated with diabetes.[1] Cutaneous complications have been associated with the duration of diabetes and with the development of other microvascular complications.[2] There is still controversy on the extent of the role played by blood glucose control in the development or progression of diabetes related cutaneous manifestations. Table 9.6 lists the clinical presentations and treatments of many common dermatologic complications associated with diabetes. (See Detection and Treatment of Foot Complications for information about foot ulcers.)

Acanthosis Nigricans

Acanthosis Nigricans is a common skin condition that has been associated with insulin resistance and type 2 diabetes. Although it can occur at any age, it is most often seen in children and early adolescents. Especially prevalent in obese individuals, it is characterized by darkening and thickening of the skin in areas of major folds (neck, arm, and axillaries). The skin thickening is believed to be associated with high circulating insulin acting as a growth hormone. The darkening pigmentation is seen most often among Hispanic, African-American, and Native American peoples. There is no treatment *per se* for the condition except to reduce weight and lessen other insulin stimulants (such as hyperglycemia).

Connective tissue complications

Limited joint mobility

Limited joint mobility (LJM) is characterized by bilateral restriction in movement of the metacarpophalangeal and interphalangeal joints of the little finger. As LJM progresses the restriction moves radially to the joint of the other fingers, resulting in the inability to press the palms of the hand together in what has been called the "prayer sign." More severe cases of LJM may include restriction in the wrist, elbow, knees, and hips. Limited joint mobility does not result in joint inflammation or significant pain. It occurs in type 1, and type 2 diabetes. The highest incidence is among postpubescent teenagers with duration of diabetes more than 5 years. The prevalence of LJM has been reported to be as high as 58 per cent in studies of individuals with type 1 diabetes[3] and shows no gender bias. Several studies have demonstrated an association of LJM with a thick waxy skin appearance as well as with long-term microvascular complications (retinopathy and nephropathy). The cause of LJM appears to be a build-up of cross linked glycosylated collagen that is resistant to degradation by collagenase. The collagen builds up so much that extension and flexion in the joint are diminished. Interestingly, LJM is apparently not related to glycemic control.[3] There is no effective treatment for the condition, and research on the effect of aldose reductase inhibitors on LJM has met with limited success. Differential diagnosis includes osteoarthritis, other inflammatory arthritic conditions, and joint trauma.

Dupuytren's disease

Dupuytren's disease (DD) or contracture is a

Table 9.6 Common dermatologic complications associated with diabetes

Dermatologic Complication	Clinical presentation	Treatment
Necrobiosis lipoidica diabeticorum (NLD)	Red to brown thickening of the skin, often with rim of raised inflamed areas and central depression, resulting in a scaly appearance; usually found bilaterally on the front of the shin, but can also be found on the chest and arms; lesions may ulcerate due to trauma; more common in women	Normally not treated unless lesion becomes ulcerated; then excision and skin graft are required
Diabetic scleredema	Thickening of skin on back, shoulders and neck; found in both type 1 and type 2 diabetes; not to be confused with scleroderma-like syndrome (SLS)	Normally left untreated
Scleroderma-like syndrome (SLS)	Sclerosis of skin on hands and fingers often found in young individuals with type 1 diabetes along with limited joint mobility (LJM); associated with other microvascular complications of diabetes	Normally left untreated, but is a warning sign to improve metabolic control to prevent other complications
Diabetic shin spots	Small brown patches on the shins of individuals with longstanding diabetes	Normally left untreated
Tinea pedis or athlete's foot	Red rash, often between the toes, caused by fungal infection	Treat with standard antifungal agents; severe cases may require griseofulvin; encourage use of cotton socks
Onychomycosis	Thickened, discolored nails due to fungal infection	Treat with griseofulvin, itraconazole, or terbinafine hydrochloride
Lipohypertrophy	Fatty deposits at the site of injection	Encourage varying injection site within an anatomic region
Xanthoma diabeticorium (eruptive xanthoma)	Small (1–3 cm) yellow raised papular skin lesions on the elbows, hips, and buttocks; often itchy; associated with poor glycemic control; develop rapidly due to extreme hypertriglyceridemia.	Lesions usually clear quickly when glycemic control is restored

fibrosis of the palmar aponeurotic space of the hands. The symptoms of DD include lumps or nodules in the palm of the hand near the base of the third, fourth, and/or fifth digits. In addition, localized indentations in the palm due to connective tissue "tethering" of the skin are often found. Serious cases of DD involve the contracture of one or more of the affected digits due to the formation of Dupuytren's cord, a long band of connective tissue that extends from the nodules in the palm into the finger. The cord causes Dupuytren's contracture of the proximal interphalangeal joint.

In a study of individuals with type 1 and type 2 diabetes, the prevalence of DD was 14 per cent, with no difference in prevalence due to gender.[4] Treatment of DD includes fasciectomy and, in severe cases, capsulotomy. Patients with significant disability due to DD should be referred to a hand surgeon.

Frozen shoulder (adhesive capsulitis)

Frozen shoulder, or adhesive capsulitis, is characterized by a gradual loss of range of motion in the glenohumeral joint due to inflammation and thickening of the joint capsule. Inflammation of the capsule leads to the formation of adhesions, which further reduce joint mobility. Patients often avoid the pain associated with moving the shoulder, exacerbating the formation of adhesions. Frozen shoulder is normally not associated with arthritis but has been associated with thyroid disease and diabetes. The pathogenesis of frozen shoulder is unknown and the exact cause-and-effect relationship between diabetes and frozen shoulder is poorly understood. It is more prevalent in individuals with diabetes compared with the general population. Initially treat with anti-inflammatory medications (aspirin, ibuprofen, naproxen, prednisone) along with physical therapy to increase the range of motion of the shoulder.

Normally, frozen shoulder resolves after 3–12 months of therapy. In cases that are more difficult, referral for local injection, arthroscopic surgery, or repair of rotator cuff injuries may be indicated.

Oral complications

Periodontal disease

Periodontal disease is the most common oral complication associated with diabetes. It has been labeled the "sixth complication of diabetes mellitus."[5] Individuals with diabetes suffer more periodontal attachment loss, alveolar bone loss and deeper pocket depths compared with people without diabetes.[6] Interestingly, undiagnosed type 2 diabetes is often discovered in the dentist's chair. Oral manifestations found in individuals with undiagnosed diabetes include excessive gingival bleeding, increased saliva production (sialorrhea), candidiasis, acetone breath, and delayed healing. In order to identify more individuals with diabetes, some communities have equipped dentists with blood glucose meters in order to screen individuals for diabetes. All individuals with elevated blood glucose levels (fasting blood glucose $\geqslant$ 100 mg/dL [5.6 mmol/L] or casual blood glucose $\geqslant$ 140 mg/dL [7.8 mmol/L]) should be referred to their physician for diagnostic tests.

The relationship between diabetes and the increase in periodontal disease is not clearly understood. Studies of periodontal flora in individuals with type 1 and type 2 diabetes have demonstrated the presence of the same microbes as in control subjects.[7] This supports the hypothesis that differences in oral flora are not a critical factor. Rather, impairment of leukocyte function associated with undiagnosed or poorly controlled diabetes results in compromised resistance to oral infection. Other possible causative mechanisms include diabetes related alterations in collagen metabolism as well as changes in the thickness of capillary basement membranes.

The maintenance of good glycemic control (HbA_{1c} within 1.0 percentage point of the upper limit of normal) is of paramount importance to prevent the development or progression of periodontal disease. Research has shown that the rate of periodontal destruction is directly related to the level of blood glucose control. Because periodontal disease is preventable, it is critical that a documented referral to a dentist be made annually. In addition, individuals with diabetes should be warned of the increased risk of periodontal disease and instructed to maintain good oral hygiene by practicing good brushing and flossing technique.

Caries, xerostomia, and candidiasis

The prevalence of coronal caries in individuals with type 1 diabetes appears to be related to glycemic control. Patients whose diabetes is in poor control tend to have more coronal caries when compared with individuals without diabetes. Much less is known about the effect of diabetes on the prevalence of caries in individuals with type 2 diabetes. The importance of good oral hygiene, maintenance of good glycemic control

(HbA_{1c} within 1.0 percentage point of the upper limit of normal), and regular visits to the dentist are the keys to preventing coronal caries.

Xerostomia (dry mouth) is associated with diabetes and the exact relationship is not clearly understood, but it may involve underlying diseases of the salivary gland such as Sjögren's syndrome. Commonly prescribed antihypertensives, antidepressants, analgesics, and antihistamines may all cause xerostomia. Left untreated, xerostomia may result in increased dental decay, oral candidiasis infections, and difficulty swallowing. Mild cases of xerostomia should be treated with maintenance of proper hydration, frequent small amounts of water, and sugarless candies or gum to increase flow of saliva. More moderate to severe cases should be treated with commercially available artificial saliva.

The most common oral fungal infection is *Candida albicans*. Diabetes is a risk factor for the development of a *C. albicans* infection, but other systemic factors such as pernicious anemia and AIDS should also be taken into account. Several medications that are currently used to treat oral fungal infections are listed in Table 9.7.

Table 9.7 Pharmacologic therapy for oral fungal infections

Drug	Dose	Comment
Fluconazole tablets	200 mg first day; 100 mg/daily 2–3 weeks	Monitor liver function; may increase levels of sulfonylurea
Clotrimazole lozenge	1 lozenge, 5 times/day for 2 weeks	Allow lozenges to dissolve slowly; monitor liver function
Nystatin pastilles	1 to 2 pastilles, 4–5/day for 2 days after symptoms disappear; 2 weeks max.	Do not chew or swallow pastille, high doses may cause gastrointestinal disturbances
Ketoconazole tablets	200 mg/day for 1 to 2 weeks	Associated with hepatic toxicity; monitor liver function before and during treatment

Polycystic ovary syndrome (PCOS)

In the United States, polycystic ovary syndrome (PCOS) is the most common cause of infertility in women. It is found at a disproportionately high incidence among women with insulin resistance (with the highest incidence among obese females). Since both obese and non-obese women with PCOS are insulin resistant with corresponding hyperinsulinemia, PCOS is thought to induce a unique form of insulin resistance that is separate from obesity related insulin resistance. PCOS is characterized by hyperandrogenism, chronic anovulation, and infertility. It is characterized by derangements in gonadotropin releasing hormone, increased luteinizing hormone, and decreased follicle stimulating hormone.

Screening, risk factors, symptoms and diagnosis

Screening for PCOS is based on the presence of risk factors and clinical signs or symptoms. All females with irregular menstrual cycles, oligomenorrhea, or amenorrhea should be screened. Additionally, excessive hair (hirsutism) should be assumed to be related to PCOS. Finally, as PCOS is part of metabolic syndrome, any other component of insulin resistance should be considered a risk factor necessitating screening for other components of the syndrome (i.e. diabetes, hypertension, dyslipidemia). The first diagnostic test for PCOS is measurement of total testosterone by radio immunoassay. If total testosterone is between 50 ng/dL and 200 ng/dL (normal < 2.5 ng/dL) PCOS is present. If > 200 ng/dL serum DHEA-S should be measured. If DHEA-S > 700 μg/dL rule out an ovarian or adrenal tumor. These tests should be followed by tests for hypothyroidism, hyperprolactinemia, and adrenal hyperplasia.

Treatment

The treatment of PCOS is directed primarily at its clinical manifestations: menstrual irregularity, infertility, and hirsutism. The choice of treatments is related to the co-morbidities associated with insulin resistance. Generally, the choices are: weight loss with medical nutrition and activity therapy. Recently, the insulin sensitizer metformin has been used effectively to enhance insulin sensitivity in the treatment of PCOS. Before metformin can be initiated the patient must be evaluated for renal, pulmonary, and cardiac disease. The presense of any of these conditions generally makes metformin contraindicated. Metformin should be started using no more than 250 mg/day given with the largest meal. If the patient is already treated for diabetes with insulin, metformin therapy may be initiated. After the first week, increase the dose by 250 mg in the morning. Thereafter weekly increases of 250 mg can continue alternating between morning and evening meals until normal menstrual cycles or 2000 mg/day of metformin is reached. If after 3 months normal menstrual cycle has not begun than oral contraceptive therapy may be added.

Note. If the insulin/glucose ratio is $\leqslant 10$ μ/mg then the treatment depends upon BMI. For obese adolescents MNT to manage weight precedes use of oral contraceptive therapy. If normal or lean body mass then the patient is given low-androgen-activity oral contraceptive therapy for 3 months. If this does not resolve symptoms, then antiandrogen therapy is initiated. If the MNT, metformin, and oral contraceptive therapies have failed to ameliorate the PCOS symptoms, refer the patient to a pediatric endocrinologist.

Targets, monitoring, and follow-up

Normal menstrual cycles and fertility are the principal targets of treatment. Close monitoring of menstrual cycles with follow-up every 3 months with testosterone and liver function tests is recommended. Annually, the patient should be evaluated for all co-morbidities of insulin resistance.

References

Detection and treatment of diabetic nephropathy

1. Jerums G, Allen TJ, Gilbert R, *et al*. Natural history of diabetic nephropathy. In: Baba S and Kaneko T, eds. *Diabetes 1994*. Amsterdam: Elsevier, 1994: 695–700 (Excerpta Medica International Congress Series 1100).
2. Coonrod BA, Ellis D, Becker DJ, *et al*. Predictors of microalbuminuria in individuals with IDDM. Pittsburgh Epidemiology of Diabetes Complications Study. *Diabetes Care* 1993; **16**: 1376–1383.
3. Diabetes Control and Complications Trial Research Group. The effect of intensive treatment of diabetes on the development and progression of long-term complications in insulin-dependent diabetes mellitus. *N Engl J Med* 1993; **329**: 977–986.
4. Raguram P, Massy ZA and Keane WF. Diabetic hyperlipidemia: vascular disease implications and therapeutic options. In: Baba S and Kaneko T, eds. *Diabetes 1994*. Amsterdam: Elsevier, 1994: 706–712 (Excerpta Medica International Congress Series 1100).
5. Nelson RG, Knowler WC, Pettitt DJ and Bennett PH. Kidney diseases in diabetes. In: Harris MI, Cowie CC, Stern MP, *et al*., eds. *Diabetes in America*. 2nd ed. National Diabetes Data Group, NIH, NIDDK, 1995. National Institutes of Health Publication 95–1468.
6. Turtle JR, Yue DK, Fisher EJ, Hefferman SJ, McLennan SV and Zilkens RR. The mesangium in diabetes. In: Baba S and Kaneko T, eds. *Diabetes 1994*. Amsterdam: Elsevier, 1994: 32–36 (Excerpta Medica International Congress Series 1100).
7. Larkins RG and Dunlop ME. The link between hyperglycemia and diabetic nephropathy. *Diabetolo-*

gia 1992; **35**: 499–504.

8. Nelson RG, Knowler WC, Pettitt DJ, Hanson RL and Bennett PH. Incidence and determinants of elevated urinary albumin excretion in Pima Indians with NIDDM. *Diabetes Care* 1995; **18**: 182–187.
9. UK Prospective Diabetes Study Group. Intensive blood-glucose control with sulphonylureas or insulin compared with conventional treatment and risk of complications in patients with type 2 diabetes (UKPDS 33). *Lancet* 1998; **352**: 837–853.
10. Mathiesen ER, Ronn B, Jensen T, Storm B and Deckert T. Relationship between blood pressure and urinary albumin excretion in development of microalbuminuria. *Diabetes* 1990; **39**: 245–249.
11. Microalbuminuria Collaborative Study Group. Microalbuminuria in type 1 diabetic patients. *Diabetes Care* 1992; **15**: 495–501.
12. American Diabetes Association. Clinical Practice Recommendations 2003. Diabetic Nephropathy. *Diabetes Care* 2003; **26**(suppl 1): S94–S98.
13. Burtis CA and Ashwood ER eds. *Tietz Textbook of Clinical Chemistry*. 2nd ed. Philadelphia, PA: Saunders, 1994: 989–990 and 1522–1538.
14. U.S. Renal Data System. *USRDS 2002 Annual Data Report: Atlas of End-Stage Renal Disease in the United States*. National Institutes of Health, National Institute of Diabetes and Digestive and Kidney Diseases, Bethesda, MD, 2002.
15. Parving HH, Lehnert H, Brochner-Mortensen J, Gomis R, Andersen S and Arner P. The effect of irbesartan on the development of diabetic nephropathy in patients with type 2 diabetes. *N Engl J Med* 2001; **345**: 870–878.
16. Lewis EJ, Hunsicker LG, Clarke WR, *et al*. Renoprotective effect of the angiotensin-receptor antagonist irbesartan in patients with type 2 diabetes. *N Engl J Med* 2001; **345**: 851–860.
17. Brenner BM, Cooper ME, de Zeeuw D, Keane WF, Mitch WE, Parving HH, Remuzzi G, Snapinn SM, Zhang Z and Shahinfar S. Effects of losartan on renal and cardiovascular outcomes in patients with type 2 diabetes and nephropathy. *N Engl J Med* 2001, **345**: 861–869.
18. ALLHAT Collaborative Research Group. Major outcomes in high-risk hypertensive patients randomized to angiotensin-converting enzyme inhibitor or calcium channel blocker vs diuretic. The Antihypertensive and Lipid-Lowering Treatment to Prevent Heart Attack Trial (ALLHAT). *JAMA* 2002; **288**: 2981–2997.

Detection and treatment of eye complications

1. Klein R, Klein B, Moss SE and Cruickshanks KJ. Relationship of hyperglycemia to the long-term incidence and progression of diabetic retinopathy. *Arch Intern Med* 1994; **154**: 2169–2178.
2. Klein R and Klein BE. Vision disorders in diabetes. In: Harris MI, Cowie CC, Stern MP, *et al*., eds. *Diabetes in America*. 2nd ed. National Diabetes Data Group, NIH, NIDDK, 1995; National Institute of Health Publication 95–1468.
3. Santiago JV, ed. *Medical Management of Insulin-Dependent (Type I) Diabetes*. 2nd ed. Alexandria, VA: American Diabetes Association, 1994.
4. Lyons TJ, Silvestri G, Dunn JA, Dyer DG and Baynes JW. Role of glycation in modification of lens crystallins in diabetic and nondiabetic senile cataracts. *Diabetes* 1991; **40**: 1010–1015.
5. Ansari N, Awasthi Y and Srirastava S. Role of glycosylation in protein disulfide formation and cataractogenesis. *Exp Eye Res* 1980; **31**: 9–19.
6. Frank RN. The aldose reductase controversy. *Diabetes* 1994; **43**: 169–172.
7. Diabetes Control and Complications Trial Research Group. The effect of intensive treatment of diabetes on the development and progression of long-term complications in insulin-dependent diabetes mellitus. *N Engl J Med* 1993; **329**: 977–986.
8. The Kroc Collaborative Study Group. Blood glucose control and the evolution of diabetic retinopathy and albuminuria. A preliminary multicenter trial. *N Engl J Med* 1984; **311**: 365–372.
9. The Kroc Collaborative Study Group. Diabetic retinopathy after two years of intensified insulin treatment. Follow-up of The Kroc Collaborative Study. *JAMA* 1988; **260**: 37–41.
10. UK Prospective Diabetes Study Group. Intensive blood-glucose control with sulphonylureas or insulin compared with conventional treatment and risk of complications in patients with type 2 diabetes (UKPDS 33). *Lancet* 1998; **352**: 837–853.
11. Klein R, Klein B, Moss SE, Davis MD and DeMets DL. The Wisconsin Epidemiologic Study of Diabetic Retinopathy. III. Prevalence and risk of diabetic retinopathy when age at diagnosis is 30 or more years. *Arch Ophthalmol* 1984; **102**: 527–532.
12. ETDRS Research Group. Photocoagulation for diabetic macular edema. *Arch Ophthalmol* 1985; **103**: 1796–1806.
13. Diabetic Retinopathy Vitrectomy Study Research Group. Early vitrectomy for severe proliferative diabetic retinopathy in eyes with useful vision: results of a randomized trial – Diabetic Retinopathy Vitrectomy Study Report 3. *Arch Ophthalmol* 1988; **95**: 1307–1320.
14. Diabetic Retinopathy Vitrectomy Study Research Group. Early vitrectomy for severe vitreous hemorrhage in diabetic retinopathy: four-year results of a randomized trial – Diabetic Retinopathy Study

Report 5. *Arch Ophthalmol* 1990; **108**: 959–964.
15. UK Prospective Diabetes Study Group. Tight blood pressure control and risk for of macrovascular and microvascular complications in type 2 diabetes: UKPDS 38. *BMJ* 1998; **317**: 708–713.
16. Estacio RO, Jeffers BW, Gifford N, Schreir RW. Effect of blood pressure control on diabetic microvascular complications in patients with hypertension and type 2 diabetes. *Diabetes Care* 2000; **23**: B54–B64.
17. American Diabetes Association. Clinical Practice Recommendations 2003. Diabetic retinopathy. *Diabetes Care* 2003; **26**(suppl 1): S99–S102.

Detection and treatment of diabetic neuropathy

1. Eastman RC. Neuropathy in diabetes. In: Harris, MI, Cowie CC, Stern MP, *et al.*, eds. *Diabetes in America.* 2nd ed. National Diabetes Data Group, NIH, NIDDK, 1995; National Institute of Health Publication 95–1468.
2. Diabetes Control and Complications Trial Research Group. The effect of intensive treatment of diabetes on the development and progression of long-term complications in insulin-dependent diabetes mellitus. *N Engl J Med* 1993; **329**: 977–986.
3. Jamal GA. Pathogenesis of diabetic neuropathy: the role of n-6 essential fatty acids and their eicosanoid derivatives. *Diabetes Med* 1990; **7**: 574–579.
4. Boulton AJ and Malik RA. Diabetic neuropathy. *Med Clin North Am* 1998; **82**: 909–929.
5. Raskin P. The relationship of aldose reductase activity to diabetic complications. In: Baba S and Kareko T, eds. Diabetes 1994. Amsterdam: Elsevier, 1994: 321–325 (Excerpta Medica International Congress Series 1100).
6. Max MB, Lynch SA, Muir J, Shoaf SE, Smoller B and Dubner R. Effects of desipramine, amitriptyline, and fluoxetine on pain in diabetic neuropathy. *N Engl J Med* 1992; **326**: 1250–1256.
7. Pfeifer MA. A highly successful and novel model for treatment of chronic painful diabetic peripheral neuropathy. *Diabetes Care* 1993; **16**: 1103–1115.
8. Santiago JV, ed. *Medical Management of Insulin-Dependent (Type I) Diabetes*. 2nd ed. Alexandria, VA: American Diabetes Association, 1994.
9. Vinik A, Maser R, Mitchell B, Freeman R. Diabetic autonomic neuropathy: Technical review. *Diabetes Care* 2003; **26**: 1553–1579.
10. Erbas T, Varoglu E, Erbas B, Tastekin G and Ahalin S. Comparison of metoclopramide and erythromycin in the treatment of diabetic gastroparesis. *Diabetes Care* 1993; **16**: 1511–1514.
11. Valdovinos MA, Camilleari M and Zimmerman BR. Chronic diarrhea in diabetes mellitus: mechanisms and an approach to diagnosis and treatment. *Mayo Clin Proc* 1993; **68**: 691–702.
12. Fedorak RN, Field M and Chang EB. Treatment of diabetic diarrhea with clonidine. *Ann Intern Med* 1985; **102**: 197–199.
13. Nakabayashi H, Fujii S, Miwa U, Seta T and Takeda R. Marked improvement of diabetic diarrhea with the somatostatin analogue octreotide. *Arch Intern Med* 1994; **154**: 1863–1867.
14. Haines ST. Treating constipation in the patient with diabetes. *Diabetes Educ* 1995; **21**: 223–232.

Detection and treatment of foot complications

1. Rith Najarian S, Branchaud C, Beaulieu O, Gohdes D, Simonson G and Mazze R. Reducing lower extremity amputations due to diabetes: application of the Staged Diabetes Management approach in a primary care setting. *J Fam Pract* 1998; **47**: 127–132.

Further reading

1. Alvarez OM, Gilson G and Auletta MJ. Local aspects of diabetic foot ulcer care: assessment, dressings, topical agents In: Levin ME, ed. *The Diabetic Foot.* 5th ed. 1993: 259–281.
2. American Diabetes Association. Foot care in patients with diabetes mellitus. *Diabetes Care* 1998; **21**: S54–S55.
3. Caputo GM, Cavanagh, PR, Ulbrecht JS, Gibbons GW and Karchmer AW. Assessment and management of foot disease in patients with diabetes. *N Engl J Med* 1994; **331**: 854–860.
4. Edmonds ME. Improved survival of the diabetic foot: the role of a specialized foot clinic. *Q J Med* 1986; **232**: 763–771.
5. Litzelman DK, Slemenda DW, Langefeld CD, Hays LM, Welch, MA, Bild DE, Ford ES and Vinicor F. Reduction of lower extremity clinical abnormalities in patients with non-insulin dependent diabetes mellitus: a randomized, controlled trial. *Ann Intern Med* 1993; **119**: 36–41.
6. Malone JM, Synder M, Anderson G, *et al.* Prevention of amputation by diabetic education. *Am J Surg* 1989; **158**: 520–524.
7. McNeely MJ. The independent contributions of diabetic neuropathy and vasculopathy in foot ulceration. *Diabetes Care* 1995; **18**: 216–219.
8. Mitchell BD, Hawthorne VM and Vinik AI. Cigarette

smoking and neuropathy in diabetic patients. *Diabetes Care* 1990; **13**: 434–437.
9. Orchard TJ and Strandness DE. Assessment of peripheral vascular disease in diabetes: report and recommendations of an international workshop. *Circulation* 1993; **88**: 819–828.
10. Osmundson PJ. Course of peripheral occlusive arterial disease: vascular laboratory assessment. *Diabetes Care*, 1990; **13**: 143–152.
111. Plummer SE and Albert SG. Foot care assessment in patients with diabetes: a screening algorithm for patient education and referral. *Diabetes Educator* 1995; **21**: 47–51.
12. Rith-Najarian S, Soluski T and Gohdes DM. Identifying patients at high-risk for lower extremity amputation in a primary care setting: a prospective evaluation of simple screening criteria. *Diabetes Care* 1992; **15**: 1386–1389.
13. Rith-Najarian S, Price M and Gohdes DM. Foot care in minorities: preventing amputations in high-risk populations. In: Levin ME, ed. *The Diabetic Foot*. 5th ed. 1993: 577–586.
14. Rith Najarian S and Gohdes DM. Foot disease in diabetes [Letter]. *N Engl J Med* 1995; **332**: 269–269.
15. Rosenblum BL. Maximizing foot salvage by a combined approach to foot ischemia and neuropathic ulceration in patients with diabetes. *Diabetes Care* 1994; **17**: 983–987.

Detection and treatment of dermatologic, connective tissue, and oral complications

1. Yosipovitch G, Hodak E and Vardi P. The prevalence of cutaneous manifestations in IDDM patients and their association with diabetes risk factors and microvascular complications. *Diabetes Care* 1998; **21**: 506–509.
2. Jelinek JE. The skin in diabetes. *Diabetes Med* 1993; **10**: 201–213.
3. Arkkila PE, Kantola IM and Viikari JS. Limited joint mobility in type 1 diabetic patients: correlation to other diabetic complications. *J Intern Med* 1994; **236**: 215–223.
4. Arkkila PE, Kantola IM and Viikari JS. Dupuytren's disease: association with chronic diabetic complications. *J Rheumatol* 1997; **24**: 153–159.
5. Loe H. Periodontal disease: the sixth complication of diabetes mellitus. *Diabetes Care* 1993; **16**: 329–34.
6. Grant-Theule DA. Periodontal disease, diabetes, and immune response: a review of current concepts. *J West Soc Periodontal Abstr* 1996; **44**: 69–77.
7. Loe H and Genco RJ. Oral complications in diabetes. In: *Diabetes in America*. 2nd ed. National Diabetes Data Group, NIH, NIDDK, 1995; National Institutes of Health Publication 95–1468.

10 Hospitalization

Individuals with diabetes are hospitalized for acute problems associated with diabetes management and for other inter-current events. Inpatient management differs significantly depending upon the type of diabetes, reason for the admission, time of the admission, current therapy, state of glycemic control, and existence of co-morbidities. In this section, protocols are presented for people with type 1 or type 2 diabetes hospitalized for diabetes related problems or for medical/surgical reasons.

Individuals with diabetes suffer disproportionately from several medical conditions that may require short or extended hospitalization. During the hospital stay, questions often arise as to how to manage diabetes, what changes in therapy may be necessary, and what level of control is optimal. Little is written about the procedures for the care of hospitalized individuals with diabetes, explaining in part the significant variation in practice within the same hospital. The material in this section is a compilation of current understanding of the approach to diabetes management within a hospital setting. A complete list of references used for this section is given at the end of the chapter. Because persons with diabetes are hospitalized frequently, the material has been divided according to three major classifications:

1. hospitalization for a diabetes related event, such as hypoglycemia, poor glycemic control, diabetic ketoacidosis (DKA), and hyperglycemic hyperosmolar syndrome (HHS)

2. hospitalization for a non-surgical event, such as an illness

3. hospitalization for surgery

The current impact of diabetes related hospitalizations

As many as 3 million individuals with diabetes are hospitalized annually with an average length of stay of 8 days.[1] While poor control of diabetes accounts for between 10 and 15 per cent of the hospitalizations, cardiovascular and peripheral vascular disease account for about another third. The key factors that predict hospitalization are duration of diabetes, presence of complications, and gender. The most likely candidate for hospitalization will be a woman with type 2 diabetes of long duration (> 10 years) treated with insulin and having vascular complications. For individuals with type 2 diabetes, insulin-treated versus non-insulin-treated hospitalization rates are 18 versus 10 per cent, respectively. With the presence of complications, these rates rise to 40 versus 30

Staged Diabetes Management: A Systematic Approach (2nd Edition) R. S. Mazze, E. S. Strock, G. D. Simonson and R. M. Bergenstal
 ISBN: 0 470 86576 8

per cent.[1] The most likely reason for an individual with type 1 diabetes to be admitted to a hospital is the presence of several complications.[1] These individuals have a hospitalization rate of 33 per cent versus eight per cent for those with no complications. The rate of admission for DKA is unknown, but it is suspected that 1–2 per cent of people with type 1 diabetes are admitted annually for DKA management. Least known is the rate of admission for "diabetes out of control." Overall, the hospitalization rates for people with diabetes are between two and three times those of age and gender matched non-diabetic individuals.

Hospitalization practice guidelines

There are no specific standards of care for hospitalization for diabetes, due to the wide variety of medical conditions. Nevertheless, there are several key principles:

1. Stabilization of blood glucose to near-normal level of glycemic control.

2. Anticipating and reacting to the changes in metabolic control due to the stress of illness.

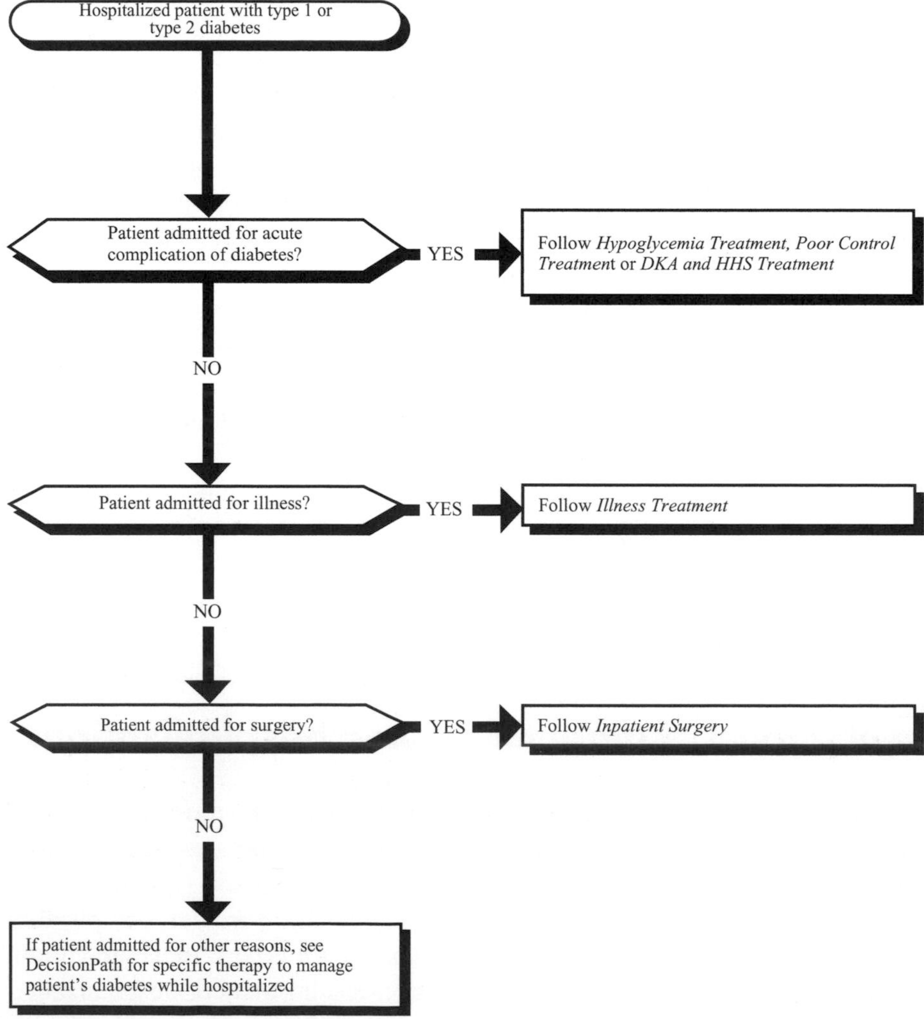

Figure 10.1 Hospitalization Master DecisionPath

3. Allowing the patient to return to self-care as soon as possible.

Staged Diabetes Management provides a Master DecisioinPath to identify the reason for hospitalization and to suggest the appropriate Specific DecisioinPath (see Figure 10.1). When more than one reason for hospitalization occurs, follow each DecisioinPath simultaneously.

Common clinical concerns

When an individual is to be hospitalized, there are two important concerns: the level of glycemic control and the current therapy. Glycemic control is an issue because it may interfere with the treatment for the current hospitalization. Current diabetes therapy makes a significant difference because most of ambulatory diabetes self-management is prospective, relying on intermediate- and long-acting drugs. This assumes a certain degree of predictability regarding when the patient is going to eat, level of activity, timing of medication, and so on. For individuals with diabetes who are hospitalized for medical emergencies and/or surgery, factors such as food intake and stress hormone level are not as predictable, which may necessitate modification to the diabetes regimen. Initiation of Physiologic Insulin Stage 4 (see Chapters 4, 5, or 6) or intravenous insulin may be required in order to establish and/or maintain glycemic control during hospitalization.

Hospitalization for problems related to glycemic control

Hospitalization for acute metabolic complications of diabetes results in a tremendous expenditure of health care resources. In many cases, development of acute metabolic complications can be prevented via utilization of the appropriate diabetes regimens and diabetes self-management education. Staged Diabetes Management DecisioinPaths for the inpatient management of diabetes related acute metabolic complications are described in the following section.

Hypoglycemia

Hospitalization for the management of hypoglycemia is becoming less frequent due to increased education and use of SMBG. However, hospitalization for severe hypoglycemia still does occur, especially when the patient is found unconscious. Hypoglycemia (non-pregnant), nominally defined as blood glucose < 70 mg/dL (3.9 mmol/L), with apparent symptoms (sweating, palpitations, blurred vision, significant hunger, confusion, or coma) is generally the result of a departure from the normal daily schedule. Often mild to moderate hypoglycemia can be self-treated, but severe hypoglycemia (< 40 mg/dL or 2.2 mmol/L) may require intravenous dextrose or glucagon. Specifically, hypoglycemia may be caused by too much insulin or oral agent (sulfonylurea, repaglinide or nateglinide), more exercise than usual, or insufficient carbohydrate intake. As many as five per cent of type 1 diabetes patients and 1–3 per cent of type 2 diabetes patients per year experience a severe hypoglycemic episode.

The first step in treating hypoglycemia is to determine the patient's status and blood glucose level. If a reflectance meter is available, measure the blood glucose to make certain that the problem is truly hypoglycemia (blood glucose < 70 mg/dL or 3.9 mmol/L). Many individuals with type 2 diabetes will experience relative hypoglycemia after consistently elevated blood glucose levels are significantly reduced with intensive diabetes management. In this case, while the symptoms may be pronounced, the patient is in no real danger.

Once hypoglycemia is verified, patients who are able to eat or drink should be given 30 grams of carbohydrate (glucose tablets, orange juice, etc.). Monitor the blood glucose every 15–30 minutes until levels are stabilized (blood glucose

> 100 mg/dL or 5.6 mmol/L). If the patient is unconscious or unable to eat or drink because of severe neuroglycopenia, two treatment options are available. The most common treatment – especially in the hospital and emergency room setting – is intravenous glucose. Administer a bolus of 10–20 ml of 50 per cent dextrose (glucose) followed by 10 per cent dextrose infused at 100 mL per hour until blood glucose levels are stabilized. Document the blood glucose levels every 30 minutes during initial intravenous treatment. The second treatment option is the subcutaneous or intramuscular administration of glucagon. Glucagon stimulates glycogenolysis and gluconeogenesis in the liver, dramatically increasing hepatic glucose output. The standard dose is 1.0 mg for adults and 0.5 mg for children. Alternatively, the dose for children may be calculated at 15 mg/kg. When the patient regains consciousness or is able to eat and drink, provide sufficient carbohydrate (fruit juice, glucose tabs, crackers, etc.) to sustain improved glycemic control. Continued blood glucose monitoring is necessary to make certain the levels remain stable (> 100 mg/dL or 5.6 mmol/L and < 200 mg/dL or 11.1 mmol/L). Figure 10.2 shows the DecisioinPath for inpatient treatment of hypoglycemia.

It is important to determine the cognitive state of the individual during and immediately following hypoglycemic episodes. If the patient cannot remember the early symptoms of hypoglycemia (possibly due to hypoglycemia unawareness induced by autonomic neuropathy) and the action taken to try to overcome the hypoglycemia, consider maintaining the patient in the hospital to re-evaluate the current diabetes therapy.

Investigation of hypoglycemic episodes

Once the patient is stabilized, the cause of the hypoglycemic episode needs to be investigated and methods for prevention put into place. In most cases the current therapy is directly related to the episode and needs to be evaluated. The therapy adjust DecisioinPaths for type 1 and type 2 diabetes in Chapters 4–6 provide guidelines for evaluating and optimizing therapies. Additionally, consider educating the patient regarding self-treatment. The patient should be instructed to ingest 15 grams of carbohydrate at the earliest signs of hypoglycemia. The blood glucose should begin to rise after 15 minutes, and this can be verified by testing the blood glucose. When the blood glucose reaches 100 mg/dL (5.6 mmol/L), it is safe to cease treatment and monitor blood glucose every 2 hours until the next meal. Self-monitoring of blood glucose, and not symptom alleviation, is the best method for determining the response to interventions that count hypoglycemia since blood glucose level is a velocity measure that constantly changes. To rapidly reach a steady state, the effect of long-acting oral agents and insulin must be counteracted with carbohydrate. Injectable glucagon may be used at home to counter more severe cases of hypoglycemia when the person does not respond to repeated treatment with carbohydrate.

Possible contributing factors to frequent hypoglycemia include high-dose oral hypoglycemic agents, overinsulinization (> 1.0–1.5 U/kg/day, especially with intermediate-acting insulin in the elderly), starvation, increased activity/exercise, alcohol intake, and inter-current illness. Additionally, some medications, such as β-blockers, may decrease hypoglycemia awareness. Self-monitoring blood glucose two to four times per day at different times (before meals, 2 hours after the start of meal, bedtime, and occasionally 3 AM) is recommended in order to identify patterns of hypoglycemia. Multiple-injection regimens that utilize both short-acting and long-acting insulin should replace single-injection regimens. Persistent hypoglycemia should be treated vigorously in consultation with an endocrinologist specializing in diabetes. See the Appendix, Figures A.6 and A.7, for more information. Table 10.1 summarizes changes in therapy when there is persistent hypoglycemia.

Poor glycemic control

The policies of hospitalizing for "diabetes out of control" vary by community and by medical insurance coverage. In general, each case must be

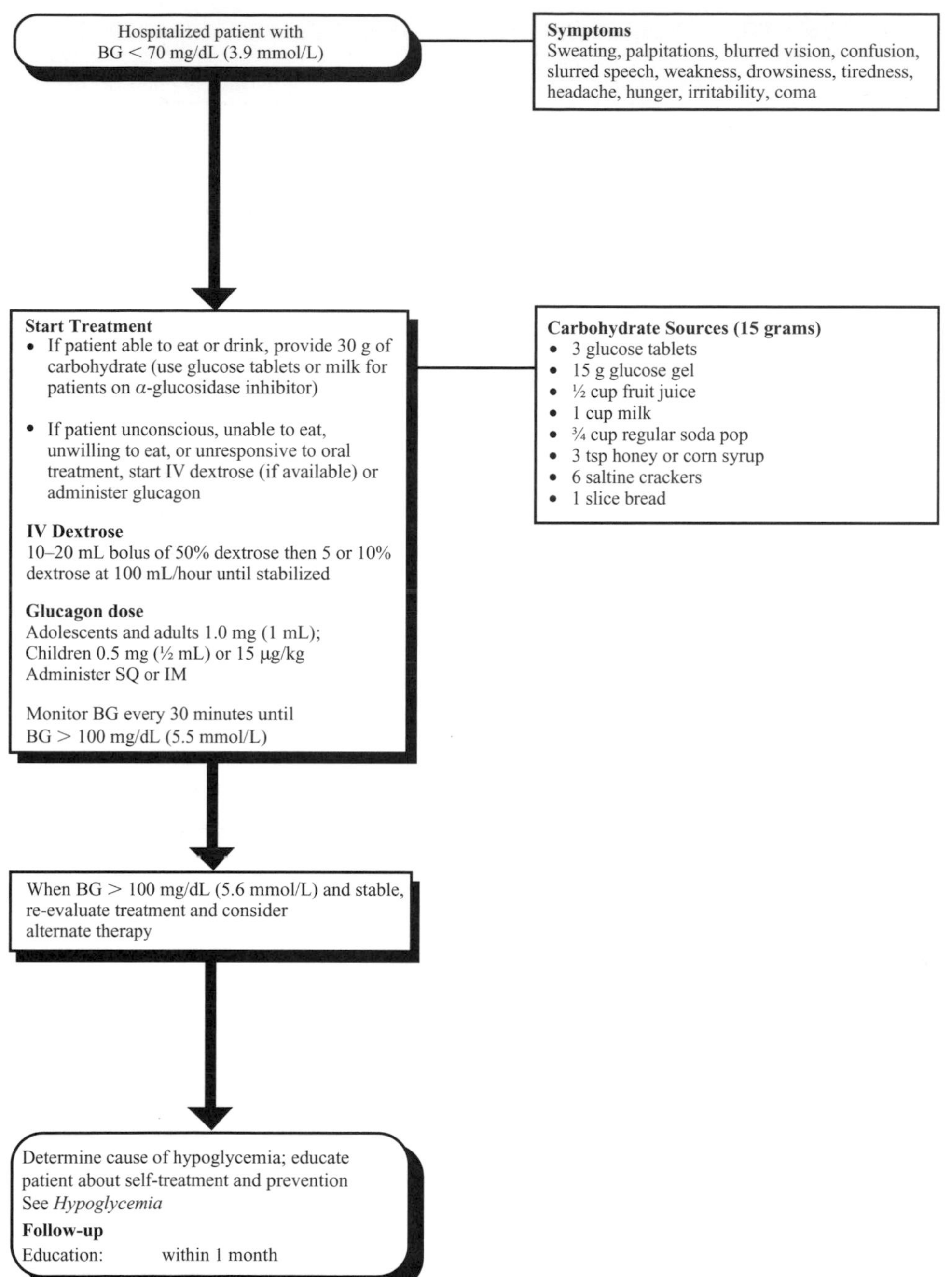

Figure 10.2 Hypoglycemia Treatment/Inpatient DecisionPath

judged individually. The critical elements are whether the patient is in imminent danger of severe hypoglycemia or hyperglycemia and to what degree self-care or ambulatory care is feasible. If there is any chance of a severe episode, or if the patient is unable to self-treat the acute situation, hospitalization should be considered. The purpose is to stabilize blood glucose levels. Since this should be a brief stay, management by subcutaneous injection rather than by intravenous insulin is appropriate (see Figure 10.3).

The first step is to determine whether the blood

Table 10.1 Changes in diabetes therapy when admitted for poor control

Current therapeutic stage	Therapy changes for hypoglycemia	Therapy changes for hyperglycemia
Type 2 diabetes: medical nutrition therapy stage	Rarely occurs; modify food plan	Start oral agent or insulin therapy
Type 2 diabetes: oral agent stage	Lower dose, switch to non-hypoglycemic agent (metformin, thiazolidinedione, alpha-glucosidase inhibitor) or switch to medical nutrition therapy	Start insulin therapy; synchronize food plan with insulin regimen
Type 2 diabetes: any insulin stage	Lower dose, increase number of injections to mimic physiologic release of insulin, or switch to non-hypoglycemic oral agent	Intensify insulin therapy; synchronize food plan with insulin regimen
Type 1 diabetes: any insulin stage	Adjust insulin regimen if not at target; adjust and synchronize nutrition therapy with insulin regimen	Intensify insulin therapy; adjust and synchronize nutrition therapy with insulin regimen; monitor for DKA

glucose level is rising or falling by SMBG monitoring every 15–30 minutes. If it is rising rapidly, there is a danger of ketoacidosis or coma and treatment should begin immediately. In such a case, initiating Physiologic Insulin Stage 4 (see Chapters 4, 5, or 6, depending on the type of diabetes) will bring the blood glucose under control. Hyperglycemic individuals with type 1 diabetes should be monitored for DKA. Individuals with type 2 diabetes should be evaluated for hyperglycemic hyperosmolar syndrome (HHS).

Once the patient is stabilized, it is incumbent upon the practitioner to determine the cause of the poor control. Likely causes include improper therapy, insufficient diabetes and nutrition education, adherence issues, drug interaction, and hypoglycemia unawareness. Table 10.1 details changes that can be made in diabetes therapies to help improve control.

Diabetic ketoacidosis

Diabetic ketoacidosis (DKA) is preceded by a relative or absolute insulin deficiency leading to increased gluconeogenesis in the liver and a reduction in glucose uptake by muscle and fat. Combined with increased counter-regulatory hormone release, this ultimately leads to hyperglycemia. Left untreated, elevated blood glucose causes dehydration and osmotic diuresis (see Figure 10.4). When levels exceed the renal threshold ($>$ 175 mg/dL or 9.7 mmol/L), electrolyte (potassium, sodium, phosphate, magnesium) loss occurs. Relative or absolute insulin deficiency also affects lipid metabolism by increasing lipolysis and serum free fatty acid levels. The liver responds by increasing oxidation of the free fatty acids, resulting in the overproduction of ketone bodies (3-hydroxybutyrate and acetoacetate). The accumulation of ketone bodies causes acidemia and a marked increase in respiration.

Diabetic ketoacidosis is diagnosed on the basis of clinical symptoms, physical examination, and laboratory data. The presence of ketones and blood glucose $>$ 250 mg/dL (13.9 mmol/L) alone does not necessarily meet the criteria for DKA. DKA is present when the pH is $<$ 7.3 and bicarbonate is $<$ 15 mEq/L. Additionally, DKA is usually accompanied by abdominal discomfort, fatigue, thirst, Kussmaul breathing (deep/heavy breathing), fruity breath, and vomiting. Diabetic ketoacidosis occurs primarily in individuals with type 1 diabetes.

Upon diagnosis of DKA, hospitalization should be considered. Dehydration should be countered immediately with 1 liter normal saline during the first hour, followed by 1 liter of normal saline

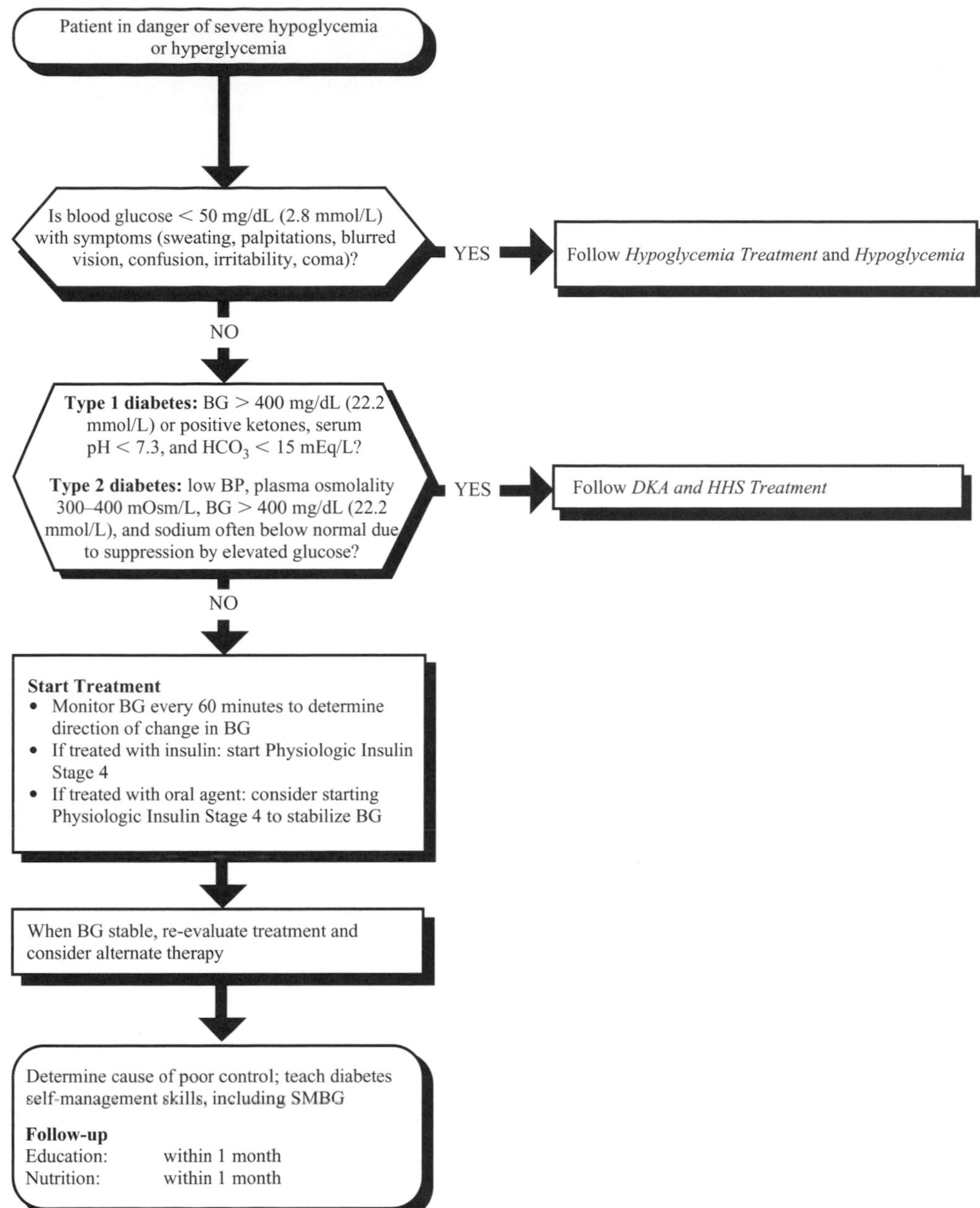

Figure 10.3 Poor Control Treatment/Inpatient DecisionPath

during the next 2 hours (see Figure 10.4). Fluid replacement should continue at approximately 250 mL per hour using 0.45 per cent (half normal) saline with maximum fluid replacement usually not exceeding 7.0 to 7.5 liters during the first 24 hour period. Next, intravenous insulin should be initiated. A bolus of 0.1 U regular insulin/kg body weight should be administered followed by 0.1 U/kg/hr intravenous insulin (10 U regular/100 mL of normal saline). Note that the 0.1 U/kg bolus of insulin is sometimes omitted in young children.

Although the normal saline will help reduce electrolyte imbalance, potassium replacement should be initiated based on initial potassium levels at presentation. Patients presenting with

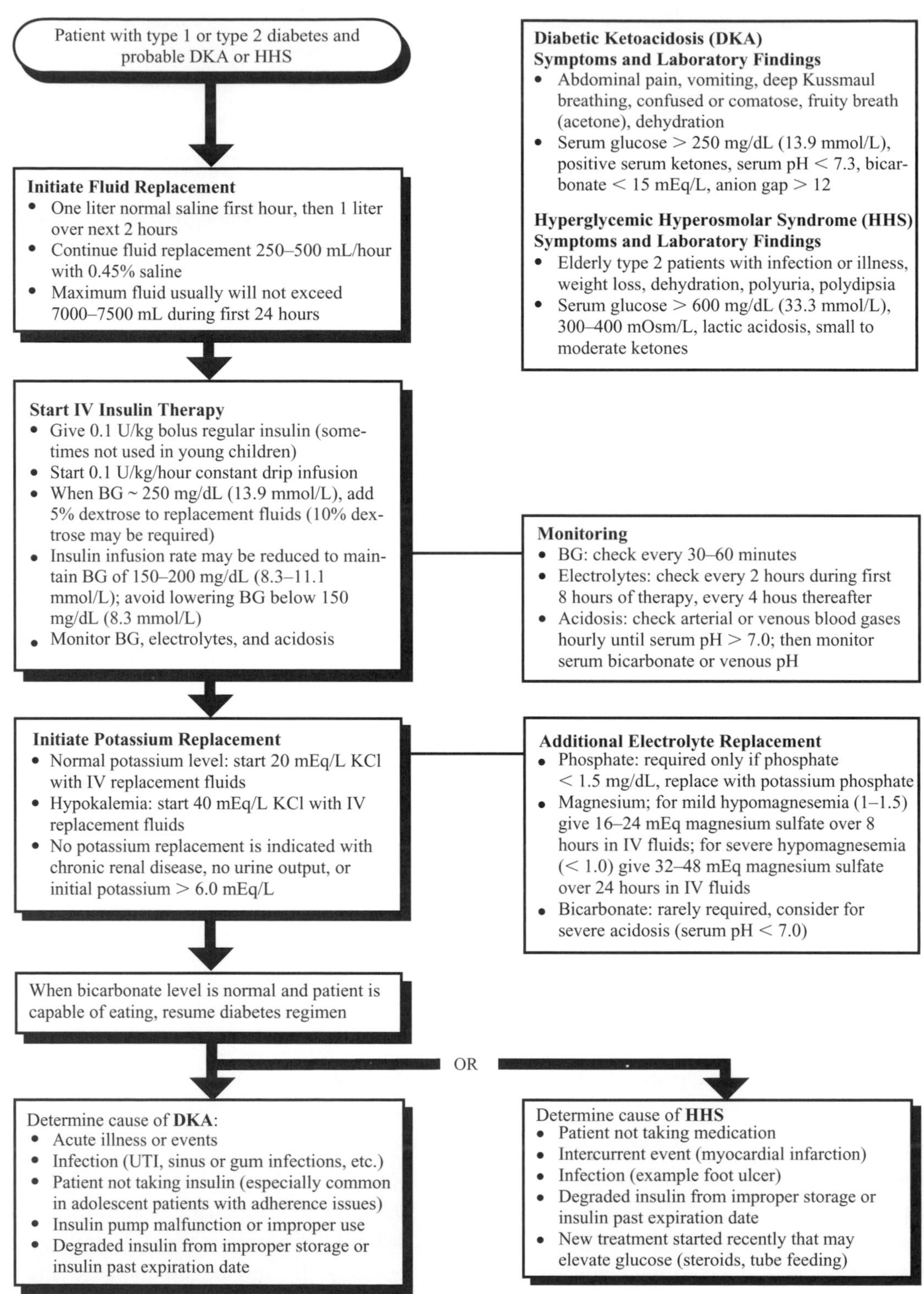

Figure 10.4 DKA and HHS Treatment/Inpatient DecisionPath

normal potassium levels should receive 20 mEq/L potassium chloride with the replacement fluids. Patients presenting with initial hypokalemia will require 40 mEq/L potassium chloride with replacement fluids. Exceptions for potassium replacement include patients with chronic renal disease and those not producing urine. Additional electrolyte replacements (phosphate, magnesium, and bicarbonate) should be considered (see Figure 10.4).

Patients require close surveillance while ketones are positive and when vomiting. Blood glucose levels should be determined at the bedside every 30–60 minutes, and electrolytes should be checked every 1–2 hours during the first 8 hours and every 4 hours thereafter. Check arterial or venous blood gases every 2–4 hours to monitor for acidosis until serum pH surpasses 7.0.

Patients with newly diagnosed diabetes should be started on insulin once the blood glucose has been stabilized in the hospital. See Insulin Stage 2/Start and Insulin Stage 3/Start in Chapter 6. Patient education should focus on survival skills before discharge and continue on an outpatient basis. Because DKA and hospitalization are traumatic experiences, learning survival skills in the hospital setting is less than optimal. Make certain that the survival skills are reiterated during the first office visit.

The most probable causes of DKA are not taking insulin, underlying infection, insulin pump malfunction, and acute illness (myocardial infarction, stroke). Skipping insulin doses is more frequent among adolescents and young adults who are struggling with adherence issues (see Appendix Figures A.19–A.23). See Table 10.1 for therapy adjustment recommendations, when required.

Hyperglycemic hyperosmolar syndrome

Diabetic hyperglycemic hyperosmolar syndrome (HHS) occurs in individuals with type 2 diabetes and results from a combination of hyperglycemia, dehydration, acidosis, and renal insufficiency. The elderly suffer disproportionately from it and have a high risk of morbidity. With HHS moderate to large ketones are absent in the presence of hyperglycemia and dehydration complicated by hyperosmolality, although this absence alone does not necessarily meet the criteria for HHS. Clinical signs and criteria include dehydration, sodium 120–140 mEq/L, low blood pressure ($< 100/60$ mmHg), high blood glucose (> 400 mg/dL or 22.2 mmol/L), and high serum osmolality (300–400 mOsm/L). In addition, the classic symptoms of weight loss, polyuria, and polydipsia are present. Renal insufficiency and lactic acidosis may also be present. Hospitalization is indicated for the administration of intravenous fluids and insulin to treat the severe dehydration and hyperglycemia.

Dehydration should be treated immediately with normal saline, which will also assist in combating electrolyte imbalance (see Figure 10.4). At the same time, intravenous insulin (10 U regular/100 mL of normal saline at a rate of 0.1 U/kg/hr) should be initiated. Although the normal saline will help reduce electrolyte imbalance, replacement should be considered for potassium, sodium, and bicarbonate. Blood glucose levels should be determined at the bedside every 1–2 hours.

Lactic acidosis is sometimes a consequence of HHS. When severe stress, injury, or coma occur, be cognizant of the risk of lactic acidosis, especially if there is liver or kidney disease. This is especially the case if the patient has been treated with metformin.

Bicarbonate therapy may be required to raise serum pH over 7. Look for acute renal failure; hemodialysis may be needed.

Once the patient is stabilized, identify possible causes of HHS, such as not taking oral agent or insulin, inappropriate therapy, underlying infection, and acute illness (e.g. myocardial infarction). Often an adjustment in therapy is needed to prevent future occurrences. Table 10.1 details the recommended changes in therapy, when required.

Hospitalization for illness

Individuals who enter the hospital for non-diabetes/non-surgical reasons are at significant risk of hyperglycemia or hypoglycemia depending on their prandial state, stress level, and current insulin therapy (see Figure 10.5). Patients who can eat and are capable of self-management should maintain their current diabetes regimen and SMBG four times per day. Patients too ill to

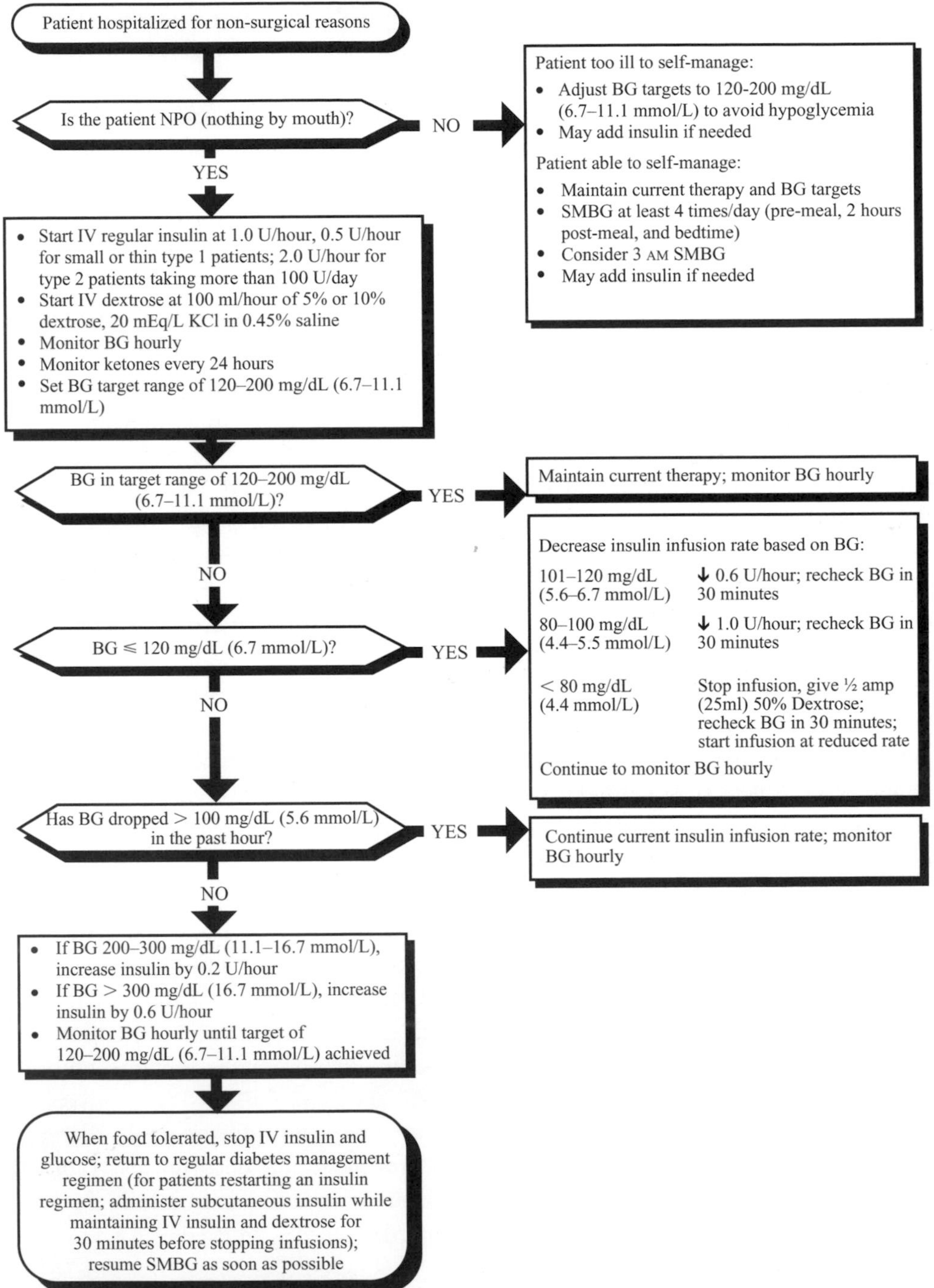

Figure 10.5 Illness Treatment/Inpatient DecisionPath

self-manage should maintain current regimen with the assistance of the nursing staff. Blood glucose targets should be temporarily increased to 120–200 mg/dL (6.7–11.1 mmol/L) in order to prevent hypoglycemia. Subcutaneous insulin should be initiated if blood glucose levels consistently rise above 200 mg/dL (11.1 mmol/L). If the patient is using intermediate- or long-acting insulin, be cognizant of action curves that may overlap with shorter-acting insulin (regular, lispro and aspart) used in the inpatient setting. It may take as long as 24 hours for the effect of long-acting insulin to completely dissipate. If the patient is NPO, intravenous insulin is strongly recommended. The major objective is to maintain blood glucose between 120 and 200 mg/dL (6.7 and 11.1 mmol/L). To accomplish this, the first step is to determine the current level of glycemic control followed by blood glucose determinations on an hourly basis. Frequent blood glucose monitoring is the only method to accurately assess glycemic control. Once the effect of intermediate- and long-acting insulin is dissipated, using short-acting insulin (either subcutaneous or intravenous) during hospitalization is advised to allow for flexibility, the unpredictability of the hospitalization, the change in diet and activity level, and the effects of stress (see Table 10.2). Because of its rapid action, lispro insulin should be considered if subcutaneous insulin administration is initiated.

Among the most common inter-current events resulting in hospitalization for illness are infections, myocardial infarction (MI), or stroke. In these instances, managing glycemic control as well as the inter-current event is important. With respect to MI, the presence of high blood glucose levels (> 300 mg/dL or 16.7 mmol/L) may contribute to increased myocardial damage. Myocardial infarction is associated with the release of counter-regulatory hormones, which destabilize blood glucose levels. With respect to infection, blood glucose control is vital to assist in the healing process.

If blood glucose is less than 240 mg/dL (13.3 mmol/L) and ketones are negative, the patient may be managed at home by telephone with frequent SMBG (1–2 hours). If the blood glucose is between 240 and 400 mg/dL (13.3 and 22.2 mmol/L) and up to moderate ketones are present, the response depends upon the patient's ability to self-treat and the absence of dehydration. If these criteria are not met, immediate hospitalization may be necessary. Since DKA can occur rapidly, this is very important in children with type 1 diabetes. In type 2 diabetes, hyperglycemic hyperosmolar syndrome can occur.

The first consideration for an individual hospitalized for an illness is to determine the ability of the patient to eat regular meals and to maintain normal diabetes self-management (SMBG, administer insulin, etc.). See the Illness Treatment/Inpatient DecisioinPath (see Figure 10.5). If the patient is able to eat, but is too ill for diabetes self-management, steps must be taken to ensure assistance with diabetes management is given. Blood glucose targets may be relaxed to 120–200 mg/dL (6.7–11.1 mmol/L) to avoid the potential for hypoglycemia. The patient who cannot

Table 10.2 Changes in diabetes therapy for illness

Current therapeutic stage	Therapy changes for illness
Type 2 diabetes: medical nutrition therapy stage	If entry fasting blood glucose > 120 mg/dL (6.7 mmol/L) or casual blood glucose > 160 mg/dL; (8.9 mmol/L)consider temporary insulin therapy
Type 2 diabetes: oral agent stage	Consider starting insulin therapy
Type 2 diabetes: any insulin stage	Intensify insulin therapy if not at target; modify food plan to synchronize with changes in insulin regimen
Type 1 diabetes: any insulin stage	Intensify insulin therapy if not at target; modify food plan to adjust for changes in insulin regimen

eat should be started on intravenous insulin (10 U regular/100 mL saline) and 100 mL per hour intravenous dextrose (5 or 10 per cent dextrose, 20 mEq/L KCl in 0.45 per cent saline). Typical insulin infusion rates are 0.5 U/hr for small or thin individuals with type 1 diabetes, 1.0 U/hr for adults with type 1 or type 2 diabetes, and 1.5 to 2.0 U/hr for individuals with type 2 diabetes taking > 100 U insulin per day. Blood glucose should be monitored every hour and maintained between 120 and 200 mg/dL (6.7 and 11.1 mmol/L). The insulin infusion rate should be titrated up or down to respond to changing blood glucose levels. Once the patient is capable of eating, the intravenous insulin and dextrose may be discontinued and the patient may resume the normal regimen.

The stress of illness may necessitate increased insulin doses; or a patient normally treated with medical nutrition therapy or oral agents may have to temporarily start insulin until the illness is completely resolved.

Hospitalization for surgery

Hospitalization for surgery raises several important glycemic control issues. Prandial state, stress, trauma, and anesthetic therapy may affect glycemic control in an unpredictable manner. Ascertaining the level of glycemic control at entry is important, as is monitoring before, during, and after surgery because the risk of complications increases as blood glucose levels rise. Drugs used in preparation for surgery, anesthetic agents used during surgery, and postoperative drugs may contribute to hyperglycemia. If severe hyperglycemia occurs, the patient may experience fluid loss, electrolyte imbalance, compromised wound healing, and susceptibility to infection.

Stress induced by surgery results in the release of counter-regulatory hormones (catecholamines, glucagon, cortisol, and growth hormone). When there is insufficient endogenous or exogenous insulin, these hormones may contribute to significant hyperglycemia, glycosuria, lipolysis, and ketogenesis. Left untreated, the result may be diabetic ketoacidosis or hyperglycemic hyperosmolar syndrome (HHS).

Changes in the diabetes therapy are usually required for surgery. In general, individuals requiring insulin prior to surgery should receive intravenous insulin and glucose during surgery in order to control blood glucose throughout surgery independent of the type of diabetes or current therapy. Exceptions may be for minor surgical procedures (i.e. cataract removal, tooth extraction, dermatological procedures, and so on) where increased subcutaneous insulin and diligent monitoring of blood glucose may be sufficient to maintain appropriate blood glucose (120–200 mg/dL or 6.7–11.1 mmol/L). Individuals in the medical nutrition therapy Stage often require no extraordinary treatment before, during, or after surgery. Individuals with type 2 diabetes treated with oral agents often have insufficient endogenous insulin production, therefore intravenous insulin will be required for major surgical procedures to overcome the effects of stress-induced counter-regulatory hormone release. The degree of surgical trauma, staff availability for closely monitoring and altering insulin, and the degree of metabolic decompensation expected are all factors that should be considered when altering therapy for either planned or emergency surgery (see Table 10.3).

Planned surgery

Preoperative modification of diabetes therapies is critical to ensure appropriate metabolic control and good patient outcomes (see Table 10.3). Patients treated with insulin should not take the morning injection of intermediate- or long-acting insulin. Patients taking second-generation sulfonylureas (glyburide, glipizide, and glimepiride) should cease taking medications on the morning of surgery. Patients taking chlorpropamide, a long-acting, first-generation sulfonylurea, should

Table 10.3 Changes in diabetes therapy for surgery

Current therapeutic stage	Therapy changes for planned surgery	Therapy changes for emergency surgery
Type 2 diabetes: medical nutrition therapy stage	Modify food plan according to preparation for surgery (i.e. only clear liquids)	Closely monitor blood glucose; use insulin as required
Type 2 diabetes: oral agent stage	Adjust to optimize control, may have to withhold dose prior to surgery	Closely monitor blood glucose; use insulin as required
Type 2 diabetes: any insulin stage	Intensify insulin therapy if not at target, modify food plan according to preparation for surgery (e.g. only clear liquids)	Closely monitor blood glucose; adjust insulin therapy if not at target; consider intravenous insulin and intravenous glucose
Type 1 diabetes: any insulin stage	Intensify insulin therapy if not at target; modify food plan according to preparation for surgery (e.g. only clear liquids)	Closely monitor blood glucose; adjust insulin therapy if not at target; consider intravenous insulin and intravenous glucose; modify food plan as required

cease taking the drug at least 36–48 hours before surgery. Patients treated with metformin should stop taking the medication at the time of, or prior to, the surgical procedure. Blood glucose should be monitored hourly. Start subcutaneous insulin injections (4–6 U of regular insulin) for blood glucose > 250 mg/dL (13.9 mmol/L). If blood glucose rises above 350 mg/dL (19.4 mmol/L), consider starting intravenous insulin and dextrose (see Figure 10.6).

In order to maintain adequate glycemic control before, during, and after major surgery, all patients treated with insulin, and many treated with oral agents, should be placed on intravenous insulin and dextrose. Intravenous dextrose (10 per cent dextrose, 20 mEq/l KCl, 0.45 per cent saline) is started at a rate of 100 mL per hour. Intravenous insulin (10 U R/100 mL saline) is started at a rate based on the patient's current total insulin dose. If the patient is taking less than 20 U/day, 20–50 U/day, or greater than 50 U/day, the initial infusion rate should be 0.5 U/hr, 1.0 U/hr, and 1.5 U/hr, respectively. The blood glucose should be monitored every 30–60 minutes in order to maintain blood glucose in the range of 120–200 mg/dL (6.7–11.1 mmol/L). The insulin infusion rate should be lowered 0.2 to 0.3 U/hr if the blood glucose dips below 120 mg/dL (6.7 mmol/L) and increased by 0.3 to 0.6 U/hr if the blood glucose exceeds 200 mg/dL (11.1 mmol/L). During recovery blood glucose monitoring should continue every 1–2 hours. Intravenous insulin and dextrose can be discontinued once the patient is able to eat and is capable of starting a normal oral agent or insulin regimen.

While patients with type 2 diabetes treated with medical nutrition therapy often require no extraordinary treatment during hospitalizations for surgery, they still require diligent blood glucose monitoring and may need exogenous insulin to overcome the effects of stress induced counterregulatory hormone release. Individuals currently treated with sulfonylureas or metformin undergoing short surgical procedures may or may not require exogenous insulin. For patients undergoing longer procedures, the likelihood of requiring exogenous insulin is substantially higher.

Emergency surgery

If possible, determine the current therapy. If treated with insulin, use caution when compensating for the current level of control since intermediate- and long-acting insulins may still be a factor. If no information regarding current therapy is available, assume that a buffered insulin or long-acting oral agent has been used and immediately determine

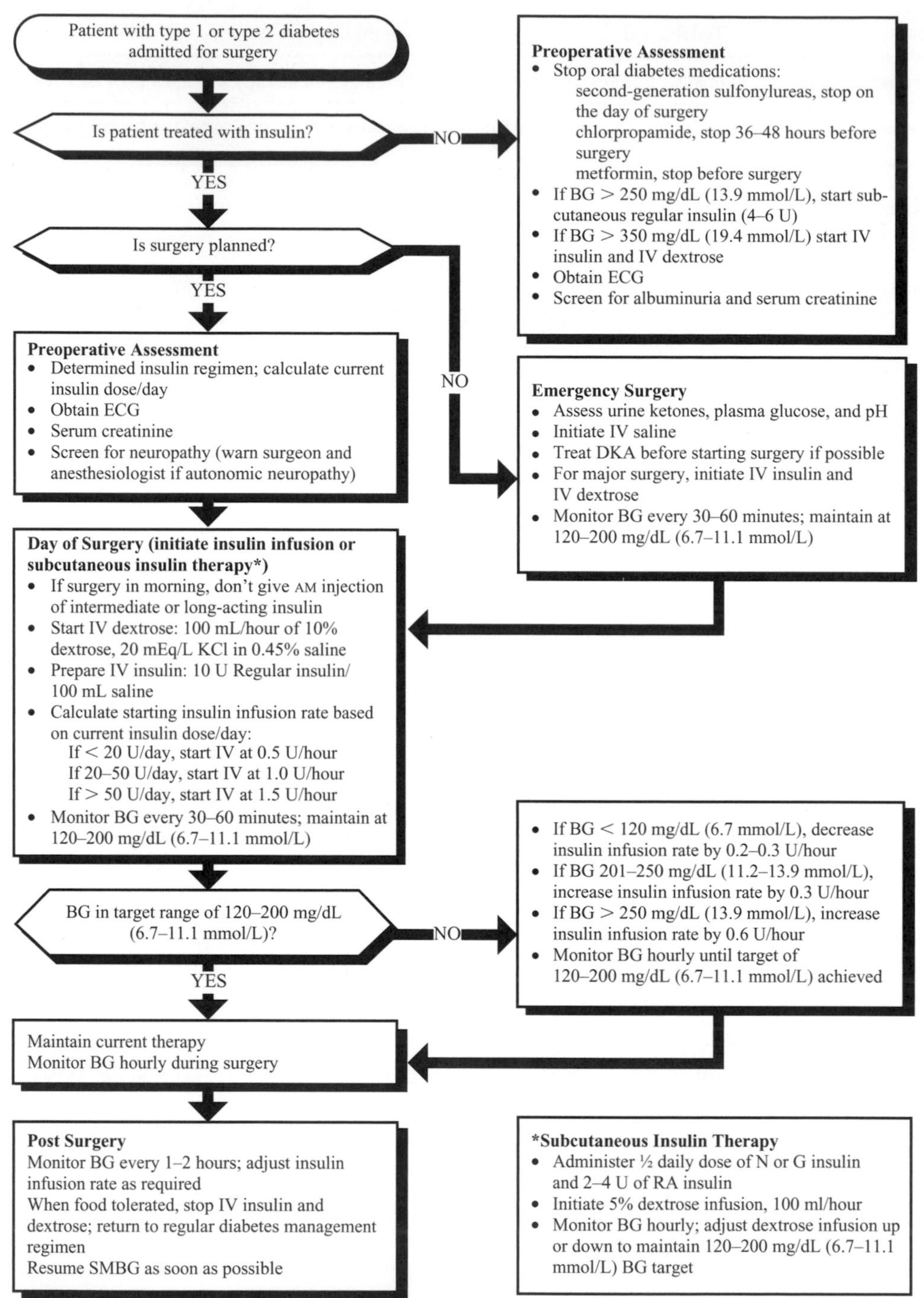

Figure 10.6 Inpatient Surgery DecisionPath

the current metabolic status of the patient, including blood glucose, urine ketones, and serum pH. For major emergency surgery, intravenous insulin (1.0 U regular insulin/hr) and intravenous dextrose (10 per cent dextrose, 20 mEq/L KCl, 0.45 per cent saline) should be initiated and blood glucose monitored every 30 to 60 minutes. The intravenous insulin rate should be titrated up or down in order to maintain blood glucose in the range of 120–200 mg/dL (6.7–11.1 mmol/L).

Post surgery

Continue to monitor blood glucose every 1–2 hours. Additional subcutaneous insulin injections or adjustments in the insulin infusion rate may be required to maintain blood glucose in the target range of 120–200 mg/dL (6.7–11.1 mmol/L). Stop the insulin and dextrose infusions once the patient is able to tolerate food and resume the usual diabetes regimen. Monitor blood glucose regularly. Make certain that the patient's usual diabetes regimen maintains blood glucose in the target range before discharging the patient.

Reference

1. Aubert RE, Geiss LS, Ballard DJ, Cocanougher B, and Herman WH. Diabetes-related hospitalization and hospital utilization. In: *Diabetes in America*. 2nd ed. NIH Publication No. 95-1468, 1995.

Further Reading

1. Alberti G. Diabetes emergencies. In Galloway J, Potvin J, Shulman C, eds. *Diabetes Mellitus*. 9th ed. Indianapolis, In: Lilly, 1988.
2. Alberti G, and Mazze R, eds. Frontiers in Diabetes Research: Current Trends in Non-Insulin Dependent Diabetes Mellitus. Amsterdam: Excerta Medica, 1989.
3. Babineau TJ, and Bothe A. General surgery considerations in the diabetic patient. *Infect Dis Clin North Am* 1995; **9**: 183–193.
4. Bergenstal R, Etzwiler D, Hollander P, Spencer M, Strock E, and Mazze R. In: Alberti G, Mazze R, eds. Frontiers in Diabetes Research: Current Trends in Non-Insulin-Dependent Diabetes Mellitus. Amsterdam: Excerpta Medica, 1989.
5. Cryer PE, Fisher JN, and Shamoon H. Hypoglycemia: technical review. *Diabetes Care* 1994; **17**: 734–755.
6. Fish LH, Weaver TW, Moore AL, and Steel LG. Value of postoperative blood glucose in predicting complications and length of stay after coronary artery bypass grafting. *Am J Cardiol*. 2003; **92**: 74–76.
7. Groop LC. Sulfonylureas in NIDDM. *Diabetes Care* 1995; **15**: 737–754.
8. Hirsch IB, and McGill JB. The role of insulin in the treatment of diabetes mellitus during surgery. *Diabetes Care* 1990; **13**: 980–991.
9. Hirsch IB, Paauw DS, and Brunzell J. Inpatient management of adults with diabetes. *Diabetes Care* 1995; **18**: 870–878.
10. *Medical Management of Type 2 Diabetes*. 4th ed. Alexandria, VA: American Diabetes Association, 1998.
11. Shulman C. Diabetes mellitus and surgery. In: Galloway J, Potvin J, Shulman C, eds. *Diabetes Mellitus*. 9th ed. Indianapolis, In: Lilly, 1988.

Appendix

Staged Diabetes Management: A Systematic Approach (2nd Edition) R. S. Mazze, E. S. Strock, G. D. Simonson and R. M. Bergenstal

ISBN: 0 470 86576 8

STAGED DIABETES MANAGEMENT
SITE ASSESSMENT SURVEY

Name and Title of Person Completing the Assessment:

Name: ________________________ **Title:** ________________ **Date:** _________

SECTION ONE: ORGANIZATIONAL INFORMATION

Name of Site/Clinic ____

Geographic Service Area of Site/Clinic ____________________________

Address: ____

____

Contact Person: __________________________ Title ________________

Address: _________________________ State: _________ Zip: _______

Phone: __________________ Fax: ________________ E-mail: _________

Name of Parent Organization if any _________________________________

Service Area of Parent Organization ________________________________

Address: ____

____

Contact Person: ____________________________ Title _________________

Address: __________________________ State: _________ Zip: ______

Phone: __________________ Fax: ________________ E-mail: ___________

Figure A.1 Diabetes needs assessment survey

Describe the setting of your facility:

a. ❒ Hospital
b. ❒ IHS Facility
c. ❒ Managed Care Organization
d. ❒ Out Patient Clinic (Ambulatory Care)
e. ❒ Teaching Hospital
f. ❒ Other

PLEASE ATTACH A COPY OF YOUR FACILITY'S ***ORGANIZATIONAL CHART*** indicating *where the Diabetes Program fits within the organization.*

SECTION TWO: DIABETES DEMOGRAPHICS

1. Estimated number of individuals by diabetes diagnosis:

AGE	Type 1 Male	Type 1 Female	Type 2 Male	Type 2 Female	Gestational (GDM)
< 18 years					
19–44 years					
45–65 years					
> 66 years					

2. Estimated number of individuals by ethnicity and type of diabetes

	Percent	Type 1	Type 2	Gestational (GDM)
African American				
Alaska Native				
American Indian				
Asian				
Caucasian				
Hispanic				
Pacific Islander				
Other				

2

Figure A.1 Continued

a) What is the number of registered patients (user population) at your site? ______

3. How many staff provide diabetes services?

Facility/Clinic	MD*	PA*	NP*	RN*	RD*	CHR/ CMA*	PHN*	Pharmacist	Other

***Medical Doctor *Physican Asst. *Nurse Practitioner *Registered Nurse**
***Registered Dietitian *Community Health Representative or Certified Medical Assistant**
***Public Health Nurse**

SECTION THREE: DIABETES CARE

1. What are the current screening and diagnostic criteria in your clinic?

Type 1 ______________________________

Type 2 ______________________________

Gestational ______________________________

2. Are practice guidelines for diabetes or other diseases in place in your organization?

❒ Yes ❒ No

If yes, please attach a copy of your guidelines.

3

Figure A.1 Continued

3. Which measures of patient glucose control do you use?

Measure	Yes	No	Frequency
Capillary blood glucose in office			
Fasting blood glucose in office			
Glycosylated Hemoglobin A1C (HbA_{1c})			
Post-prandial blood glucose			
Self-monitored blood glucose			

Comments:

4. Are individuals with diabetes routinely screened for the following?

Screening	Yes	No	Frequency	Comments
Depression				
Drugs and or alcohol				
Dyslipidemia				
Foot Complications				
Hypertension				
Microalbuminuria				
Neuropathy				
Periodontal Disease				
Retinopathy				
Urine protein by UA				

4

Figure A.1 Continued

5. Which of the following services/programs are available for your patients and community?

Service	Yes	No	Frequency or Comments
Activity/Exercise education			
Community Education			
Diabetes Specialty Clinic			
Follow-up/reminder calls			
In Patient Education			
Nutrition Education			
On Site Pharmacy			
Outpatient Education			
Prevention Program			
Screening for Diabetes			
Self Management Skills			

6. Which of the following referral sources are available to your program?

Specialty	Yes	No	Where - Location
Adult Endocrinology			
Cardiology			
Diabetes Nurse Educator			
Dietitian or Nutritionist			
Drug/Alcohol Counseling			
Exercise Specialist			
Mental Health			
Nephrology			
Obstetrics			
Optometry			
Ophthalmology			
Pediatric Endocrinology			
Pedorthist			
Perinatology			
Podiatry			
Smoking Cessation			
Urology			

5

Figure A.1 Continued

7. What diabetes supplies are available and/or covered in your system?

Supplies Footcare products	On Formulary yes	On Formulary no	Off Formulary yes	Off Formulary no	Who Pays ______ Self	3rd Party	Medicare	Medicaid	Capitation
Insulin									
Insulin Pens									
Ketone strips									
Lancets									
Lancet devices									
Meters									
Meter strips									
Oral Agents									
Record books									
Syringes									
Visual strips									
Other									

8. Which pharmaceutical agents are used at your site(s). Rank in order of use – 1 = (most frequent use) to 10 = (Less frequently used)

INSULINS	*On Formulary*	*Off Formulary*	*SITE NAME*	*SITE NAME*
Glargine				
NPH				
Ultra Lente				
Regular				
Lispro/Aspart				
70/30				
50/50				
Mix 75/25, Mix 70/30				
Other				
ORAL AGENTS				
Metformin				
Sulfonylureas				
Thiazolidinediones				
α-Glucosidase inhibitors				
Repaglinide/Nateglinide				
Other				

6

Figure A.1 Continued

9. At which point are patients referred for diabetes education?

Check all that apply	Who provides diabetes education?					
	CDE	CHR	NP/PA	Pharm	RD	RN
Newly Diagnosed type 1						
Newly Diagnosed type 2						
Type 1 Continuing Education						
Type 2 Continuing Education						
Impaired Glucose Tolerance						
Inpatient						
Gestational Diabetes						
At Onset of Complications						
Pre-conception Counseling						
Other						

SECTION FOUR: DIABETES EDUCATION SERVICES

1. Do you have a diabetes education curriculum in place in your facility? ❐ Yes ❐ No.
   If yes, please describe or attach summary.

2. What diabetes patient education materials do you use?: ❐ ADA ❐ Drug Co ❐ IDC
   ❐ IHS ❐ In House ❐ Ministry of Health ❐ Other

7

Figure A.1 Continued

SECTION FIVE: SYSTEM ASSESSMENT

1. Is there a diabetes committee or team? ❒ Yes ❒ No
   - Chairperson: ______________________________
   - Members: (by discipline and role)

     ____
     ____
     ____
     ____
     ____
     ____

   - Will this committee/team be responsible for the implementation of SDM?

     ❒ Yes ❒ No

2. How will you evaluate success of the SDM program?

   ____
   ____

   a) What process/outcome inidcators will you use? ______________

   b) How often will you measure outcomes? ______________

3. Are you currently auditing diabetes care? ❒ Yes ❒ No

8

Figure A.1 Continued

4. Do you have the following processes to enhance your diabetes care in place?

	Yes	No	Comments
Diabetes Flowsheet on chart			
Case Reviews/Grand Rounds			
Diabetes Support Group(s)			
Community Awareness Program			
Patient Satisfaction Survey			
Rapid HbA_{1c} available at time of patient visit			
Foot Care Clinic			

5. How will you involve/inform others of the SDM program, its content and implementation process
   a. Medical staff and employees:

      ____

   b. Health care professionals outside the facility:

      ____

   c. Patients and their families: ____

   d. Community and/or community agencies: ______________________________

6. What strengths does your community bring to the diabetes program?

   ____

   ____

7. What barriers to improved diabetes care do you have, or expect to experience?

   ____

9

Figure A.1 Continued

8. What questions do you have to assist you with the Site Preparation or training for SDM?

____

____

____

Thank you for your assistance.

10

Figure A.1 Continued

SDM Patient Chart Audit Form

1. Site Name ______________________________

2. Abstraction Date: *(mm/dd/yy)* ______________________________

3. Abstractor Name: ______________________________

4. Abstractor Title: ______________________________

5. Patient Gender: ☐ **1 = Female** ☐ **2 = Male**

6. Patient Date of Birth: *(mm/dd/yy)* ______________________________

7. Pre-Diabetes:
Type of glucose abnormality diagnosed

- ☐ **1 = Impaired Glucose Tolerance**
- ☐ **2 = Impaired Fasting Glucose**
- ☐ **3 = Other**

8. Diabetes Type:

☐ **0 = Not documented**	☐ **3 = Gestational Diabetes**
☐ **1 = Type 1 Diabetes**	☐ **4 = Prior Gestational Diabetes**
☐ **2 = Type 2 Diabetes**	☐ **5 = Other**

9. Year Diabetes Diagnosed: ______________________________

10. Race:

☐ **1 = Asian**	☐ **5 = White**
☐ **2 = American Indian/Alaska Native**	☐ **6 = Other**
☐ **3 = Black/African-American**	☐ **7 = Unknown**
☐ **4 = Native Hawaiian/ Other Pacific Islander**	

11. Ethnicity:
Does patient self-identify as Spanish, Hispanic, or Latino?

- ☐ **1 = No**
- ☐ **2 = Yes**

12. Visit Date: *(mm/dd/yy)* ______________________________

13. Blood Pressure Date: *(mm/dd/yy)* ______________________________

14. Most Recent Blood Pressure Systolic: ______________________________

15. Most Recent Blood Pressure Diastolic: ______________________________

16. Most Recent HbA_{1c} Date: *(mm/dd/yy)* ______________________________

17. Most Recent HbA_{1c} Value: ______________________________

18. HbA_{1c} Lab Normal Range: ______________

19. Total Serum Cholesterol Date: *(mm/dd/yy)* ______________________________

20. Total Serum Cholesterol Value: ______________________________

21. LDL Date: *(mm/dd/yy)* ______________________________

22. LDL Value: ______________________________

International Diabetes Center
Park Nicollet

Figure A.2 SDM patient chart audit form

23. HDL Date: *(mm/dd/yy)* ______________________

24. HDL Value: ______________________

25. Serum Triglyceride Value: *(mm/dd/yy)* ______________________

26. Serum Triglyceride Value: ______________________

27. Gross Protein Present:

- ☐ **0 = Not documented**
- ☐ **1 = Yes, or previously diagnosed**

OR

28. Microalbumin Test Date *(mm/dd/yy)* ______________________

OR

29. Urine Albumin Creatinine Ratio Date *(mm/dd/yy)* ______________________

AND

30. Urine Albumin Creatinine Ratio *(mg/g)*: ______________________

31. Self-Management Education:

- ☐ **0 = Not documented**
- ☐ **1 = Yes**

32. Nutritional Education:

- ☐ **0 = Not documented**
- ☐ **1 = Yes**

33. Self-Monitoring Blood Glucose:

- ☐ **0 = Not documented**
- ☐ **1 = Yes**

34. Foot Exam Date: *(mm/dd/yy)* ______________________

35. Tobacco Status Documented:

- ☐ **1 = Not documented** ☐ **2 = Yes, documented in chart**
- ☐ **3 = Previous tobacco user**

36. If smoker, was referral for Tobacco Cessation made?:

- ☐ **0 = Not documented**
- ☐ **1 = Yes**

37. Retinal Exam Date: *(mm/dd/yy)* ______________________

38. Metabolic syndrome: *is patient diagnosed with any type of Metabolic Syndrome in addition to the above diabetes types?*

- ☐ **1 = No** ☐ **2 = Yes**

International Diabetes Center
Park Nicollet

Figure A.2 Continued

Medical History

- Symptoms/laboratory tests at diagnosis
- Previous and current diabetes therapy and control (SMBG and HbA_{1c})
- Weight history/especially previous diets
- Nutrition and exercise pattern assessment
- Medications: assess those that may affect BG (β-blockers, steroids, thiazides)
- Growth and development in children and adolescents
- Acute or chronic complications including hypoglycemia/hyperglycemia; neuropathy; sexual dysfunction; retinopathy; nephropathy; foot problems; cardiovascular disease; gastrointestinal symptoms
- Prior or current infections including skin, dental, genitourinary
- History of other conditions, including endocrine and eating disorders
- Smoking and/or alcohol use
- Lifestyle, cultural, psychosocial, abuse, occupational, and economic issues
- Previous education about diabetes

Physical Exam

- Determine body mass index (BMI = weight/height^2 = kg/m^2)
- BP (sitting and standing)
- Examinations: funduscopic; dental; thyroid; cardiovascular; abdominal; neuro/vascular; feet; insulin injection sites
- Growth and development in children (plot on growth charts)
- Sexual maturation in children

Laboratory Evaluation

- Fasting (preferred) or casual plasma glucose, if there is a question as to the validity of SMBG results or for meter quality assuarance
- Hemoglobin A_{1c} (HbA_{1c})
- Fasting lipid profile within 6 months of diagnosis
- Urinalysis (urine culture if sediment)
- Urine microalbumin (timed or random albumin/creatinine ratio) if dip stick negative for proteinuria; after 5 years of duration in postpubertal type 1; at diagnosis and then annually in type 2
- Serum creatinine in adults; in children if proteinuria present
- Thyroid functions in all type 1, in type 2 when thyroid disease is suspected
- Other lab assessments as indicated by history (chem profile, CBC)
- EKG (adults)

Management Plan

- Set short- and long-term goals (weight control, exercise, food plan, medications, monitoring)
- Determine SMBG and HbA_{1c} targets
- Record current medications
- Address lifestyle changes such as activity level and smoking cessation
- Educate about preventive care (foot, eye, dental)
- Plan contraception and pregnancy with women of childbearing age
- Refer patient to registered dietitian for nutrition recommendations (exercise plan) and instruction
- Refer patient to diabetes educator for self-management training, BG and urine ketone monitoring and record-keeping instructions
- Plan follow-up schedule with patient
- Refer patient for special services as necessary

Figure A.3 Medical Visit/Initial DecisionPath

Follow-up Visit
Every 1–2 months during adjust phase; every 3–4 months during maintain phase

Interim History

- Note current stage (food plan, oral agent, etc., particularly self-adjustment of insulin/oral agent)
- Review current medications and illnesses
- Review SMBG and HbA_{1c} targets
- Discuss episodes of hypoglycemia/hyperglycemia (frequency, cause, severity, symptoms, treatment)
- Address presence of intercurrent illness/ketonuria
- Assess nutrition; exercise; lifestyle changes; psychosocial issues; complications
- Evaluate patient's adherence issues
- Assess sexual activity beginning with puberty
- Birth control/pregnancy planning for women of childbearing age
- Review record book
- Assess frequency of monitoring; SMBG ranges; patterns of hypoglycemia/hyperglycemia; validate meter accuracy annually; response to exercise; illness
- If memory meter used, compare with record book or download into computer for analysis

Physical Exam

- Determine body mass index (BMI = weight/height^2 = kg/m^2)
- BP (sitting and standing)
- Examinations: funduscopic; dental; thyroid; cardiac; abdominal; neuro/vascular; feet; injection sites for patients on insulin
- Growth and development in children (plot on growth charts)
- Sexual maturation in children
- Examine previous abnormal findings

Laboratory Evaluation

- Fasting (preferred) or casual plasma glucose, if there is a question as to the validity of SMBG results or for meter quality assurance
- HbA_{1c}

Management Plan

- Refer patient to diabetes educator and/or regisitered dietitian for review of self-management and/or medical nutrition therapy as indicated
- Consult with specialists as indicated (ophthalmologist, nephrologist, neurologist, podiatrist)

Yearly Check-Up

- Complete eye examination with dilation by ophthalmologist: annually after 5 years duration in post-pubertal type 1; at diagnosis and then annually in type 2
- Lipid profile: every 5 years if normal; annually if abnormal
- Albuminuria: each visit
- Urine microalbumin (time or random albumin/creatinine ratio) if dip stick negative for proteinuria: after 5 years duration in postpubertal type 1; at diagnosis and then annually in type 2
- Thyroid: age < 18 if growth problems, enlarged thyroid, or symptoms; age $\geqslant 18$ if suspected problems
- EKG: all adults
- Foot examination (pulses, nerves and inspection)

Figure A.4 Medical Visit/Follow-up DecisionPath

Weight (lb)

Height	130	135	140	145	150	155	160	165	170	175	180	185	190	195	200	205	210	215	220	225	230	235	240	245	250	255	260	265	270	275	280	285	290	295	300	305
5'0"	25	26	27	28	29	30	31	32	33	34	35	36	37	38	39	40	41	42	43	44	45	46	47	48	49	50	51	52	53	54	55	56	57	58	59	60
5'1"	25	26	26	27	28	29	30	31	32	33	34	35	36	37	38	39	40	41	42	43	43	44	45	46	47	48	49	50	51	52	53	54	55	56	57	58
5'2"	24	25	26	27	27	28	29	30	31	32	33	34	35	36	37	37	38	39	40	41	42	43	44	45	46	47	48	48	49	50	51	52	53	54	55	56
5'3"	23	24	25	26	27	27	28	29	30	31	32	33	34	35	35	36	37	38	39	40	41	42	43	43	44	45	46	47	48	49	50	50	51	52	53	54
5'4"	22	23	24	25	26	27	27	28	29	30	31	32	33	33	34	35	36	37	38	39	39	40	41	42	43	44	45	45	46	47	48	49	50	51	51	52
5'5"	22	22	23	24	25	26	27	27	28	29	30	31	32	32	33	34	35	36	37	37	38	39	40	41	42	42	43	44	45	46	47	47	48	49	50	51
5'6"	21	22	23	23	24	25	26	27	27	28	29	30	31	31	32	33	34	35	36	36	37	38	39	40	40	41	42	43	44	44	45	46	47	48	48	49
5'7"	20	21	22	23	23	24	25	26	27	27	28	29	30	31	31	32	33	34	34	35	36	37	38	38	39	40	41	42	42	43	44	45	45	46	47	48
5'8"	20	21	21	22	23	24	24	25	26	27	27	28	29	30	30	31	32	33	33	34	35	36	36	37	38	39	40	40	41	42	43	43	44	45	46	46
5'9"	19	20	21	21	22	23	24	24	25	26	27	27	28	29	30	30	31	32	32	33	34	35	35	36	37	38	38	39	40	41	41	42	43	44	44	45
5'10"	19	19	20	21	22	22	23	24	24	25	26	27	27	28	29	29	30	31	32	32	33	34	34	35	36	37	37	38	39	39	40	41	42	42	43	44
5'11"	18	19	20	20	21	22	22	23	24	24	25	26	26	27	28	29	29	30	31	31	32	33	33	34	35	36	36	37	38	38	39	40	40	41	42	43
6'0"	18	18	19	20	20	21	22	22	23	24	24	25	26	26	27	28	28	29	30	31	31	32	33	33	34	35	35	36	36	37	38	39	39	40	41	41
6'1"	17	18	18	19	20	20	21	22	22	23	24	24	25	26	26	27	28	28	29	30	30	31	32	32	33	34	34	35	36	36	37	38	38	39	40	40
6'2"	17	17	18	19	19	20	21	21	22	22	23	24	24	25	26	26	27	28	28	29	30	30	31	31	32	33	33	34	35	35	36	37	37	38	39	39
6'3"	16	17	17	18	19	19	20	21	21	22	22	23	24	24	25	25	26	27	27	28	29	29	30	31	31	32	32	33	34	34	35	36	36	37	37	38
6'4"	16	16	17	18	18	19	19	20	21	21	22	23	23	24	24	25	26	26	27	27	28	29	29	30	30	31	32	32	33	33	34	35	35	36	37	37

Patients with BMI > 25 kg/m^2 have a higher risk of adverse effects on health

BMI is defined as body weight (kg) divided by height squared (m^2) (BMI = kg/m^2)

1 meter = 39.37 inches, 1 kilogram = 2.2 pounds

Figure A.5 BMI chart

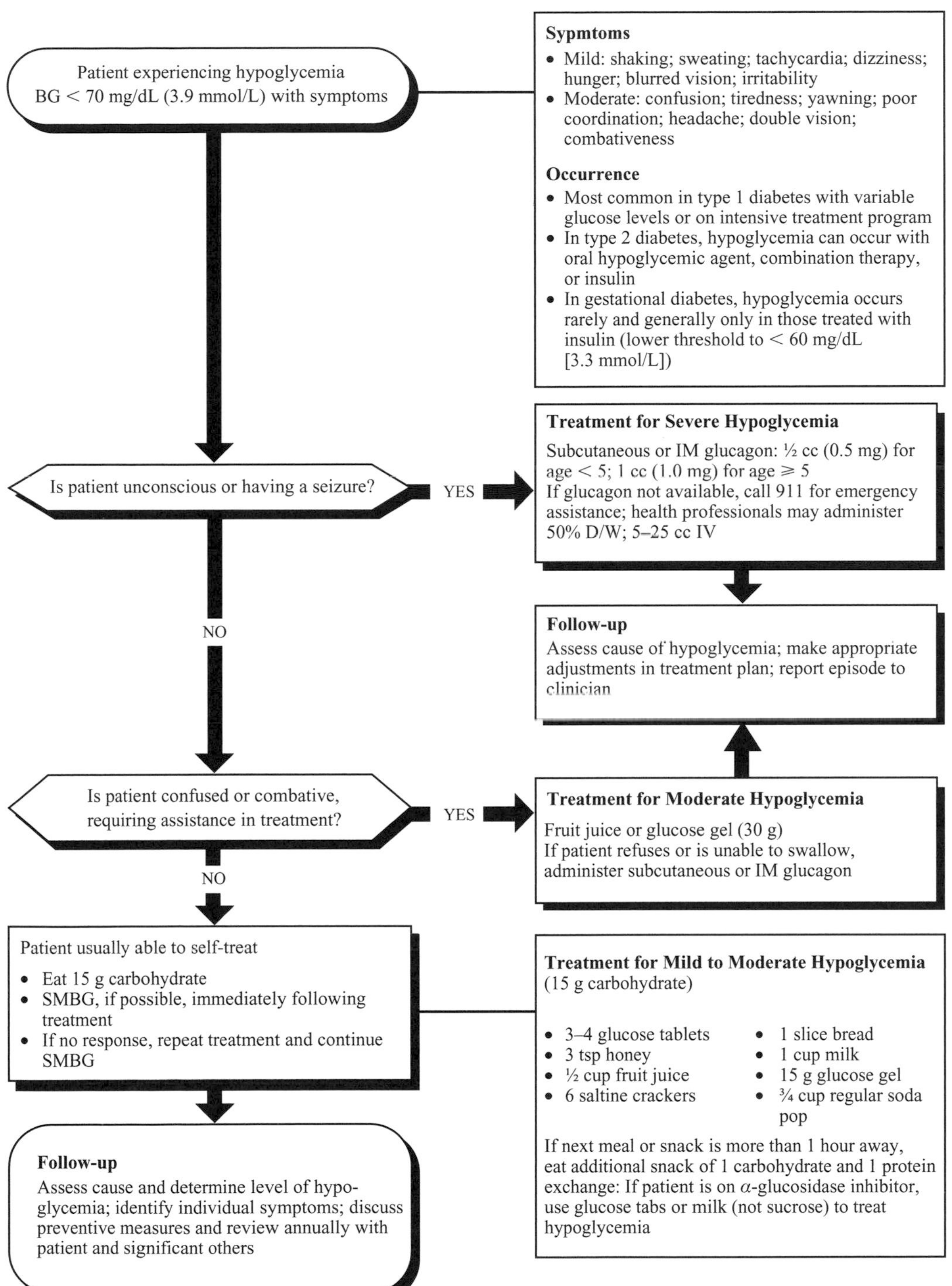

Figure A.6 Hypoglycemia/Treatment DecisionPath

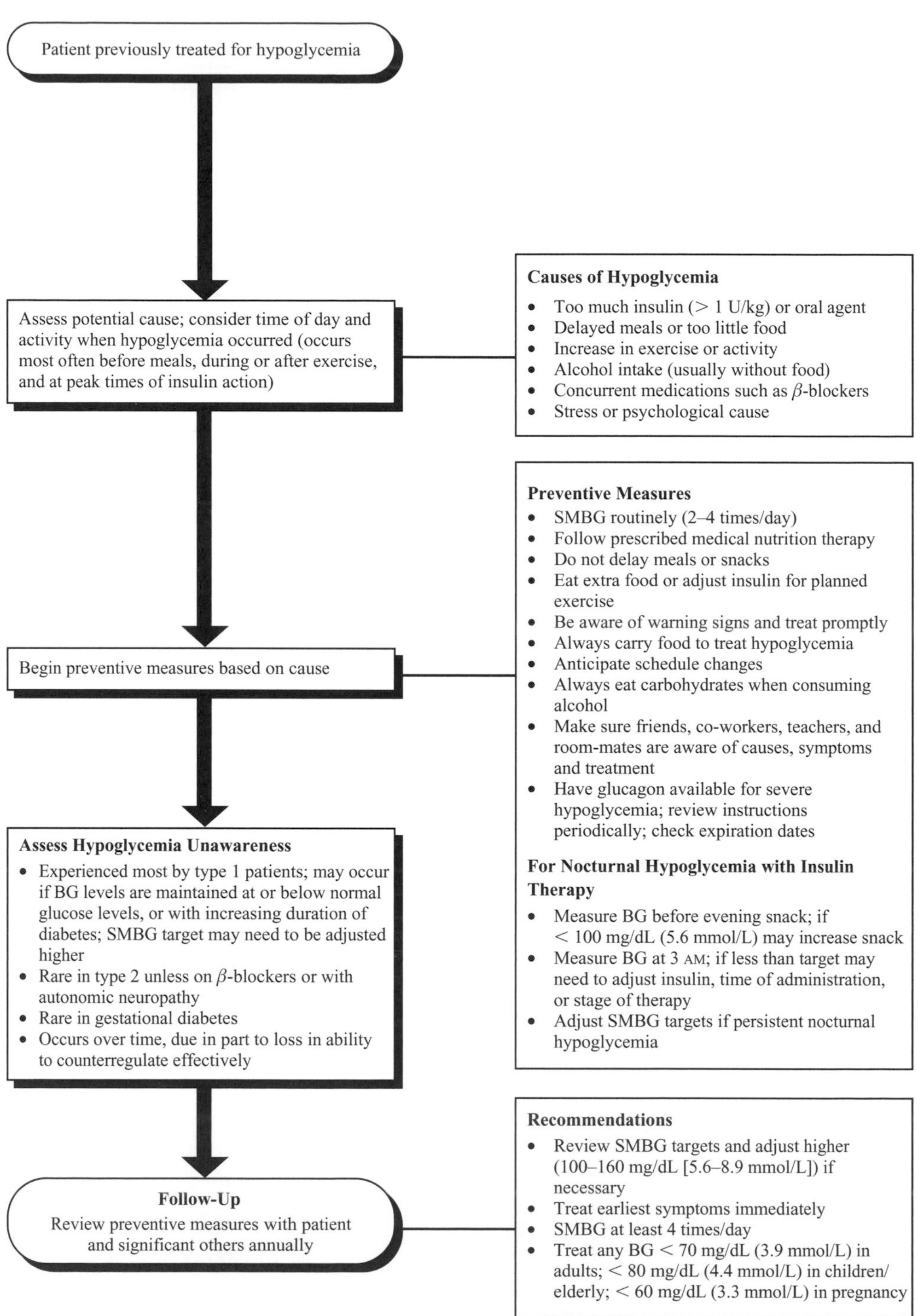

Figure A.7 Hypoglycemia/Prevention DecisionPath

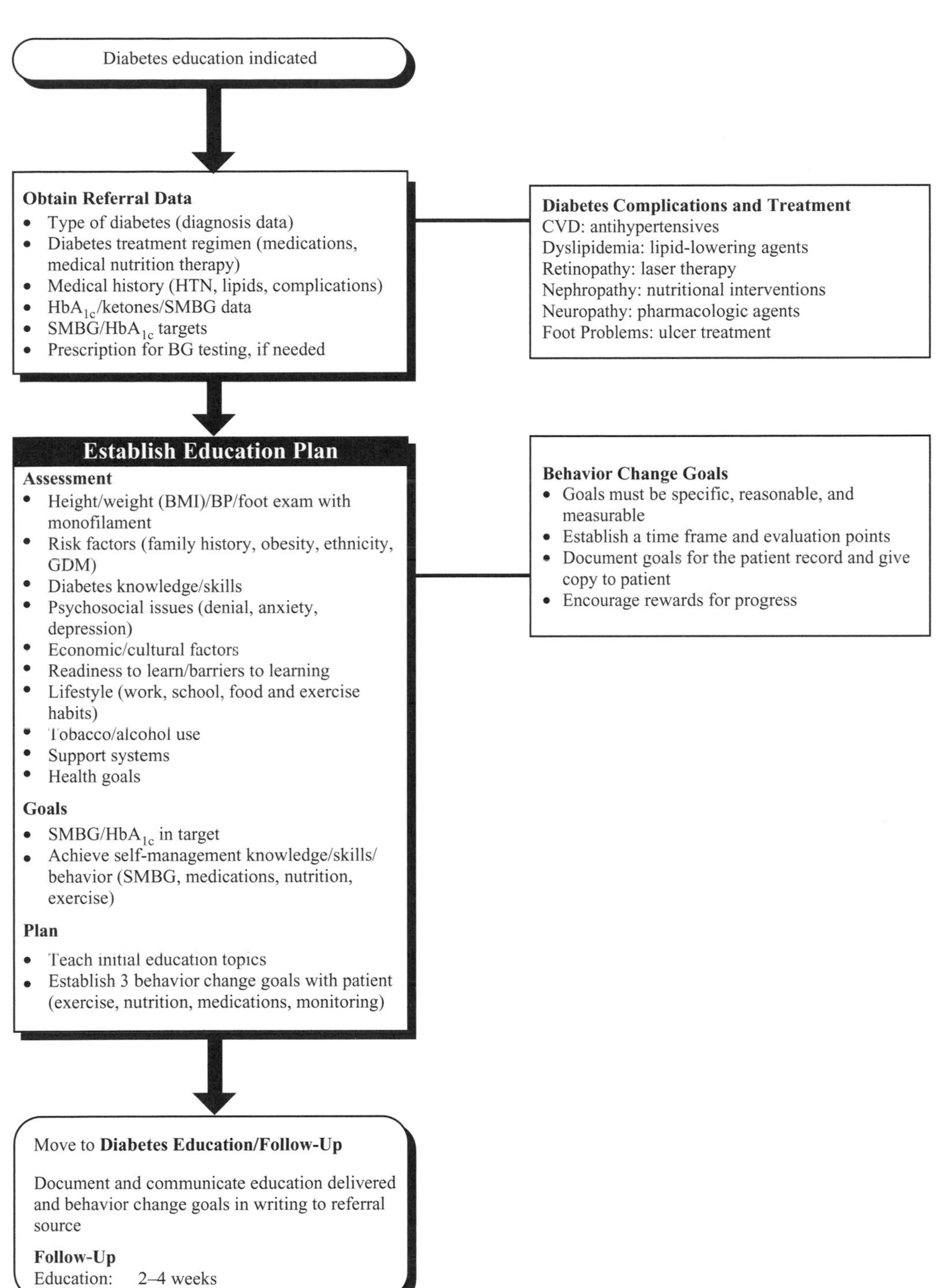

Figure A.8 Diabetes Education/Initial DecisionPath

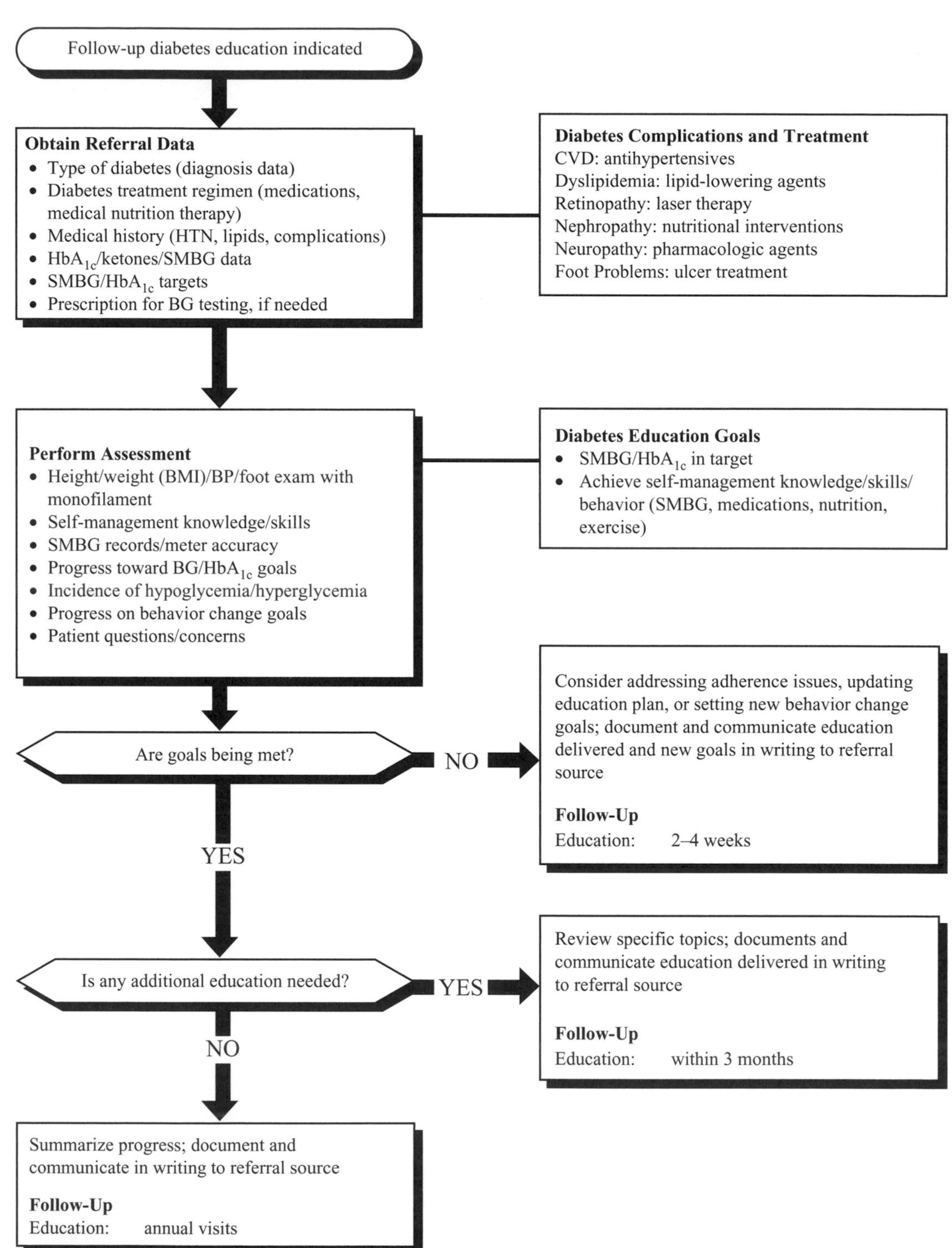

Figure A.9 Diabetes Education/Follow-up DecisionPath

Initial Visit

General Information
- Diabetes pathophysiology (definition and causes of hyperglycemia, type 1 vs. type 2)
- Interaction of food/exercise/medication
- Insulin resistance/obesity (type 2)
- Target goals (SMBG, HbA_{1c}, weight)
- Medication administration/adjustment
- SMBG technique/record-keeping
- Daily schedule (testing, medication, meals, snacks)
- Hypoglycemia signs (dizziness, sweating, confusion, loss of consciousness)
- Hyperglycemia signs (fatigue, acetonic, polyuria, polydipsia, polyphagia)
- Prevention/treatment of hypoglycemia/hyperglycemia
- Emergency phone numbers
- Patient education materials

Add for Insulin Users
- Insulin action
- Daily injection schedule/site rotation
- Insulin injection technique (site, angle, drawing and mixing)
- Insulin storage
- Syringe/lancet disposal
- Hypoglycemia/glucagon use
- Urine ketone monitoring (type 1)
- Medical identification

Add for Insulin Pump Users
- Pump operation and care
- Site care (change site every 24–48 hours)
- Use of algorithm for bolus/basal ratio
- Record-keeping

Follow-up Visits

General Information
- New topics based on assessment
- Review first-visit topics/re-educate as needed
- Check SMBG skills/meter accuracy
- Precautions when driving
- Illness management
- Benefits/responsibilities of self-care

Added for Insulin Users
- Pattern control
- Compensatory/anticipatory insulin adjustments
- Hypoglycemia unawareness
- Review injection technique
- Travel/schedule changes and effect on insulin

Added for Insulin Pump Users
- Review hypoglycemia signs (dizziness, sweating, confusion, loss of consciousness)
- Unexplained hyperglycemia (causes, recognition, treatment)
- Exercise (insulin adjustments, pump care)
- Problem-solving skills

Add as Needed
- Foot/skin/dental care
- Recognition of complications (numbness, persistent ulcers, blurry vision, frequent urination)
- Healthy lifestyle (weight management, exercise, tobacco and alcohol use, stress management)
- Travel/schedule changes
- Sexuality (impotence, contraception, pregnancy planning)
- Psychological adjustments
- Community diabetes resources

Figure A.10 Diabetes education topics

Nutrition intervention indicated

Obtain Referral Data
- Type of diabetes (diagnosis data)
- Diabetes treatment regimen (medications, medical nutrition therapy)
- Medical history (HTN, lipids, complications)
- HbA_{1c}/ketones/SMBG data
- SMBG/HbA_{1c} targets
- Medical clearance for exercise (adults)

Diabetes Complications and Treatment
CVD: antihypertensives
Dyslipidemia: lipid-lowering agents
Retinopathy: laser therapy
Nephropathy: nutritional interventions
Neuropathy: pharmacologic agents
Foot Problems: ulcer treatment

Establish Food Plan

Assessment
- Food history or 3 day food record (meals, times, portions)
- Nutrition adequacy
- Height/weight/BMI
- Weight goals/eating disorders
- Psychosocial issues (denial, anxiety, depression)
- Economic/cultural factors
- Nutrition/diabetes knowledge
- Readiness to learn/barriers to learning
- Work/school/sports schedules
- Exercise (times, duration, types)
- Tobacco/alcohol use
- Vitamin/mineral supplements

Goals
- SMBG/HbA_{1c} in target
- Achieve desirable body weight (adults)
- Normal growth and development (children)
- Consistent carbohydrate intake

Plan
- Establish adequate calories for growth and development/reasonable body weight
- Set meal/snack times
- Integrate insulin regimen with medical nutrition therapy (insulin users)
- Set consistent carbohydrate intake
- Encourage regular exercise
- Establish adequate calories for pregnancy/lactation/recovery from illness

Medical Nutrition Therapy Guidelines
- Total fat = 30% total calories; less if obese and high LDL
- Saturated fat < 10% total calories; < 7% with high LDL
- Cholesterol < 300 mg/day
- Sodium < 2400 mg/day
- Protein reduced to 0.8 g/kg/day (~10% total calories) if macroalbuminuria
- Calories decreased by 10–20% if BMI > 25 kg/m^2

Calorie Requirements
Adults
Most men/active women: weight (lb) × 15 kcal
Most women/inactive men/most adults > age 55: weight (lb) × 13 kcal
Inactive women/obese adults/inactive adults > age 55: weight (lb) × 10 kcal

Children/Method 1
First year: 1000 kcal/year
Ages 1–10: add 100 kcal/year
Age 11–15: boys add 200 kcal/year; girls add 100 kcal/year
Age > 15: Boys add for activity (23 kcal/lb very active, 18 kcal/lb normal, 16 kcal lb inactive); girls calculate as adult

Children/Method 2
First year: 1000 kcal
Ages 1–3: add 40 kcal/inch
Age > 3: Boys 125 kcal × age; girls 100 kcal × age; add up to 20% kcal for activity

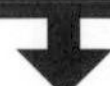

Move to **Nutrition Education/Follow-Up**
Document and communicate medical nutrition therapy and education delivered in writing to referral source

Follow-Up
Nutrition: within 1 month

Figure A.11 Nutrition Education/Initial DecisionPath

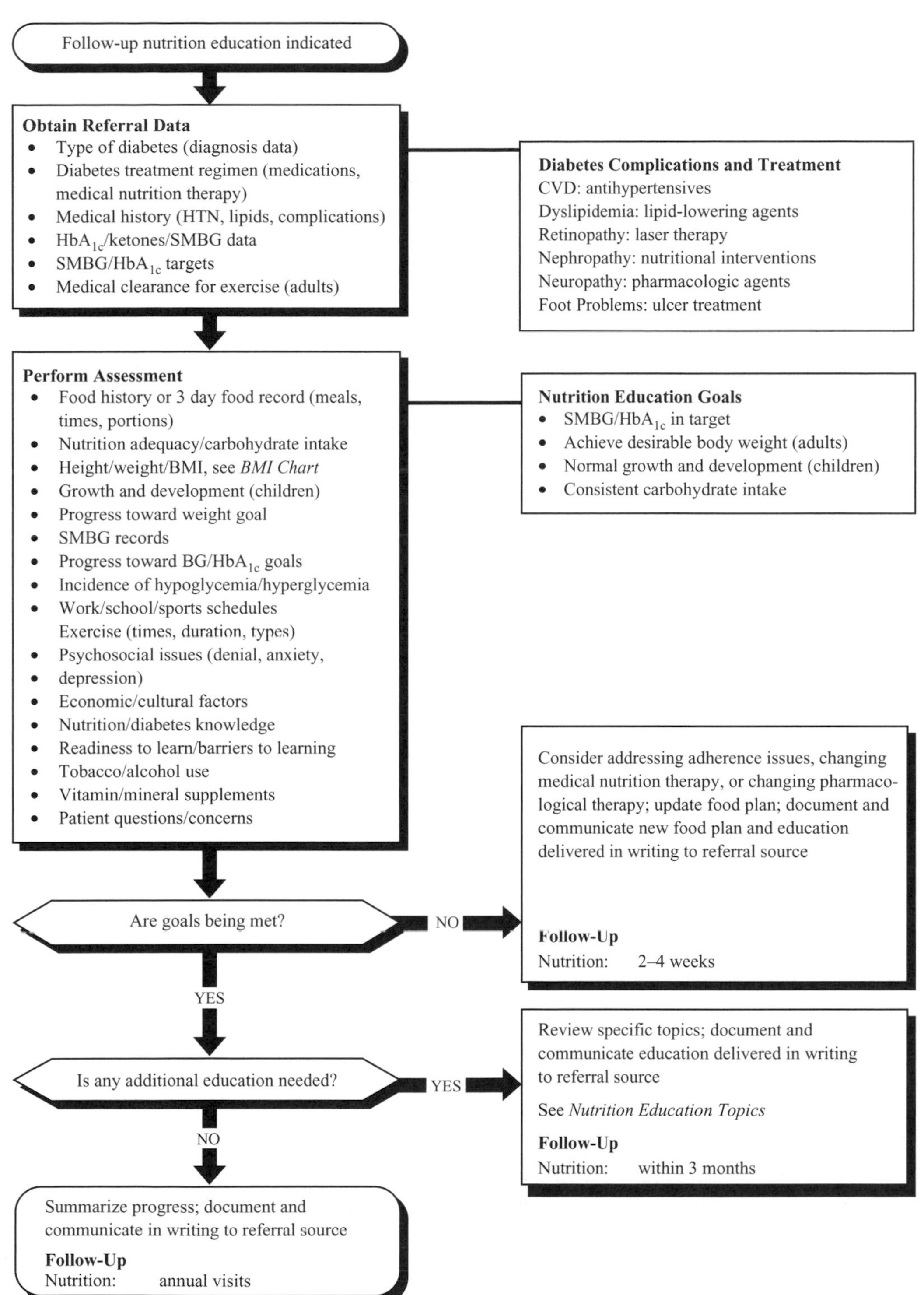

Figure A.12 Nutrition Education/Follow-up DecisionPath

Initial Visit

General Information

- Food components (carbohydrate, protein, fat)
- Effect of food on BG levels (carbohydrates have greatest effect)
- Portion control (average servings, measuring, estimating)
- Realistic weight goals (achievable, maintainable)
- Guidelines for fat intake
- Guidelines for exercise
- Guidelines for treatment of hypoglycemia
- Individualize medical nutrition therapy

Add for Insulin Users

- Synchronization of insulin with food
- Consistency in timing of meals and snacks
- Prevention and treatment of hypoglycemia (food or beverage choices and amounts)
- Adjusting food intake/insulin for exercise

Follow-up Visits

General Information

- Review first visit topics and short-term goals
- Carbohydrate counting
- Nutrition management during short-term illness
- Food nutrition labels/healthy food choices
- Use of food with higher sugar content
- Reset short-term goals
- Food related questions/problem-solving

Add for Insulin Users

- Pattern control for adjusting insulin/food
- Anticipatory insulin adjustments for changes in basic medical nutrition therapy
- Travel/schedule changes; effect on insulin
- Review SMBG/food and insulin adjustments
- Food/insulin adjustments for short-term illness

Add as Needed

- Sources of carbohydrate/protein/fat; effects on BG/other health factors (blood lipids, CHD)
- SMBG to problem solve/identify patterns related to food intake
- Adjusting meal times or delayed meals
- Travel/schedule changes
- Holidays/special occasions; restaurant/fast food choices
- Alcohol guidelines/effect on BG
- Recipes/menu ideas/cookbooks
- Dietetic foods/sweeteners
- Exchanges and equivalencies
- Behavior modification/problem-solving tips
- Vitamin/mineral/nutritional supplements

Figure A.13 Nutrition education topics

For All Patients

General Information

- Method of meal planning that takes into account only carbohydrate content of foods
- May be used in people with type 1 diabetes, type 2 diabetes, and in pre-gestational and gestational diabetes
- Individualize carbohydrate intake for each patient
- 15 g carbohydrate = 1 carbohydrate choice
- 1 carbohydrate choice is provided in one serving of food from the starch, fruit, or milk food exchange lists
- "Simple" and "complex" carbohydrate absorption rates are similar
- Emphasize total carbohydrate content of foods, rather than the source
- Carbohydrate is the first and primary nutrient that affects BG levels
- Consistency of carbohydrate intake will promote consistency in BG control
- Serves as a guideline for how much carbohydrate to consume at meals and snacks
- Provides flexibility in food choices

Sugar

- Sugar (sucrose) affects BG levels in a similar way as other carbohydrate foods
- Sugar and foods high in sugar must be counted into the food plan or substituted for other carbohydrate
- Foods that are high in sugar are often high in fat and low in nutrients, making them a source of "empty calories"
- Sugar and foods high in sugar should not be encouraged, rather worked into the food plan appropriately

Considerations

- Potential for weight gain if too many foods high in fat are consumed
- Nutritional inadequacy of the diet if the food plan is not well balanced with a variety of foods

Additional Considerations

Intensive Management

- May be be used to teach people how to make adjustments in regular or rapid-acting insulin for adding or subtracting food from their usual food plan
- Normally 1 unit bolus insulin for each 15 g of carbohydrate (or 1 carbohydrate choice)
- Add 1 unit of short-acting insulin to cover 1 extra carbohydrate choice to be eaten at that meal
- Subtract 1 unit of short-acting insulin from usual dose if 1 less carbohydrate choice is to be eaten at that meal
- Frequent monitoring and diligent record keeping are required

Type 2 Diabetes

- Typically 3–4 carbohydrate choices at meals and 1–2 choices at snacks
- Spread carbohydrate choices throughout the day to promote BG control
- Avoid high-fat foods to prevent possible weight gain

Figure A.14 Carbohydrate counting

Carbohydrate Servings (15 g carbohydrate; 60–90 calories)			
Starch Group		**Fruit Group**	
Bagel or English muffin	1 half or 1 oz	Banana	½ medium
Bread, slice or roll	1 or 1 oz	Berries or melon	1 cup
Cereal, cooked	½ cup	Canned fruit in juice or water	½ cup
Cereal, dry, unsweetened	¾ cup	Dried fruit	¼ cup
Corn, cooked	½ cup	Fresh fruit	1 medium
Crackers, snack	4–5	Fruit juice	⅓ to ½ cup
Dried beans, cooked	½ cup	Grapes or cherries	12 to 15
Graham crackers	3 squares	Raisins	2 tbsp
Hamburger or hot dog bun	1 half or 1 oz		
Lima beans, cooked	⅔ cup	**Milk Group**	
Muffin, small	1	Milk, skim or low-fat	1 cup
Pancakes, 4" across	2	Yogurt, low-fat, artificially sweetened (6–8 oz)	¾ to 1 cup
Pasta, cooked	½ cup		
Peas, cooked	⅓ cup	Yogurt, plain, low-fat (6–8 oz)	¾ to 1 cup
Popcorn, plain, unbuttered	3 cups		
Potato, small	1		
Potato, mashed	½ cup		
Rice, cooked	½ cup		
Squash, winter, cooked	1 cup		
Taco shells, 6" across	2		
Tortilla, 6" across	1		
Waffles, 4½" across	1		

Meat and Meat Substitutes Servings (7 g protein; 5 g fat; 50–100 calories)		
Meats	**Meat Substitutes**	
Beef, lamb, pork, seafood, ham, veal	Cottage cheese	¼ cup
Poultry with skin removed	Cheese	1 oz
	Egg	1
Meats should be baked, broiled, roasted, or grilled	Peanut butter	2 tbsp
Average serving size is 3 oz	Tuna or salmon packed in water	¼ cup

Fat Servings (5 g fat; 45 calories)			
Butter	1 tsp	Peanut butter	2 tsp
Cream cheese	1 tbsp	Reduced-calorie margarine	1 tbsp
Cream, table or light	2 tbsp	Reduced-calorie mayonnaise	1 tbsp
Gravy	2 tbsp	Reduced-calorie salad dressing	2 tbsp
Margarine	1 tsp	Salad dressing	1 tbsp
Mayonnaise	1 tsp	Sour cream	2 tbsp
Nuts	1 tbsp	Sunflower seeds	1 tbsp
Oil	1 tsp		

Excerpted from *My Food Plan*

Figure A.15 Food choices

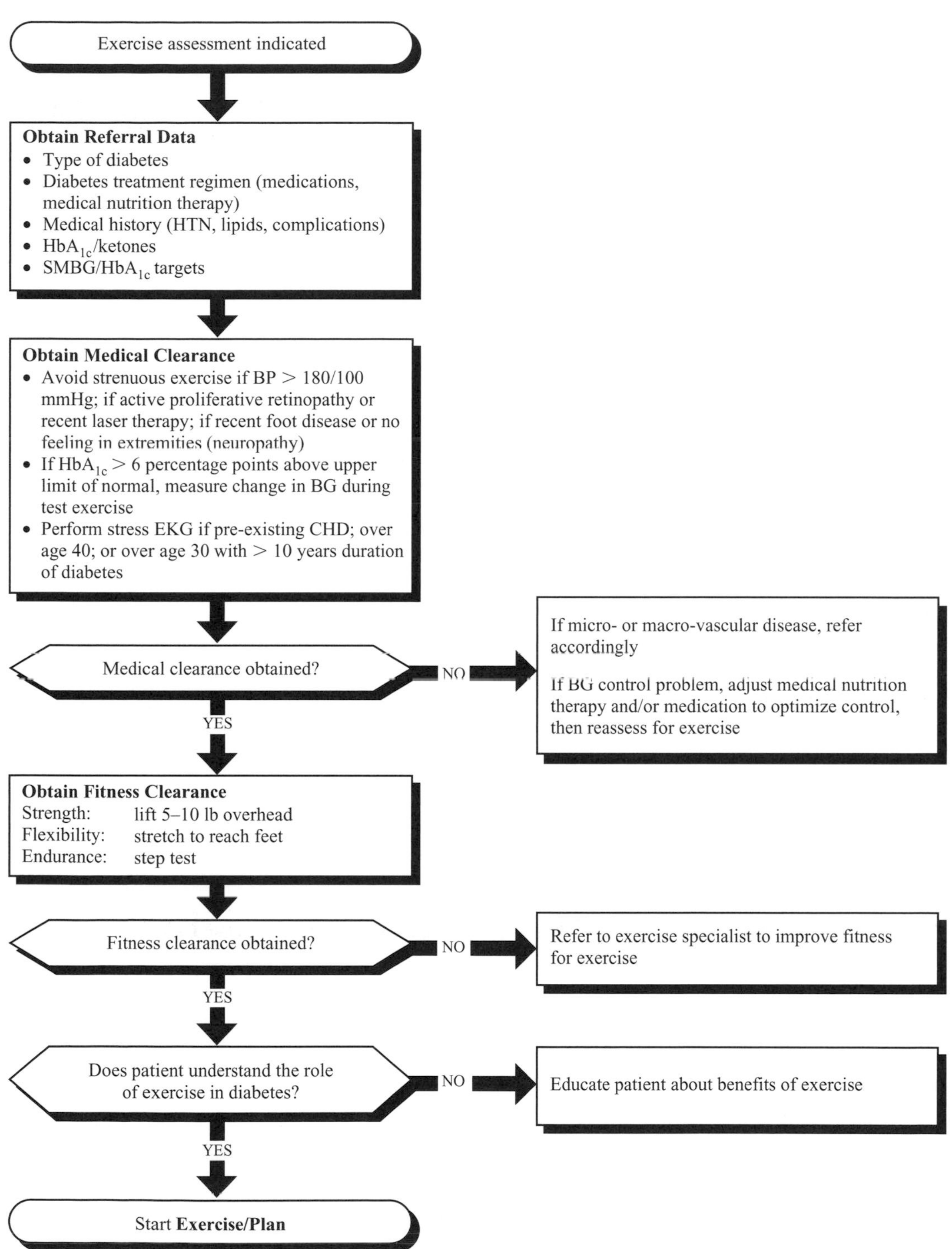

Figure A.16 Exercise/Assessment

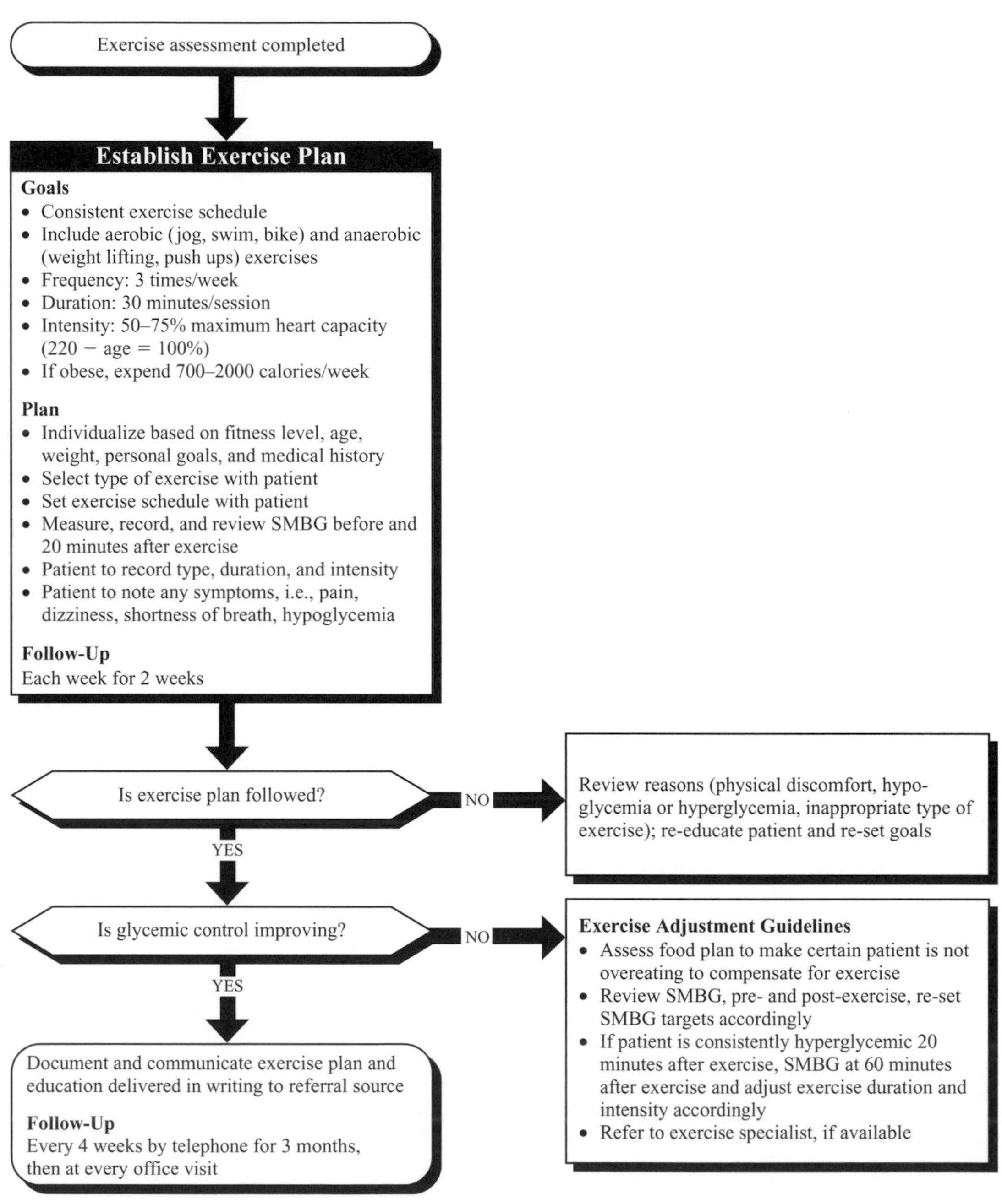

Figure A.17 Exercise/Plan DecisionPath

Initial Visit

General Information
- Food components (carbohydrate, protein, fat)
- Effect of food on BG levels (carbohydrates have greatest effect)
- Portion control (average servings, measuring, estimating)
- Realistic weight goals (achievable, maintainable)
- Guidelines for fat intake
- Guidelines for exercise
- Guidelines for treatment of hypoglycemia
- Individualize food plan

Add for Insulin Users
- Synchronization of insulin with food
- Consistency in timing of meals and snacks
- Prevention and treatment of hypoglycemia (food or beverage choices and amounts)
- Adjusting food intake/insulin for exercise

Follow-Up Visits

General Information
- Review first-visit topics and short-term goals
- Carbohydrate counting
- Nutrition management during short-term illness
- Food nutrition labels/healthy food choices
- Use of food with higher sugar content
- Reset short-term goals
- Food related questions/problem-solving

Add for Insulin Users
- Pattern control for adjusting insulin/food
- Anticipatory insulin adjustments for changes in basic food plan
- Travel/schedule changes; effect on insulin
- Review SMBG/food and insulin adjustments
- Food/insulin adjustments for short-term illness

Add as Needed
- Sources of carbohydrate/protein/fat; effects on BG/other health factors (blood lipids, CHD)
- SMBG to problem solve/identify patterns related to food intake
- Adjusting meal times or delayed meals
- Travel/schedule changes
- Holidays/special occasions; restaurant/fast food choices
- Alcohol guidelines/effect on BG
- Recipes/menu ideas/cookbooks
- Dietetic foods/sweeteners
- Exchanges and equivalencies
- Behavior modification/problem-solving tips
- Vitamin/mineral/nutritional supplements

Figure A.18 Exercise education topics

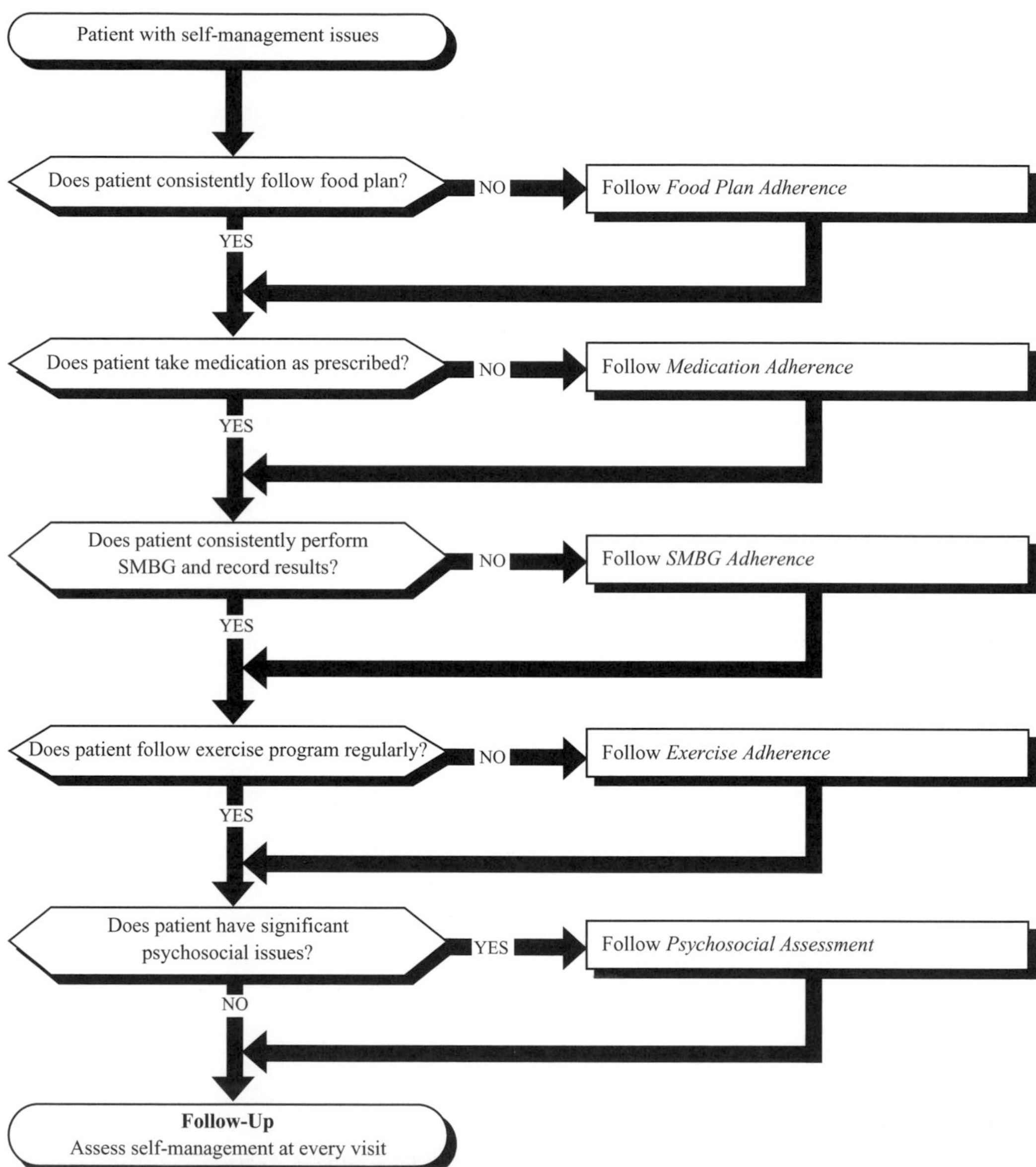

Figure A.19 Diabetes Management Patient Adherence DecisionPath

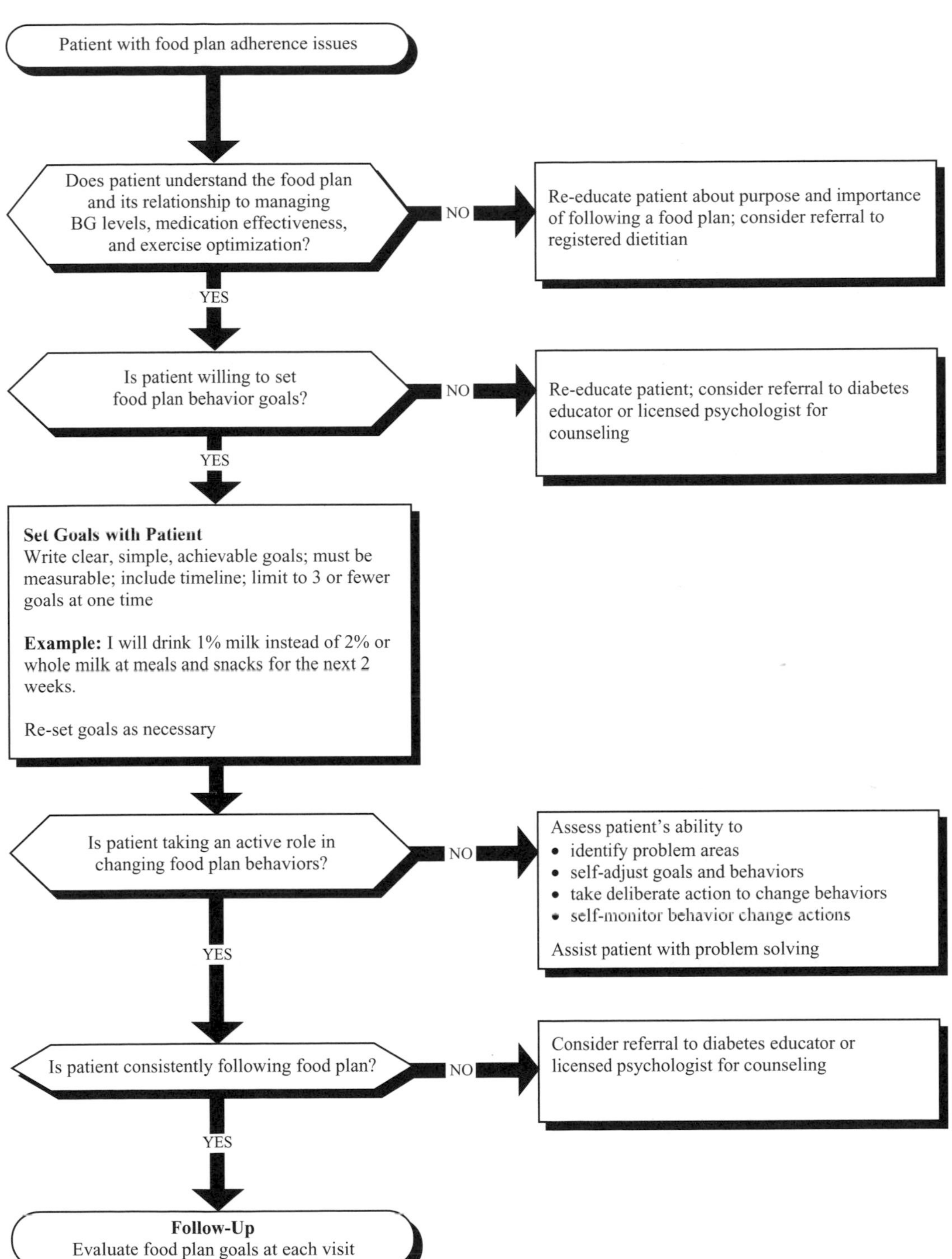

Figure A.20 Food Plan Adherence DecisionPath

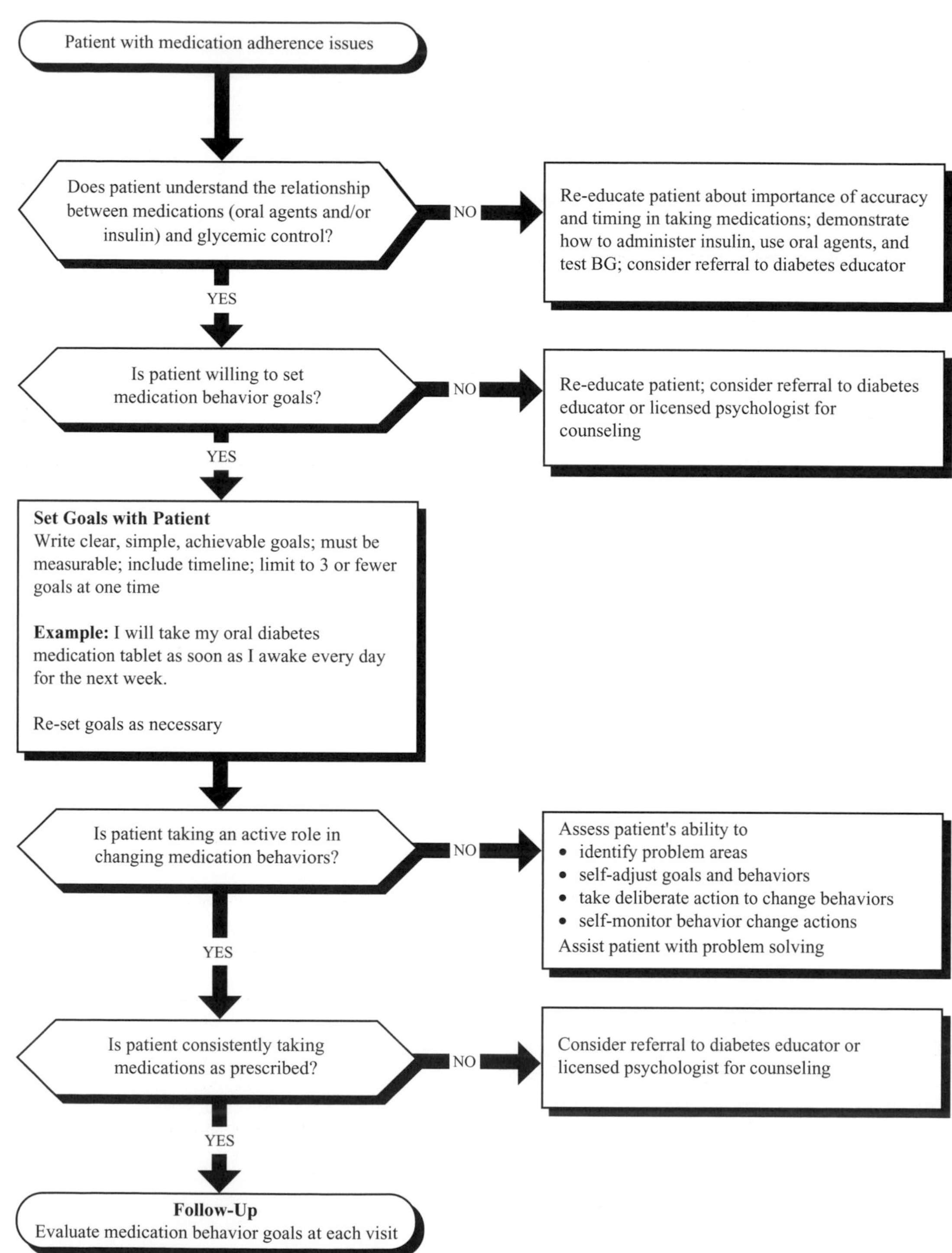

Figure A.21 Medication Adherence DecisionPath

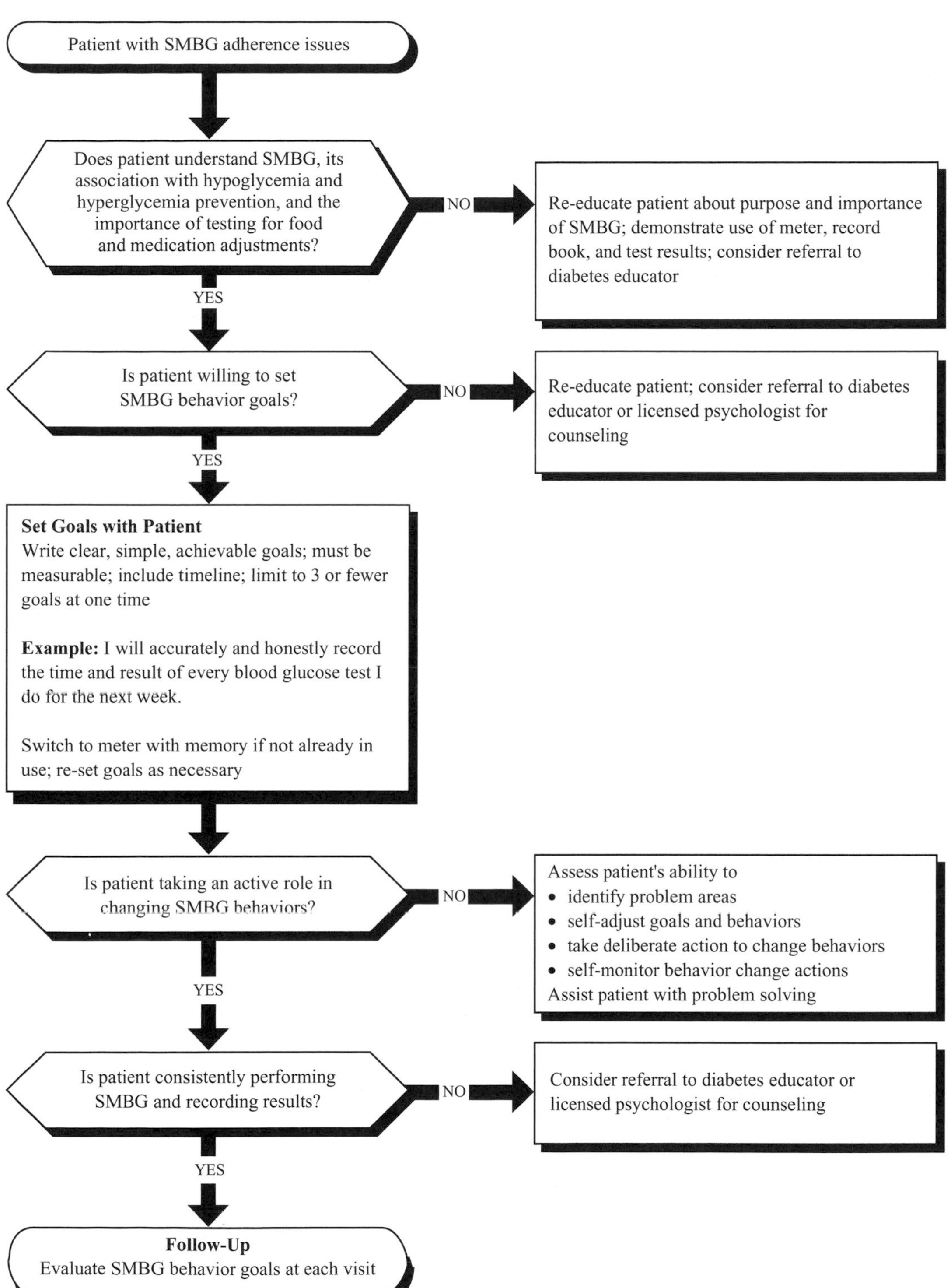

Figure A.22 SMBG Adherence DecisionPath

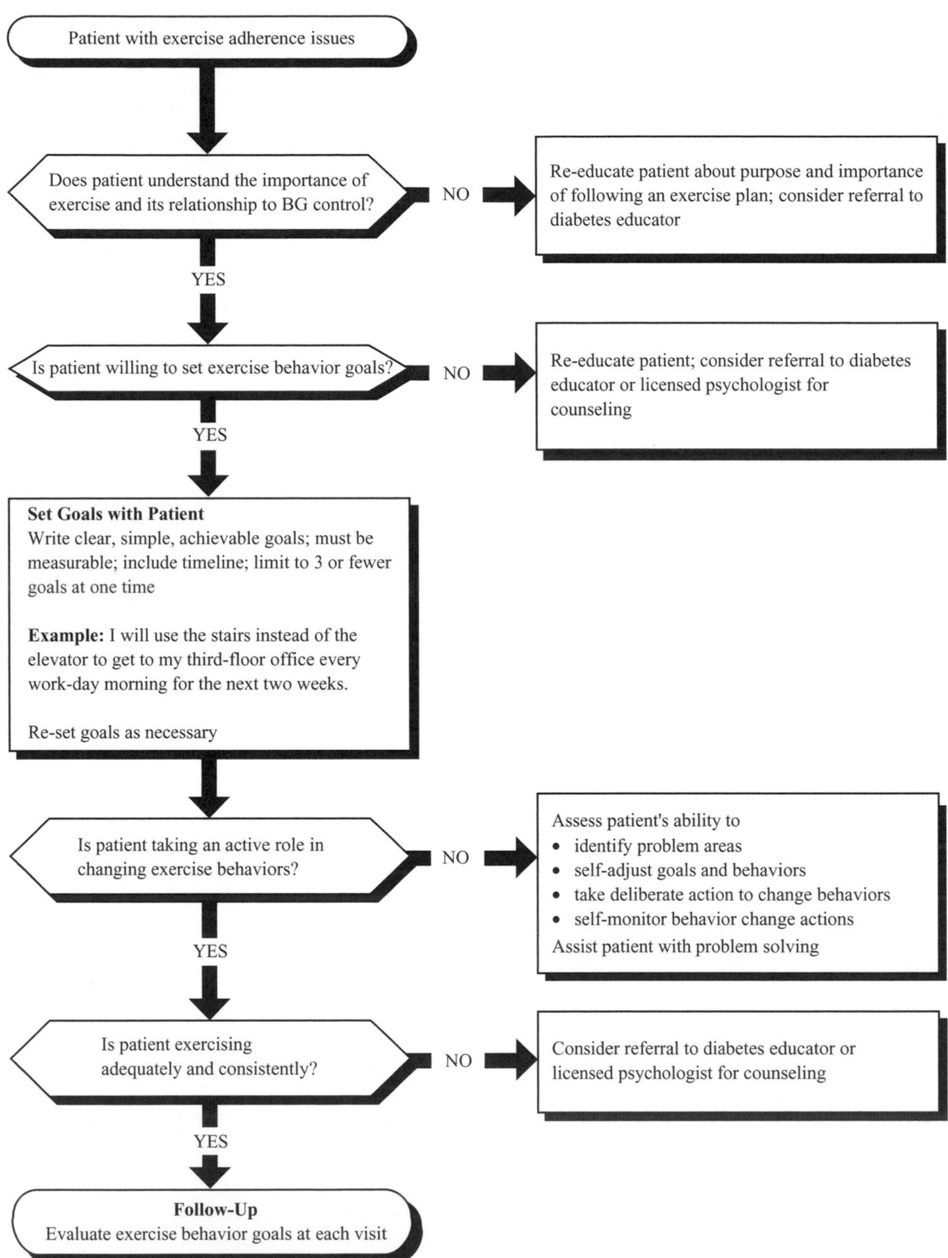

Figure A.23 Exercise Adherence DecisionPath

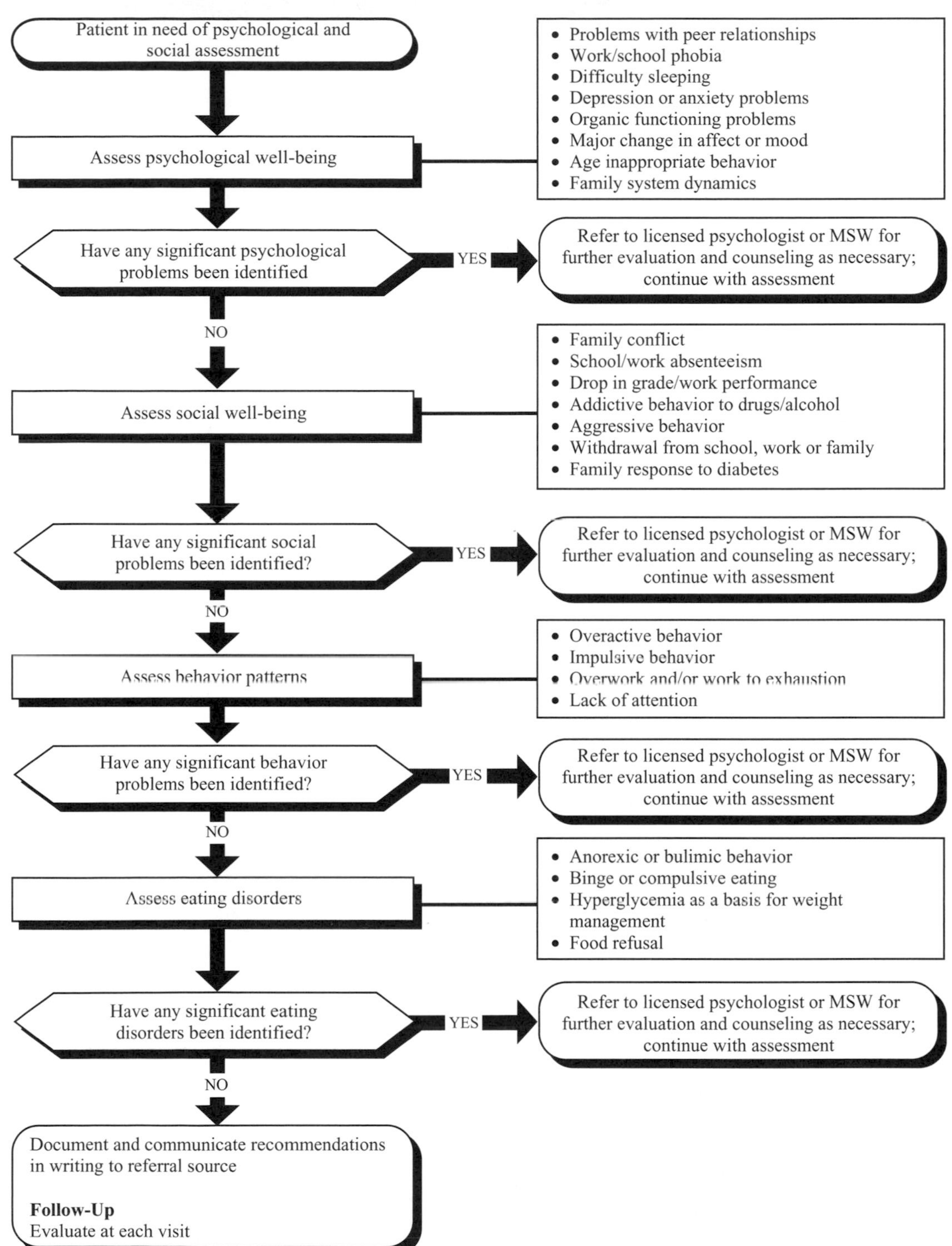

Figure A.24 Psychological and Social Assessment DecisionPath

Complication	Patient Complaints	Clinical Evidence	Action
Hypertension and dyslipidemia	Often none; may be blurred vision, fatigue	**Hypertension** BP ⩾ 130/80 mmHg **Dyslipidemia** LDL ⩾ 100 mg/dL (2.6 mmol/L) HDL < 40 mg/dL (1.0 mmol/L) Triglycerides ⩾ 150 mg/dL (1.7 mmol/L)	Follow *Hypertension and Dyslipidemia Practice Guidelines*
Nephropathy	Usually no symptoms	**Microalbuminuria:** 30–300 mg Alb/g creatinine 30–300 mg Alb/24 hr 20–200 μg Alb/min (AER) **Macroalbuminuria:** > 300 mg Alb/g creatinine > 300 mg Alb/24 hr > 200 μg Alb/min (AER)	Follow *Nephropathy Practice Guidelines, Kidney Disease Assessment,* and *Microalbuminuria Screening, Diagnosis, and Treatment*
Retinopathy	Blurred vision in undiagnosed and poorly controlled patients; often no symptoms with early nonproliferative diabetic retinopathy; dramatic changes in the field of vision (spots, cobwebs, flashing, lights); sudden loss of vision with more severe diabetic retinopathy	**Early Nonproliferative Diabetic Retinopathy:** microaneurysms, dot hemorrhages, hard (lipid) exudates **Moderate to Severe Nonproliferative Diabetic Retinopathy:** cotton wool spots, venous and intraretinal microvascular abnormalities, severe dot and blot hemorrhages **Proliferative Diabetic Retinopathy:** neovascularization, vitreous hemorrhage, retinal detachment	Follow *Diabetic Retinopathy Screening and Diagnosis*
Neuropathy	Diffuse burning pain in feet and legs; unsteady walking; loss of sensitivity to hot and cold; "pins and needles" sensations in hands and feet;	**Distal Symmetrical Sensorimoter Polyneuropathy:** paresthesia and dysethesia, diminished thermal discrimination, ataxic gait	Follow *Distal Symmetrical Sensorimotor Polyneuropathy, Gastroparesis, Diabetic Diarrhea,* and *Genitourinary Autonomic Neuropathy*
	Early satiety, nausea, vomiting; erectile dysfunction; vaginal dryness;	**Autonomic Neuropathy:** persistent tachycardia, orthostatic hypotension, gastroparesis, recurring bladder infections, penile impotence and retrograde ejaculation marked by infertility	
	Pain while moving wrist or hands; isolated pain behind eye	**Focal Neuropathies:** Sudden diplopia and pain behind eye, Bell's palsy, carpal tunnel syndrome, foot drop	
Foot complications	Hot or burning sensation; sore(s) that does not heal or is infected; change in shape of foot; localized reddening at pressure points; no feeling in feet; tingling feeling in feet	**Low-Risk Normal Foot:** no ulcers or deformities; sensate to 10 g, 5.07 monofilament **High-Risk Abnormal Foot:** insensate to 10 g, 5.07 monofilament; foot deformities present **High-Risk Simple Ulcer:** ulcer < 2 cm wide and < 0.5 cm deep; no infection **High-Risk Complex Ulcer:** ulcer ⩾ 2 cm wide and/or ⩾ 0.5 cm deep; infection present	Follow *Diabetic Foot Management Practice Guidelines, Foot Assessment and Treatment,* and *Foot Ulcer Treatment*
Dermatological, connective tissue and oral complications	Patches of discolored and/or thickened skin; athletes foot; lumps at injection sites; restricted movement in joints, small lumps or pits in palms; bad breath; dry mouth; infection in mouth	**Dermatological:** necrobiosis scleredema on back and shoulders; sclerosis of skin on hands; diabetic shin spots; onychomycosis; lipohypertrophy; eruptive xanthoma **Connective Tissue:** limited joint mobility in fingers and elbows; Dupuytren's disease; frozen shoulder **Oral:** periodontal disease; delayed healing; xerostomia; oral fungal infection	Follow *Dermatological, Connective Tissue, and Oral Complications* section

Figure A.25 Annual comprehensive diabetes review

Index

Page numbers in *italics* indicate figures and tables.

Staged Diabetes Management: A Systematic Approach (2nd Edition) R. S. Mazze, E. S. Strock, G. D. Simonson and R. M. Bergenstal

ISBN: 0 470 86576 8